www.bma.org.uk/li

WITHDRAWN
FROM LIBRARY

BRITISH MEDICAL ASSOCIATION
0531712

COMPLICATIONS IN ORAL AND MAXILLOFACIAL SURGERY

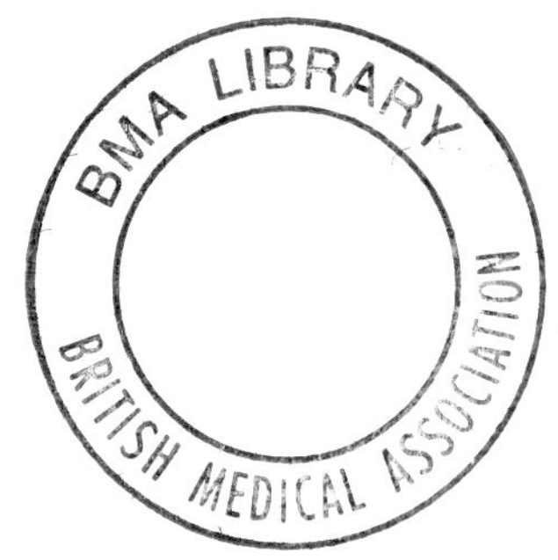

COMPLICATIONS IN ORAL AND MAXILLOFACIAL SURGERY

Leonard B. Kaban, DMD, MD, FACS
Walter C. Guralnick Professor and Chairman
Department of Oral and Maxillofacial Surgery
Massachusetts General Hospital and
Harvard School of Dental Medicine
Boston, Massachusetts

M. Anthony Pogrel, MB, ChB, BDS, FDSRCS, FRCS, FACS
Professor and Chairman
Department of Oral and Maxillofacial Surgery
University of California, San Francisco, School of Dentistry,
San Francisco, California

David H. Perrott, DDS, MD, FACS
Associate Professor
Department of Oral and Maxillofacial Surgery
Harvard School of Dental Medicine
Unit Chief and Residency Program Director
Department of Oral and Maxillofacial Surgery
Massachusetts General Hospital
Boston, Massachusetts

BMA LIBRARY BRITISH MEDICAL ASSOCIATION

W.B. SAUNDERS COMPANY
A Division of Harcourt Brace & Company
Philadelphia London Toronto Montreal Sydney Tokyo

W.B. SAUNDERS COMPANY
A Division of Harcourt Brace & Company

The Curtis Center
Independence Square West
Philadelphia, Pennsylvania 19106

Library of Congress Cataloging-in-Publication Data

Complications in oral and maxillofacial surgery / [edited by] Leonard B. Kaban, M. Anthony Pogrel, David H. Perrott.

p. cm.

ISBN 0–7216–4861–4

1. Mouth—Surgery—Complications. 2. Jaws—Surgery—Complications. 3. Face—Surgery—Complications. I. Kaban, Leonard B. II. Pogrel, M. Anthony. III. Perrott, David H. [DNLM: 1. Surgery, Oral. 2. Intraoperative Complications. 3. Postoperative Complications. WU 600 C737 1997]

RK529.C65 1997 617.5′ 22059—dc20

DNLM/DLC 95–41999

COMPLICATIONS IN ORAL AND MAXILLOFACIAL SURGERY ISBN 0–7216–4861–4

Copyright © 1997 by W.B. Saunders Company.

All rights reserved. No part of this publication may be reproduced or transmitted in any form or by any means, electronic or mechanical, including photocopy, recording, or any information storage and retrieval system, without permission in writing from the publisher.

Printed in the United States of America.

Last digit is the print number: 9 8 7 6 5 4 3 2 1

To our patients who have endured the complications described herein
LBK

To my wife and best friend, Ann
MAP

To my parents
DHP

CONTRIBUTORS

Jeffery W. Armstrong, DDS
Staff, Oral and Maxillofacial Surgery Residency Program, Wilford Hall Medical Center, Lackland Air Force Base, Texas
Complications of Temporomandibular Joint Surgery

G. William Arnett, DDS, FACD
Clinical Instructor and Lecturer, Oral and Maxillofacial Surgery, Loma Linda University, Loma Linda; Valley Medical Center at Fresno, Fresno; University of California, Los Angeles, and University of Southern California, Los Angeles; St. Francis Medical Center of Santa Barbara, and Santa Barbara Cottage Hospital, Santa Barbara, California
The Long-Term Unfavorable Result in Orthognathic Surgery II: Injury to the Temporomandibular Joint and Trigeminal Nerve

Meredith August, DMD, MD
Instructor, Oral and Maxillofacial Surgery, Harvard School of Dental Medicine; Massachusetts General Hospital, Boston, Massachusetts
Complications Associated with Treatment of Head and Neck Cancer

Robert A. Bays, DDS
Professor and Chief, Division of Oral and Maxillofacial Surgery, Department of Surgery, Emory University School of Medicine; Chief, Oral and Maxillofacial Surgery/Dentistry, Emory University Hospital, Crawford Long Hospital, Grady Memorial Hospital, Egleston Children's Hospital at Emory University; Consultant, Veterans Affairs Medical Center, Atlanta, Georgia
Complications of Orthognathic Surgery

Charles N. Bertolami, DDS, DMedSc
Professor and Dean, University of California, San Francisco, School of Dentistry, San Francisco, California
Complications Associated with Wound Healing

Jon P. Bradrick, DDS
Associate Professor, Case Western Reserve University School of Medicine; MetroHealth Medical Center, Cleveland, Ohio
Complications in the Treatment of Midface Fractures

Daniel Buchbinder, DMD
Associate Professor, Oral and Maxillofacial Surgery and Otolaryngology; Director, Residency Training Program (Oral and Maxillofacial Surgery), Mount Sinai School of Medicine; Chief, Division of Oral and Maxillofacial Surgery, Mount Sinai Medical Center, New York, New York
Long-Term Complications After Vascularized Bone Grafts

Robert Campbell, DDS
Professor, Oral and Maxillofacial Surgery, and Professor, Anesthesiology, Virginia Commonwealth University, Medical College of Virginia, Richmond, Virginia
Ambulatory (Office) Anesthesia Complications

Thomas B. Dodson, DMD, MPH
Associate Professor, Department of Surgery, Division of Oral and Maxillofacial Surgery, Emory University School of Medicine, Atlanta, Georgia
Donor Site Morbidity: Diagnosis, Treatment, and Prevention

M. Franklin Dolwick, DMD, PhD
Professor and Director of Residency Program, Department of Oral and Maxillofacial Surgery, University of Florida, College of Dentistry, Gainesville, Florida
Complications of Temporomandibular Joint Surgery

G. E. Ghali, DDS, MD
Assistant Professor of Surgery, Division of Oral and Maxillofacial/Head and Neck Surgery, Louisiana State University School of Medicine, Shreveport, Louisiana
The Long-Term Unfavorable Result in Orthognathic Surgery I: Mandibular, Maxillary, and Combined Deformities

Richard H. Haug, DDS
Associate Professor, Case Western Reserve University School of Medicine; Director of Oral and Maxillofacial Surgery, MetroHealth Medical Center, Cleveland, Ohio
Complications in the Treatment of Midface Fractures

John F. Helfrick, DDS, MS
Professor and Chairman, Department of Oral and Maxillofacial Surgery, University of Texas Health Science Center; University of Texas Dental Branch, Houston, Texas
The Long-Term Unfavorable Result in Cleft Lip and Palate Surgery

Martin B. Hirigoyen, MBBS
Microvascular Fellow, Mount Sinai School of Medicine; Microvascular Research Laboratory, Mount Sinai Medical Center, New York, New York
Long-Term Complications After Vascularized Bone Grafts

David A. Keith, BDS, FDS RCS, DMD
Associate Professor of Oral and Maxillofacial Surgery, Harvard School of Dental Medicine; Visiting Oral and Maxillofacial Surgeon, Massachusetts General Hospital; Chief, Oral and Maxillofacial Surgery, Harvard Community Health Plan, Boston, Massachusetts
The Long-Term Unfavorable Result in Temporomandibular Joint Surgery

Michael E. Koury, DDS
Assistant Clinical Professor, Department of Oral and Maxillofacial Surgery, University of California, San Francisco, School of Dentistry, San Francisco, California
Complications in the Treatment of Mandibular Fractures

Peter E. Larsen, DDS
Associate Professor, Director of Oral and Maxillofacial Surgery Residency, Ohio State University, Department of Oral and Maxillofacial Surgery; Chief of Pediatric Oral and Maxillofacial Surgery, Columbus Children's Hospital, Columbus, Ohio
Dentoalveolar Trauma

Robert B. Layzer, MD
Professor of Neurology, University of California, San Francisco, School of Medicine, San Francisco, California
Nitrous Oxide Abuse and Its Neurologic Complications

Diana V. Messadi, BDS, MMSc, DMSc
Assistant Adjunct Professor, Section of Oral and Maxillofacial Surgery and Section of Diagnostic Sciences of Orofacial Pain, University of California, Los Angeles, School of Dentistry, Los Angeles, California
Complications Associated with Wound Healing

Roger A. Meyer, MD, DDS, MS, FACS
Assistant Clinical Professor, Division of Plastic, Reconstructive, and Maxillofacial Surgery, Emory University School of Medicine; Active Staff, Department of Surgery, Northside Hospital; Consultant, Cleft Lip and Palate, Maxillofacial and Craniofacial Surgery, Children's Medical Services, State of Georgia, Department of Human Resources, Atlanta, Georgia
Evaluation and Management of Neurologic Complications

Stephen Milam, DDS, PhD
University of Texas Health Science Center, San Antonio, Texas
The Long-Term Unfavorable Result in Orthognathic Surgery II: Injury to the Temporomandibular Joint and Trigeminal Nerve

Michael Miloro, DMD, MD
Assistant Professor, Oral and Maxillofacial Surgery, Ohio State University, Department of Oral and Maxillofacial Surgery; Director, Dentofacial Deformities Program, Ohio State University, College of Dentistry, Columbus, Ohio
Dentoalveolar Trauma

Jackson P. Morgan III, DDS
Assistant Professor of Surgery, University Medical Center of Florida, The University of Florida, Jacksonville, Florida
Complications in the Treatment of Midface Fractures

David H. Perrott, DDS, MD, FACS
Associate Professor, Department of Oral and Maxillofacial Surgery, Harvard School of Dental Medicine; Unit Chief and Residency Program Director, Department of Oral and Maxillofacial Surgery, Massachusetts General Hospital, Boston, Massachusetts
Complications Associated with the Use of Rigid Internal Fixation in Maxillofacial Surgery

M. Anthony Pogrel, MB, ChB, BDS, FDSRCS, FRCS, FACS
Professor and Chairman, Department of Oral and Maxillofacial Surgery, University of California, San Francisco, School of Dentistry, San Francisco, California
Complications of Third Molar Surgery

Douglas P. Sinn, DDS
Professor and Chairman, Division of Oral and Maxillofacial Surgery, University of Texas Southwestern Medical Center at Dallas; Professor and Chairman, Parkland Memorial Hospital and Its Affiliates, Dallas, Texas
The Long-Term Unfavorable Result in Orthognathic Surgery I: Mandibular, Maxillary, and Combined Deformities

William A. Shapiro, MD
Associate Clinical Professor, Department of Anesthesia, University of California, San Francisco, School of Medicine, San Francisco, California
Anesthetic Complications: Avoidance and Management

Richard A. Smith, DDS
Clinical Professor, Oral and Maxillofacial Surgery, University of California, San Francisco, School of Dentistry, San Francisco, California
Long-Term Complications of Osseointegrated Implants

John R. Werther, DMD, MD, FACS
Assistant Professor, Oral and Maxillofacial Surgery, Vanderbilt University School of Medicine; Assistant Chief, Oral and Maxillofacial Surgery, Nashville Veterans Affairs Medical Center, Nashville, Tennessee
Complications of Facial Cosmetic Surgery

Michael F. Zide, DMD
Associate Director of Oral and Maxillofacial Surgery, John Peter Smith Hospital, Fort Worth, Texas
The Long-Term Unfavorable Result in Midface Trauma

PREFACE

In the fall of 1989, the senior editor was asked to be a guest editor of an early issue (Vol. 2, No. 3) of a new W.B. Saunders Company periodical: *Oral and Maxillofacial Surgery Clinics of North America.* Although somewhat skeptical of the necessity for yet another periodical and the ability to present new and useful information in the format suggested, the project was completed and published under the title Complications, Poor Results and Treatment Failures in Oral and Maxillofacial Surgery.[1] The *Oral and Maxillofacial Clinics of North America* has since become a widely read and an important resource for surgeons interested in the oral and maxillofacial region.

The subject of complications was selected because it had not been previously addressed in an organized manner in a single volume. This period preceded the publication of Parameters of Care for Oral and Maxillofacial Surgeons.[2] Oral and maxillofacial surgeons were not comfortable and forthcoming in addressing adverse outcomes for a variety of reasons. For example, it was believed that, perhaps, outlining and discussing a series of complications and poor results would simply be ammunition for plaintiffs' attorneys and would add to already serious litigation problems.

On the other hand, a discussion of complications, treatment failures, and poor results encountered by surgeons and presented in a dignified, academic, honest, and objective manner was thought to be extremely useful for the practicing surgeon. It would also provide the opportunity for our profession to analyze common complications, to determine how they occurred, and to consider prevention and management—all to the good of our patients and future surgeons in training.

The response to the issue was very positive. Subsequently, the subject of complications was addressed at several national oral and maxillofacial surgery meetings, including one sponsored by the American Association of Oral and Maxillofacial Surgeons and one by the University of California, Los Angeles. Anecdotal feedback from readers indicated that there was no resultant surge in malpractice litigation. In fact, the volume was helpful to some defendants, as it demonstrated that complications without negligence do indeed occur even in the best of hands. Based on this experience, we made plans to expand this project into a book.

Why a book? The larger format allowed us to increase the number and breadth of subjects and to discuss them in greater detail. In addition, more time made it feasible to approach additional senior surgeons, who are recognized experts in oral and maxillofacial surgery, for their contributions. Because of the magnitude of the project, it was not possible for LBK to complete it as a single editor. We were fortunate to recruit Drs. Tony Pogrel and David Perrott to be co-editors.

All were faculty members in the Department of Oral and Maxillofacial Surgery at the University of California, San Francisco, under the chairmanship of LBK. As a group we became interested in the area of complications and carried out a number of projects on various aspects of this subject: diagnosis and management of complications related to third molar extractions and inferior alveolar and lingual nerve injury, and complications of mandibular fractures and rigid internal fixation.

Complications in Oral and Maxillofacial Surgery is divided into three major sections. The first deals with general considerations, including the anesthetic complications in the operating room and ambulatory (office) settings, the history and current status of nitrous oxide abuse and toxicity, and the effects of normal and abnormal wound healing on the occurrence and management of surgical complications.

We then discuss problems and adverse outcomes in the early phases of treatment, i.e., intraoperative and early postoperative complications. Although some contributors have chosen to provide lists of complications of varying lengths, the emphasis is on diagnosis, prevention, and management. Special emphasis is on preoperative planning and complication avoidance. For example, in the chapter Complications of Orthognathic Surgery, Dr. Robert Bays analyzes the most common mishaps in mandibular and maxillary surgery. He discusses, in each case, how the complications most often occur and, most importantly, how accurate preoperative diagnosis and treatment planning will, in most cases, prevent these problems. If a complication does occur, he discusses its diagnosis and management.

In the chapter Complications in the Treatment of Mandibular Fractures, Dr. Michael E. Koury reviews some controversial aspects of fracture management, including retention of teeth in the line of fracture, optimum duration of maxillomandibular fixation, effects of delay in treatment, and advantages and disadvantages of rigid internal fixation. These subjects are discussed in the context of prevention and management of complications.

The combination of chapters on complications of third molar surgery by Dr. Pogrel and neurologic complications by Dr. Roger Meyer deals with diagnosis, prevention, and current concepts of management of the most common nerve injuries seen by the oral and maxillofacial surgeon. The information regarding types of injury and timing and results of microsurgical repair of the inferior alveolar and lingual nerves is particularly relevant for practicing surgeons at this time.

The last part of the book is a presentation of the unfavorable long-term result. The emphasis may be on the patient who has had one or more operations for a particular problem with a poor final outcome. There may or may not have been specific acute complications along the way; however, the final result is less than ideal. The senior authors of these chapters have illustrated that despite the best we have to offer, there are occasional unfavorable outcomes. In other cases, inaccurate diagnosis and misguided treatment planning have led to inevitable adverse outcomes. For example, in the chapter on the long-term unfavorable result in temporomandibular joint (TMJ) surgery, Dr. David A. Keith discusses the outcomes of patients with chronic pain who have had multiple TMJ operations. Many of these patients have experienced not only the persistence of pain but also multiple operative scars, hypomobility/ankylosis, and other iatrogenic complications from inadequate diagnosis and treatment planning.

Dr. Richard A. Smith has compiled one of the most thorough chapters dealing with long-term complications of osseointegrated implants. This chapter is written in an impartial and objective way, with no particular bias toward implant type.

The editors would especially like to thank the contributors for their enthusiasm and courage in participating in this project. It is one thing to write a traditional book chapter, which is essentially an unrefereed document usually highlighting the author's best results. It is quite a different matter to write a chapter that highlights complications or unfavorable outcomes for all the readers to see and evaluate. Each of the contributors is well known to the editors, and although the subject of this book is complications and unfavorable outcomes, we all have also obtained an occasional excellent result.

We would like to thank Larry McGrew at W.B. Saunders Company for his help and guidance in this project. His availability and his competence as a facilitator without interference was a tremendous asset to the editors and contributors. We hope that the readers of this book derive some benefit from the information we have worked so hard to communicate. Finally, we hope that this benefit to our readers translates into improved patient care and to improved education for our trainees, for these are the ultimate goals of any academic exercise.

Leonard B. Kaban
Boston, Massachusetts

M. Anthony Pogrel
San Francisco, California

David H. Perrott
Boston, Massachusetts

1. Kaban LB (Editor): Complications, poor results and treatment failures. Oral and Maxillofacial Surgery Clinics of North America, Volume 2, Number 3, August, 1990.
2. Parameters of Care for Oral and Maxillofacial Surgeons. J Oral Maxillofac Surg 53(Supplement), September, 1995.

CONTENTS

Section 1
General Considerations

Chapter 1
ANESTHETIC COMPLICATIONS

Avoidance and Management

by

William A. Shapiro

Introduction

In a managed care environment, sick patients continue to require surgery. As cost-effective care through capitated reimbursement takes hold, all physicians will become "gatekeepers" to hold down costs. Not only will anesthesiologists be expected to continue to deliver safe state-of-the art care, they will be assuming an increasing role in minimizing perioperative costs. They will ask for the minimum necessary preoperative laboratory tests, choose less expensive premedication and anesthetic agents whenever possible, carefully evaluate the utility of expensive monitoring devices, and determine whether postoperative care will require recovery in a more expensive, monitored care setting. These challenges will be greatest in the sickest patients. Our current and future goal will be safe anesthesia and state-of-the-art surgery delivered at a fraction of previous costs. As scientists, we want our results to continue to improve. Although the hope is that we can achieve these aims, the new reality is that we *must* succeed.

By preparing patients for surgery, we believe we accomplish two functions: increased safety and improved efficacy. When systemic medical problems are brought under control, patients experience less perioperative morbidity and mortality. They also require less expensive postoperative care and can be discharged from the hospital sooner. With these goals in mind, this chapter focuses on preoperative preparation of the patients with the most common significant systemic diseases, and then discusses the recognition and management of the most serious intraoperative problems. These are the patients who most often, if not always, require surgery in a hospital operating room and not an outpatient or same-day surgery setting. Because one chapter cannot cover all preoperative medical conditions, I discuss those most commonly encountered. Anesthetic considerations and intraoperative management of rare diseases are reviewed in a number of texts.[1, 2]

THE SUBJECTS DISCUSSED IN THIS CHAPTER ARE:

- Team approach
- Closed-claim statistics related to mortality and serious morbidity
- How to prepare the patient for surgery
  Preoperative evaluation
  Primary care physician consultation
  Cardiac diseases
  Pulmonary diseases and airway abnormalities
  Hepatic diseases
  Renal diseases
  Endocrine diseases
- Perioperative management of the patient in intermaxillary fixation
- Anesthetic complications and their management
  Malignant hyperthermia
  Anaphylaxis
  Cardiac arrest
  Ventricular fibrillation and rapid ventricular tachycardia
  Pulseless electrical activity
  Asystole

Team Approach

Health care providers working as a team represent the only acceptable approach to the perioperative management of high-risk patients. The expertise of clinicians from a number of specialties, including anesthesia, medicine (e.g., cardiology, pulmonary medicine), and surgery, overlap when high-risk patients undergo anesthesia and surgery. Clinicians must be confident that their specialist colleagues are the best qualified: Each specialist provides a unique clinical perspective with expert knowledge. The expectation is that the patient will have the best chance for a successful outcome. However, each specialty also must acknowledge its own limitations—it is inappropriate and counterproductive for a specialist in one field to presume to tell a specialist in another how to proceed or perform. Rather, each must provide the information unique to his or her specialty to optimize the performance of other team members and patient outcome. Descriptors such as "cleared for surgery" offer no valuable information; the recommendation to "avoid hypotension" identifies a lack of understanding of the intraoperative environment.

Closed-Claim Statistics Related to Mortality and Serious Morbidity

Complications related to anesthesia continue to occur and, unfortunately, always will. Mortality due to anesthesia has been recognized since the introduction of inhalation anesthesia in 1844.[3] Current estimates are 1 per 10,000 anesthetics.[4–6] Overall mortality related to anesthesia varies from study to study and depends upon several factors. These factors are at work in the preoperative, intraoperative, and postoperative periods. *Preoperative* factors that appear to predict outcome are patient age, the American Society of Anesthesiologists (ASA) physical status classification, intensity and location of surgery (major versus minor), and the nature of surgery as elective or emergent.[7–10] None of these four "predictors" appears to be altered by intraoperative anesthetic management (i.e., anesthetic agents or technique—regional versus general).[8] Closed-claim analysis of factors responsible for *intraoperative* catastrophes identifies failure to recognize a problem, such as esophageal intubation or breathing circuit disconnection, and the inability to manage a difficult airway.[11] Because patients are known to suffer postoperative cardiac, pulmonary, and embolic complications, as yet unidentified *postoperative* risk factors also are surely at work. When preoperative, intraoperative, and postoperative statistics are combined, overall anesthetic mortality may be as low as 1 per 50,000 to 1 per 100,000 in healthy patients having elective minor surgery and as high as or higher than 1 per 1,000 in medically compromised older patients having extensive emergency surgery. Combining all anesthetics places the risk of mortality in the range of 1 in 10,000.

How to Prepare the Patient for Surgery

Preoperative Evaluation

Preoperative preparation begins with a complete medical history, including a review of the patient's chart and current medications and a physical examination, after which an ASA physical status class category is assigned (Table 1–1). In 1961, Dripps and colleagues[9] modified a previously developed physical status classification to standardize a patient's preoperative medical status. This classification is independent of the type of surgery to be performed and is not altered even if the surgery focuses on the organ system determining the ASA classification.

The ASA physical status classification was developed not to assess anesthetic risk nor to predict outcome. It has always been intended to summarize the preoperative history and physical findings into a simplified classification for planning anesthetic management and facilitating communication between health-care providers. Despite these limitations, several investigators have found a relationship between the ASA classification and postoperative outcome. Postoperative mortality is higher in patients assigned ASA III and IV classifications.[9, 10, 12] Cardiac arrest is three times more frequent in patients designated as ASA III and IV than in those assigned to class I or II, and ASA III and IV patients are less likely to survive cardiac arrest.[13] The complication rate for adverse events other than mortality is also higher for ASA III and IV patients.[9, 10, 14, 15]

Primary Care Physician Consultation

Most patients with systemic diseases are under the care of an internist or specialist who has determined the degree of cardiovascular and respiratory dysfunction and prescribed appropriate medication. This information must be made available to those responsible for the administration of the anesthesia. The primary care physician's most recent assessment of the patient's medical status should be incorporated into the preop-

Table 1–1. American Society of Anesthesiologists (ASA) Physical Status Classification of Preoperative Patients*

Classification	Description of the Patient's Physical Condition
I	Healthy patient
II	Mild systemic disease—no functional limitation
III	Severe systemic disease—functional limitation
IV	Severe systemic disease that is life-threatening
V	A moribund patient not expected to survive 24 hours with or without surgery

*An *E* after a number designates an emergency operation.

erative history. Whenever necessary, the primary care physician and anesthesia provider(s) should consult. A preoperative consultation with another physician must not, however, be a request for "clearance" for surgery. Rather, it provides the opportunity to better define the extent of the disease or nature of any recent changes to reduce the risks associated with anesthesia and surgery. The history, appropriate laboratory examinations, and physician consultation (if required) allow the anesthesiologist to choose the best anesthetic agents and technique as well as intraoperative monitors for the scheduled operation.

Preoperative preparation should include continuation of all medication that treats any medical condition up to and including the day of surgery. Medication that inhibits coagulation may be discontinued at the discretion of the surgeon. Historically, monoamine oxidase inhibitors were discontinued 2 weeks prior to elective surgery, but this practice has been challenged.[16]

Cardiac Diseases

Ischemic Heart Disease

Background

More than half of all postoperative deaths are cardiac in origin.[17] Patients with known coronary artery disease (CAD) and those with risk factors for CAD constitute 10% to 15% of the non–cardiac surgery population. When the risk associated with age (over 65 years) is added, approximately 30% of the 20 to 25 million patients undergoing noncardiac surgery each year have at least one risk factor known to be associated with higher perioperative cardiac morbidity or mortality. Therefore, approximately 7 million surgical patients each year have identifiable preoperative cardiac risk factors.

Several investigators have attempted to pinpoint objective preoperative findings to identify patients at increased risk for postoperative cardiac morbidity and mortality. The preoperative risk factors associated with increased cardiac morbidity and mortality currently are (1) recent (within the last 6 months) myocardial infarction (MI), (2) signs or symptoms of congestive heart failure (CHF), (3) angina, (4) valvular heart disease, (5) frequent premature ventricular contractions (PVCs), (6) type of operation, (7) patient age, and (8) overall medical condition as assessed by laboratory values for liver, kidney, and lung disease.[18, 19]

The rate of perioperative MI in adult patients without cardiac disease is approximately 0.15% to 0.5%.[20] It has long been recognized that patients with cardiovascular disease, particularly those who experience angina or those who have had a prior myocardial infarction, have a higher perioperative risk of infarction, averaging 5% to 6%.[21, 22] Those patients who have had a documented myocardial infarction within the prior 6 months are at an even greater risk for re-infarction—up to 37% for a recent infarction—and the mortality rate for members in this group who suffer re-infarction averages approximately 50%.[21, 22]

The hope is that the preoperative identification of cardiac risk factors will lead to treatment before and management during surgery that reduce the risk of postoperative cardiac morbidity. Unfortunately, objective data remain limited.

Preoperative Preparation

History. After reviewing the patient's chart, the anesthesia provider must obtain a history directly from the patient scheduled to undergo surgery. Most patients are likely to be preoccupied with their upcoming surgery and therefore may neglect to mention recent, subtle changes in symptoms that may be important. All newly presenting cardiovascular symptoms must be addressed prior to surgery. Changes in the frequency or intensity of previous cardiac symptoms must be investigated, and if appropriate, surgery must be postponed pending adjustment in medical therapy or surgical intervention if required.

Patients with cardiac disease may be assigned by their cardiologist to a New York Heart Association (AHA) classification of cardiac reserve.[23] This classification, which ranges from 1 (no limitation) to 4 (discomfort with any activity), is based on an evaluation of the level of effort required to produce symptoms that limit patients' physical activity. Changes in the AHA classification may indicate an evolving or acute process further limiting cardiac reserve. Preoperatively, patients should be questioned about changes in exercise tolerance and the nature of the symptoms that limit exercise. Postponing surgery until additional information can be obtained from more sophisticated cardiac examinations can be important to further define the extent of disease and to identify areas of myocardium at risk. This information is critical to anesthesia planning and may help minimize cardiac risk, regardless of the location of surgery.[24] For some patients, cardiac valve surgery, coronary artery bypass graft surgery (CABG), or percutaneous transluminal coronary angioplasty (PTCA) may be recommended prior to elective noncardiac surgery.[25, 26]

Because patients who have suffered an MI within the previous 6 months are at increased risk, elective surgery should be postponed, whenever possible, until the risk of re-infarction is reduced. One study suggests that invasive hemodynamic monitoring reduces the risk of re-infarction in patients undergoing noncardiac surgery who have had a myocardial infarction within the previous 6 months.[27]

Physical Examination. Physical examination of the cardiovascular system should focus primarily on risk factors. Abnormal physical findings related to cardiac rhythm, central venous pressure (CVP), cardiac murmurs or gallops, and evidence of CHF are associated with increased risk. Any abnormal finding detected during physical examination should be investigated and corrected or stabilized before elective surgery.

Laboratory Examination. All patients known to have cardiovascular disease should present a recent preoperative chest radiograph (CXR) and electrocardiogram (ECG). In addition to hemoglobin or hematocrit values, laboratory screening should focus on obtaining the information relevant to the patient's preexisting medical condition or appropriate for anesthetic/surgical management. For example, the presence of diabetes warrants measurement of glucose; the use of chronic pharmacologic therapy indicates screening of plasma electrolytes; and the use of regional anesthesia requires serum coagulation parameters. Abnormalities in laboratory values should be investigated and corrected whenever possible before elective surgery is undertaken.

Medication. With few exceptions, all cardiac medication should be continued up to and on the day of surgery. Patients using sublingual nitroglycerin should be instructed to bring medication to the preoperative area to use if necessary. In addition to reassuring the patient, the use of nitroglycerin minimizes the duration of any preoperative ischemic event. Some anesthetists suggest avoiding diuretic medication on the day of surgery when use of a Foley catheter is not anticipated. Antibiotic prophylaxis is recommended for patients with valvular heart disease or mitral valve prolapse. Because choice of drugs, doses, and duration of antibiotic prophylaxis can change periodically, it is important to consult with the appropriate specialist to determine the prophylactic regimen. For patients receiving anticoagulation for previous cardiac valve surgery, a cardiologist should be consulted to guide management of perioperative coagulation therapy.

Intraoperative Preparation

All inhalation and intravenous agents used to induce anesthesia cause hypotension. Narcotics and benzodiazepines further reduce blood pressure in patients who are hypovolemic or are placed in reverse Trendelenberg position to reduce blood loss during head and neck procedures. No single drug or combination has proved superior in reducing cardiovascular morbidity or mortality; the choice of agents is based on the procedure and the experience of the anesthesiologist.

Because patients with cardiovascular disease have limited reserve, the goal of intraoperative monitoring is to diagnose quickly and accurately, thereby limiting periods of hypotension, arrhythmias, or myocardial ischemia. Current monitoring practice includes ECG, blood pressure monitoring, pulse oximetry, and measurement of inspired and exhaled airway gases. Most ECG monitors are equipped to monitor ST segments during surgery. Intraoperative arrhythmias occur frequently and may indicate myocardial ischemia in patients with cardiac disease. It is important to determine whether the arrhythmia is the cause or the effect of ischemia to ensure appropriate therapy. Direct measure of arterial or pulmonary artery pressure (PAP) or transesophageal echocardiography (TEE) evaluation of overall cardiac function, regional wall motion, and valvular function facilitates management of patients with significant cardiac disease, particularly for long or complicated surgery.[28]

Some groups of patients may require close monitoring of intravascular volume by measurement of CVP or PAP and urine output. Patients on diuretic therapy may begin surgery with a reduced intravascular volume. During major head and neck surgery, blood loss with consequent fluid and electrolyte administration can be associated with shifts in intravascular volume. Such patients may benefit from direct central venous and arterial pressure monitoring. ASA III or IV patients scheduled for major head and neck surgery who have symptoms of CHF would benefit from close monitoring of intravascular volume. TEE has been recognized as an additional monitor of intracardiac volume.[29]

Postoperative Preparation

The postoperative period is risky, and some patients may require postoperative monitoring in an intensive care unit (ICU) setting after surgery. Ischemia often is silent, and arrhythmias, although common postoperatively, also may indicate primary myocardial dysfunction. Of the approximately 7 million patients known preoperatively to be at high risk, approximately 50,000 suffer a perioperative myocardial infarction each year, 3 days after surgery being the peak time for postoperative myocardial infarction. The factors contributing to and the timing of infarction are not well understood. Myocardial oxygen supply and demand, the autonomic nervous system (particularly as it affects heart rate and the coronary circulation), coagulation factors, and the effects of pain have been proposed.

Treatment of postoperative cardiac morbidity can range from intravenous antiischemic agents to diagnostic catheterization followed by percutaneous transluminal coronary angioplasty (PTCA) or administration of streptokinase or other blood-thinning agents. The use of anticoagulants remains controversial in patients who have just undergone surgery, however, because it places them at increased risk for postoperative hemorrhage. Medical therapy usually is sufficient to treat postoperative myocardial dysfunction.

Hypertension

An estimated 60 million Americans have hypertension.[30] Forty-five percent of patients more than 65 years old have a systolic blood pressure greater than 160 mm Hg or a diastolic pressure greater than 95 mm Hg.[31] A significant number of treated hypertensive patients arrive in the operating room with elevated blood pressure.

Preoperative hypertension is associated with major fluctuations in intraoperative blood pressure, whether or not the patient is under treatment for hypertension,[32] and has been associated with postoperative cardiac morbidity.[33, 34] Although some investigators have recommended preoperative treatment of hypertension to reduce perioperative morbidity,[32, 35] not all believe that hypertension per se affects outcome.[36]

Whether or not treatment of hypertension improves perioperative outcome, patients with long-standing hypertension have end-organ disease affecting the cardiovascular and renal systems and the brain. Hypertensive cardiovascular disease is the most common cause of left ventricular hypertrophy and is commonly associated with congestive heart failure, an established risk factor for postoperative cardiac morbidity.

For the preceding reasons, the discovery of unsuspected hypertension during the preoperative examination indicates a thorough cardiac and renal examination to identify abnormalities. For those patients being treated for chronic hypertension, medication should be continued up to and on the day of surgery.

Most anesthesiologists believe that intraoperative blood pressure values should be maintained within 20% to 30% of the awake value obtained preoperatively, with pharmacologic intervention as necessary. Minimal delay in intraoperative treatment above or below these levels is recommended. Elevation in blood pressure often occurs during intubation and extubation of the trachea[32, 37] and during surgical stimulation. Profound decreases in blood pressure may occur after induction of anesthesia and upon initiation of positive-pressure ventilation.[38] A number of pharmacologic agents are available to blunt these stressful periods.

The early postoperative period (immediately after extubation and for the first several hours of recovery) also is stressful, and aggressive treatment of hypertension should continue as long as necessary into the postoperative period.

It is not clear when elective surgery should be postponed for asymptomatic elevated blood pressure. Diastolic blood pressure above 110 mm Hg is clearly abnormal and likely requires further therapy before elective surgery; however, no recommendation for elevated systolic pressure has been made.

Valvular Heart Disease

Patients with symptomatic aortic or mitral valve disease require a complete examination by a cardiologist prior to elective surgery. Severely symptomatic patients may need corrective heart surgery before undergoing elective surgery. Some patients with valvular heart disease require special intraoperative monitors, including direct arterial pressure and PAP pressure monitoring as well as TEE. Intraoperative management should include maintenance of sinus rhythm and pharmacologic intervention as indicated to maintain adequate preload and systemic arterial blood pressure. For asymptomatic mitral valve prolapse, no special considerations are necessary other than antibiotic prophylaxis.[39]

Pacemakers

More than 1 million persons in the United States have temporary or permanent pacemakers. Perioperative management of these patients is reviewed extensively elsewhere.[40] A unique consideration deserves discussion, however; the disruption of pacemaker function during electrosurgical cautery.

When a pacemaker is programmed to function in the demand mode, cardiac pacing is *synchronized* to occur when the patient's intrinsic heart rate falls below the pacemaker's preset rate. When the patient's intrinsic heart rate is above the preset pacemaker rate, the pacemaker is *inhibited* or turned off. During surgery, a demand pacemaker may become inhibited for prolonged periods owing to electrosurgical cautery interference. The pacemaker interprets *intermittent* interference as intrinsic patient cardiac electrical activity and temporarily ceases to function. This event can easily induce long periods of little or no cardiac stimulation and, consequently, no cardiac output. When intermittent electrosurgical interference occurs or is anticipated, placing a strong magnet over the pacemaker generator will convert the pacemaker function to fixed-rate mode, thereby eliminating the pacemaker interpretive function. (Programmed in the fixed-rate mode, cardiac pacing is carried out at a preset, fixed rate that is independent of intrinsic cardiac electrical activity.) Preoperatively, the "magnet" mode of the pacemaker should be tested prophylactically to ensure that it will respond appropriately to the magnet—in some permanent pacemakers, the "magnet" mode can serve to activate other pacemaker modalities. *Continuous* interference usually is not disruptive of pacemaker function, because most demand pacemakers default into a fixed-rate mode in response to continuous electrical interference.

If a pacemaker malfunctions during surgery or does not respond as predicted to placement of a magnet over the generator, a cardiologist should be called to the operating room to evaluate and ensure proper pacemaker function.

Pulmonary Diseases and Airway Abnormalities

Managing the airway and interacting with the pulmonary system is a primary function of the anesthesiologist. The most common cause of intraoperative mortality is inadequate delivery of oxygen,[11] and respiratory causes are second only to cardiac causes of postoperative mortality. Normal pulmonary physiology, the effects of anesthetic agents and muscle relaxants on the respiratory system, and the impact of positive-pressure ventilation on gas exchange and the circulatory system are not discussed here; the interested reader is referred to any number of texts on these subjects.[41, 42] Instead, this section discusses how to prepare patients with pulmonary disease for anesthesia and surgery, how to avoid intraoperative complications related to the respiratory system, and how to minimize postoperative respiratory dysfunction.

Preoperative Evaluation of Patients with Pulmonary Disease

Respiratory function and pulmonary reserve can be assessed preoperatively using a dyspnea scale developed by Boushy and colleagues[43] (Table 1–2). This classification can also be useful in planning perioperative management. The Boushy classification is particularly important, because all patients in dyspnea class 1 and most in class 2 are unlikely to experience perioperative pulmonary problems. For symptomatic patients (dys-

Table 1–2. Grade of Dyspnea due to Pulmonary Problems (Walking on Level Ground at a Normal Cadence)

Classification	Description of Breathing Effort
0	No dyspnea walking on level ground.
I	"I can walk forever if I take my time."
II	Dyspnea with moderate exertion. "I get short of breath after (a number) of blocks."
III	Dyspnea with even exertion. "I get short of breath walking to the bathroom."
IV	Dyspnea at rest.

Modified from Boushy SF, Billing DM, North LB, et al: Clinical course related to preoperative pulmonary function in patients with bronchogenic carcinoma. Chest 1971;59:383.

pnea classes 3 and 4), preoperative pulmonary function testing may be useful to furnish a baseline if it is anticipated that postoperative therapy or measures to improve pulmonary function will be required.[44]

Smoking

The incidence of postoperative respiratory and cardiac complications is higher in those who use tobacco.[44, 45] Many of the studies documenting perioperative respiratory problems associated with smoking were conducted in patients undergoing thoracic or abdominal surgery.[46] Smoking, however, produces cardiopulmonary abnormalities that affect *all* patients undergoing anesthesia and surgery. Smoking produces respiratory system abnormalities that begin early,[47] and lung architecture and function continue to deteriorate as long as smoking continues. Therefore, all patients who smoke are placed into ASA class II or higher. The amount and duration of tobacco use should be documented as part of every preoperative evaluation.

Respiratory abnormalities associated with smoking have anesthetic implications. Smokers are prone to respiratory infections and often produce sputum even when not suffering an active infection. They have "irritable" airways and are prone to cough and to produce copious secretions during tracheal intubation and extubation. Tracheal suctioning confers risk because it may lead to coughing, with subsequent low lung volumes, wheezing, and gas exchange abnormalities producing oxygen desaturation. Smokers may also be at increased risk for perioperative aspiration.[48]

Patients who smoke are likely to have other factors increasing anesthetic risk. Long-term smokers often are elderly and have hypertension and other manifestations of cardiovascular disease. Obesity further increases risk for postoperative pulmonary problems.[49]

Preoperative Preparation of Patients Who Smoke

Respiratory infections, bronchitis, sputum production, and wheezing are common preoperatively in smokers and, whenever possible, should be treated and corrected prior to surgery. Patients may be instructed preoperatively to stop smoking but are unlikely to do so. The longer the discontinuation of smoking prior to surgery, the better (i.e., lower) carbon monoxide levels will be. Cessation of smoking for 1 or 2 days preoperatively, however, does not significantly reduce postoperative respiratory complications.[50] Patients must be informed of their increased risk for postoperative complications to allow them to participate actively in measures to facilitate recovery. Preoperative instruction in techniques that encourage postoperative deep breathing and coughing (e.g., incentive spirometry) require follow-up instruction postoperatively to be successful.[51]

Some long-term smokers develop cor pulmonale with right heart failure and pulmonary hypertension. Many have progressed to blood gas abnormalities, including carbon dioxide retention and hypoxemia. These patients are at very high risk for perioperative complications. Preoperative pulmonary and cardiac consultations are necessary to define the extent of the disease and to determine optimal perioperative management.[52] Intraoperative management usually requires invasive monitoring and frequent arterial blood gas analysis. Postoperative management typically requires monitoring in an ICU setting and prolonged intubation.

Smokers manifesting stridor preoperatively should be evaluated for signs of impending airway obstruction. Because tobacco use is associated with cancer of the upper airway and larynx, a history of difficulty breathing in the supine position, problems swallowing, airway problems after previous surgery, or audible stridor on physical examination warrants consultation with an otolaryngologist to define the extent of airway obstruction.

Asthma

Asthma is the most common respiratory disease in children. Overall, it affects approximately 3% of the population of the United States.[53] Perioperative respiratory complications are higher in these patients.[54]

Preoperative review of the medication taken by an asthmatic patient is critical. Patients should be instructed to continue medication, including inhalers, up to and on the day of surgery. Inhalers should be brought to the operating room, because many anesthesiologists require that they be used immediately before surgery, even when lungs are clear.

The etiology of preoperative wheezing must be identified, care being taken to differentiate cardiac from pulmonary causes.[54, 55] This step helps determine appropriate treatment. Cardiac-induced wheezing may confer greater risk of perioperative morbidity and mortality.

Chronically asthmatic patients who are not wheezing at the time of surgery generally do well. Those who routinely use an inhaler, as well as those with minimal preoperative wheezing, should be encouraged to use additional inhalation treatments just prior to induction of anesthesia, particularly when endotracheal intubation is anticipated.

Chronic Obstructive Pulmonary Disease

Chronic obstructive pulmonary disease (COPD) is a progressive pulmonary disease, often caused by excessive smoking, that results in obstruction to airflow, frequent infections, and, ultimately, alterations in gas exchange, including chronic hypoxemia and subsequent hypercarbia. Eventually, lung architecture is destroyed, and pulmonary reserve becomes severely limited.

In long-standing COPD, the severity of the lung disease must be quantified through preoperative pulmonary function testing. Every effort should be made to improve the patient's preoperative status. Pulmonary infection should be treated with antibiotics. Bronchodilator therapy should be administered (if necessary) to improve gas flow, and patients should be instructed preoperatively in postoperative measures (e.g., incentive spirometry) that can decrease respiratory complications. Planning for postoperative recovery in an intensive care unit may be prudent for patients with advanced COPD.

Airway Mass Lesions

Approximately 2% to 3% of surgical patients prove to present difficulty in intubation.[56] Most of these cases can be anticipated from preoperative history or physical examination. Several investigators have attempted to define upper airway anatomy predisposing to difficult intubation. Unfortunately, all methods appear to have an uncomfortable rate of both false-negative and false-positive predictions. One of the more commonly used techniques is the Mallampati scale.[57] According to Mallampati and colleagues,[57] findings suggestive of difficult intubation are: small mouth opening, narrow mandible, "overbite," short distance between the mandible and the thyroid cartilage, limited range of neck motion, large tongue or neck, and visibility of only the hard palate during full mouth opening with maximal tongue extension. Difficult intubation usually is managed by awake fiberoptic intubation of the trachea. Retrograde intubation from the larynx to the mouth or nose is an alternative technique for the difficult case.[57a]

All patients who describe having a hoarse voice for more than 2 weeks or a change in voice in the absence of an upper respiratory infection should undergo an otolaryngologic examination prior to elective surgery to exclude or define abnormal upper airway anatomy, including the presence of any lesion.

Difficulties tend to arise when an unsuspected difficult intubation is encountered. The ASA has developed an algorithm for management of the difficult airway that has become part of routine anesthesia resident training.[58] Because emergency management of the airway may require the use of a laryngeal mask airway or transtracheal jet ventilation, these devices should be available in every operating room. If several attempts at laryngoscopy fail, it is best to awaken the patient and reschedule surgery, if possible. Multiple attempts at intubation are likely to induce edema of the tongue and posterior pharynx, making it difficult to ventilate the patient.

Upper Respiratory Infection (URI): To Proceed with Surgery or Not?

Whether to proceed with surgery in the patient with a URI is a common dilemma. The decision is also influenced by age, financial, and emotional factors. Conflicting data exist. One study of patients ranging in age from newborn to 20 years found no difference in perioperative respiratory complications in patients with and without preoperative URI.[59] A study of pediatric patients alone, however, reported significant increases in adverse respiratory events in those with a preoperative URI.[60] Tait and Knight[59] found no difference whether or not the patient was intubated, whereas Cohen and Cameron[60] showed an 11-fold increase in respiratory complications if the trachea was intubated.

Because the decision to proceed with or postpone surgery is in doubt, it should be made in consultation with the surgeon and patient after all physical findings and laboratory data have been obtained. If the chest radiograph shows an acute active process, surgery should be postponed. In an ASA II or III patient with a productive cough and fever whose blood analysis shows a left shift in white cell count, surgery should probably be postponed.

Hepatic Diseases

Hepatic disease may contribute to abnormal pharmacokinetics of anesthetic agents or alterations in coagulation and may increase the risk of postoperative morbidity and mortality in patients with moderate or severe hepatitis, particularly acute hepatitis from any cause.[61]

All anesthetics cause transient abnormalities in liver function tests (LFTs).[62] Patients with preexisting hepatic disease have a higher incidence of postoperative abnormal LFT results, and thus a higher incidence of postoperative morbidity and mortality.[63]

There is no consensus on the utility or cost-effectiveness of routine preoperative serum LFTs in asymptomatic patients, even though some patients with no history of liver disease have abnormal LFT values.[64] The goal of preoperative testing is to identify patients with abnormal values so that the cause can be identified and surgery postponed (if possible) for treatment. If surgery cannot be delayed, the goal is to avoid further injury to the liver by careful selection of anesthetic agents.

Preoperative evaluation of patients with jaundice or ascites should include LFTs. In all ASA III patients and in ASA II patients with a history of alcohol ingestion, baseline LFTs should be obtained preoperatively, whether or not ascites is present. LFTs should also be performed in patients with a history of previous liver disease to verify return of normal liver function prior to surgery.

Much has been written about the anesthetic halothane and its association with postoperative liver disease. Review of the literature suggests that the development of postoperative liver dysfunction after anesthesia and surgery should not be routinely ascribed to "anesthesia," because the rate of other causes such as viruses and nonanesthetic drugs is higher.[65, 66]

Renal Diseases

Anesthesia and surgery decrease urinary output and the concentrating ability of the kidney.[67] These parameters of renal function return to baseline after surgery. Patients with mild kidney disease, determined by elevation in the blood urea nitrogen (BUN) and creatinine concentration, are at risk for further compromise of renal function and acute tubular necrosis. These measures of renal function vary widely and may not change until there is a 50% reduction in glomerular filtration rate. Because patients with renal disease often also have additional systemic disease(s), preoperative preparation should address all affected organ systems.

Preparation and perioperative management of these patients requires careful attention to maintenance of intravascular volume and urinary output. Nephrotoxic drugs should be avoided. Patients receiving diuretic therapy and those who have a recent history of vomiting or diarrhea must be evaluated carefully for intravascular hypovolemia and electrolyte abnormalities. Perioperative maintenance of urinary output may require continuous monitoring with a Foley catheter and measurement of intravascular volume via CVP or PAP. Periodic measurement of serum electrolytes and pH may also be required.

Patients on Dialysis

Most patients with end-stage renal disease (ESRD) require periodic dialysis and typically have concurrent heart disease, hypertension, and diabetes. They are routinely classified as ASA III or higher. By the time they first present for fistula placement for dialysis, they often have electrolyte and glucose abnormalities, low hemoglobin concentrations, and chronic metabolic acidosis and are at increased risk for perioperative morbidity as well as both fatal and nonfatal cardiac arrest.[68]

Preoperatively, intravascular volume should be evaluated, particularly if dialysis has been completed within 1 to 2 hours prior to surgery. Medications should be reviewed. Minimal preoperative laboratory examination should include measurement of hemoglobin, serum potassium, glucose, and carbon dioxide concentrations. Because serum magnesium and phosphate abnormalities can occur, baseline values should be obtained preoperatively if prolonged surgery is anticipated. Acid-base and electrolyte abnormalities should be corrected prior to surgery.

Intraoperative management should include periodic measurement of electrolytes, including pH and glucose concentration. Hemoglobin measurements are required if blood loss and blood replacement are anticipated. Vascular shunts placed for hemodialysis should be checked periodically during surgery to confirm patency.

Acid-base abnormalities must be detected and treated early to avoid adverse effects of acidosis on myocardial performance as well as peripheral vascular responsiveness. If spontaneous ventilation is allowed, affected patients may develop respiratory acidosis following intravenous sedation or inhalation anesthesia. Acidosis also alters drug effects and metabolism.

Postoperatively, patients on kidney dialysis are prone to infection, and care must be taken to minimize the risk of infection during vascular access or drug infusion.

Hypokalemia, particularly if acute, has been associated with cardiac arrhythmias.[69] For patients with chronic hypokalemia, most anesthesiologists would postpone elective surgery if serum potassium level is less than 3.5 to 4.0 mEq/L. Others consider 3.0 mEq/L the threshold for postponing elective surgery.[70] It is important to remember that a 1.0-mEq/L decrease in serum potassium represents a body deficit of approximately 100 mEq without any change in pH or glucose metabolism. Restoration of appropriate potassium levels must be achieved slowly to ensure patient safety.[71]

Hyperkalemia adversely affects the cardiac conduction system. Most anesthesiologists recommend postponing surgery when serum potassium levels equal 6.0 to 6.5 mEq/L. At these values, an ECG should be obtained. ECG changes secondary to hyperkalemia can be related to both total body potassium level and the rate of change as serum potassium increases. When ECG changes accompany hyperkalemia, treatment must be initiated to reduce the serum potassium concentration.

Endocrine Diseases

Diabetes

Approximately 10 million patients in the United States suffer from diabetes, an endocrine disorder characterized by an absolute or relative deficiency of insulin. Diabetes is commonly divided into two types characterized by clinical features, with some overlap. Type I diabetes, believed to be an autoimmune disease, results in the loss of pancreatic insulin-producing beta cells (absolute lack of insulin) and is associated with episodes of ketoacidosis. Type I diabetes generally begins at an early age, and exogenously administered insulin is required to maintain normal serum glucose levels and to avoid ketoacidosis. In type II diabetes (present in over 90% of all diabetics), pancreatic beta cells continue to produce insulin, but glucose level in the blood remains high. Type II diabetic patients generally are older and obese, do not require insulin (glucose is controlled by diet or oral hypoglycemic agents), and, although hyperglycemic, rarely experience hypoglycemic ketoacidosis. When insulin is deficient, these patients are prone to hyperosmolar, nonketotic hyperglycemia and subsequent coma.

Perioperative complications in diabetic patients may be related to the disease per se or to associated systemic diseases.[72] Acute complications include hypoglycemia and coma from either ketoacidosis or a nonketotic hyperglycemic hyperosmolar state. Long-term complications include autonomic and peripheral neuropathies, as well as ocular, renal, and cardiovascular manifestations. Diabetic patients are prone to episodes of "silent" cardiac ischemia. Some of these complications can also produce serious morbidity, eventually resulting in the need for surgery.

Preoperative management of these patients must include review of the medications used to manage glucose levels and their efficiency. The extent of end-organ damage due to diabetes should be documented, and cardiovascular function and cardiac reserve must be determined. Autonomic neuropathies can result in shortened gastric emptying times, placing these patients at increased risk for gastric aspiration.[73]

"Tight" control of glucose includes continuous insulin infusion, whereas "classic" control utilizes an intermittent regimen. The intraoperative impact of "tight" control of glucose and the long-term effects of both regimens are controversial and beyond the scope of this chapter. Both approaches require frequent measurement of glucose levels and adjustment in insulin administration. Portable compact devices are now available to accurately measure whole blood glucose concentration. Fluctuations in glucose levels should be avoided perioperatively and probably occur less often than in the past with the use of these devices. "Tight" control may incur risk of hypoglycemia more frequently than "classic" control—any occurrence of hypoglycemia intraoperatively is unacceptable while a patient is under general anesthesia or sedated with intravenous agents.

Infection is common postoperatively in diabetic patients and can be lethal. Glucose and insulin management is important. The cardiovascular and renal systems must be monitored closely in the recovery period because alterations in these organ systems often cause serious postoperative morbidity.

Obesity

Obesity affects the cardiovascular and respiratory systems, increasing perioperative morbidity and mortality.[74] Obesity also affects every aspect of anesthetic care, from choice of invasive or noninvasive blood pressure monitoring (intravascular monitoring of arterial pressure often is required, because patient size precludes accurate reading from blood pressure cuffs) to increased ventilator work to exchange respiratory gases.[75] Commonly, obese patients develop hypertension, cardiac hypertrophy, and type II diabetes. Deep vein thromboses, pulmonary emboli, and strokes are common. Gastric emptying is delayed. Smoking and alcohol intake further increase the risk associated with anesthesia and surgery. Postoperative respiratory complications are common.

Morbid obesity generally is defined as more than twice the predicted weight. These patients are often referred to as "pickwickian." They are hypoxemic and hypercarbic at rest, typically having right heart failure and polycythemia. Unfortunately, little can be done preoperatively to improve their condition. Their perioperative management usually includes invasive hemodynamic monitoring and postoperative care in an ICU.

Patients should be informed preoperatively of their increased perioperative risk and of strategies that may be used to decrease it. For example, awake fiberoptic intubation of the trachea may be the safest way to secure the airway, and postoperative intubation, perhaps in an intensive care setting, may be necessary to facilitate the work of breathing. Obesity also makes it difficult to position the patient ideally for the anesthesiologist and the surgeon. Alternative strategies, such as positioning in the postanesthesia care unit (PACU) to avoid hypoxemia, may help to reduce the risk of perioperative morbidity and mortality in obese patients.[76]

Perioperative Management of the Patient in Intermaxillary Fixation

Intermaxillary fixation is part of the treatment for several oral and maxillofacial surgery procedures. Airway management after surgery and, in particular, the period immediately after tracheal extubation deserves discussion, because affected patients may later develop airway obstruction or have difficulty clearing material from their oral cavity if they vomit.

Plans for extubation should include knowledge of the patient's preoperative pulmonary status, a plan for postoperative pain management, and equipment to remove the intermaxillary fixation, if necessary. Emergency release may be questionable. An oral and maxillofacial surgeon can release an internal fixation in 35 seconds; other health care professionals, over 2 minutes.[78a]

Before extubation is considered, the patient's mental status should have returned to the preoperative level. In most cases, they should be awake and alert and should understand all instructions given by the PACU or ICU nurses. Pharmacologic agents used to manage pain and decrease anxiety must be titrated in anticipation of extubation. While intubated, the patient should be instructed on how to mobilize secretions and how to use a suction device to remove debris from the oral cavity. Prior to extubation, the patient should suction the oral cavity and remove or swallow all accumulated secretions.

Devices to remove the intermaxillary fixation and personnel skilled in their use must be immediately available. If a nasogastric or orogastric tube is in place, it should be attached to suction and the stomach decompressed. Some suggest removal of the gastric tube before extubation; however, others remove it within a few hours after extubation.

A bag and mask system to deliver positive-pressure ventilation and a source to administer 100% oxygen should be available and confirmed to function properly before extubation of the trachea is attempted.

In some cases, direct visualization of the posterior pharynx prior to extubation may facilitate the decision about when to extubate the trachea. This approach may be accomplished via fiberoptic insertion through the nose. Inspection of the upper airway for swelling, bleeding, or other abnormalities may influence the plan for extubation.

At least 5 minutes before planned extubation, the inspired oxygen concentration should be increased to

100% ("preoxygenation") to provide the patient with several minutes of oxygen reserve in case postextubation airway problems develop. Unless a patient has copious pulmonary secretions, suctioning through the endotracheal tube prior to extubation should not be necessary and, in fact, can lead to unwarranted hypoxemia and systemic hypertension.[77, 78] In addition, pulmonary secretions are more efficiently mobilized by having the patient cough than by suctioning through endotracheal tubes. Some suggest deflating the endotracheal tube cuff and occluding the orifice of the endotracheal tube while asking the patient to take a breath, in order to evaluate potential airway obstruction in the posterior pharynx at the level of the base of the tongue and entrance to the larynx. Most anesthesiologists judge that if the patient can "breathe around the endotracheal tube," airway obstruction after extubation is unlikely. After "preoxygenation," the endotracheal tube cuff should be deflated and the tube removed while the patient is taking a deep breath of 100% oxygen. Once extubated, the patient should be instructed to take another deep breath to confirm airway patency.

No matter how well prepared, any plan for extubation may fail, resulting in postextubation airway obstruction or hypoxia. Therefore, a plan for resecuring the airway must be part of the extubation process. In some patients, extubation plans may include the presence of a surgeon who can perform a tracheostomy if the airway is lost after extubation.

Anesthetic Complications and Their Management

Malignant Hyperthermia

Malignant hyperthermia (MH) associated with anesthesia is a disorder of skeletal muscle inherited as an autosomal dominant trait. Human studies have identified the genetic linkage.[79] In patients who have inherited MH, triggering agents such as halothane and succinylcholine cause a massive increase in intracellular calcium, which produces sustained skeletal muscle activity, muscular rigidity, tachycardia, and fever.[80]

Massive skeletal muscle activity produces an increase in CO_2 production and oxygen consumption. Once the process is initiated, the following changes ensue: tachycardia with PVCs, temperature elevation, increasing end-tidal CO_2 ($ETCO_2$) tension, acidosis (both metabolic and respiratory), hyperkalemia, and, finally, muscle destruction with rhabdomyolysis and myoglobinuria. Death occurs if untreated. The only anesthetic triggering agents identified thus far are the inhalation agents, except nitrous oxide, and the muscle relaxant succinylcholine. Propofol does not appear to trigger MH.

Diagnosis must proceed with a high index of suspicion. No one sign is pathognomonic for MH. An unexpected rapid increase in temperature may be one of the late signs that MH is in progress. Increases in $ETCO_2$ may occur from faulty equipment, sepsis, or hyperthermia secondary to devices used to warm the patient. Other conditions producing some of the symptoms common to MH are pheochromocytoma, thyroid storm, and neuroleptic malignant syndrome.

Treatment of MH begins by discontinuing administration of the triggering agent(s). Dantrolene, 2.5 mg/kg IV, should be administered immediately, and repeated as frequently as every 5 minutes (if necessary) up to a total of 10 mg/kg. This drug is safe and must be administered while the circulation is still intact in order to reach the affected skeletal muscle. Without dantrolene, patients suffering from MH die. Increased carbon dioxide production should be treated by hyperventilation with 100% oxygen. Patients must be actively cooled by all methods available, including gastric lavage with iced saline whenever possible. Serum electrolytes and arterial blood gases should be measured early, with measurements repeated as often as necessary after therapy has begun. Hyperkalemia should be treated early, before it affects cardiac rhythm. Successful treatment is indicated by reductions in temperature, carbon dioxide production, and PVCs. Patient monitoring should continue for 2 to 3 days after resolution of an acute episode to detect signs of renal failure from myoglobin.

Patients who have experienced a prior episode of MH and patients with a strong family history of MH should receive dantrolene, 2.0 to 2.5 mg/kg IV, immediately prior to induction of anesthesia.

The Malignant Hyperthermia Association of the United States recommends calling a 24-hour hotline (Medic Alert, US) from which current information and immediate physician consultation for MH emergencies may be obtained 7 days a week; the phone number is (209) 634-4917.

Anaphylaxis

An excellent review of intraoperative anaphylactic reactions by Moss appears in the 1994 ASA Refresher Course Lectures.[81] Anaphylaxis most often occurs in response to administration of pharmacologic agents but also may occur with graft material, latex, or adjuvants used as preservatives for drugs. True anaphylaxis is an immunologically (immunoglobulin E [IgE])–mediated, severe, life-threatening allergic reaction. In a true anaphylactic hypersensitivity reaction (also known as an antigen-antibody reaction), IgE antibodies cause a massive release of pharmacologically active substances from within mast cells throughout the body. These substances produce urticaria, bronchospasm and upper airway edema, peripheral vasodilatation, alterations in capillary permeability, tachycardia, and changes in cardiac contractility.

Anaphylactoid is the term applied to non–IgE-mediated reactions. Non–IgE-mediated reactions are more common than IgE reactions, and their clinical manifestations typically are not as severe. In most anaphylactoid reactions, the mast cells release primarily histamine, and do so in much smaller quantities than in response to a true anaphylactic reaction. These smaller amounts of histamine result in a slow-developing, usually less severe, often limited clinical reaction. However, the clinical presentation of a severe anaphylactoid reaction may be indistinguishable from that of an anaphylactic reaction.

Ninety percent of all severe drug reactions occur within 10 minutes of administration.[82] The first signs of a severe reaction may be an unexplained or unexpected increase in heart rate of more than 30 beats per minute and a decrease in blood pressure of more than 30 torr. Bronchospasm occurs in a minority (less than 30%) of full-blown anaphylactic or anaphylactoid reactions. Similarly, cutaneous manifestations may or may not be present. If bronchospasm and urticaria accompany the cardiovascular changes just described, however, a severe allergic drug reaction (or an allergic reaction from some other cause) is under way.

Once the diagnosis of an anaphylactic or severe anaphylactoid reaction has been made, all inhalation anesthetics must be discontinued, and the lungs must be ventilated with 100% oxygen. Therapy is twofold: First, liberal administration of isotonic fluids through large-bore intravenous catheters must begin immediately. Large amounts of intravenous fluids, occasionally up to 4 to 6 liters, may be required. Second, epinephrine *must* be given intravenously to reverse the effects of the vasoactive substances causing cardiovascular collapse.[83] If the reaction is diagnosed early, the first dose of epinephrine may be small—0.1 mg; however, if blood pressure is already low, an initial dose of up to 0.4 mg may be required. Potentially, an initial bolus dose of epinephrine can be followed by a continuous infusion that can be adjusted to changes in blood pressure. Antihistamines (both H_1 and H_2 blockers) and steroids also may be administered, but they are not first-line treatment and should be considered only after administration of epinephrine and fluid.

Transient periods of hypotension during routine surgery are common. Treatment with ephedrine and a small bolus of isotonic fluid almost always resolves the hypotension. In a true anaphylactic reaction, ephedrine and small fluid boluses do not suffice; in fact, a lack of response to these agents is one indicator that anaphylaxis may be in progress. Epinephrine, not ephedrine, is the only acceptable treatment for anaphylactic or profound anaphylactoid reactions and must be administered immediately to ensure a successful outcome.

Following an anaphylactic or severe anaphylactoid reaction, patients should be observed in a monitored setting for 24 hours postoperatively. After resolution of an acute episode, skin testing can be performed to identify the cause.

Patients with a history of anaphylactic or severe anaphylactoid reactions should be treated preoperatively with H_1 and H_2 blockers. Though steroids do not have a place in the treatment of an acute reaction, their prophylactic use is advocated by some.[83] Intravenous access with large-bore intravenous catheters should be established in case a reaction occurs and fluid administration is required.

Cardiac Arrest[84]

Cardiopulmonary resuscitation and Advanced Cardiac Life Support (ACLS) protocols are revised periodically.[85, 86] Although intraoperative cardiac arrest and appropriate treatments have never been evaluated in a manner similar to that in emergency rooms, coronary care or intensive care units and cardiac electrophysiology laboratories, anesthesiologists, and surgeons understand the propensity of patients with cardiac disease for myocardial ischemia, infarction, arrhythmias, and cardiac arrest.

The current ACLS recommendations for treatment of cardiac arrest were presented at the 1992 National Conference on Cardiopulmonary Resuscitation and Emergency Cardiac Care and subsequently published in *JAMA* (October 1992). Because each case of cardiac arrest varies according to the clinical context, the 1992 recommendations encourage flexibility in decision-making and offer their algorithms as summaries to be used wisely, not blindly. The National Conference concluded that their protocols represent guidelines that may be modified to suit the clinical setting and the patient's symptoms. Table 1–3 is a list of the recommended dosages of commonly used antiarrhythmic agents.

Because the ACLS protocols are based on studies of

Table 1–3. Recommended Doses for Antiarrhythmic Agents*

Drug	Dosage
Adenosine	6–12 mg through a central vein; 12 mg may be repeated
Amiodarone	5–10 mg/kg loading dose over 30 min
Atropine	0.4–1.0 mg up to a total of 0.04 mg/kg
Bretylium	5–10 mg/kg loading dose over 20 min, followed by 0.5–2.0 mg/min infusion
Digitalis	0.25–1.0 mg up to a total dose of 2.0 mg
Esmolol	5–20 mg IV or infusion of 25–200 μg/kg/min
Ephedrine	5–10 mg
Epinephrine	0.1–1.0 mg; "high-dose" (up to 0.1 mg/kg); acceptable infusion dose is 2–10 μg/min
Glycopyrrolate	0.2–0.4 mg
Isoproterenol	1–4 μg/min infusion
Lidocaine	1.5 mg/kg loading dose followed by 1–4 mg/min infusion
Magnesium	1–2 g
Nitroglycerin	10 μg/min up to 5 μg/kg/min, as indicated
Procainamide	500 mg loading dose (slowly) followed by 1–4 mg/min infusion (total loading dose up to 17 mg/kg)
Propranolol	0.25–1.0 mg every 1–2 min up to a total of 0.15 mg/kg
Sodium bicarbonate	1 mEq/kg; arterial blood gases should guide therapy
Verapamil	0.25–5.0 mg up to a total dose of 20 mg

*All dosage recommendations are for intravenous administration in adults.

out-of-hospital cardiac arrest and of in-hospital cardiac arrest of patients *outside* the operating room, the ACLS recommendations must be modified to address the unique clinical conditions associated with surgery. For example, most, if not all, surgical patients already have intravenous lines, supplemental oxygen, and an intubated trachea, all of which are part of ACLS resuscitation efforts.

Cardiac arrest scenarios fit into two categories. Heart rate is either too rapid or too slow. Although simplistic, categorizing life-threatening arrhythmias in this way provides a basis for treatment. That is, all tachycardias resulting in inadequate blood pressure or organ hypoperfusion require immediate defibrillation. Conversely, any bradycardia too slow to produce adequate cardiac output requires immediate cardiac pacing. Devices for administering cardiac pacing and defibrillation should be immediately accessible wherever anesthesia and surgery are performed.

Once a life-threatening intraoperative cardiac arrhythmia is recognized, airway management must include the administration of 100% oxygen, and the patient's trachea immediately intubated (if not already done). If pulse oximetry verified adequate peripheral oxygen saturation immediately preceding the arrest, hypoxemia is not likely the cause. Equally critical and time dependent is determining whether an anesthetic overdose is the possible cause of the arrest. All operating rooms in which high-risk surgery is performed should be equipped with gas analyzers to sample both inspired and exhaled gases from the patient's airway. Exhaled anesthetic gas concentrations should be reviewed and the anesthetic concentration reduced if indicated by analysis of the information. Continuous infusions of intravenous anesthetics should be stopped until cardiac stability is restored.

Blood gas analysis should begin early in all cases of intraoperative cardiac arrest and continue often enough to evaluate treatment. Blood gas analysis should direct therapy of acid-base abnormalities and verify adequate oxygenation. The use of sodium bicarbonate to correct acidosis during cardiac arrest continues to be evaluated.[86] Although this agent is recommended for use in a number of arrest scenarios, it is important to remember that sodium bicarbonate can decrease aortic pressure[87] and does increase total body carbon dioxide content. Both changes are counterproductive during conditions requiring cardiopulmonary resuscitation (CPR).

Ventricular Fibrillation and Rapid Ventricular Tachycardia

Unexpected ventricular fibrillation or pulseless ventricular tachycardia (Fig. 1–1) should be treated by immediate defibrillation (Fig. 1–2). Early defibrillation is critical and is the major determinant of survival in cardiac arrest due to ventricular fibrillation. There can be no delay in diagnosis. If a defibrillator is not immediately available when ventricular fibrillation or pulseless ventricular tachycardia is first noted, CPR must be initiated at once and continued until a defibrillator arrives. Once the defibrillator is at hand, the first shock should be conducted at 200 joules (J). If the arrhythmia persists, a second shock of 200 to 300 J should follow, with subsequent shocks conducted at 360 to 400 J. Some clinicians believe that if the first external shock of 200 J is unsuccessful, all subsequent defibrillation attempts should occur at the highest energy level available. If three attempts at defibrillation are not successful and the patient remains pulseless, CPR must be started (or continued) and pharmacologic therapy initiated.

Guidelines recommend administration of epinephrine, 1.0 mg IV every 3 to 5 minutes. Higher doses (3 to 5 mg IV every 3 to 5 min) may be considered if the lower dose is ineffective. The positive effects of epinephrine derive from its α_1-adrenergic stimulatory properties, which induce arterial vasoconstriction, thereby increasing coronary artery perfusion pressure. Large doses (2 to 2.5 times the IV dose) are recommended if epinephrine is to be delivered through an endotracheal tube, although the optimal endotracheal tube dose for treating cardiac arrest has not been defined.[88] A continuous infusion of epinephrine also may be considered.

If pharmacologic therapy is to be effective, the cellular environment must be evaluated. Electrolyte (particularly hyperkalemia) and acid-base (particularly acidosis) abnormalities must be corrected, and hypoxia must be eliminated. Arterial blood gas analysis should guide bicarbonate therapy. Sodium bicarbonate administration should not be withheld on theoretic grounds but used to correct a metabolic acidosis when deemed appropriate. If ST segment changes precede the arrest, myocardial ischemia may be the cause, and pharmacotherapy may be necessary.

Data demonstrating improvement in outcome when doses higher than the recommended epinephrine dose (1.0 mg) are given are conflicting.[89, 90] There are no studies evaluating the use of epinephrine during intraoperative cardiac arrest. Other drugs recommended to assist defibrillation after three unsuccessful shocks include bretylium, administered in a 5-mg/kg bolus followed 5 minutes later by a 10-mg/kg bolus. In the operating room, some clinicians prefer to initiate pharmacologic defibrillation with lidocaine (1.5-mg/kg IV bolus followed by a constant infusion of 1 to 4 mg/min), reserving epinephrine for later use if defibrillation remains unsuccessful.

Other recommendations to facilitate defibrillation are procainamide, administered at 30 mg/min up to a 500-mg loading dose followed by a constant infusion of 2 to 4 mg/min, and magnesium sulfate at 1 to 2 g IV. When none of these agents succeeds, intravenous administration of amiodarone has been suggested, but studies of the efficacy of this drug during cardiac arrest are lacking, and this agent is not addressed in the ACLS guidelines.[91] Whether any antiarrhythmic agent can alter the outcome of ventricular fibrillation or pulseless ventricular tachycardia when defibrillation and epinephrine administration fail is unclear.[86]

Even a short, easily terminated episode of intraoperative ventricular fibrillation or pulseless ventricular

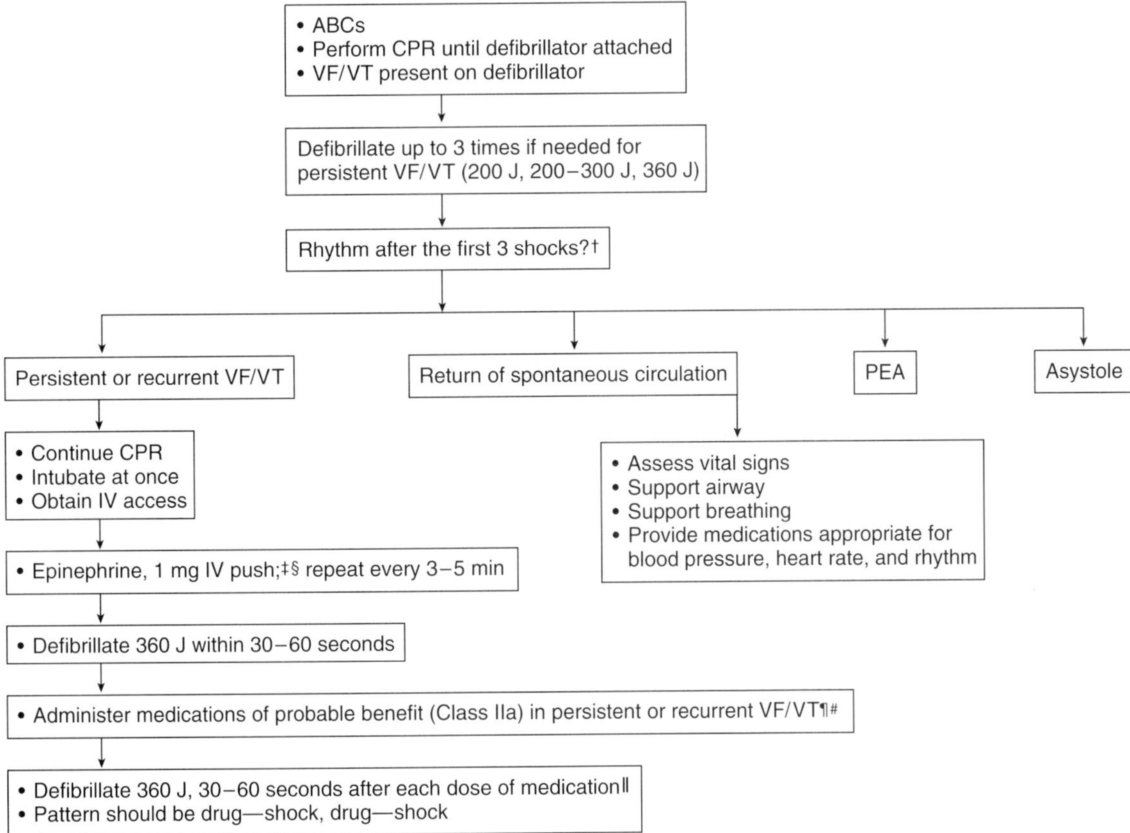

Class I: definitely helpful.
Class IIa: acceptable, probably helpful.
Class IIb: acceptable, possibly helpful.
Class III: not indicated, may be harmful.
* Precordial thump is a Class IIb action in witnessed arrest, no pulse, and no defibrillator immediately available.
† Hypothermic cardiac arrest is treated differently after this point. See section on hypothermia.
‡ The recommended dose of epinephrine is 1 mg IV push every 3–5 min. If this approach fails, several Class IIb dosing regimens can be considered:
- Intermediate: epinephrine, 2–5 mg IV push, every 3–5 min
- Escalating: epinephrine, 1–3–5 mg IV push, 3 min apart
- High: epinephrine, 0.1 mg/kg IV push, every 3–5 min.

§ Sodium bicarbonate (1 mEq/kg) is Class I if patient has known preexisting hyperkalemia.
‖ Multiple sequenced shocks (200 J, 200–300 J, 360 J) are acceptable here (Class I), especially when medications are delayed.
¶ • Lidocaine, 1.5 mg/kg IV push. Repeat in 3–5 min to total loading dose of 3 mg/kg; then use:
- Bretylium, 5 mg/kg IV push; repeat in 5 min at 10 mg/kg
- Magnesium sulfate, 1–2 g IV in torsades de pointes or suspected hypomagnesemic state or severe refractory VF
- Procainamide, 30 mg/min in refractory VF (maximum total 17 mg/kg).

• Sodium bicarbonate, 1 mEq/kg IV:
Class IIa
- If known preexisting bicarbonate-responsive acidosis
- If overdose with tricyclic antidepressants
- To alkalinize the urine in drug overdoses.

Class IIb
- If intubated and continued long arrest interval
- On return of spontaneous circulation after long arrest interval.

Class III
- If hypoxic lactic acidosis.

Figure 1–1. Algorithm for the treatment of ventricular fibrillation *(VF)* and pulseless ventricular tachycardia *(VT)*. *ABCs*, airway, breathing, circulation; *PEA*, pulseless electrical activity;

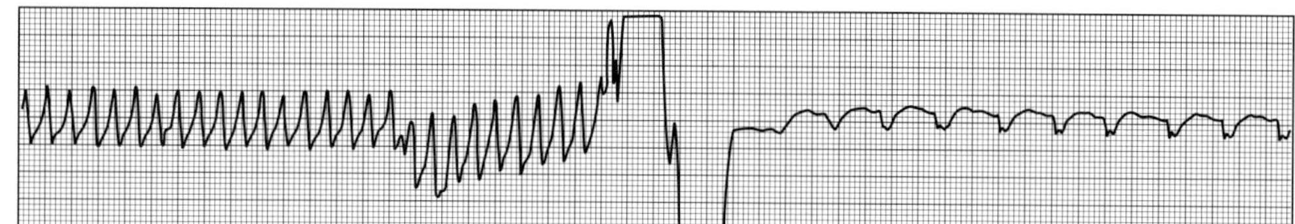

Figure 1–2. Ventricular flutter/fibrillation. After the rhythm is defibrillated, sinus rhythm with a wide QRS complex returns.

tachycardia should stimulate a search for the cause. If the cause is not treated, the condition is likely to recur.

Pulseless Electrical Activity

Pulseless electrical activity (PEA) replaces the former term, *electromechanical dissociation*. The new term incorporates electromechanical dissociation and a group of ECG rhythms (other than ventricular tachycardia and ventricular fibrillation) associated with an absence of a detectable pulse. These rhythms include idioventricular rhythms, ventricular escape rhythms, postdefibrillation idioventricular rhythms, and bradysystolic rhythms. These arrhythmias often are associated with specific clinical conditions that are reversible when identified early and treated appropriately. The complete list of causes is presented in the treatment algorithm (Fig. 1–3). Intraoperatively, the most common causes are likely to be related to the type of surgery performed.

During major head and neck surgery, blood loss is likely to be the most common cause. Tension pneumothorax, particularly if the site of operation is near the diaphragm, also may be a cause. Pulmonary barotrauma may result in a tension pneumothorax in patients undergoing such procedures, because most have a long history of smoking and associated lung disease. Other causes of pulseless electrical activity are pulmonary embolism and cardiac tamponade due to air or a pericardial effusion. Although PEA is a dramatic event, prognosis is favorable if the cause is identified and treated early. When the cause of pulseless electrical activity is not quickly identified and corrected, intravenous epinephrine, 1 mg every 3 to 5 minutes, may be required to restore blood pressure. Higher epinephrine doses also may be indicated.

Atropine, 1 mg every 3 to 5 minutes up to a total dose of 0.04 mg/kg, or transcutaneous pacing may be indicated for bradycardia.

Asystole

Asystole is a rhythm associated with poor prognosis and survival. However, this conclusion is based largely on studies of out-of-hospital patients and nonsurgical patients in the wards or intensive care units. If asystole is the result of *prolonged unsuccessful* attempts at terminating ventricular fibrillation or pulseless ventricular tachycardia, further resuscitation attempts to treat asystole will almost always fail. If asystole follows *early termination* of ventricular fibrillation or other pulseless tachyarrhythmias, then cardiac pacing or CPR alone or in combination with epinephrine is more likely to restore an effective cardiac rhythm. The treatment algorithm for asystole is shown in Figure 1–4.

Intraoperative treatment of asystole appears to have a better outcome than treatment given outside the operating room, but studies to verify this clinical impression are lacking. The 1992 ACLS guidelines for treatment of asystole place more emphasis on identifying and eliminating the causes, and encourage the early use of emergency transcutaneous pacing. The list of possible causes of asystole is presented in the algorithm. Interventions are determined by the causes. Routine use of defibrillation to treat asystole is discouraged.

The immediate goal when intraoperative asystole is suspected is twofold: (1) verify the arrhythmia using at least two ECG leads and (2) initiate maneuvers to produce a cardiac rhythm (Fig. 1–5). If asystole is confirmed by observing two ECG leads or by direct observation of the heart, then cardiac pacing, preferably transcutaneous, should be instituted as soon as possible.

If a pacemaker is not immediately available, CPR should continue until cardiac pacing can be instituted. Fine ventricular fibrillation may masquerade as asystole; if the diagnosis is *uncertain*, immediate defibrillation with 200 J is acceptable therapy, although studies of shocks for asystole have detected no improvement in survival. Recommended treatment strategies include intravenous pharmacologic agents likely to stimulate cardiac pacemaker cell discharge. The suggested drugs include epinephrine (1.0 mg) and atropine (1.0 mg up to a total of 0.04 mg/kg) every 3 to 5 minutes. Larger doses of epinephrine may also be appropriate. Isuprel (IV infusion of 2 to 10 μg/min) is no longer recommended. However, the effect of this agent on cardiac pacemaker cells is well-established.

Again, it is important to remember that neither cardiac pacing nor pharmacologic therapy will be successful unless the patient has a normal acid-base balance and is not hypoxic. Therefore, analysis of an arterial blood sample should be conducted early in the evaluation and treatment of asystole.

Conclusion

Preoperative preparation, intraoperative vigilance, and postoperative care are the foundations of a successful surgical outcome. A good working relationship among the patient's primary physician, anesthesiologist, and surgeon is essential. Each must be able to talk to the other whenever necessary. Questions and subsequent responses written on the chart should be preceded by discussion whenever an important issue is identified. In the operating room, the surgeon and anesthesiologist must know what the other is doing,

PEA includes
- Electromechanical dissociation (EMD)
- Pseudo-EMD
- Idioventricular rhythms
- Ventricular escape rhythms
- Bradyasystolic rhythms
- Postdefibrillation idioventricular rhythms

- Continue CPR
- Intubate at once
- Obtain IV access
- Assess blood flow using Doppler ultrasound

↓

Consider possible causes (Parentheses indicate possible therapies and treatments):
- Hypovolemia (volume infusion)
- Hypoxia (ventilation)
- Cardiac tamponade (pericardiocentesis)
- Tension pneumothorax (needle decompression)
- Hypothermia
- Massive pulmonary embolism (surgery, thrombolytics)
- Drug overdoses such as tricyclics, digitalis, β-blockers, calcium channel blockers
- Hyperkalemia*
- Acidosis†
- Massive acute myocardial infarction

↓

- Epinephrine, 1 mg IV push,*‡ repeat every 3–5 min

↓

- If absolute bradycardia (<60 beats/min) or relative bradycardia, give atropine, 1 mg IV
- Repeat every 3–5 min up to a total of 0.04 mg/kg§

Class I: definitely helpful.
Class IIa: acceptable, probably helpful.
Class IIb: acceptable, possibly helpful.
Class III: not indicated, may be harmful.
* Sodium bicarbonate, 1 mEq/kg, is Class I if patient has known preexisting hyperkalemia.
† Sodium bicarbonate, 1 mEq/kg:
Class IIa
- If known preexisting bicarbonate-responsive acidosis
- If overdose with tricyclic antidepressants
- To alkalinize the urine in drug overdoses.

Class IIb
- If intubated and long arrest interval
- On return of spontaneous circulation after long arrest interval.

Class III
- If hypoxic lactic acidosis.

‡ The recommended dose of epinephrine is 1 mg IV push every 3–5 min. If this approach fails, several Class IIb dosing regimens can be considered:
- Intermediate: epinephrine, 2–5 mg IV push, every 3–5 min
- Escalating: epinephrine, 1–3–5 mg IV push (3 min apart)
- High: epinephrine, 0.1 mg/kg IV push, every 3–5 min.

§ Shorter atropine dosing intervals are possibly helpful in cardiac arrest (Class IIb).

Figure 1–3. Algorithm for pulseless electrical activity *(PEA)*.

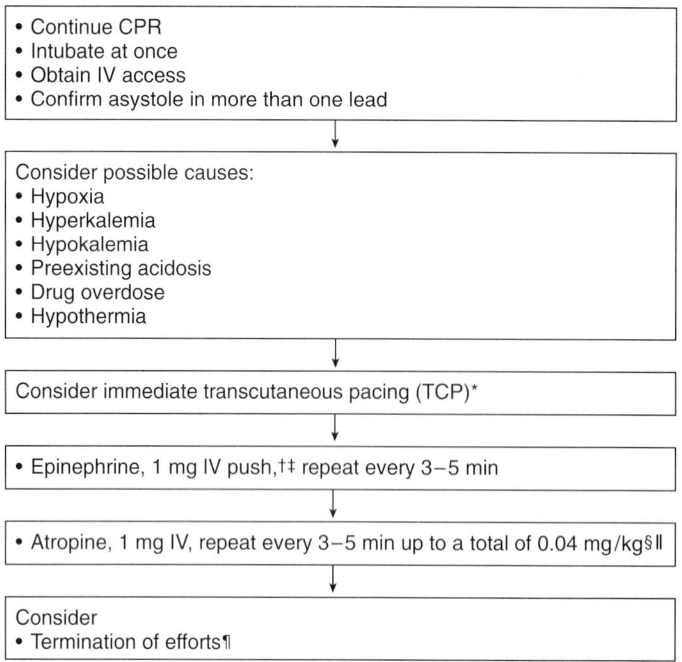

Class I: definitely helpful.
Class IIa: acceptable, probably helpful.
Class IIb: acceptable, possibly helpful.
Class III: not indicated, may be harmful.

* TCP is a Class IIb intervention. Lack of success may be due to delay in pacing. To be effective, TCP must be performed early, simultaneously with drugs. Evidence does not support routine use of TCP for asystole.

† The recommended dose of epinephrine is 1 mg IV push every 3–5 min. If this approach fails, several Class IIb dosing regimens can be considered:
- Intermediate: epinephrine, 2–5 mg IV push, every 3–5 min
- Escalating: epinephrine, 1–3–5 mg IV push, 3 min apart
- High: epinephrine, 0.1 mg/kg IV push, every 3–5 min.

‡ Sodium bicarbonate, 1 mEq/kg, is Class I if patient has known preexisting hyperkalemia.

§ Shorter atropine dosing intervals are Class IIb in asystolic arrest.

‖ • Sodium bicarbonate, 1 mEq/kg:
  Class IIa
  - If known preexisting bicarbonate-responsive acidosis
  - If overdose with tricyclic antidepressants
  - To alkalinize the urine in drug overdoses.

  Class IIb
  - If intubated and continued long arrest interval
  - On return of spontaneous circulation after long arrest interval.

  Class III
  - If hypoxic lactic acidosis.

¶ If patient remains in asystole or other agonal rhythms after successful intubation and initial medications and no reversible causes are identified, consider termination of resuscitative efforts by a physician. Consider interval since arrest.

Figure 1–4. Algorithm for asystole.

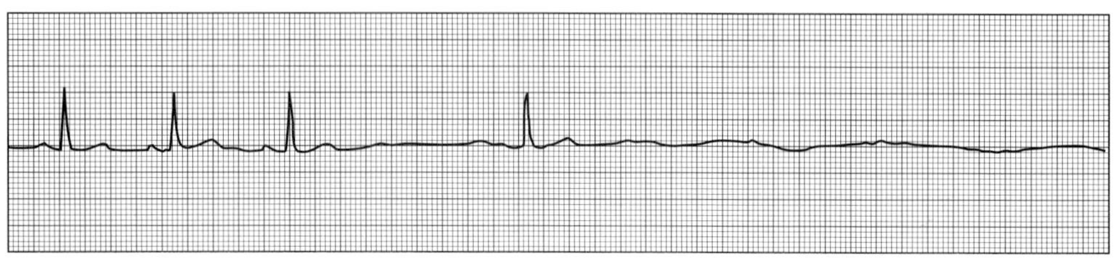

Figure 1–5. The first three beats are sinus rhythm. After the fourth beat, there is a period of no cardiac electrical activity, consistent with asystole.

and intraoperative communication must occur freely, particularly when problems with blood pressure or cardiac rhythm are encountered. Staying out of trouble is always preferred to getting out of trouble. Working together is the only method that offers the best outcome. Anything less should not be tolerated.

Acknowledgment

The author gratefully acknowledges the assistance of Winifred von Ehrenburg, M.A., for editorial advice.

References

1. Katz J, Benumof J, Kadis L: Anesthesia and Uncommon Diseases, ed 3. Philadelphia, WB Saunders, 1990.
2. Stolting RK, Dierdorf SF: Anesthesia and Co-Existing Disease, ed 3. New York, Churchill Livingstone, 1993.
3. Snow J: On the inhalation of the vapour of ether in surgical operations. London, John Churchill, 1847.
4. Derrington MC, Smith G: A review of studies of anaesthetic risk, morbidity, and mortality. Br J Anaesth 1987;59:815.
5. Lunn JN, Mushin WW: Mortality Associated with Anaesthesia. London, Nuffield Provincial Hospitals Trust, 1982.
6. Buck N, Devlin HB, Lunn JN: Report of the Confidential Enquiry into Perioperative Deaths: Nuffield Provincial Hospitals Trust. London, The King's Fund Publishing House, 1987.
7. Tiret L, Hatton F, Desmonts JM, et al: Prediction of outcome of anaesthesia in patients over 40 years: A multifactorial risk index. Stat Med 1988;7:947.
8. Cohen MM, Duncan PG, Tate RB: Does anesthesia contribute to operative mortality? JAMA 1988; 260:2859.
9. Dripps RD, Lamont A, Eckenhoff JE: The role of anesthesia in surgical mortality. JAMA 1961;178:261.
10. Marx GH, Matteo CV, Orkin LR: Computer analysis of post anesthetic deaths. Anesthesiology 1973;39:54.
11. Caplan RA, Posner KL, Ward RJ, et al: Adverse respiratory events in anesthesia: A closed claim analysis. Anesthesiology 1990;72:828.
12. Vacanti CJ, Van Houten RJ, Hill RC: A statistical analysis of the relationship of physical status to postoperative mortality in 68,388 cases. Anesth Analg 1970;49:564.
13. Keenan RL, Boyan CP: Cardiac arrest due to anesthesia: A study of incidence and causes. JAMA 1985;253:2373.
14. Cohen MM, Duncan PG, Pope WDB, et al: Postoperative complications: Factors of significance to anaesthetic practice. Can Anaesth Soc J 1987;34:2.
15. Forrest JB, Rehder K, Cahalan MK, Goldsmith CH: Multicenter study of general anesthesia. III: Predictors of severe perioperative adverse outcomes. Anesthesiology 1992;76:3.
16. Wong KC: Preoperative discontinuation of monoamine oxidase inhibitor therapy: An old wives' tale? Semin Anesth 1986;5:145.
17. Mangano DM: Perioperative cardiac morbidity. Anesthesiology 1990;72:153.
18. Goldman L, Caldera DL, Nussbaum SR: Multifactorial index of cardiac risk in noncardiac surgical procedures. N Engl J Med 1977;297:845.
19. Detsky AS, Abrams HS, Forbath N, et al: Cardiac assessment for patients undergoing noncardiac surgery: A multifactorial clinical risk index. Arch Intern Med 1986;146:2131.
20. Knorring JV: Postoperative myocardial infarction: A prospective study in a risk group of surgical patients. Surgery 1981;90:55.
21. Tarhan S, Moffitt EA, Taylor WF, Guiliani ER: Myocardial infarction after general anesthesia. JAMA 1972;220:1451.
22. Steen PA, Tinker JH, Tarhan S: Myocardial reinfarction after anesthesia and surgery. JAMA 1978;239:2566.
23. Criteria Committee, New York Heart Association, Inc: Diseases of the Heart and Blood Vessels: Nomenclature and Criteria for Diagnosis, ed 6. Boston, Little, Brown, 1964, p 114.
24. Raby KE: Reducing cardiac risk in patients undergoing peripheral vascular surgery. J Myocard Ischemia 1994;6:37.
25. Crawford ES, Morriss GC, Howell JF, et al: Operative risk in patients with previous coronary artery bypass. Ann Thorac Surg 1978;26:215.
26. Huber KC, Evan MA, Bresnahan JF, et al: Outcome of noncardiac operation in patients with severe coronary disease successfully treated preoperatively with coronary angioplasty. Mayo Clin Proc 1992;67:15.
27. Rao TLK, Jacobs KH, El Etr AA: Reinfarction following anesthesia in patients with myocardial infarction. Anesthesiology 1983;59:499.
28. Crawford MH: Transesophageal echocardiography. Cardiol Clin 1993;11:1.
29. Leung LM, Levine EH: Left ventricular end-systolic cavity obliteration as an estimate of intraoperative hypovolemia. Anesthesiology 1994;81:1102.
30. Subcommittee on Definition and Prevalence of the 1984 Joint National Committee: Hypertension prevalence and the status of awareness, treatment, and control in the United States. Hypertension 1985;7:457.
31. Working Group on Hypertension in the Elderly: Statement on hypertension in the elderly. JAMA 1986;256:70.
32. Prys-Roberts C, Meloche R, Foex P: Studies of anaesthesia in relation to hypertension. I: Cardiovascular responses of treated and untreated patients. Br J Anaesth 1971;43:122.
33. Stone JG, Foex P, Sear JE, et al: Risk of myocardial ischemia during anesthesia in treated and untreated hypertensive patients. Br J Anaesth 1988;61:675.
34. Mauney FM, Ebert PA, Sabiston DC: Postoperative myocardial infarction: A study of predisposing factors, diagnosis and mortality in a high risk group of surgical patients. Ann Surg 1970;172:497.
35. Asiddao CB, Donegan JH, Whitesell RC, et al: Factors associated with perioperative complications during carotid endarterectomy. Anesth Analg 1982;61:631.
36. Goldman L, Caldera DL: Risks of general anesthesia and elective operation in the hypertensive patient. Anesthesiology 1979; 50:285.
37. Bedford RF, Feinstein B: Hospital admission blood pressure: A predictor for hypertension following endotracheal intubation. Anesth Analg 1980;59:367.
38. Prys-Roberts C, Foex P, Green LT, et al: Studies of anaesthesia in relation to hypertension. IV: The effects of artificial ventilation on the circulation and pulmonary gas exchange. Br J Anaesth 1972;44:335.
39. Durack DT: Prevention of infective endocarditis. N Engl J Med 1995;332:38.
40. Shapiro WA: Practical management of the pacemaker patient. (Refresher Course Abstracts, p 19.) Society of Cardiovascular Anesthesiologists, Montreal, Canada, April 23–27, 1994.
41. Benumof JL: Respiratory physiology and respiratory function during anesthesia. *In* Miller RD (ed): Anesthesia. New York, Churchill Livingstone, 1994, p 577.
42. Schwartz DE, Katz JA: Delivery of mechanical ventilation during general anesthesia. *In* Tobin MJ (ed): Principles and Practice of Mechanical Ventilation. New York, McGraw-Hill, 1994, p 529.
43. Boushy SF, Billing DM, North LB, et al: Clinical course related to preoperative pulmonary function in patients with bronchogenic carcinoma. Chest 1971;59:383.
44. Tisi GM: Preoperative evaluation of pulmonary function. Am Rev Respir Dis 1979;119:293.
45. Robinson K, Conroy RM, Mulcahy R: When does the risk of acute coronary heart disease in ex-smokers fall to that in non-smokers? Br Heart J 1989;62:16.
46. Warner MA, Offerd KP, Warner ME, et al: Role of preoperative cessation of smoking and other factors in postoperative pulmonary complications: A blinded prospective study of coronary artery bypass patients. Mayo Clin Proc 1989;64:609.
47. Neiwoehner DE, Kleinerman J, Rice DB: Pathologic changes in the peripheral airways of young cigarette smokers. N Engl J Med 1974;291:755.
48. Wright DJ, Pandya A: Smoking and gastric juice volume in outpatients. Can Anaesth Soc J 1979;26:328.
49. Gould AB: Effect of obesity on respiratory complications following general anesthesia. Anesth Analg 1962;41:448.
50. Pearce AC, Jones RM: Smoking and anesthesia: Preoperative abstinence and postoperative morbidity. Anesthesiology 1984; 61:576.
51. Celli BR, Rodriguez KS, Snider GL: A controlled trial of intermit-

tent positive pressure breathing, incentive spirometry, and deep breathing exercises in preventing pulmonary complications after abdominal surgery. Am Rev Respir Dis 1984;130:12.
52. Matthay MA, Niederman MS, Wiedemann HP: Cardiovascular-pulmonary interaction in chronic obstructive pulmonary disease with special reference to pathogenesis and management of cor pulmonale. Med Clin North Am 1990;74:571.
53. Barnes PJ: A new approach to the treatment of asthma. N Engl J Med 1989;321:1517.
54. Kingston HGG, Hirshman CA: Perioperative management of the patient with asthma. Anesth Analg 1984;63:844.
55. Fishman AP: Cardiac asthma—a fresh look at an old wheeze. N Engl J Med 1989;320:1346.
56. William KN, Carli F, Cormack RS: Unexpected, difficult laryngoscopy: A prospective survey in routine general surgery. Br J Anaesth 1991;66:38.
57. Mallampati SR, Gatt SP, Gugino LD, et al: A clinical sign to predict difficult tracheal intubation: A prospective study. Can Anaesth Soc J 1985;32:429.
57a. Dhara A: Retrograde intubation: a facilitated approach. Br J Anaesth 1992;69:631–633.
58. American Society of Anesthesiologists Task Force on Management of the Difficult Airway: Practice guidelines for management of the difficult airway. Anesthesiology 1993;78:597.
59. Tait AR, Knight PR: Intraoperative respiratory complications in patients with upper respiratory tract infections. Can J Anaesth 1987;34:300.
60. Cohen MM, Cameron CB: Should you cancel the operation when a child has an upper respiratory tract infection? Anesth Analg 1991;72:282.
61. Strunin L: Preoperative assessment of the patient with liver dysfunction. Br J Anaesth 1978;50:25.
62. Clark R, Doggart J, Tavery T: Changes in liver function after different types of surgery. Br J Anaesth 1976;48:119.
63. Farman JV: Anaesthesia in the presence of liver disease and for hepatic transplantation. Br J Anaesth 1972;44:946.
64. Wataneeyawech M, Kelly KA Jr: Hepatic diseases: Unsuspected before surgery. N Y State J Med 1975;75:1278.
65. Alter MJ: Non-A, non-B hepatitis: Sorting through a diagnosis of exclusion. Ann Intern Med 1989;110:583.
66. Bunker JP, Forrest WH, Mosteller F, et al (eds): The National Halothane Study: A Study of the Possible Association Between Halothane Anesthesia and Postoperative Hepatic Necrosis. National Institute of General Medical Sciences, Washington, DC, US Government Printing Office, 1969.
67. Sladen RN: Effect of anesthesia and surgery on renal function. Crit Care Clin 1987;3:373.
68. Solomonson KD, Johnson ME, Ilstrup D: Risk factors in patients having surgery to create an arteriovenous fistula. Anesth Analg 1994;79:694.
69. Cohen JD, Neaton JD, Prineas RJ, Daniels KA: Diuretics, serum potassium, and ventricular arrhythmias in the multiple risk factor intervention. Am J Cardiol 1987;60:548.
70. Hirsch IA, Tomlinson DL, Slogoff S, Keats AS: The overstated risk of preoperative hypokalemia. Anesth Analg 1988;67:131.
71. Harrington JT, Isner JM, Kassirer JP: Our national obsession with potassium. Am J Med 1982;73:155.
72. Hirsch IB, McGill JB, Cryer PE, White PF: Perioperative management of surgical patients with diabetes mellitus. Anesthesiology 1991;74:346.
73. Mulhall BP, O'Fearghail M: Diabetic gastroparesis: Case report and review of the literature. Anaesthesia 1984;39:468.
74. Morray JP, Geiduschek JM, Caplan RA, et al: A comparison of pediatric and adult anesthesia closed malpractice claims. Anesthesiology 1993;78:461.
75. Buckley FP: Anesthetizing the Morbidly Obese Patient. (ASA Refresher Course Lectures, pp 53–67.) American Society of Anesthesiologists, Philadelphia, JB Lippincott, 1990.
76. Vaughan RW, Bauer S, Wise L: Effect of position (semirecumbent versus supine) on postoperative oxygenation in markedly obese subjects. Anesth Analg 1976;55:37.
77. DePew CL, Noll ML: Inline closed-system suctioning: A research analysis. Dimensions of Critical Care Nursing 1993;13:73.
77a. Goss AN, Chau KK, Mayne LH: Intermaxillary fixation: how practical in emergency jaw release? Anaesth Intens Care 1979;7: 253–257.
78. Stone KS, Bell SD, Preusser BA: The effect of repeated endotracheal suctioning on arterial blood pressure. Appl Nurs Res 1991;4:152.
79. Levitt RC, Olckers A, Meyers S, et al: Evidence for the localization of malignant hyperthermia susceptibility locus (MHS2) to human chromosome 17q. Genomics 1992;14:562.
80. Gronert GA: Malignant hyperthermia. Anesthesiology 1980; 53:395.
81. Moss J: Anaphylactoid and anaphylactic reactions in the operating room. (ASA Refresher Course Lectures, p 145.) American Society of Anesthesiologists, San Francisco, California, Oct.: 15–19, 1994.
82. Delage C, Irey NS: Anaphylactic deaths: A clinicopathologic study of 43 cases. J Forensic Sci 1972;17:525.
83. Barach EM, Nowak RM, Lee TG, et al: Epinephrine for treatment of anaphylactic shock. JAMA 1984;251:2118.
84. Shapiro WA: Management of intraoperative cardiac arrhythmias and cardiac arrest. *In* White RA, Hollier LH (eds): Vascular Surgery: Basic Science and Clinical Correlations. Philadelphia, JB Lippincott, 1994, p 597.
85. American Heart Association: Standards and guidelines for cardiopulmonary resuscitation (CPR) and emergency cardiac care (ECC). JAMA 1992;268:2171.
86. Niemann JT: Cardiopulmonary resuscitation. N Engl J Med 1992;327:1075.
87. Kette F, Weil MH, Gazmuri RJ: Buffer solutions may compromise cardiac resuscitation by reducing coronary perfusion pressure. JAMA 1991;266:2121.
88. Intratracheal drugs. Lancet 1988;1:743.
89. Koscove EM, Paradis NA: Successful resuscitation from cardiac arrest using high-dose epinephrine therapy. JAMA 1988;259:3031.
90. Brown CG, Martin DR, Pepe PE, et al: A comparison of standard-dose and high-dose epinephrine in cardiac arrest outside the hospital. N Engl J Med 1992;327:1051.
91. Kutalek SP, Horowitz LN, Spielman SR, et al: Emergent use of intravenous amiodarone for refractory ventricular tachyarrhythmias [abstract]. Circulation 1985;72(suppl 3):274.

Chapter 2

AMBULATORY (OFFICE) ANESTHESIA COMPLICATIONS

by

Robert Campbell

Introduction

The administration of ambulatory anesthesia in free-standing surgicenters, hospital outpatient departments, and offices has been one of the most cost-efficient advancements in the modern health care system. Despite the advantages of being able to perform surgery and to send a patient home at minimal cost, however, the surgeon and the anesthesiologist both must be cognizant of complications that may occur within 24 to 48 hours of discharge. Careful selection of patients, although important, is no guarantee of a successful outcome. An ASA I (American Society of Anesthesiologists classification; see Chapter 1, Table 1–1) patient may have a serious complication if either the surgical procedure or the anesthetic technique is flawed. In the case of the former, excessive bleeding, pain, or airway obstruction could be fatal. These are some examples of "delayed" (after discharge from the facility) surgical complications with postanesthesia implications. Faulty anesthesia technique can be expected to result in *intraoperative* or *early postoperative* (i.e., in the recovery room) consequences, but a seemingly benign intraoperative anesthetic event (e.g., difficult airway maintenance, excessive tachycardia, hypertension) can also result in "delayed" complications (e.g., airway edema, myocardial infarction, pneumonia, respectively).

THE SUBJECTS DISCUSSED IN THIS CHAPTER ARE:

Preanesthesia Considerations

Patient Selection

The evaluation of ASA I patients who are going to receive *local anesthesia alone* does not need to be as thorough as for ASA II or III patients. Nevertheless, a medical history that includes recent hospitalizations, all previous surgical procedures, all existing medications, including exact amounts currently being used, allergies to medications, including the seriousness of the reaction, use of illegal drug substances, and postanesthesia experiences is still very useful and may affect even a local anesthetic administration. Vital signs should be recorded at the initial visit and before the use of local anesthesia at each visit. When local anesthesia alone is used, an updated medical history at 6-month intervals seems adequate.

For patients who are candidates for intravenous anesthetic agents of any type, additional attention should be given to the cardiovascular and respiratory system review. The ASA classification allows the risk level to be established on the basis of a simple definition of the extent of organ system disease.

Careful consideration should be given as to whether laboratory tests are necessary, specific, and cost-effective. Certainly, tests that are neither selective for a specific disease (i.e., mild to moderate anemia) nor sensitive enough to be conclusive (less than 75% to 90% confidence level) may not be warranted.[1] For example, the likelihood of a severe hypotensive event during anesthesia induction, caused by fasting, in anemic males under the age of 40 years with no history of risk factors, is extremely low. Tests in this type of patient should be requested only if the planned type of surgery or anesthesia is likely to lead to a morbid complication according to the medical history. For example, if the likelihood of abnormal potassium values in anyone not taking diuretics for any reason is slim, electrolyte tests do not need to be ordered. At present, there is a general trend to eliminate unnecessary laboratory testing for anesthesia, unless a clinical finding suggests that further tests are needed.

Preoperative Preparation

Both deep sedation and general anesthesia techniques have the potential to diminish or completely eliminate protective reflexes, including swallowing, coughing, and laryngospasm. The potential for a sedated patient to "slip into" a state of general anesthesia when sedation was intended certainly emphasizes the necessity to have all patients refrain from solid food for 6 hours (children) to 8 hours (adults). Some patients may either forget or deliberately conceal important information regarding food intake, particularly children or mentally handicapped patients, who may ingest food unless properly supervised. Although vomiting or aspiration is rare, the chance of aspiration increases if airway obstruction occurs.[2] Despite the fact that aspiration of gastric contents is more rare in the outpatient than in hospitalized patients, it has been shown that outpatients have greater gastric acidity and residual gastric fluid.[3]

Pediatric patients 2 to 6 years of age are required to be *nil per os* (NPO) for solid food for 6 or more hours before deep sedation or general anesthesia, although changes in these restrictions allow for 2 to 3 mL/kg of clear fluid (i.e., water, apple juice, ginger ale) up to 3 hours prior to induction.[4] Relaxation of the previous standards requiring complete intake prohibition is based upon the infrequency of significant airway obstruction and aspiration and the need to satisfy the needs of the pediatric patient. Fluid restriction from the previous evening to the time of surgery can produce a state of relative hypovolemia in children, who cannot be fluid loaded by the intravenous route prior to mask induction. Inhalation induction can result in rapid onset of hypotension in the hypovolemic child. Children who will accept an intravenous line are less likely to become hypovolemic with this anesthetic technique. If children are kept on NPO status for long periods before induction, a state of relative hypoglycemia may also occur. Although this is considered significantly less of a risk than years ago, the hypoglycemic patient is still at risk for delayed awakening after anesthesia and lethargy after discharge. Allowing preoperative *oral* fluids, especially with a glucose-containing solution, can help guard against these complications without the risk of worsening gastric fluid volumes or increasing gastric acidity.[4] In fact, allowing clear fluid intake decreases acidity *and* intragastric volume. In addition, the stimulation of adrenaline, aldosterone, and antidiuretic hormones from the physiologic stress of anesthesia is likely to be delayed by allowing preoperative fluids, especially in children.

Prior to discharge, written and oral postoperative and postanesthesia instructions should be relayed to the responsible adult attending to the patient at home. Because some sedatives and anesthetic agents have prolonged psychomotor and memory effects, written instructions specifically disallowing certain postanesthesia activities should be considered. Two cases, one involving an accident while driving an automobile and a second resulting in quadriplegia from a fall down stairs, have been related verbally to me as postanesthesia complications in patients within 24 hours of discharge from the office.

Patients taking prescribed medications should continue to do so the morning before anesthesia in most situations. Interruption of most medications (e.g., birth control pills, psychotropic drugs, antihypertensives) is usually unnecessary and in some cases counterproductive. The stability of the patient under general anesthesia can be affected, particularly if drugs used to control hypertension and cardiac rhythm are not taken even on the day of surgery. It is also important that postoperative pain medications be taken with careful instructions to avoid the possibility of overdose, especially on the first postoperative evening, when anesthetic drugs or active breakdown products may still be circulating and partially therapeutically effective. During medical history assessment, particular attention should be directed to patients who snore at night. Such a patient already exhibits some degree of airway obstruction that could be worsened on the first postoperative night.

Airway Assessment

Although the presence of a heavily muscled or fat neck, large circumferential diameter of the abdomen, and receding mandible has been traditionally labeled as a harbinger of difficulty in airway management, the accuracy of this "clinical hunch" has never been scientifically proven.[5] Airway assessment techniques have been advanced to a more formal examination rather than relegated to a "hunch." Under the assumption that the base of the tongue played an important role for the visualization of the larynx, Mallampati and associates[6] developed a relatively simple grading system. These researchers designed and tested a preoperative technique assessing the ability to visualize the soft palate, tonsillar fauces, and the uvula to predict the ease or difficulty of glottic exposure during laryngoscopy.[6] During oral examination in the seated position with the mouth fully open, inspection of the oral pharynx is performed. The classification is described as follows: soft palate, fauces, and uvula all visible (class I); fauces and soft palate visible (class II); and soft palate alone, but no tonsillar fauces or uvula visible (class III). With the higher classification, it was presumed, there would be more difficulty in exposing the laryngeal structures and, subsequently, the intubation would be more difficult. In this study, class II patients were nearly evenly distributed in laryngoscopic difficulty (excellent, good, fair, poor), whereas class I patients were generally easy to manage. Although most office anesthesia uses a nasal inhaler, preinduction assessment of the airway utilizing the Mallampati classification might also be a predictor of airway difficulty during deep sedation or general anesthesia. The major advantage in knowing how to objectively assess the difficulty of laryngoscopy might also be important in planning to avert airway complications during nasal inhaler anesthesia.

Other methods that have been used successfully involve assessments of body weight, neck flexion, mandibular retrognathism, prominence of maxillary incisors, mandibular range of opening, and thyromental distance.[7] These techniques are probably more useful if endotracheal intubation is definitely considered for the surgery.

Cardiopulmonary Assessment

Much attention is given to ASA II or III patients with a history of cardiac or pulmonary disease. Some ASA I patients, however, have *subtle* symptoms that can be overlooked. Despite the utilization of good techniques and appropriate drug selection, two conditions can occur during anesthesia that have a high rate of mortality in a presumably healthy patient: bronchospasm and hypoxia-related multifocal ventricular arrhythmia.

The patient with seasonal hay fever and multiple drug allergies could be considered an ASA I candidate even if according to the history the patient had "outgrown" asthma. In this situation, auscultation of the chest should be performed even for those who are going to receive deep sedation, because mild wheezing can be overlooked. Asthma is the most common pulmonary condition and has been on the rise in the past 10 years. Brief auscultation over the dorsal surface of the chest in all five lung fields, particularly at the bases, is useful regardless of whether the patient is to be intubated. A serious intraoperative attack can occur, particularly if wheezing is overlooked in this situation. At the very least, auscultation establishes a baseline. Consider the following case:

Case 1

A 17-year-old female presented for the extraction of four third molars. After induction with nalbuphine, 10 mg, midazolam, 5 mg, and thiopental, 25 mg (1 mL), local anesthesia with 2% xylocaine 1:100,000 epinephrine was injected in all four quadrants, and surgery was begun. After the extraction of the maxillary third molar, another 2 mL of Pentothal (50 mg) was given, and the mandibular surgery was begun. Within minutes of the Pentothal injection, the patient coughed and began bucking. Positive pressure was attempted to ventilate the lungs, without success. Succinylcholine was administered to facilitate airway control, but the patient could not be ventilated. An endotracheal tube was placed, but ventilation was still impossible. Bradycardia and cyanosis ensued. When the emergency medical team arrived, proper positioning of the endotracheal tube was verified and further resuscitation was continued, but the patient expired.

Analysis

This patient had a history of mild allergy to penicillin. The drugs used indicate most likely a planned deep sedation rather than a general anesthetic. The patient developed a coughing episode after the second injection of the barbiturate. When the emergency team arrived, the accuracy of placement of the endotracheal tube verified by direct vision essentially meant that the obstruction or high resistance to breathing was caused by either endobronchial intubation or bronchospasm. When epinephrine was given, the patient could be ventilated, but cardiac activity could not be restored. The diagnosis was probable anaphylactoid reaction to the barbiturate.

When a patient appears by medical history to be an obvious ASA I candidate, cardiac and pulmonary examination is frequently not conducted with the same intensity as for a patient in whom review of systems indicates possible problems. The absence of wheezing is no guarantee against drug-induced bronchospasm, but patients with a history of multiple drug allergy are prime candidates for an allergic response of any degree of severity. Patients with an existing hyperreactive airway from a recent upper respiratory tract infection or from smoking may not be classified ASA II by definition, but may have subtle abnormal bronchial sounds that could be missed prior to anesthesia induction.

During the brief cardiac evaluation, auscultation for murmurs could reveal valuable information. Although the intricacies of murmur diagnosis are difficult for the inexperienced listener, gross murmurs (i.e., holosystolic, grade III or higher, and loud diastolic) can be discovered in the apparent ASA I candidate. Patients with a history of exercise intolerance and increased frequency of upper respiratory tract signs and symptoms should be more closely evaluated. Consider the following case:

Case 2

A 16-year-old male presented for the extraction of four third molars. After induction with fentanyl, 0.1 mg, midazolam, 3 mg, and several 1-ml increments of 1% methohexital, local anesthesia with 2% xylocaine, 1:100,000 epinephrine dilution, was injected in all four quadrants. The anesthesia was maintained with halothane by nasal endotracheal tube at an acceptable clinical dose. After the surgical removal of the third wisdom tooth, the patient demonstrated a drop in oxygen saturation as measured by pulse oximetry, to approximately 90%. The inspired oxygen concentration was increased from 50% to 100%, and the procedure continued. There was no apparent respiratory impairment (i.e., obstruction or hypoventilation during the surgery). Within minutes, the electrocardiogram was flat and quickly recognized. Attention was directed to the leads, which were thought to have been disconnected. Cyanosis quickly ensued, however, and full cardiac arrest was diagnosed. All resuscitative efforts failed despite rapid, successful endotracheal intubation and intravenous administration of epinephrine.

Analysis

Retrospectively, the patient was not an athletic type, so no history regarding *exercise intolerance* or easy fatigability was obtainable. There was a history of frequent "bronchial conditions" that were treated by routine medical care. There was no history of heart murmur, but auscultation was not done in the office before induction of anesthesia. Autopsy reported a severe nonobstructive, hypertrophic cardiomyopathy. The decreased oxygen saturation was the first sign of trouble, and "brady-asystole" the second.

It has been conservatively estimated that there are 15 to 20 cases of sudden death in young athletes per year.[8] Routine physical examinations ("school physicals") are not likely to reduce the incidence of sudden death, unless murmurs are discovered that can be followed up by echocardiography. Obstruction to the left ventricular outflow tract generally creates a loud holosystolic ejection murmur at the left sternal border, and the grading and duration may well indicate the severity of the condition. Stress associated with increased heart rate or hypotension at any time during anesthesia may precipitate cardiovascular collapse. Dilated or nonobstructive cardiomyopathy can be much more clandestine and difficult to diagnose by physical examination alone. Frequently, there are no abnormal cardiac sounds to help make the diagnosis during the preoperative office evaluation until heart failure is near.

Table 2–1. Timing of Cardiovascular and Respiratory Collapse in 52 Patient Deaths Under Dental Office General Anesthesia

Phase of Anesthesia	Cases of Cardiovascular Collapse	Cases of Respiratory Collapse
Induction	2	2
Maintenance	1	16
Recovery	19	12
Total	22	30

Data from Coplans MP, Curson I: Deaths associated with dentistry. Br J Dent 1982;153:357.

Intraoperative Anesthesia Considerations and Complications

Prevention of Complications

Adverse effects of intravenous sedation and general anesthesia in the dental office are commonly associated with the pharmacologic effects (expected or unexpected), the physiologic body responses (normal or abnormal), and the presence of underlying diseases that were not previously recognized. With respect to the decision-making processes associated with complications of anesthesia, *human error* has been implicated in approximately 86% of hospital anesthesia mishaps: of these, 42% occurring immediately prior to or shortly after induction, 42% occurring during maintenance, and 12% during the recovery period.[9] This breakdown differs from office-type anesthesia. Analyzing 52 deaths during dental anesthesia, Coplans and Curson[10] found that 4 (7.5%) occurred during induction, 17 (32.5%) during maintenance, and 31 (60%) during the final phase of surgery or shortly thereafter, during recovery (Table 2–1). In the office setting, the two categories of adverse effects that most patients suffer are cardiovascular and respiratory (Table 2–2). In contradistinction to hospital-based anesthesia, the recovery phase appears to be the time period where the mortality rate is the highest in dental office anesthesia.

Table 2–2. Causes of Complications Leading to Morbidity and Mortality in Office Anesthesia

Cardiovascular	Arrhythmia (pain, intrinsic) Hypotension (postural, hypovolemia) Syncope (rare)
Respiratory	Spasm (bronchial, laryngeal) Hypoventilation (obstruction) Apnea (drug-induced) (rare)

Knowing the general types of complications and the phases of anesthesia during which they are likely to occur allows one to be alert for changes in vital signs and to take appropriate precautions if possible. Prevention of complications is directly related to decreasing the likelihood of making technical and pharmacologic mistakes and taking unnecessary chances. Consider the following case:

Case 3

A 6-year-old boy presents for the extraction of deciduous teeth I and J. General anesthesia is induced with halothane, nitrous oxide, and oxygen. Oxygen saturation is monitored by pulse oximetry alone. During the extraction, the patient moves, begins to buck, and starts to show oxygen desaturation. Within 30 seconds, despite attempts to ventilate the patient, cyanosis occurs, and severe bradycardia ensues.

Analysis

The induction of anesthesia was performed with an inhalation agent that has a high arrhythmogenic potential, particularly if pain stimulates the sympathetic nervous system. Although performing surgery using light anesthesia in children is a risky technique, there was also little backup in monitoring and "salvage potential" by fluid resuscitation without an intravenous line in place. An electrocardiogram would allow one to judge the anesthetic depth and would sound an audible warning if premature ventricular arrhythmias or bradycardia were occurring prior to complete cardiovascular collapse. An intravenous line would have been a useful backup to administration of a muscle relaxant for laryngospasm or a vasoactive agent for bradycardia or other ventricular arrhythmias. The anticipated brevity and simplicity of the procedure seemed to dictate the technical aspects of the anesthesia.

Although several medical institutions routinely perform minor procedures with only mask inhalation agent and no intravenous line access (IV), full monitoring with a sphygmomanometer or electrocardiograph at least allows early warning for impending problems before they become complications. Still, not starting an IV during surgery can invite problems, especially in the recovery room, if there is a need for antiemetics or fluids. Prevention of complications in either the hospital or office setting is probably related more to avoiding judgmental errors than to ASA classification. In the ASA II or III patient, there is generally more concern for the medical condition and the tendency to be conservative, whereas in the ASA I patient with no discernible risk factors, there may be less planning.

Office Preparation

Serious complications rarely occur in office anesthesia practice. Despite one's best efforts to have all the necessary monitoring equipment available and in place, however, potentially serious complications *do* occur even if not recognized as such. In the hospital operating room or free-standing surgicenter, life-threatening events occur frequently enough that staged practice sessions are generally not needed. In the office this probably is not the case, however, and preparedness becomes more difficult to achieve and maintain. Practice emergency sessions can be regularly scheduled for less busy times of the year. Review of basic and advanced life-support protocols, as well as formal certification, is most useful. Slow "walk-through" scenarios with the assignment of special tasks to each team member can precede a full-scale actual-time drill session. In addition, an impromptu, simulated emergency can be staged spontaneously by the surgeon to assess preparedness of the office staff. These are best attempted at a less busy time of the day. Staged sessions held while they are completing a single office procedure can even take the form of the surgeon's *asking the anesthesia team personnel* what they would do if a particular complication occurred. Such question and answer sessions add to office preparedness.

Prior to the first case of the day, all anesthesia equipment should be checked except for the defibrillator, which can be checked weekly. *Backup* positive-pressure ventilator, suction equipment, and adequate gas oxygen supply systems should be identified and adequate function verified. Treatment drugs should be readily available for the most common types of emergencies. Even the establishment of a "mini-med pack" of the five most needed drugs is strongly recommended; it should be kept separate from the other emergency equipment and drugs and perhaps set up for each operating room that is used for general anesthesia or sedation (Table 2–3). Although there may be situations in which other drugs or devices are needed and even preferred, having these *five* drugs and *three* syringes in one container enables them to be mobilized from one location to another quickly and used while other agents (e.g., aminophylline, dantrolene, nitroglycerin) are being readied.

Monitoring

General Aspects

The collection of information about a range of normal physiologic functions is important during surgery

Table 2–3. Mini-Med Pack: Drugs for Early Treatment of Five Most Common Complications in Office Anesthesia

Drug	Syringe Size Needed (mL)	Complication(s) Used For
Atropine	3	Bradycardia
Lidocaine	5	Ventricular arrhythmia
Succinylcholine	5	Laryngospasm
Ephedrine*	10	Hypotension
Epinephrine*	10	Allergy (bronchospasm, anaphylaxis)

*Dilution of 1 mL to 10 mL.

under general anesthesia and, occasionally, local anesthesia as well. The intensity of the monitoring process and the range of equipment used to monitor often depend upon the patient's preoperative status. Even in a healthy ASA I patient who has a history of "palpitations," the administration of vasoconstrictors in local anesthesia may warrant continuous blood pressure and heart rate monitoring for the first 10 to 15 minutes of the procedure or visit. Certainly, patients taking antihypertensives or antiarrhythmics might benefit from monitoring throughout the office surgery. In patients with known cardiovascular disease, taking a good medical history is not a substitute for monitoring, which allows for prompt recognition of adverse events. The type and intensity of monitoring vital signs should be individualized. For example, if a surgical procedure is likely to produce sympathetic stimulation despite good pain control, routine electrocardiographic monitoring may be indicated, especially if the procedure is done under local anesthesia alone. Routine monitoring of cardiac rhythm in young athletes who have a high incidence of generally benign cardiac arrhythmias can be as important as in those with coronary artery disease (CAD) if deep sedation or general anesthesia is planned.[11] Even in young, seemingly healthy patients, it is possible to produce a situation in which protective reflexes, such as swallowing and coughing, are obtunded to varying degrees through the use of small amounts of drugs with enteral or parenteral techniques, including rectal, oral, intramuscular, and intravenous routes of delivery. Vigilance on the part of the individual monitoring the patient is still very important.

In 1986, the American Society of Anesthesiologists (ASA) developed standards for basic intraoperative monitoring that consist of five principal elements: clinical observation by trained personnel, oxygenation, ventilation, circulation, and body temperature. Subsequent modifications were made in a few areas: Pulse oximetry was mandated for all patients undergoing general anesthesia, and later, capnography was required for all endotracheally intubated patients. The perceived benefits of adding those two modalities are early warning of adverse physiologic events (e.g., hypoxemia and inadequate ventilation) and better technical vigilance of vital signs during anesthesia. Though these are considered important adjuncts, mechanical monitors should not substitute for clinical observation by a trained person whose sole function is to monitor the patient. The secondary benefits of adding pulse oximetry and capnography are a reduction of malpractice premiums[12] and of the number of monetary awards paid on malpractice claims.[13]

The quality of monitoring for an office outpatient should be the same as for an ambulatory care center outpatient. Mandatory equipment for monitored anesthesia care (MAC) should be essentially the same as for full general anesthesia, as follows: sphygmomanometer, electrocardiograph, stethoscope, and pulse oximeter, to monitor blood pressure, heart rhythm, breath sounds, and arterial oxygen concentration, respectively. Both the depth of anesthesia and the type of surgery play a role in choosing to add or to delete a monitor. For example, temperature monitoring is fairly routine in hospital operating rooms and ambulatory care centers attached to hospitals, where a patient can frequently become hypothermic. In the office, hypothermia is seldom a problem, and temperature monitoring is unnecessary. The added cost of such equipment does not justify the minimal return in valuable information. Also, the risk of malignant hyperthermia, which has a high mortality rate even if treated with dantrolene (8%), is considerably less likely to occur in office anesthesia, because inhalation trigger agents (e.g., halothane, isoflurane, succinylcholine) are used less frequently. When total intravenous anesthesia (TIVA) is used in the office, temperature monitoring is not crucial. As previously mentioned, however, when inhalation agents are warranted to improve the stability of the anesthesia, skin temperature monitors should be used, particularly if multiple triggering agents are used in combination or if an inhalation agent is used for any longer than 30 minutes.

The utilization of endotracheal intubation is less common in office anesthesia, because most minor office procedures can be accomplished under deep or conscious intravenous sedation. Even though the airway may be in less jeopardy, complications such as laryngospasm, vomiting, and aspiration are still a concern, and clinical monitoring should be continuous and even more intensified in an airway unprotected by an endotracheal tube. Monitoring of skin color, unpredictable patient movement, and reservoir bag activity are more crucial monitors, and no mechanical monitor can replace these clinical observations. If a patient moves while surgery is being performed under anesthesia by nasal inhaler mask, quick response to deepen the level is important to avoid the perils of the patient's being in anesthesia stage 2. If the airway is controlled with an endotracheal tube, however, deepening anesthesia, usually by increasing the inhalation agent concentration, is less worrisome and in some respects easier to accomplish. Auscultation of breath sounds is also more crucial during nasal inhaler anesthesia than during endotracheal anesthesia. A stethoscope properly positioned above the suprasternal notch is very helpful in diagnosing upper airway obstruction. Airway obstruction can occur during deep sedation (e.g., with chloral hydrate in children) or during general anesthesia with TIVA (e.g., methohexital infusion). Operations in the lower jaw in nonintubated patients are particularly liable to result in obstruction of the airway by depressing the mandible downward (e.g., during extraction) or retracting the tongue. Auscultation is more important in such cases, as it can detect an early airway obstruction prior to any undesirable changes in oxygen saturation.

Pulse Oximetry

Although few controlled studies have been conducted to undisputably support using pulse oximetry routinely, clinical experience has persuaded most anesthetists and surgeons that early detection of hypoxemia has indeed prevented serious accidents. During conscious sedation with nitrous oxide alone in children or adults, or with the use of oral sedatives alone in adults, pulse oximetry is not likely to be useful in terms of time or cost-effectiveness. Indeed, some studies utilizing pulse oximetry routinely have shown that there is not a statistically significant reduction of anesthesia-related deaths.[14, 15] Analysis of critical incidents during general anesthesia, however, has indicated that arterial desaturation occurred frequently during maintenance of anesthesia.[16] Because a high percentage of respiratory-related deaths in dental surgery patients in the study by Coplans and Curson[10] occurred during the maintenance phase (nearly 33%), pulse oximetry could be most useful in avoiding tragedy. Arterial oxygen desaturation was more frequent, but it was also milder (e.g., SaO_2 value of 85% to 92%) compared with induction of and recovery from anesthesia.[16]

The routine utilization of pulse oximetry during general anesthesia has been universally accepted. The two main advantages are evaluations of hemoglobin oxygen saturation and heart rate. When applied *during* anesthesia, its usefulness may be greater than in the postanesthesia recovery phase.[17] Errors associated with body movement, including light anesthesia shivering, are minimal. The number of false alarms, however, is estimated at approximately 1 per 8 minutes to 14 per hour.[14] In fact, during one study with chloral hydrate sedation in pediatric dental patients, up to 90% of the alarms sounded were false and only 10% were significant.[18] When high false alarm rates occur, there is a serious risk of "desensitizing" the staff to a point of decreased alertness when the oximeter sounds. This is especially true when a clip-on finger probe rather than the bandage-taped type is used that cannot be as easily dislodged.

During recovery, apnea has been estimated to occur frequently (1 episode per 37 minutes) and to last 30 seconds or longer.[19] If the patient has been well oxygenated with a face tent or mask, apnea may go unnoticed by a pulse oximeter. In fact, studies have shown that periods of apnea and desaturation can and frequently do increase as the recovery stay lengthens. Perhaps this is due to the greater attention the patient receives early on admission to the recovery area and less observation later. Incidence of these events (desaturation below 90% and apnea) was increased from 2% on admission to the recovery room to 9% at the time of *anticipated* discharge.[17] Patients breathing room air during the first 10 minutes of recovery average a 90% SaO_2. In over 40% of the patients, *moderate* (75% to 84% SaO_2) to *severe* (75% or less) hypoxemia was observed. Administration of 35% oxygen dramatically improved these measures without further ventilatory assistance.[20]

The routine use of oxygen during recovery has not gone without challenge, however. Some experts advocate a "room air challenge" to ascertain whether the residual effects of anesthetic agents, particularly narcotics and muscle relaxants are present and impairing ventilation and air exchange *prior* to transfer to the recovery room.[14, 21] *Mild* episodes of desaturation (85%–92% SaO_2) are rarely dangerous. Indeed, patients afflicted with central or obstructive sleep apnea generally survive night episodes at these levels, probably because the oxygen consumption and metabolic processes decrease during sleep. Similarly, in the postanesthesia period, *mild* desaturation is generally innocuous. It does present as a concern, however, if a pediatric patient has mild desaturation and is still obtunded and not moving around after a stir-up regimen (e.g., pressing on the angle of the mandible) or after verbalizing (e.g., patient crying). Adults, who have larger functional residual volumes than children, are at less risk during recovery. Because hypoxemia is more likely to produce bradycardia and hypotension in children, pediatric patients should be evaluated more closely.

Capnography

The measurement of exhaled carbon dioxide depends on gas movement and its analysis by an infrared sensor. The mere presence of a carbon dioxide waveform generally indicates that breathing is occurring. There are cases, however, in which an endotracheal tube accidentally placed into the esophagus demonstrates small amounts of carbon dioxide on the capnograph for a few breaths.[22] In some respects, the capnograph is a more useful indicator of the adequacy of ventilation than the pulse oximeter, primarily because of its nearly instantaneous measure of gas exchange. In contradistinction, before a pulse oximeter sounds a warning, many seconds or minutes of abnormal events (e.g., obstruction, hypoventilation, decreased cardiac output) may have transpired. These complications could be more readily picked up by a capnograph.

With its present technology, a sensor gives digital and/or graphic information. Its usefulness in office outpatient anesthesia is limited in nonintubated patients. Because a semi-open system is being utilized and air dilution under a nasal inhaler or through-the-mouth breathing occurs, the numeric function is all but useless. For example, if exhaled air containing 4.5% carbon dioxide (e.g., 35 to 40 mm Hg at end exhalation) is diluted, the capnograph registers significantly *lower* peak exhalation values than 35 to 40 torr. In the intubated patient with a semi-closed system, however, the values would be more indicative of ventilation-related events. In this situation, a higher than normal value may indicate hypoventilation or a hypermetabolic state such as malignant hyperthermia, and a lower than normal value may indicate lowered cardiac output and subsequent decrease in pulmonary perfusion. Yet the presence of a waveform does have some advantages. For example, in pediatric patients undergoing deep sedation (e.g., chloral hydrate, ketamine), both oxygen supplementation and carbon dioxide analysis can be observed. When a nasal cannula with a side-stream sampling line is utilized, the presence of *any* level of carbon dioxide produces a waveform and indicates air movement out of the nose. Complete airway obstruction or apnea can be detected *immediately* by the absence of a waveform. Hypoventilation, however, produces a smaller waveform, rendering this technique less informative in patients with depressed respiration rather than apnea or total obstruction.

In several respects, capnography and pulse oximetry are equally useful but independent noninvasive tools. Hypoxemia is the most proximate cause of neurologic damage or adverse cardiovascular events, and measures of end-tidal carbon dioxide can forecast conditions that would be picked up by pulse oximetry only later. Therefore, if capnography is used appropriately in certain situations, it gives an *earlier* warning sign of impending arterial oxygenation problems. Prospective evaluation of closed-claim cases showed that capnography added to pulse oximetry could have avoided 93% of preventable mishaps that were potentially life-threatening.[23] Respiratory events alone accounted for 34% of the adverse events. Inadequate ventilation, esophageal intubation, and difficult airway problems accounted for 73% of the respiratory problems.[24]

The capnograph is more complicated than the pulse oximeter in its interpretation of the data, including numbers and waveforms. In addition to its advantages in generally measuring *exhaled* carbon dioxide, the absolute measure of *inhaled* carbon dioxide may be useful. For example, if inhaled CO_2 is known to be essentially zero and there is some CO_2 rebreathing, there may be a failure in the gas delivery system from the gas machine through the circuit to the patient. If a Bain (Mapleson D) system is used and inadequate total fresh gas flow (FGF) is administered, potentially dangerous rebreathing can be suspected from the characteristics of the capnograph waveform. Detection may allow adjustment in FGF before serious CO_2 retention develops. An elevation of CO_2 is diagnosed by observing the waveform and is useful regardless of whether intubation or nasal anesthesia is used. In general, lower end-tidal carbon dioxide levels are *less* diagnostic than excessive levels or the total absence of waveform. Over-interpretation of the numbers presented on capnograph is a common mistake.

Additionally, as with pulse oximetry, an alarm system is part of the capnograph and is frequently susceptible to false-positive alerts. Adjustable high and low limits are generally a feature of the equipment, but when the capnograph is used along with pulse oximetry, sound pollution from false alarms with two monitors in the operatory is common. For this reason, capnography would probably be most useful in preventing complications associated with office anesthesia when endotracheal intubation is utilized. Another clinical situation in which capnography would be very useful is in nonintubated children undergoing restorative dentistry or surgery under deep sedation while covered with drapes. A nasal cannula can be used to administer oxygen and simultaneously produce a carbon dioxide waveform indicating the patient is breathing (Fig. 2–1). This monitoring technique is particularly useful during continuous infusion of hypnotics (e.g., propofol, methohexital).

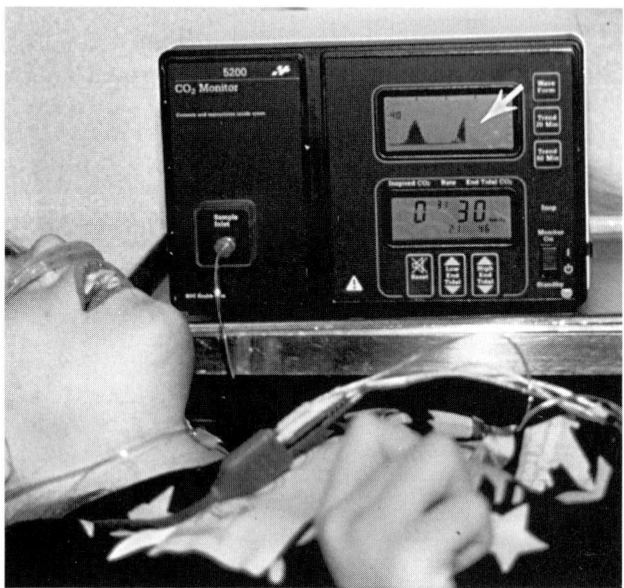

Figure 2–1. Carbon dioxide wave form *(arrow)* generated by a sidestream sampling line from the nasal cannula.

Electrocardiography

The continuous display of heart rate and rhythm on the oscilloscope is useful in detecting (1) ventricular rate by audible signal, (2) R–R periodicity, (3) P wave presence, and (4) QRS configuration. Abnormalities in these measures are rather easy for those with advanced cardiac life support (ACLS) training to detect. The most useful aspect of continuous electrocardiographic (ECG) monitoring is the audible QRS signal. The most common and potentially serious office anesthesia complications picked up by the ECG, especially during surgery, are tachycardia and premature ventricular contractions in adults and bradycardia during halothane induction in children. Both can be recognized by oscilloscopic observation and seldom require a graphic printout for diagnosis.

Other, more subtle changes can occur but are rarely of clinical importance in ASA I patients. Although myocardial ischemia can occur in presumably young healthy adults, a myocardial infarction is very rare. Because myocardial ischemia during anesthesia most commonly occurs secondary to tachycardia or hypotension, watching for ST segment depression would seem plausible. Even expert clinicians, however, often fail to detect intraoperative ischemic changes when viewing oscilloscopes alone.[25] Even with use of a modified three–chest lead system to view a V_5 area, significant ischemic events are missed without a printout.

There is a lack of concordance of different monitoring devices for intraoperative myocardial ischemia. In comparisons of different techniques (e.g., transesophageal echocardiography [TEE] and Holter monitors), there is often considerable discrepancy, especially when ischemia is mild to moderate.[26] When TEE and Holter monitoring are compared with the printed rhythm strip, further disagreement in interpretation is common. Studies showing that postoperative myocardial ischemia occurs more frequently than intraoperative or preoperative ischemia suggest that the capacity to diagnose intraoperative ischemia may be of limited value in predicting patients' outcome.[27] Perhaps the only exception is when new-onset T-wave inversion occurs during a procedure that was not present at the beginning of surgery.

Drug Technique–Specific Mechanical Monitoring

As previously mentioned, when conscious sedation with nitrous oxide is utilized, the need to use even a minimally invasive technique like pulse oximetry is very questionable. As the level of consciousness changes (i.e., from conscious to deep sedation or to general anesthesia), so should the intensity and type of mechanical monitoring system. Even when it is *possible* that a patient can enter into a deeper stage of anesthesia, the monitors placed should be predictive of this possibility. Knowledge of the most common causes of serious morbidity and mortality (see Table 3–2) should be applied to selection of mechanical monitors, and their *sequence* of placement should be in a proximate relationship to the drug or technique used.

For example, when halothane is used for pediatric patients, a situation in which the incidence of arrhythmia may be as high as 35%, an electrocardiographic monitor should be used and more carefully observed than perhaps the blood pressure.[28] Cardiac output in children is more dependent upon heart rate than blood pressure. In this case the sequence of monitor placement after induction, according to importance from first to last, is as follows: pulse oximetry, ECG, intravenous line placement (IV), and sphygmomanometer. If ketamine is administered intramuscularly, the pediatric patient becomes unresponsive within 5 minutes. Problems associated with induction using this technique are few, but two—namely breath-holding, which can occur in the very young (1 to 3 years old), and limited working time—are to be expected. The best monitor placement sequence for this technique would be pulse oximeter, followed by IV placement, then ECG, and sphygmomanometer last. The early establishment of an IV line is facilitated by the good analgesic quality of ketamine. If a procedure longer than 5 to 10 minutes is planned, either a continuous intravenous technique or supplementation with inhalation agents (e.g., halothane) is required. If halothane is added after intramuscular (IM) ketamine, arrhythmias, breath-holding, and laryngospasm should be anticipated, and appropriate precautions taken. For this reason, IV placement for the delivery of drugs is very important and could be life-saving even in very short procedures.

In adults, all the monitoring systems should be placed prior to the induction of anesthesia and, if possible, prior to or simultaneous with IV line placement. Baseline pulse oximetry values may be helpful, especially in cigarette smokers, who may have elevated carboxyhemoglobin levels. When anesthetic agents are administered that could produce malignant hyperthermia (e.g., volatile inhalation agents and succinylcholine), skin temperature monitoring should be considered as previously mentioned. Because succinylcholine is the most reliable and predictable muscle relaxant available and is effective in 60 seconds, a nerve stimulator is *not* important, at least for intubation.

The use of mechanical monitors should not be a substitute for clinical monitoring. After anesthesia induction of pediatric patients, the first nonmechanical monitor recommended to monitor airway patency is the stethoscope, placed over the trachea just above the sternum. Assessing breath sounds to verify a smooth transition through anesthesia stage 2, in which several complications can occur, to stage 3 is even more important than placing a pulse oximeter. If respiration is regular and unobstructed, one can usually assume that the $Sa{O_2}$ is normal.

Monitoring inspired oxygen concentrations is mandated by the ASA standards. The motivating factor behind this recommendation is the frequent use of closed-system anesthesia and low-flow techniques. The sensor is placed on either the exhalation or inhalation limb of the anesthetic breathing system. Certainly, when low-flow (FGF less than 2 L/min) techniques are used with a circle system with nitrous oxide, there is a greater potential for error in inspired oxygen concentration.[29] This becomes important mostly for office anesthesia in intubated patients. In techniques using a semi-open technique (i.e., nasal inhaler), in which FGF can be potentially diluted with ambient air, in-line oxygen analyzers become less important. If the oxygen flowmeter on the gas machine breaks, however, the potential for significant reductions in oxygen delivery are possible.

Ideal Monitoring System

The ultimate objective of monitoring is to prevent anesthesia-related morbidity and mortality. Respiratory complications appear to be the most common cause of mortality during and after dental anesthesia, whereas cardiovascular complications are more common during recovery. Although the existing capnography technology *does* furnish nearly instantaneous waveform and numeric information, a better alarm system to prevent false alarms would be useful. Also, a method of using the system more accurately for the semi-open techniques typically found in the office would be an advantage. Similarly, pulse oximetry is plagued with a high rate of false alarms. It seems difficult, however, to improve on a technique that probably by itself has reduced malpractice premiums and morbidity, and has instilled a great deal of confidence.

Perhaps the biggest strides could be made in ECG monitoring of all patients. Oscilloscopes that can sense myocardial ischemia with more reliability and deliver an audible warning of impending danger would be useful. Indeed, computer technology may also play a role. Composite rather than multiple-component systems with a computer-generated record, if cost containable, would be a major contribution to monitoring. Adding voice instructional response warning systems could essentially replace part of the anesthesia team and be helpful in verbalizing to the anesthetist and surgeon when either side effects of drugs or medical emergencies occur.

Anesthetic Agents

Methohexital was commonly used as a sole induction and maintenance agent in the early 1970s. Owing to excessive elevation of heart rate and cardiac output, the search for methods of "taming" barbiturate anesthesia included using benzodiazepines alone or in conjunction with narcotics. By the mid-1970s, a technique using fentanyl and diazepam prior to methohexital was presented as a potential adult technique for office anesthesia in adults.[30] Over the years, modifications of a strictly barbiturate technique have become very popular and generally include a narcotic and sedative-hypnotic given in any sequence to achieve deep sedation. If complete general anesthesia is desired, smaller doses of barbiturate can be used to induce anesthesia with less tachycardia and less overall sympathetic stimulation of the body.

Another advantage of using a multiple-drug technique as opposed to an entirely "barbiturate anesthetic" is to avoid the "roller coaster" effect of this technique, with its brief periods of apnea and frequent emergence into anesthesia stage 2, resulting in delirium or excitement. Commonly, coughing, bucking, and laryngospasm also occur, necessitating temporary interruption of the operation and deepening of the level of anesthesia. Narcotics and sedatives smooth the induction and emergence by potentiating the effects of methohexital, thiopental, or propofol and producing longer-lasting effects compared with barbiturates alone. The frequent disruption of surgery associated with the "pure barbiturate anesthetic" is probably the single most common reason that today the majority of office surgery is completed using deep sedation rather than full general anesthesia.

Alternatives to a TIVA technique include the addition of inhalation agents via nasal inhaler to ensure a deeper level of anesthesia and the use of endotracheal intubation to avoid upper airway complications during surgery. Although both techniques solve some of the intraoperative upper airway complications, they require a greater knowledge of anesthetic drugs and techniques and more time to achieve an acceptable level of anesthesia prior to beginning surgery. The importance of achieving a flawless anesthesia course should take precedence over the need to complete the operation.

Side effect liability increases when narcotics are used along with benzodiazepines and barbiturates. When a combination is given, however, surgeons are more than four times as likely to have excellent versus good, fair, or poor sedation and working conditions.[31] The literature on the topic of drug interactions, including undesirable and frequently unpredictable effects of combining several drugs, is vast. Hospital anesthesia is commonly conducted with 10 or more drugs.[32] Excess morbidity, including a 24% chance of having an adverse interaction, can occur when 10 to 15 drugs are administered concurrently. Multiple drugs are utilized safely by anesthesiologists, however, and most agree that the practice greatly *improves* patient safety.

Preoperative Drug Interactions

A number of pharmacodynamic interactions function during anesthesia induction, maintenance, and recovery to control the depth of sedation and anesthesia. To evaluate this response, the most often-used endpoints are: hypnosis (i.e., loss of response to voice command), analgesia (i.e., minimal autonomic response to a well-defined stimulus), and muscle relaxation (i.e., limitation of controlled and uncontrolled body movement). Intravenous sedatives and narcotics and inhalation agents potentiate one another to varying degrees. Generally, the resultant respiratory depression can be controlled and, in some instances, used as an advantage *if* the interactions are known, regardless of whether they are predictable or not. For example, narcotics decrease respiratory rate in a dose-dependent manner. When a nasal inhaler is placed over the nose and a patient becomes hyperpneic during the process, the limited volume of air in the mask (30 to 40 mL) would impede full inhalation. Combining narcotics and sedatives would decrease minute ventilation and tidal volumes and allow for smooth respiratory airflow through the breathing hose leading to the mask. Mild elevation of arterial carbon dioxide with this general approach of using narcotics as "advantageous respiratory depressants" does not produce serious cardiovascular effects in the healthy ASA I patient.[33]

Narcotic-Benzodiazepine Interactions

Diazepam and midazolam are the two most commonly administered benzodiazepines used in ambulatory anesthesia. More than 80 deaths have been associated with the administration of midazolam to sedate patients for diagnostic or therapeutic procedures in the United States alone.[34] Although midazolam used alone produces minimal respiratory depression and arterial oxygen hemoglobin desaturation, the effects are quite variable.[35, 36] Seventy-eight percent of the deaths associated with midazolam were respiratory in nature, and in 57%, an opioid was added. When midazolam alone is used at doses as high as 0.2 mg/kg, more significant depression of ventilatory response to CO_2 was measured.[37] In addition, elderly patients are more prone to respiratory depression at much lower doses. A pharmacodynamic effect on a reduced number of benzodiazepine-,Dd (receptors) in the cortex of the brain may be the reason for greater sensitivity in this age group.

Low-dose fentanyl (i.e., 50 μg) has little hypnotic effect by itself but is effective in potentiating benzodiazepine-induced hypnosis. Thus, when used for conscious sedation, the opioid is useful for effects other than analgesia. Not all opioids have the same pharmacodynamics. Midazolam and morphine are additive. When midazolam is added to fentanyl, however, a potentiation occurs, whereby 25% of a dose of fentanyl and 25% of a dose of midazolam produce the same endpoint as a 100% dose of midazolam alone.[38]

Butorphanol is an agonist-antagonist opioid believed to have analgesic but "ceiling-like" respiratory depressant effects. It commonly produces sedation (κ-receptor effect) unlike other purely agonist agents. Marked sedation with butorphanol is characteristically different from that with fentanyl or meperidine and other μ-receptor agonists. In the presence of pain, butorphanol can cause dysphoria, whereas this reaction is quite infrequent with fentanyl. Other agents, such as nalorphine and pentazocine, have been reported to have similar unpleasant mental effects (e.g., depersonalization and hallucinations) postoperatively. The respiratory depressant effects were synergistic when added to midazolam but less than those seen with fentanyl and midazolam.

Benzodiazepine-Hypnotic Interactions

Commonly, narcotics are omitted from the sedation technique in favor of hypnotic agents like methohexital and propofol. When drugs act similarly but not identically, mechanisms of action produce additive effects. For example, benzodiazepines such as midazolam increase chloride conduction in postsynaptic membranes by potentiating the effects of gamma-aminobutyric acid (GABA), whereas barbiturates like methohexital bind at or near chloride channels to produce similar membrane hyperpolarization.[39] Midazolam-induced athetoid movements of the lower extremities (similar to those seen with methohexital) have been reported and thought to be related to this mechanism.[40] The sedative response to either drug alone (midazolam or methohexital) is similar, and together they produce a synergistic hypnosis. With the combination of the two drugs, the potency is 1.8 times that expected for either given individually.[41] Midazolam has an anticholinergic activity on the central nervous system. Symptoms include tachycardia, mydriasis, disorientation, and hyperpyrexia. In attempts to tame the stimulatory effects of methohexital on cardiac conduction, benzodiazepines are only minimally useful. Indeed, pretreatment with midazolam or diazepam decreases the total induction doses, but during maintenance, its effects decrease. The benzodiazepines are no longer considered helpful in decreasing *maintenance* doses of methohexital, which is given in a 100 to 200 μg/kg/min continual infusion or in increments for general anesthesia.

Propofol is a diisopropylphenol with a minimal excitatory effect similar to that of methohexital (i.e., myoclonus). Clinically, a skeletal motor control lack of coordination can occur when propofol is used as a sole induction agent. Methohexital is commonly associated with hiccups, whereas propofol can produce more of a clonic movement of extremities that can be mistaken during recovery or induction for low-frequency seizure activity. The most common side effect of propofol is burning upon intravenous injection, which can be minimized by giving 0.1 to 0.2 mg/kg lidocaine as IV pretreatment. When propofol is given alone for sedation or induction of general anesthesia, dose-dependent hypoventilation occurs. Its potential to produce apnea is greater than that of barbiturates. In contradistinction to a barbiturate, propofol produces a slight decrease in heart rate and a similar 20% or more decrease in blood pressure. Overall, propofol produces more depression of cardiac output and systemic vascular resistance than barbiturates. Propofol is such a potent adrenergic inhibitor that it obtunds but does not completely eliminate hemodynamic responses to laryngoscopy and pharyngeal stimulation.

Several advantages of propofol make it a very useful agent. Its concentration, 1% solution, induction dose, and maintenance dose are exactly the same as for methohexital. The use of propofol with benzodiazepines and narcotics is similar to that of methohexital. However, a slightly more depressed level of vital signs, including heart rate, blood pressure, and respirations, occurs with propofol infusion. Its major advantage is decreasing pharyngeal reactivity to secretions; subsequently, fewer incidences of laryngospasm and bucking occur during the lighter levels of anesthesia. Secondarily, whenever tachycardia is clinically undesirable (e.g., coronary artery disease, hypertension), propofol is a better choice than methohexital, even when the latter is preceded by narcotics. The major disadvantage of propofol is its minimal shelf-life after its container is opened. Several deaths were reported soon after the FDA release; they were due to bacterial growth in the fat emulsion vehicle that dissolves the active drug. Propofol cannot be kept more than 6 hours, nor will refrigeration extend the shelf-life. When propofol is added to midazolam, a hypnotic synergism occurs similar to that when methohexital is added to midazolam.[42] The only pharmacodynamic difference is that the barbiturate has an antianalgesic effect, whereas propofol does not possess analgesic qualities. Midazolam has more reliable amnestic qualities than propofol given alone.

Narcotic-Hypnotic Interactions

The combination of narcotic and hypnotic is the most commonly administered two-drug regimen in hospital-type anesthesia for induction, yet the one least used in office anesthesia. In the hospital operating room, opioids such as fentanyl are frequently front-loaded, being given prior to barbiturate, phenol, or imidazole induction agents. Pretreatment with narcotics decreases the induction dose for all hypnotics by about 20%. A low dose of fentanyl (100 μg) used to decrease propofol induction results in an ultrashort recovery and is a very useful combination in brief surgical procedures. Its use is primarily designed to control the airway and "take over" respiration for the patient prior to the administration of a muscle relaxant and subsequent intubation. The combination of fentanyl and propofol often produces a more profound respiratory depression, and spontaneous respiration may frequently cease for as long as 60 to 90 seconds when full induction doses of propofol are given. For an office outpatient, nonintubation nasal inhaler technique, a better choice would be a narcotic followed by a benzodiazepine, because then much smaller doses of propofol or methohexital (i.e., 1 to 3 mL) would be needed to complete induction. When spontaneous respiration is desirable right from the outset, this combination of three agents for office anesthesia is more controllable than a hypnotic-narcotic combination alone. Nalbuphine and propofol have a synergism similar to that of butorphanol and propofol. The major difference is the longer duration of the narcotic effect of nalbuphine (3 to 6 hours) compared with butorphanol (2 to 4 hours). The slight stimulatory effect of agonist-antagonist opioids and hypnotics on blood pressure makes them an attractive combination in certain clinical situations.

Volatile-Intravenous Agent Interactions

The "methohexital-resistant" patient has been described as requiring gradually escalating doses in an often desperate attempt to keep the patient asleep. This condition is frequently signified by tachycardia, hypertension, and a pattern of light anesthesia. In one study, approximately 9% of 513 patients who received fentanyl, diazepam, and methohexital still had excessive heart rates.[43] Enflurane was used to lower the heart rates and decrease the need for excessive doses of methohexital. Narcotic agonists produce a dose-dependent reduction in minimum alveolar concentration (MAC) for all inhalation agents. If a steady state of narcotic infusion is used, MAC for isoflurane can be decreased by 50% to 70%. Narcotic and volatile anesthetics are often combined to stabilize the intraoperative vital signs by decreasing wide fluctuations in heart rate and blood pressure. A patient with a difficult airway (e.g., heavy neck) who is "barbiturate resistant" has a smoother anesthetic course, and surgical conditions are better, when an inhalation agent is added that allows more laminar, slower airflow as well as neck and tongue muscle relaxation. The chances of a patient's waking up unexpectedly and developing laryngospasm are far less when volatile agents are used.

In adults the combination of narcotic and inhalation anesthesia is better tolerated than inhalation alone. Reducing MAC clearly leads to lower end-tidal concentrations at the end of surgery and inspired concentrations during surgery. Minimum alveolar concentration can also be reduced by midazolam and propofol infusion. When propofol is used alone as a maintenance agent, there is less nausea than when enflurane is added. The recovery time is essentially the same, however, for brief (30 to 50 minute) procedures.[44]

Drug Abuse Interactions

Chronic abuse of prescription drugs can present anesthetic complications with little warning. Medications that affect the formation of adrenergic neurotransmitters (e.g., clonidine), prevent reuptake of norepinephrine (e.g., tricyclic antidepressants), or delay the breakdown of catecholamines (e.g., aminophylline) can cause a number of expected or less common symptoms. Whether a serious complication occurs frequently depends on the dose of the prescription drug. High doses of anticholinergic agents or tricyclic antidepressants can produce persistent elevations in blood pressure and heart rate, and even ventricular ectopy at any point in anesthesia, especially during postoperative emergence, when the sympathetic tone is increased. A patient who has tachycardia prior to induction that does not convert to a normal rate after intravenous narcotic and sedative are given may be manifesting a prescription drug effect rather than merely signs of anxiety about the impending surgery. Patients using amphetamine-type drugs for dieting purposes, phenylpropanolamine or pseudoephedrine for decongestion, or excessive thyroid replacement may also demonstrate similar cardiovascular symptoms that, if left untreated, may have serious consequences *during* or *after* anesthesia.

Ethanol abuse generally produces resistance to sedatives and hypnotics. However, cardiovascular disturbances, including hypertension, elevated triglyceride levels, cardiac conduction disturbances (e.g., changes in T wave or PR interval, bundle branch blocks), and depressed cardiac function (e.g., cardiomyopathy) are uncommon but should be expected in patients undergoing office surgery. Many alcoholic patients may not be readily recognizable on clinical appearance alone.

Abuse of nonprescription drugs is an ever-increasing problem, especially among young, seemingly healthy patients needing simple office surgery. Chronic cocaine use affects the central nervous system (e.g., behavior disorders, hallucinations) as well as the cardiovascular system. Arrhythmias, myocardial ischemia, and infarction have occurred postoperatively in cocaine users. Whether these reactions are caused by foreign substances adulterating the cocaine supply or are due to myocardial ischemia and scarring, coronary artery spasm, or catecholamine-platelet aggregation is not completely known. Marijuana use within 24 hours before anesthesia may produce somnolence or severe tachycardia during recovery from barbiturate anesthesia.[45] Narcotic abuse generally does not produce intraoperative complications other than narcotic resistance, but the abuse of some agents (e.g., pentazocine, meperidine) has been the cause of postoperative seizures. The major concern with these agents is the habit-seeking behavior that could be a factor in the early postanesthesia phase (within 24 hours). Self-administration of narcotic-like substances in this period can result in severe cardiorespiratory depression and death.

Treatment of excessive cardiovascular stimulation should be considered when heart rate exceeds 140 beats/min and does not appear to be decreasing after any apparent cause (e.g., pain, drug effects) has been ruled out. If this condition lasts well into the recovery period (e.g., 20 minutes or more), esmolol, 0.3 mg/kg bolus over 1 minute, should be given. With a 9-minute therapeutic half-life, the effects dissipate quickly, making esmolol very safe and overdose very unlikely. If little or no effect is observed in 5 minutes, a second dose, of 0.2 mg/kg, should be given. If the heart rate decreases by 10 to 20 beats after the first dose, a second dose at half the original level should be given 5 minutes after the first. Hypertension associated with tachycardia often responds to esmolol. Hypertension alone of more than 220 mm Hg systolic associated with drug interactions may be treated, but the urgency is less than if hypertension is accompanied by tachyarrhythmias. Blood pressure can usually be controlled slowly, with less serious concern if it occurs postoperatively. However, nifedipine, 10 mg either sublingual (with a hole in the capsule) or swallowed, is frequently accompanied by a reduction of blood pressure in 15 to 20 minutes. The sublingual route may be more responsive than the enteral route but is less sustained. The major concern is that the peak effect of the enteral route takes 20 to 45 minutes to occur, and its duration of 4 hours or more requires careful postoperative monitoring. The best clinical technique for office use would be to place a hole in the capsule and have the patient keep it sublingual for 10 minutes, and then *discard* it. Provided that the patient is not hypovolemic, this practice allows partial control of hypertension if its cause is anesthesia related (e.g., vasoconstrictors, drug interaction).

Complications

Treatment of complications that occur in the office takes on a slightly different perspective from that in the hospital operating room, where several other anesthesia, medical, and nursing personnel are readily available. Generally, the complications are of a wider variety in the hospital environment, the anesthetic management even of ASA I patients is more complex, and the rescue technology available is different. Nevertheless, some considerations should be discussed even if the treatment is essentially the same.

Laryngospasm

The recognition and management of either partial or full laryngospasm are basic and should be frequently practiced by the anesthesia team. The causes are associated with a light level of anesthesia or foreign material (e.g., blood, saliva, emesis) on the vocal cords. Deepening the level of anesthesia as quickly as possible (unless the operation is completed) along with appropriate suctioning and airway support is also routine and needs little discussion. If, however, laryngospasm occurs during anesthesia induction in a child with an inhalation agent prior to intravenous line placement, there are fewer treatment alternatives. If partial obstruction occurs, deepening anesthesia with halothane and 50% oxygen is usually curative but may take several minutes to complete. If full laryngospasm occurs without an IV line in place, either chest compressions with full-face mask and positive-pressure ventilation or muscle relaxant given intramuscularly is warranted. The intramuscular route via a submental transcutaneous injection is the easiest and has the quickest onset (Fig. 2–2). Approximately 3 mg/kg of succinylcholine with 3-mL maximum volume can be safely given through the skin into the tongue by a 25-gauge needle with this technique.[46] The heaviest pediatric patient-candidate for this administration route would have a 20-kg body weight, which would require 60 mg IM. Other muscular areas (e.g., shoulder, thigh) do not allow as rapid absorption. Transtracheal administration of drugs is useful, but unless sufficient airflow into the trachea is available to spread the fluid deeper into the more vascular areas, the absorption may be much slower. This option is not likely during complete laryngospasm with little or no airflow, nor should one take the chance of administering transtracheal succinylcholine in such a serious situation.

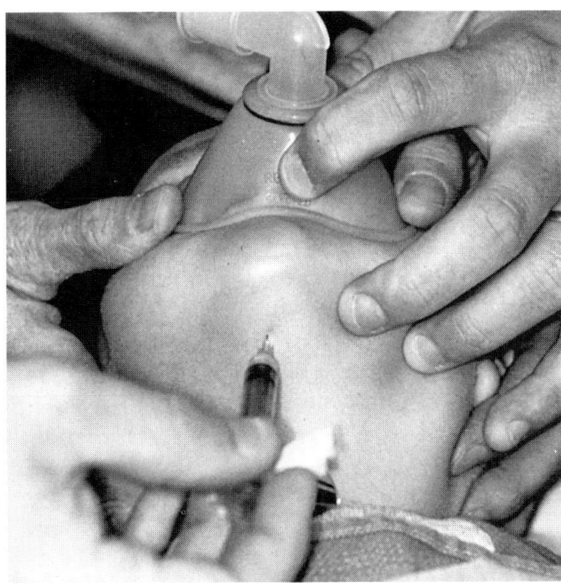

Figure 2–2. Intramuscular succinylcholine administered through the submental, transcutaneous route to treat laryngospasm.

Aspiration

If emesis or silent regurgitation occurs and the lung is soiled, pneumonitis can occur. The incidence of serious aspiration is approximately 0.05% (1 in 2,131).[2] Of 185,358 cases in one study, 87 showed either radiographic or clinical signs of aspiration, but less than 50% of these had radiographic evidence.[2] The clinical diagnosis was based upon chest auscultation. Aspiration of five different types of materials can occur, and treatment should be individualized. Liquid acid (e.g., gastric fluid), if aspirated in quantities greater than 0.3 to 0.5 ml/kg,[47] may cause more serious signs and symptoms than a nonacid nonsolid (e.g., blood). If a liquid nonacid (e.g., pus) is aspirated, lung infection may occur and needs to be treated appropriately with antibiotics in addition to other support care. Aspiration of a solid acid (e.g., food) can cause problems similar to those of liquid acid but also requires hospitalization for bronchoscopy if strongly suspected. Aspiration of a solid nonacid (e.g., dental materials) also requires bronchoscopic examination, but patients can usually be discharged more quickly. The most benign aspirate is blood, which generally requires no treatment.

Treatment of aspiration pneumonitis has changed over the years. Steroids and antibiotics are no longer considered the standard of care. The former generally delay the healing process, and the latter are useful only if aspiration of pus from an intraoral wound is suspected. Current therapy consists of continuous positive airway pressure ventilation (CPAP) to maintain

PaO_2 above 70 torr and $PaCO_2$ below 50 torr. If hypotension occurs during CPAP, vasopressors (e.g., dobutamine) should be given under the monitoring of a pulmonary artery catheter, especially because chemical pneumonitis can cause large volumes of plasma to translocate into the lung and produce systemic hypovolemia. Not all patients, however, need full treatment or hospitalization. Consider the following case:

Case 4

A 58-year-old male had deep sedation in an oral surgery office for multiple tooth extractions. At the completion of the operation, the patient was recovering on nasal inhaler oxygen. When the oxygen was removed, the SaO_2 decreased to 89% on room air, and the patient looked "grayish" and felt weak. Oxygen was restarted, and the SaO_2 increased to 96% with a pulse of 100 beats/min. A second attempt to remove the oxygen 10 minutes later was accompanied by a similar response. Auscultation of the chest revealed mild rales bilaterally. The patient was transferred to a hospital emergency room with a diagnosis of either aspiration or early congestive heart failure. Electrocardiogram and chest film were normal. After 3 hours of emergency room observation, the patient was discharged home.

Analysis

Not all patients who aspirate during surgery need hospitalization or full medical treatment.[48] Stable SaO_2 values on room air in the low 90% range are acceptable. This, however, is not always the case. If a patient is breathing 100% oxygen and the SaO_2 stays at 90% or slightly above (e.g., greater than PaO_2 60 torr), intubation can probably be avoided. If the SaO_2 is 85% (e.g., PaO_2 50 torr) or less on 100% oxygen *and* the patient is clinically depressed or obtunded, re-induction of general anesthesia and the administration of a muscle relaxant to achieve paralysis and place an endotracheal tube is probably life-saving. The "gray area" is when SaO_2 is greater than 85% but the patient is being assisted with positive-pressure ventilation. Also to be considered is the need for high fluid volumes of balanced salt solution to offset the large translocation of fluids that can occur after aspiration.

Bronchospasm

Perhaps the most feared respiratory complication (with the possible exception of malignant hyperthermia) is bronchospasm with severe, life-threatening hypoxemia. Although this is a rare office complication, ASA I patients who have legitimate multiple drug allergies or history of asthma attacks requiring adrenergic agents should be carefully considered. However, these ASA II–type patients can be safely operated in the office under either deep sedation or general anesthesia. Even a laryngospasm during light anesthesia can trigger a bronchospasm in this situation. In fact, laryngospasm may be the first sign of bronchospasm, followed by cardiovascular collapse in the allergic patient. Nonallergic causes (psychogenic asthma) may be exacerbated by severe anxiety prior to dental surgery. If preoperative wheezing is confined to only small areas of the lung, pretreatment with the patient's supply of bronchodilator is warranted. Anesthesia should not be induced until the patient shows signs of psychological *and* respiratory stability and an acceptable SaO_2 on room air. Most β_2-selective adrenergic drugs also have some cardiovascular effects. If possible, deep sedation should be considered without using barbiturates such as methohexital and Pentothal. Maintaining some verbal contact with the patient enables early diagnosis of worsening bronchospasm, which may be easier to treat. Narcotics that are essentially non–histamine-releasing agents (e.g., fentanyl) should be used in lieu of most other narcotics (e.g., meperidine). Although some anaphylactoid reactions to midazolam have been reported as rare, even this drug should be carefully titrated in patients with multiple drug allergies and a history of asthma.[49]

Cardiovascular Complications

Induction of anesthesia is generally accompanied by peripheral vasodilation, resulting in a decrease in systemic vascular resistance (SVR). If normal autonomic sympathetic reflexes are active, the greater the decrease in SVR, the more likely that the accompanying decreases in blood pressure will stimulate the baroreceptor reflex in the carotid and aortic bodies. An acceleration of heart rate usually occurs, the magnitude of which is variable and, in most cases, unpredictable. Because all patients are slightly hypovolemic after an overnight fast and minimal, if any, oral fluids are taken prior to induction, a tachycardia generally results after induction. Some drugs (e.g., methohexital and ketamine) by their drug-specific pharmacodynamics cause more cardioacceleration than others (e.g., propofol and etomidate).

If tachycardia develops in order to maintain a normal or slightly elevated cardiac output and proper filling of peripheral blood vessels to meet the challenge of decreased SVR, myocardial oxygen consumption will rise. In a healthy heart with minimal coronary artery disease (CAD) and minimal or no cardiac valvular stenoses, tachycardia can be well tolerated even if sustained for moderately long periods (greater than 20 minutes). A good preanesthetic medical history and brief chest auscultation are likely to be preemptive in decreasing the chance of unexpected cardiopulmonary complications, but patients with occult CAD may still be at risk. Even utilizing local anesthesia alone for those with definitive cardiac conditions carries a certain degree of risk. Consider the following case:

Case 5

A 74-year-old male with three-vessel CAD, including the right coronary artery, who was mildly hypertensive and taking diltiazem, required extraction of eight maxillary teeth. A total of 8 mL of lidocaine 2% with 1:100,000 epinephrine dilution was injected. Within 5 minutes, the patient developed moderate chest pain and tachycardia (over 130 beats/min) and became hypertensive (190 mm Hg systolic). Despite the sublingual administration of nitroglycerin, the chest pain persisted. After this patient was transported to a hospital emergency room, cardiac enzyme changes suggesting acute myocardial infarction were found.

Analysis

This patient was later treated with an intravenous narcotic (0.1 mg fentanyl), sedative (midazolam, 1.0 mg), oxygen, and nitroglycerin at 0.5 μg/kg/min, and the operation was completed with approximately *12 mL* of the same local anesthetic solution. The cardiac rate was maintained below 80 beats/min by the anesthetic drugs (particularly the fentanyl) before the administration of the local anesthetic with vasoconstrictor. The patient was discharged from the office with a suitable postoperative pain control regimen to diminish the potential for pain-induced tachyarrhythmias. The nitroglycerin was given at coronary artery–protective doses and did not decrease preload significantly or cause hypotension. For this patient's weight, the dose was equivalent to 0.4 mg of sublingual nitroglycerin every 10 minutes for the duration of surgery.

Painful stimulation of the orofacial tissues can activate the trigeminal-sympathetic system. If supraventricular arrhythmias occur, the cardiac output may decrease as much as 35%.[8] Frequent premature ventricular contractions (PVCs) and ventricular tachycardia can also result in 25% and 65% reductions, respectively, in cardiac output. If tachycardia and decreased ventricular filling occur in patients with CAD, valvular stenosis, or low cardiac output conditions (e.g., cardiomyopathy), the decrease in myocardial blood flow may cause myocardial ischemia. Exactly how long myocardial ischemia can be allowed to continue untreated before myocardial infarction occurs is unknown. Although the rate-pressure product (systolic blood pressure multiplied by heart rate) and the pressure-rate quotient (mean arterial pressure divided by heart rate) have been proposed as risk indicators and potential monitors, their role as ischemia predictors is controversial. Regardless, methods of pain control, particularly the use of appropriate doses of intravenous narcotics, is quite useful in limiting excessive tachycardia. Benzodiazepines (e.g., midazolam) in young patients are very predictable in decreasing anxiety-induced endogenous catecholamine secretion, but their use in the elderly is less effective than narcotics in producing the same result. Indeed, the prolonged elimination half-life of all benzodiazepines, especially diazepam, should be considered when attempting to reduce anxiety in an elderly patient.

The administration of multiple drugs has a definite role in the delivery of safe, predictable anesthesia. In the elderly, moderate loading with narcotics (e.g., 1 to 1.5 μg/kg fentanyl) and mild loading with sedatives (e.g., 20 μg/kg midazolam) will likely decrease the possibility of undesirable fluctuation in vital signs from the baseline, despite the use of epinephrine in local anesthesia. The elimination or significant limitation of exogenous epinephrine does *not* preclude the possibility of adverse effects (e.g., arrhythmias). Judicious use of pain control drugs is probably safer in certain instances than eliminating local anesthetics with vasoconstrictors.

The presumably healthy young or older ASA I patient with undiscovered serious CAD or cardiomyopathy can still occasionally escape detection. Therefore, cardiorespiratory monitoring should be strongly emphasized, as well as a goal of maintaining baseline "office admission" vital signs throughout the surgical procedure, even if it is performed with local anesthesia alone. The administration of methohexital as the sole or predominant anesthetic drug to healthy adults commonly causes an increase in heart rate to as much as 50% above preinduction levels.[10] Although significant elevations of heart rate (i.e., to 140 beats/min or more), which are common during exercise, can be tolerated for short oral surgery procedures, they may also be accompanied by myocardial ischemia not always seen on the electrocardioscope or even a standard three-lead rhythm strip. Narcotics, especially fentanyl and its analogs, are more useful in controlling tachycardia or hypertension than sedatives alone. Although bradycardia is a common sign of "athletic training," its finding may indicate either syncope or heart block.[11] Consider the following case:

Case 6

A 17-year-old male requiring dental rehabilitation was resistant to treatment under local anesthesia alone. He appeared anxious and pale, his heart rate ranged from 60 to 80 beats/min, and his systolic blood pressure was 120 mm Hg. Diazepam, 7.5 mg, was injected intravenously at a rate of 2.5 mg every 30 seconds. After only 2.5 mg, the patient lost consciousness and was pale; the heart rate fell to 30 beats/min, and the P wave disappeared from the electrocardioscope. The heart rate fluctuated from 35 to 60 beats/min, and P waves reappeared intermittently. Systolic blood pressure was 80 mm Hg. The heart rate responded to 0.5 mg of intravenous atropine, but only after the dose was being repeated within 2 minutes of the first dose. The patient's color then improved, and he regained consciousness. The heart rate was 95 beats/min.

Analysis

Four possible explanations should be considered for this collapse: acute adrenal insufficiency, unfavorable reaction to diazepam, heart block, and vasovagal syncope. Although the clinical events are similar, symptoms of adrenal insufficiency usually develop in the postoperative period, and hypotension is accompanied by a rise in heart rate.[50] Benzodiazepines have been used extensively, even up to 50 mg of diazepam parenterally, with remarkable cardiovascular stability in healthy patients. In this case, the heart rate fell about 30 seconds after the drug administration began, which resulted in a dose of only about 2.5

mg. The electrocardiogram during the event showed intermittent suppression of the sinus node with ventricular escape, suggesting powerful vagal activity. Although heart block can respond to multiple doses of atropine, this patient's preoperative and postoperative electrocardiograms showed no evidence of heart block.

Vasovagal faint can happen with the patient in either the sitting or the supine position and may occur postoperatively (i.e., in the recovery room).[50] Fainting in the recumbent position can be particularly severe and often protracted, and it is frequently associated with brief sinus arrest. Although fear ("vasodepression syncope") is the most common cause, other conditions in the otherwise healthy patient should be considered: depression of cardiac output, congenital defects of the conduction system (cardiac syncope), and orthostatic hypotension (induced by drugs, electrolyte imbalance). Vasovagal syncope can be accompanied by decreases in all cardiovascular parameters—heart rate, blood pressure, cardiac return, and arterial oxygen saturation. If intravenous narcotics and sedatives are administered at their normal infusion rates and given too soon after syncope, serious cardiovascular collapse may occur. If syncope occurs prior to induction, atropine can be given and the response noted. If a second dose is necessary to restore the vital signs to a normal range, surgery should be delayed, if possible, for further investigation. If the heart rate returns to normal spontaneously without drug treatment or after only one dose of atropine (0.4 mg), a slower anesthesia induction can be accomplished successfully under continuous monitoring with ECG, pulse oximetry, and blood pressure. Heart rate or pulse oximetry should be carefully monitored, and any adverse effects treated early and more aggressively (i.e., ephedrine, 10 to 30 mg IV). Rather than deep sedation or general anesthesia, a lighter level of sedation would be considered safer.

Hypotension is another major cause of cardiovascular complications (see Table 2–2). If tachycardia is present (i.e., in the recovery phase), decreased cardiac filling (preload) may cause hypotension. Either drug effects or fluid volume depletion can be responsible. Patients vary in sensitivity and vascular reactivity to prolonged states of relative hypovolemia, even from an overnight fast extending into an afternoon appointment. With induction of deep sedation or general anesthesia later in the day, accompanied by intraoperative fluid restriction, hypotension may manifest initially as accentuated drops in blood pressure, which usually result in reflex tachycardia. Certain anesthetic agents (e.g., propofol), however, produce a negative chronotropic effect by their very nature; therefore, the hypotension observed may not stimulate a typical tachycardia reflex response. The elderly or volume-depleted patient may be particularly responsive to this drug if it is given at full induction doses (i.e., 1 to 2 mg/kg).

Hypotension accompanied by tachycardia is generally observed with barbiturate induction but can occur either during surgery (albeit rare) or during recovery (more common). If patients are transferred to the recovery area by standing up to facilitate either walking or wheelchair transport, several precautions should be considered. Certain maneuvers can be helpful to minimize orthostatic hypotension. Inhaling deeply before standing momentarily increases the volume of blood in the right heart by pushing the blood above the diaphragm into the right atrium. Prolonged breath holding does the opposite. During the process of standing, contraction of the leg muscles will momentarily increase intravascular blood volume by pushing more blood into the central circulation. Also, increasing the intravenous fluids for a minute or two before the patient stands can increase the blood volume by 50 to 125 mL, depending on the gauge of the intravenous catheter in place. With a mini-drip system run wide open, the maximum fluid volume that can be given through intravenous catheters of 20, 18, 16, and 14 gauge are 50, 75, 100, and 125 mL/min, respectively.[8]

When vital signs are first measured in the operating room, the mean arterial pressure is more indicative of cerebral perfusion, but the most practical measure to follow and record is the systolic blood pressure. Some patients, particularly those taking tricyclic antidepressants or other vasoactive drugs (e.g., marijuana), develop a sustained tachycardia (i.e., greater than 140 beats/min) during recovery. If the tachycardia persists for more than 15 to 20 minutes and is accompanied by nearly normal or higher than preoperative blood pressure, a short-acting β_1-selective adrenergic blocking agent should be considered. In the absence of pain, if tachycardia continues in a patient who is reclining in a chair, even a healthy patient, hypotension can occur early after discharge, which could be very serious. If the heart rate is already elevated, orthostatic hypotension can occur. Consider the following case:

Case 7

A 24-year-old female who had three third molars extracted under general anesthesia had normal vital signs throughout the operation except for moderate elevations of heart rate and blood pressure. In the recovery room she seemed to wake up without complications, but the heart rate was 130 to 140 beats/min for 20 minutes; blood pressure was near preoperative values at 116/60. Before discharge, she could stand with her eyes closed and feet together without vertigo, but the tachycardia persisted. Vital signs were heart rate 134 beats/min, blood pressure 100/60. After the patient sat back down, esmolol 0.3 mg/kg was given intravenously over 1 minute along with another 100 mL of isotonic saline solution. The heart rate decreased to 100 beats/min, and blood pressure improved to 120/70. Esmolol, 0.15 mg/kg/min, was given 5 minutes after the first dose, to achieve a more *sustained* effect, and the heart rate was stable at 75 to 80 beats/min for the next 20 minutes prior to an uneventful discharge.

Analysis

According to the history, this patient was taking amitriptyline, 75 mg at night, for chronic pain. Approximately 8 mL of lidocaine, 2% with 1:100,000 epinephrine dilution, was used for the anesthesia. A period of 40 minutes elapsed between administration of the local anesthetic and the patient's arrival in the recovery room. Tachycardia presented long after the epinephrine should have peaked and its effects terminated. As the narcosis from general anesthesia dissipated upon awakening, the sympathetic system responded more vigorously than anticipated postoperatively, perhaps related to drug-interactive effects with the amitriptyline. The treatment of the tachycardia with esmolol enabled two occurrences: the administration of a safe, rapid-onset, quickly redistributed β-selective adrenergic blocker and the resetting of the adrenergic output, resulting in a lower heart rate and allowing for better ventricular filling and improved blood pressure, especially after the intravenous infusion of a crystalloid solution. If administration of a beta blocker is considered, a fluid-loading process should also be considered if the blood pressure is normal or lower than preoperative values to protect against undesired (albeit rare) hypotension.

Respiratory Complications

The most common but a generally easily treatable respiratory complication is laryngospasm. Although this complication occurs more commonly during the induction and transition from anesthesia stage 1 to stage 3, it can also occur during emergence (i.e., from stage 3 to stage 1). The simplest approach to this complication *during induction* is to deepen the anesthetic level with an inhalation agent (e.g., halothane or isoflurane) and small enough increments of intravenous anesthetic to maintain spontaneous respiration without producing apnea. Large boluses and infusion of an intravenous agent may produce apnea. If apnea occurs, positive-pressure ventilation is necessary, but it can cause inflation of the stomach with air. Because laryngospasm may be an early sign of silent regurgitation, clearing the airway with suction and deepening the anesthetic level should precede any thought of administering a peripheral muscle relaxant (e.g., succinylcholine). Partial laryngospasm allows acceptable oxygenation, and decreases in pulse oximetry measurements should be "essentially ignored" as long as (1) the patient is breathing and receiving at least 50% oxygen and (2) the drop in oxygen saturation is modest (i.e., is still above 85%).

If either cyanosis, full laryngospasm, or a drop in pulse oximetry values to 75% (Pa_{O_2} 40 torr) occurs, the administration of succinylcholine should be strongly considered. If full muscle relaxation is obtained, intubation should be considered as long as there is a capability of continuing the anesthesia with either a total intravenous technique *and* continuous muscle relaxation or an inhalation agent, after which spontaneous respiration can return. This is essentially the same technique used in the hospital operating room setting. Clear breath sounds should be obtained after appropriate suctioning of the endotracheal tube or pharynx. If endotracheal anesthesia is not chosen after full muscle paralysis is obtained, the patient should be allowed to wake up with face mask ventilation assistance, and the procedure should be completed using deep or conscious sedation. Auscultation of the lungs for fluid should be performed, and pulse oximetry levels observed before the operation is resumed.

The major concern of laryngospasm is aspiration, but a delayed condition called *postobstructive pulmonary edema* (POPE) can occur.[51] Generally, this condition (albeit rare) occurs after extubation. The cause is probably related to the generation of very high negative intrapulmonic pressures while the patient is attempting to inhale against a closed or obstructed glottis. It is characterized by the presence of a frothy, pink sputum and rales generally in all lung fields, rather than just the basilar fields, which are more commonly the affected areas after aspiration. Treatment of POPE is generally easily accomplished with diuresis or positive-pressure mask ventilation support, but only rarely is re-intubation required.

Although stiff chest syndrome (SCS) has received considerable attention, the condition is rare but can occur with any narcotics in high enough doses. The entire fentanyl drug family, including sufentanil and alfentanil, has been implicated. When doses of fentanyl are administered slowly (e.g., 1 to 2 μg/kg) at 0.03 to 0.08 mg/min (e.g., 1 mL/1–2 min), SCS is extremely rare.[52] Should it occur, 5 to 10 mg of succinylcholine (if the patient is nearly unconscious) or 0.4 mg of naloxone (if the patient is awake) intravenously quickly reverses SCS. The fear of this complication should not overshadow the significant benefits of adding fentanyl to a sedation or general anesthesia technique. Sufentanil and alfentanil have a more rapid onset and are more lipophilic and more likely to cause SCS than fentanyl. However, there certainly may be a role for these drugs as well in the consideration of anesthesia for orthognathic or temporomandibular joint (TMJ) surgery in the office.

Bronchospasm is a serious condition that can occur secondary to drug administration (i.e., anaphylaxis-like reactions) or from other causes unrelated or co-related to anesthetics. In patients without endotracheal intubation, aspiration and drug allergy are the most common causes of bronchospasm, which occurs more often during the induction or early maintenance phase of anesthesia. Drug-induced signs and symptoms vary from full rapid cardiovascular collapse soon after the administration of a drug to more delayed, protracted coughing spells during spontaneous or assisted inspiration. Consider the following case:

Case 8

A 16-year-old male received meperidine and diazepam to facilitate the removal of four third molars. Within 10 minutes of receiving the two agents, the patient coughed several times and became apneic. The blood pressure was stable, ranging from 90 to 125 mm Hg systolic; the heart rate was 115 to 120 beats/min. When the patient was assisted with full face mask during an apneic period, he would cough several times and then begin spontaneous respiration. Any attempts to assist respiration during lung inflation caused more coughing. As the patient breathed easily at 14 to 18 breaths/min, coughing ceased. The patient remained deeply sedated but arousable by verbal or pain stimulation for about 30 minutes. Auscultation of the chest after 30 minutes revealed slight wheezing, primarily in the lower lung fields. The condition slowly resolved over the next 30 minutes. Inspection of the intravenous site revealed a redness that extended proximally to the needle entry over several venous branches.

Analysis

Meperidine produces a histamine reaction more frequently than the fentanyl-type drugs but still less frequently than morphine. The release of histamine can cause tachycardia and hypotension shortly after drug administration. The presence of cutaneous changes is common but is not always an early sign. Protracted coughing or bucking after the injection of a drug is of particular concern if a patient has a history of drug allergy, especially to penicillin or aspirin. Treatment may range from methylprednisolone or hydrocortisone to epinephrine, depending on the severity of the reaction. The crucial decision whether to deepen the level of anesthesia, *perhaps inadvertently with the offending agent* (e.g., thiopental or propofol), should be based upon the blood pressure. Unexpected severe hypotension and tachycardia should be considered signs of impending cardiovascular collapse and bronchospasm until proven otherwise by chest auscultation.

Hypoventilation can occur during maintenance or recovery from anesthesia. Nearly all drugs used for sedation, whether narcotics or sedatives used in combination or alone, produce a decrease in minute ventilation and in the normal physiologic response to hypercarbia or hypoxia. When ambient air is supplemented with higher concentrations of oxygen to produce an inhaled mixture containing 30% oxygen or more, hypoxemia is rare.[8] Even when benzodiazepines are given alone without narcotics, an average decrease in arterial oxygen partial pressure ($Pa{O_2}$) of 13 torr will occur. Without adding the narcotics, $Pa{CO_2}$ will increase approximately 3.5 torr on average.[53] When narcotics are administered with benzodiazepines while the patient is breathing room air, even though there may be no vital sign changes of clinical significance, conscious patients can have an average decrease in $Pa{O_2}$ of 30 torr and an elevation in $Pa{CO_2}$ of 7 torr.[53] The studies reporting these results were conducted before it was standard to administer oxygen and probably could not be ethically repeated today using midazolam. On the basis of similar respiratory effect profiles, however, the results would probably be similar.

Respiratory depression and subsequent hypercarbia are generally well tolerated during anesthesia for brief periods (i.e., 30 to 60 minutes). If $Pa{CO_2}$ rises above 55 torr and the pH goes below 7.25, cardiac myocardial irritability increases. During total intravenous anesthesia (TIVA) in the absence of irritating inhaled agents (e.g., halothane), however, vital signs are still generally very stable. Hypoventilation can also occur with the administration of oral sedatives that have nonnarcotic but strong hypnotic properties (e.g., chloral hydrate). At doses of 50 to 75 mg/kg, pediatric patients breathing room air frequently have decreases in oxygen saturation percentages ranging from the high 80s to the low 90s.[54] Although several deaths have been attributed to chloral hydrate, the cause is probably co-related to airway obstruction rather than the respiratory effects alone.

The maintenance phase of general anesthesia is the time when a high percentage of patients have adverse respiratory events leading to death.[10] Intravenous narcotics given early during induction generally produce respiratory depression and hypoventilation soon after administration even if short-acting narcotics (e.g., fentanyl) are given. Several narcotics (e.g., meperidine, nalbuphine, morphine) have longer therapeutic half-lives, and respiratory depression can occur later with their use, especially if sedatives are given incrementally throughout the surgical procedure. When narcotics and sedative drugs are *front-loaded*, the most vulnerable period is 10 to 15 minutes after administration, but serious respiratory problems rarely occur if the patient "drifts" through the surgery while receiving no other drugs. *Incremental techniques* with hypnotic agents carry the risk that respiratory complications may occur during maintenance of anesthesia, especially if there is accompanying hypoxemia associated with decreased attentiveness to breathing functions (i.e., depth and rate).

Periodically, closed-claim cases or public news releases reveal situations in which patients (frequently children) "failed to wake up" at the end of a dental procedure. Generally, the precipitating event, usually airway obstruction, was noticed at the end of surgery but actually occurred during the *maintenance* phase of anesthesia, accounting for the high incidence of deaths during this period.[10] Airway obstruction is common during deep sedation or general anesthesia. In one study of 550 patients given fentanyl, diazepam, and methohexital, 8.5% exhibited overt signs or symptoms of obstruction or hypoventilation.[33] Hypoventilation (less than 8 breaths/min) was more common than sustained (greater than 5 minutes) partial airway obstruction (37 and 10 patients, respectively), but none of the patients in the study who had a $Pa{CO_2}$ above 55 torr or a $Pa{O_2}$ below 70 torr ($Sa{O_2}$ values 90% to 95%) showed abnormal vital signs indicating physiologic distress. In fact, the respiratory values *averaged* $Pa{O_2}$ 132 to 143 torr and $Pa{CO_2}$ 47 to 54 torr *during* either hypoventilation or partial airway obstruction. All the patients in this study were breathing at least 35% oxygen. Conversely, if complete airway obstruction or prolonged apnea occurs during procedures *without* supplemental oxygen, a severe and unacceptable rise in carbon dioxide tension and drop in oxygen saturation can be expected.

In one study, nearly 60% (31 of 52) of the deaths occurred during recovery, but the exact causes were not well understood.[10] Theoretically, when the operation is completed and the surgical stimulus diminished or eliminated, the recovery process begins. If the level of anesthesia is light and the surgical stimulus "drives" the heart rate, blood pressure, and respirations, larger increments of intravenous anesthetics are frequently given in an attempt to maintain a deeper level of anesthesia. After discontinuation of the surgical stimulus, vital signs may drop precipitously. Therefore, in this situation, the recovery phase becomes more perilous than the induction and maintenance phases. Relative drug overdose may become more apparent, and close observation is imperative. Consider the following case:

Case 9

A 38-year-old, 170-lb, 6-ft-tall female had general anesthesia with a total of 20 mg of diazepam and 125 mL (1.25 g) of 1% methohexital to remove several teeth. When one tooth was lost into the maxillary sinus, and attempts to retrieve it were futile, the procedure was discontinued. Later that afternoon, when the second oral surgeon arrived in the office, the tooth was successfully removed using a second general anesthesia with 25 mg of diazepam and 150 mL (1.5 g) of methohexital. At the end of the second operation, as the surgeons were walking out of the operatory, the patient collapsed. Although successfully ventilated and intubated, the patient expired. Autopsy revealed hypoxic brain damage but no other body abnormalities.

Analysis

An overdose of anesthetic agents can take two forms—relative and absolute. Head-injured patients are frequently intentionally put into a "barbiturate coma" (to rest the brain activity) with 10 to 15 g of thiopental per day for a week or more, but their survival depends on adequate control of ventilation. In this case, unrecognized respiratory depression and subsequent hypercarbia occurred either throughout or after completion of the second operation, resulting in significant peripheral vascular dilation, decreased SVR, and perhaps cardiac depression from acute respiratory acidosis. Additionally, the heart rate was probably elevated during the operation by catecholamine secretion; for this reason, large amounts of methohexital were needed to keep the patient asleep. At the end of the procedure, when the endogenous catecholamine levels decreased and the heart rate and cardiac output dropped precipitously along with reduced SVR, the amount of blood being returned to the right side of the heart decreased even further, rendering the patient severely hypotensive and unresuscitatable.

During the operation, the respiratory function and perhaps the vital signs were probably driven by the surgical stimulation. Although this case occurred prior to the advent of pulse oximetry technology, it illustrates the importance of maintaining vital signs as near as possible to baseline preoperative values without overstimulation of the adrenergic system, which would result in undesirable elevations of heart rate and blood pressure. Pushing one or two drugs too far played a role in this death. An inhalation agent would have been very useful in allowing the administration of normal doses of methohexital and utilizing the lung as an uptake and excretion organ for the anesthetic. Unacceptable accumulation of barbiturate probably caused severe respiratory depression in a spontaneously breathing patient at the end of the operation.

During anesthesia induction in children with an inhalation agent, respiratory rate and rhythm should be carefully observed. Some agents are inhaled rather smoothly (e.g., halothane and nitrous oxide), and side effects such as breath-holding, excessive salivation, and laryngospasm are less common. Other agents (e.g., enflurane, isoflurane, desflurane) are more irritating to the airway, so these adverse effects are more likely to occur. If *any* of the inhalation agents is delivered too rapidly and at initially high doses (referred to as "overpressure technique"), apnea and spasm may occur, requiring controlled mask ventilation to accelerate the induction through the excitement stage (stage 2). Most pediatric airways respond during recovery as they do during induction; if airway difficulties are encountered during induction, they are likely to occur during emergence. Emergence can be *quite eventful* and may include airway obstruction (if the head assumes a flexed position with the chin down on the chest), vomiting, or laryngospasm. In rare instances, laryngospasm and mild hypoxia can precipitate postobstructive pulmonary edema or bronchospasm,[50] but this is more frequently an adult complication.

Major Office Surgery

Elective orthognathic surgery has been performed as an outpatient procedure for the past few years in ambulatory care centers and dental schools and may soon be commonplace in offices. Several surgical considerations must be addressed, including length of surgery, blood loss, and pain control.

Procedures that can be completed in 4 hours or less can usually be done in an ambulatory facility. Although time is not the final determining factor, ample time for the patient's recovery, ambulation, and discharge is necessary. It is difficult, if not impossible, to predict how an individual patient will awaken from general anesthesia. If a patient is large (either muscular or obese), it generally takes more anesthetic agent to produce the same state of stage 3 anesthesia. Some volatile agents are more fat soluble than intravenous agents, and patients anesthetized primarily with isoflurane and enflurane emerge more slowly from anesthesia. Isoflurane has an intermediate fat/blood coefficient of 45, which is comparable to that of enflurane (36). A low fat/blood coefficient is more compatible with more rapid removal of the agent from the blood and vascular poor areas. However, because isoflurane requires less metabolic degradation (0.2% as compared to 2% for enflurane), it is a more suitable agent for ambulatory anesthesia. Isoflurane has minimal reductive metabolism activity and minimal fluoride accumulation from metabolism, making it less likely than enflurane to produce hepatotoxicity, nephrotoxicity, and somnolence.

Desflurane is a newer agent with an even lower fat/blood coefficient (18.7), classifying it as a low-solubility agent compared with isoflurane. Theoretically, desflurane would be the best agent for more rapid awakening from anesthesia. The major disadvantage to using this agent is the high cost of the specialized, heated vaporizer (three times that of an isoflurane vaporizer). Total intravenous anesthesia using propofol and sufentanil infusions with low-dose isoflurane appears to be the best combination for rapid recovery.

Postoperative pain control is seldom a problem after osteotomy surgery and is related more to tissue swelling than to bone sectioning near nerves that are partially anesthetized by the operation. Intravenous ketorolac can be administered along with steroids prior to surgery to minimize swelling and postdischarge narcotic needs. If necessary, oral agents (e.g., demerol, phenergan, synthetic hydrocodones) can be prescribed. Postoperative contact can be made with the patient within 24 hours to further instruct patient and home caregivers on management of pain and nausea.

Contingencies for admission to the hospital (i.e., ambulance transfer) from either the office or the home must be planned. *Expected* causes for admission include bleeding, nausea or vomiting, need for prolonged intubation, and slow awakening. When patients have intermaxillary fixation, the complications of airway management should also be considered. Before discharge, the patient should be very alert and capable of swallowing clear liquids to ensure normal deglutition function and should demonstrate the ability to swallow in case emesis occurs during maxillomandibular immobilization.

Certain *unexpected* complications should be considered. They include urinary retention, fever, and orthostatic hypotension. Instructions for postoperative care should always be given both verbally and in written form. Contact phone numbers for the surgeon and anesthesiologist should be given to the patient's home caregivers. Telephone "rounds" should be standard practice the first postoperative evening. Patients should be discharged with enough time to allow 6 to 8 hours of home adaptation prior to retiring for the evening. This means that discharge in middle afternoon generally is advisable.

Obviously, the risks of performing major oral and maxillofacial surgery on an outpatient basis should be considered case by case. A short procedure (i.e., 3 to 4 hours), skilled operators (anesthesiologist and surgeon), and appropriate short-acting anesthetic agents should be considered. The patient's socioeconomic status, the intelligence of the home caregivers, and the distance of the patient's home from the office and a hospital emergency room should be major factors in the decision. For the patient and home caregiver who are ambivalent about assuming some responsibility in the decision to undertake this type of risk, surgery of this nature should *not* be attempted in the office.

References

1. Biery KA, Shamaskin RG, Campbell RL: Analysis of preoperative laboratory values prior to outpatient dental anesthesia. Anesth Prog 1987;34:58.
2. Olsson SL, Hambroeus-Jonzon K: Aspiration during anaesthesia: A computer-aided study of 185,358 anaesthetics. Acta Anaesthesiol Scand 1986;30:84.
3. Ong BY, Palahniuk RJ, Cummings M: Gastric volume and pH in outpatients. Can Anaesth Soc J 1978;25:36.
4. Splinter WM, Stewart JA, Muir JG: The effect of preoperative apple juice on gastric contents, thirst, and hunger in children. Can J Anaesth 1989;36:55.
5. White A, Kander PL: Anatomical factors in difficult direct laryngoscopy. Br J Anaesth 1975;47:468.
6. Mallampati SR, Gatt SP, Gugino LD, et al: A clinical sign to predict difficult tracheal intubation: A prospective study. Can Anaesth Soc J 1985;32:429.
7. Wilson ME, Spiegelhalter JA, Robertson JA, et al: Predicting difficult intubation. Br J Anaesth 1988;61:211.
8. Campbell RL: Prevention of complications associated with intravenous sedation and general anesthesia. J Oral Maxillofac Surg 1986;44:289.
9. Cooper JB, Newbower RS, Long CD, et al: Preventable mishaps: A study of human factors. Anaesthesia 1978;49:399.
10. Coplans MP, Curson I: Deaths associated with dentistry. Br J Dent 1982;153:357.
11. Huston TP, Puffer JC, Rodney WM: The athletic heart syndrome. N Engl J Med 1985;313:24.
12. Pierce EC: Anesthesia: Standards of care and liability. JAMA 1989;261:773.
13. Cheney FW, Posner K, Caplan RA, et al: Standard of care and anesthesia liability. JAMA 1989;261:159.
14. Wiklund L, Hok B, Stahl K, et al: Post anesthesia monitoring revisited: Frequency of true and false alarms from different monitoring devices. J Clin Anesth 1994;6:182.
15. Moller JT, Johannesson NW, Epersen K, et al: Randomized evaluation of pulse oximetry in 20,802 patients. II: Perioperative events and postoperative complications. Anesthesiology 1993;78:445.
16. McKay WP, Noble H: Critical incidents detected by pulse oximetry during anesthesia. Can J Anaesth 1988;35:265.
17. Tremper KK: Necessary monitoring in the post anesthesia care unit. J Clin Anesth 1994;6:178.
18. Wilson S: Conscious sedation and pulse oximetry: False alarms? Pediatr Dent 1990;12:228.
19. Stock MC, Downs JB, McDonald JS, et al: The carbon dioxide rate of rise in awake apneic humans. J Clin Anesth 1988;1:96.
20. Canet J: Early postoperative arterial oxygen desaturation: Determining factors and response to oxygen therapy. Anesth Analg 1989;69:207.
21. Downs JB: Prevention of hypoxemia: The simple, logical, but incorrect solution. J Clin Anesth 1994;6:180.
22. Sun-Ping ST, Mehta MP, Anderson JM: Comparative study of methods of detection of esophageal intubation. Anesth Analg 1989;69:627.
23. Tinker JH, Dull DL, Caplan RA: Role of monitoring devices in prevention of anesthetic mishaps: A closed claims analysis. Anesthesiology 1989;71:541.
24. Caplan RA, Posner RL, Ward RJ, et al: Adverse respiratory events in anesthesia: A closed claims analysis. Anesthesiology 1990;72:828.
25. Coriat P, Doloz M, Bousseau D: Prevention of intraoperative myocardial ischemia during noncardiac surgery with intravenous nitroglycerin. Anesthesiology 1984;61:193.
26. Ellis JE, Shah MN, Briller JE, et al: A comparison of methods for the detection of myocardial ischemia during non-cardiac surgery: Automated ST-segment analysis systems: Electrocardiography and transesophageal echocardiography. Anesth Analg 1992; 75:764.
27. Mangano DT, Browner WS, Hollenberg M, et al: Association of perioperative myocardial ischemia with cardiac morbidity and mortality in men undergoing noncardiac surgery. N Engl J Med 1990;323:1781.
28. Campbell RL, Werner M, Stewart LM: General anesthesia for the pediatric patient. J Oral Maxillofac Surg 1982;40:497.
29. Forbes AR: Inspired oxygen concentrations in semi-closed circle absorber circuits with low flows of nitrous oxide and oxygen. Br J Anaesth 1972;44:1081.

30. Campbell RL, Gregg JM, Levin KJ: Cardiorespiratory effects of a balanced anesthesia technique in outpatient general anesthesia. J Oral Surg 1976;34:399.
31. Milgram P, Beirne OR, Fiset L, et al: The safety and efficacy of outpatient midazolam intravenous sedation for oral surgery with and without fentanyl. Anesthesia Progress 1993;40:57.
32. Smith JW, Seidl LG, Cluff LE: Studies on the epidemiology of adverse drug reactions. Ann Intern Med 1966;65:629.
33. Campbell RL, Saxen MA: Respiratory effects of a balanced anesthetic technique—revisited fifteen years later. Anesthesia Progress 1994;41:1.
34. Bailey PL, Pace NL, Ashburn MA, et al: Frequent hypoxemia and apnea after sedation with midazolam and fentanyl. Anesthesiology 1990;73:826.
35. Bailey PL, Andriano KP, Goldman M, et al: Variability of the respiratory response to diazepam. Anesthesiology 1986;64:460.
36. Power SJ, Morgan M, Chakrabarite MK: Carbon dioxide response curves following midazolam and diazepam. Br J Anaesth 1983;55:837.
37. Gross JB, Zebrowski ME, Carel WD: Time course of ventilatory depression after thiopental and midazolam in normal subjects and in patients with chronic obstructive pulmonary disease. Anesthesiology 1983;58:540.
38. Ben-Shlomo I, Abd-El-Khalim H, Ezry J, et al: Midazolam acts synergistically with fentanyl for induction of anaesthesia. Br J Anaesth 1990;64:45.
39. Haefely W, Pole P: Physiology of GABA enhancement by benzodiazepines and barbiturates. *In* Olsen RW, Venter JC (eds): Benzodiazepine GABA Receptors and Chloride Channels: Structure and Function Properties. New York, Alan R Liss, 1986, pp 97–133.
40. Vorsanger GT, Roberts JT: Midazolam-induced athetoid movements of the lower extremities during epidural anesthesia reversed by physostigmine. J Clin Anesth 1993;5:494.
41. Tverskoy M, Ben-Shlomo I, Ezry J, et al: Midazolam acts synergistically with methohexitone for induction of anesthesia. Br J Anaesth 1989;63:109.
42. McClune S, McKay AC, Wright MC: Synergistic interaction between midazolam and propofol. Br J Anaesth 1992;69:240.
43. Campbell RL, Shamaskin RG, Saunders VW: Analysis of cardiovascular changes and arterial blood gases in patients resistant to methohexital anesthesia. Anesthesia Progress 1987;34:51.
44. Ding Y, Fredman B, White PF: Recovery following outpatient anesthesia: Use of enflurane versus propofol. J Clin Anesth 1993;4:447.
45. Beaconsfield P, Gensbing J, Ramsbing R: Marijuana smoking: Cardiovascular effects in man and possible mechanisms. N Engl J Med 1972;287:209.
46. Redden RJ, Miller M, Campbell RL: Submental administration of succinylcholine in children. Anesthesia Progress 1990;37:296.
47. Cote CJ: NPO after midnight for children—a reappraisal. Anesthesiology 1990;72:589.
48. Campbell RL, Paulette SW: Pulmonary aspiration in a pediatric dental patient. Anesthesia Progress 1986;33:98.
49. Fujita Y, Ishikawa H, Yokota K: Anaphylactoid reaction to midazolam. Anesth Analg 1994;79:811.
50. Verrill PJ, Aellig WH: Vasovagal faint in the supine position. Br Med J 1970;4:348.
51. Jenkins JG: Pulmonary edema following laryngospasm. Anesthesiology 1984;60:611.
52. Grell FL, Koons RA, Denson JS: Fentanyl in anesthesia. Anesth Analg 1970;49:523.
53. Campbell RL, Dionne RA, Gregg JM, et al: Respiratory effects of fentanyl, diazepam and methohexital sedation. J Oral Surg 1979;37:555.
54. Moody EH, Mourino AP, Campbell RL: The therapeutic effectiveness of nitrous oxide and chloral hydrate administered orally, rectally, and combined with hydroxyzine for pediatric dentistry. J Dent Child 1986;43:425.

Chapter 3
NITROUS OXIDE ABUSE AND ITS NEUROLOGIC COMPLICATIONS

by

Robert B. Layzer

Introduction

Unlike the others in this book, this chapter is primarily concerned with complications affecting health practitioners rather than patients. Prolonged exposure to nitrous oxide has well-documented neurologic toxicity and less well-established risks of promoting malignancy and fetal malformations.[1] For obvious reasons, such prolonged exposure rarely occurs in patients. In fact, among health practitioners, neurologic toxicity from nitrous oxide is encountered almost exclusively in those who abuse the agent for recreational purposes. There are, however, rare instances of neurotoxicity in health practitioners from chronic occupational exposure as well as in patients who had a single exposure to nitrous oxide during anesthesia.

THE SUBJECTS DISCUSSED IN THIS CHAPTER ARE:

- History of the medical use of nitrous oxide
- Prevalence of nitrous oxide abuse
- Addictive properties of nitrous oxide
- Neurotoxicity of nitrous oxide
  - Neurotoxicity from prolonged exposure to nitrous oxide
  - Neurotoxicity due to occupational exposure to nitrous oxide
  - Neurotoxicity of nitrous oxide in cases of subclinical vitamin B_{12} deficiency
- Biochemical mechanism of nitrous oxide neurotoxicity
- Treatment of nitrous oxide neurotoxicity

History of the Medical Use of Nitrous Oxide

The medical properties of nitrous oxide were first studied by Humphry Davy in 1799 and 1800.[2, 3] He discovered that the gas had both analgesic and euphoriant properties; the latter provided entertainment to Davy's friends, and the gas was then taken up by the fashionable public in the form of recreational nitrous oxide parties, which enjoyed some popularity in the early nineteenth century. (They were later replaced by "ether frolics.") In 1844, the American dentist Horace Wells began to promote the use of nitrous oxide as an anesthetic agent, but widespread use of nitrous oxide in dentistry did not begin until two decades later.[2] Because nitrous oxide is a weak anesthetic agent, attempts to achieve anesthesia with high concentrations of the gas often resulted in accidental asphyxia. Early in the twentieth century, this problem was addressed by the invention of anesthesia machines that provided safe levels of oxygen, but they were not entirely reliable. In the 1950s, the concept of administering low-dose nitrous oxide–oxygen mixtures, in order to provide analgesia and sedation rather than anesthesia, finally eliminated the danger of asphyxia.[4] From that time, the use of nitrous oxide in dentistry and oral and maxillofacial surgery was enthusiastically taught in schools of dentistry. By 1977, approximately one third of dentists in the United States used nitrous oxide in their practice.[5] At the same time, the problem of nitrous oxide abuse among dentists and oral surgeons began to come to medical attention. This development coincided with a great increase in recreational drug use in the general population.

Prevalence of Nitrous Oxide Abuse

Health practitioners may be especially prone to chemical dependency, and it has been claimed that 10% to 14% of physicians are impaired by substance abuse.[6] Because dentists, oral and maxillofacial surgeons, and anesthesiologists have easy access to nitrous oxide, they are probably at greatest risk of succumbing to nitrous oxide abuse. Even among those practitioners, however, nitrous oxide abuse is infrequent compared with abuse of other drugs. Exact incidence figures are not known, but a survey of chemical dependency among Oregon dentists disciplined for drug abuse (1979–1984) implicated nitrous oxide in 7% of the cases, compared with alcohol in 18% and meperidine in 25%.[7] Among 26 drug-dependent surgery residents identified by a 1986 survey of oral and maxillofacial training programs, meperidine was involved in ten cases, fentanyl in eight, nitrous oxide in three, and morphine, diazepam, ketamine, and cocaine each in one case.[8] A survey of drug abuse in anesthesia training programs (1970–1980) also showed meperidine and fentanyl to be the most popular drugs, but nitrous oxide was not even mentioned.[9] Likewise, nitrous oxide was not listed among the drugs used by 1,000 chemically dependent physicians in Georgia.[10]

Nitrous oxide abuse is not limited to health care workers who have access to medical gas cylinders. Nitrous oxide is also available in the form of compressed gas cartridges used in restaurants to make whipped cream and can even be obtained by expelling the propellant from whipped cream cans sold in grocery stores. In the 1960s and 1970s, there were many anecdotal reports suggesting that recreational use of nitrous oxide was popular among college students. A 1979 survey reported experience with recreational use of nitrous oxide in 14% to 20% of dental students and 9% to 17% of medical students.[11] The National Household Survey of Drug Abuse, carried out in 1991, reported a lifetime history of recreational use (not habitual abuse) of nitrous oxide in 4.8% of people aged 18 to 25 years, in 3.1% of those aged 26 to 34 years, and in 0.5% of those aged 35 years or older. For comparison, lifetime use of cocaine was reported by 18% of persons aged 18 to 25 years.[12]

Addictive Properties of Nitrous Oxide

Patients generally find nitrous oxide pleasant, and the agent has genuine (though mild) analgesic[13] and anxiolytic[14] effects. Furthermore, there are well-documented cases of chronic abuse of nitrous oxide, though they are few in number. Indeed, even Humphry Davy[15] noticed symptoms of drug dependency in himself and others after repeated "experiments" with inhaling the gas. "The desire of some individuals acquainted with the pleasure of nitrous oxide for the gas has been so strong as to induce them to breathe with eagerness, the air remaining in the bags after the respiration of others."[15] Nevertheless, there is general agreement that nitrous oxide has a very low abuse potential.

There are several reasons for this. One is that nitrous oxide gas is very inconvenient to use, being bulky and cumbersome. Second, nitrous oxide is a very weak intoxicant. Third, tolerance to the euphoriant effects of nitrous oxide develops with repeated use.[6] Fourth, under experimental conditions, most subjects do not prefer nitrous oxide to oxygen, indicating that the substance has little or no "reinforcing" effect.[16, 17]

Nitrous oxide does have certain advantages as a recreational drug. It has a pleasant, sweetish odor. Used in low concentrations (30% to 50%), it is mildly euphoriant but does not cause confusion or other mental side effects. The effects of the drug dissipate rapidly after use. Its low addictive properties may be appealing to members of the health professions. Most importantly, the gas was widely regarded until recently as being chemically inert and harmless to the user.

As it happens, nitrous oxide is not chemically inert. It very rapidly inactivates the vitamin B_{12}–dependent enzyme methionine synthase, producing a state of functional vitamin B_{12} deficiency, which causes a neurologic disorder known as subacute combined degeneration of the spinal cord. These facts came to light when patients with neurologic symptoms attributable to nitrous oxide abuse began to appear in the late 1970s.

Neurotoxicity of Nitrous Oxide

Neurotoxicity From Prolonged Exposure to Nitrous Oxide

In 1956, Lassen and associates[18] reported severe bone marrow suppression, with megaloblastic features, in tetanus patients treated with prolonged inhalation of nitrous oxide. This observation led to extensive animal research on the hematologic toxicity of nitrous oxide. A link with vitamin B_{12} metabolism was first proposed by Amess and colleagues,[19] who reported abnormalities of DNA synthesis in erythroblasts, resembling those seen in vitamin B_{12} deficiency, in patients receiving nitrous oxide continuously for 24 hours after open heart surgery. Serum vitamin B_{12} levels were normal, and Amess and colleagues[19] postulated that nitrous oxide had inactivated vitamin B_{12} by oxidizing the cobalt in cyanocobalamin, as had previously been shown to occur in vitro.

In the same year, my colleagues and I[20] reported an unusual combination of spinal cord and peripheral nerve abnormalities (myeloneuropathy) in three patients who gave a history of nitrous oxide abuse. Two were dentists, and the third was a hospital operating room technician. Simultaneously, others reported a similar syndrome in a college student who had abused nitrous oxide obtained from whipped-cream cartridges.[21] In a short time, 12 additional cases came to my attention, and the clinical features of neurotoxicity from prolonged exposure to nitrous oxide were better defined.[22] Other case reports confirmed this clinical picture.[23–31]

The initial symptoms, which appear after frequent use of nitrous oxide (several times a week for several hours at a time) for at least 3 months, consist of numbness and tingling in the hands or legs. (Interestingly, Davy described similar symptoms in himself after repeated inhalation of nitrous oxide.[3, 15]) Over the next several weeks or months, if abuse continues, most patients develop more serious signs and symptoms of a combined spinal cord and peripheral nerve disorder, with Lhermitte sign (an electric shock sensation in the limbs or trunk produced by flexion of the neck), loss of dexterity in the fingers, ataxia of gait, weakness of the legs, and even impairment of bladder and bowel control. Nearly half of the patients also experience mental changes, with altered mood or difficulty in thinking. At the height of their disability, two thirds of the patients are unable to work.[22]

Neurologic examination in typical cases discloses a sensory ataxia of gait with a positive Romberg sign, loss of vibration and position sense in the legs and hands, a stocking-pattern loss of skin sensation in the legs, and diminished ankle jerks and extensor plantar reflexes. The spinal fluid is usually normal, and electrodiagnostic tests point to the presence of an axonal, length-dependent polyneuropathy. These findings are indistinguishable from those seen in vitamin B_{12} deficiency, but B_{12} levels are normal in most cases, and the Schilling test for absorption of B_{12} from the gastrointestinal tract is normal. Some patients, however, do have subnormal serum vitamin B_{12} levels. Most patients do not have overt hematologic abnormalities, but macrocytosis of red blood cells[27] and even frank megaloblastic anemia[31] are occasionally seen.

Following the cessation of nitrous oxide abuse, most patients begin to improve in a few weeks. Some recover completely, but many are left with permanent neurologic deficits, such as ataxia of gait, leg weakness, and numbness of the feet. The outcome is similar to that seen in patients treated for subacute combined degeneration due to vitamin B_{12} deficiency, many of whom retain a significant impairment of neurologic function despite adequate doses of vitamin B_{12}.

Neurotoxicity Due to Occupational Exposure to Nitrous Oxide

Two of the original 15 patients reported in 1978[22] were oral surgeons who were heavily exposed to nitrous oxide in their practice owing to faulty anesthesia equipment. They denied any recreational use of nitrous oxide. No other cases of overt neurotoxicity from occupational exposure to nitrous oxide have been reported. In a survey of dentists and chairside assistants, however, Brodsky and coworkers[32] reported that symptoms of numbness, tingling, or weakness occurred in 1% to 2% of persons with heavy exposure to nitrous oxide, a three to four times greater incidence than for unexposed persons. It is difficult to guess how many of the symptomatic subjects had actually suffered neurotoxicity from nitrous oxide, but the incidence of "diagnosed neurologic disease" in those subjects was only one tenth the incidence of neurologic symptoms. In order to estimate the true risk of neurotoxicity from occupational exposure to nitrous oxide, a prospective study would be required, including neurologic examinations in symptomatic persons.

Neurotoxicity of Nitrous Oxide in Cases of Subclinical Vitamin B_{12} Deficiency

Five patients with subclinical vitamin B_{12} deficiency, subsequently documented by abnormal Schilling tests, developed overt symptoms of combined system disease following general anesthesia that included the use of nitrous oxide.[33–35] The interval between surgery and the onset of neurologic symptoms ranged from 17 days to 6 weeks.

It is difficult to know whether this association was more than coincidental. In anesthesia patients exposed to nitrous oxide in concentrations of 50% to 70%, the activity of the vitamin B_{12}–dependent enzyme methionine synthase in liver falls by 50% in 1 to 2 hours.[36] Because inactivation of vitamin B_{12} by nitrous oxide occurs so quickly, it is reasonable to suppose that patients already deficient in vitamin B_{12} may be at increased risk of neurologic toxicity from even a single exposure to nitrous oxide. Low-normal serum B_{12} levels did not, however, exaggerate the postoperative increase of formiminoglutamic acid excretion (a sign of inactivation of methionine synthase) in surgical patients exposed to nitrous oxide for 5 to 16 hours.[37] Neurotoxicity from ordinary use of nitrous oxide during anesthesia must be extremely rare, if it occurs at all.[38]

Biochemical Mechanism of Nitrous Oxide Neurotoxicity

In mammals, including humans, only two vitamin B_{12}–dependent enzymes have been identified. One is the cytosolic enzyme methionine synthase, which uses methylcobalamin as a cofactor; the other is the mitochondrial enzyme methylmalonyl CoA mutase, which depends on deoxyadenosylcobalamin. As shown in Figure 3–1, methionine synthase converts homocysteine to methionine, which is the precursor of S-adenosylmethionine, an important methyl-group donor; it also generates tetrahydrofolate, a necessary precursor for the conversion of deoxyuridine to thymidine in the synthesis of DNA (Fig. 3–2). Methylmalonyl CoA mutase catalyzes the conversion of succinyl-CoA to methylmalonyl-CoA, which is involved in the synthesis of odd-chain and branched-chain fatty acids.

The generation of tetrahydrofolate by the action of methionine synthase links vitamin B_{12} to folic acid metabolism and accounts for the hemopoietic abnormalities common to folate deficiency and vitamin B_{12} deficiency. For many years, however, the biochemical pathogenesis of the neurologic disorders caused by vitamin B_{12} deficiency (but not by folate deficiency) remained hidden. It was not known whether the disorder was linked to one or both of the vitamin B_{12}–dependent enzymes. Research was hampered by the difficulty of inducing neurologic changes in laboratory animals by means of dietary vitamin B_{12} deficiency alone.[39] Then, just as the first human cases of nitrous oxide neurotoxicity were discovered, Dinn and associates[40, 41] reported that monkeys exposed to nitrous oxide for 10 weeks developed pathologically verified subacute combined degeneration of the spinal cord identical to that seen in human vitamin B_{12} deficiency.

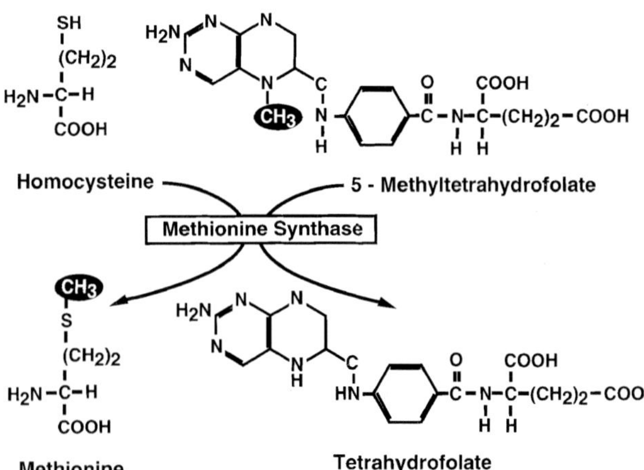

Figure 3–1. The methionine synthase reaction is a transmethylation step using methylcobalamin and S-adenosylmethionine as cofactors.

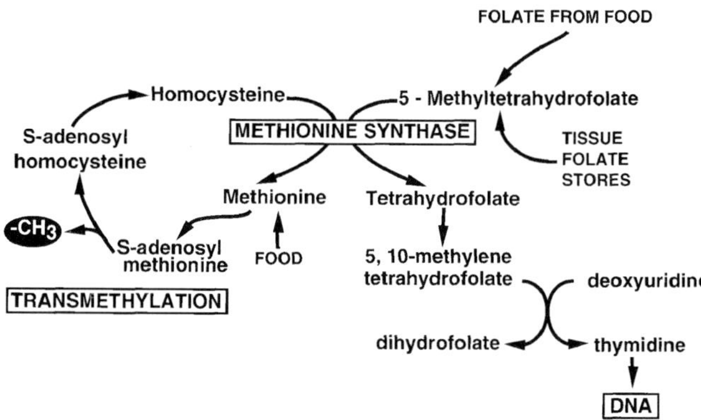

Figure 3–2. The products of the methionine synthase reaction are methionine, a precursor of S-adenosylmethionine, an important methyl-group donor; and tetrahydrofolate, necessary for the synthesis of DNA.

It was soon shown that nitrous oxide totally inactivates methionine synthase but has little effect on methylmalonyl CoA mutase. Furthermore, dietary supplementation with methionine largely prevented the neurotoxicity of nitrous oxide.[42] Subsequently, similar results were obtained in fruit bats[43] and in pigs.[44]

These experiments strongly support the concept that a diminution of methionine synthase activity is responsible for the neurologic abnormalities caused by vitamin B_{12} deficiency as well as by nitrous oxide. They also suggest that deficiency of methionine (or S-adenosylmethionine) may be crucial in causing neurologic damage. This idea gains support from the fact that cycloleucine, a methionine analog that inhibits the synthesis of S-adenosylmethionine, causes neuropathologic changes similar to subacute combined degeneration in mice.[45] The precise neuropathologic role of methionine deficiency is still a subject of speculation. Scott and colleagues[46, 47] have championed the view that impairment of transmethylation reactions in the nervous system, potentially affecting the methylation of proteins, lipids, and nucleic acids, may be the fundamental problem (Fig. 3–2). There is little direct confirmation of this hypothesis, however.

Treatment of Nitrous Oxide Neurotoxicity

As mentioned, administration of oral methionine dramatically prevents nitrous oxide neurotoxicity in monkeys[42] and in pigs.[47] Unfortunately, no experiments have been reported in which methionine was given to animals *after* neurologic symptoms appeared. In human cases, methionine has rarely been given,[31] and it is difficult to know whether such treatment has any effect on the rate of recovery. Even so, it would be prudent to give methionine supplements to any patient affected by nitrous oxide toxicity. Scott and colleagues[42] gave monkeys 2 g of DL-methionine daily, equivalent to one gram of L-methionine. For patients, a dose of 2 g of L-methionine a day for 10 days seems reasonable.

Health food stores stock L-methionine in 500-mg capsules.

Some patients with nitrous oxide neurotoxicity have been treated with vitamin B_{12}, but again, it is difficult to know whether the treatment had any effect. Stacy and associates[31] observed continued neurologic deterioration in two patients treated with vitamin B_{12}. Unusually, both patients had low serum B_{12} levels and overt megaloblastic anemia, which responded promptly to B_{12} therapy even as their neurologic status declined. (A Schilling test showed normal vitamin B_{12} absorption in the one case in which it was performed.) Fruit bats, unlike pigs and monkeys, develop low serum vitamin B_{12} levels under conditions of simultaneous dietary B_{12} deficiency and prolonged exposure to nitrous oxide. Bats given vitamin B_{12} supplements do not develop either low serum B_{12} levels or neurotoxicity from nitrous oxide.[43] Considering the ambiguous nature of this information, it seems reasonable to give both vitamin B_{12} and methionine supplements to patients affected by nitrous oxide neurotoxicity.

Summary

1. Abuse of nitrous oxide is uncommon compared with other kinds of substance abuse, occurring most often in dentists and oral surgeons, who have ready access to nitrous oxide.
2. Neurologic toxicity is a predictable consequence of prolonged nitrous oxide abuse and may also result from heavy occupational exposure to the gas.
3. The neurotoxicity of nitrous oxide is attributable to inactivation of the vitamin B_{12}–dependent enzyme methionine synthase and is clinically identical to the neurologic disorder associated with vitamin B_{12} deficiency.
4. After cessation of nitrous oxide exposure, most patients improve but permanent neurologic sequelae are common.
5. Treatment with methionine and vitamin B_{12} is indicated, but the efficacy of treatment has not been demonstrated.

References

1. Brodsky JB: Toxicity of nitrous oxide. *In* Eger EI (ed): Nitrous Oxide/N_2O. New York, Elsevier, 1985, pp 259–279.
2. Frost EAM: A history of nitrous oxide. *In* Eger EI (ed): Nitrous Oxide/N_2O. New York, Elsevier, 1985, pp 1–22.
3. Layzer RB: Nitrous oxide abuse. *In* Eger EI (ed): Nitrous Oxide/N_2O. New York, Elsevier, 1985, pp 249–257.
4. Smith RA, Beirne OR: The use of nitrous oxide by dentists. *In* Eger EI (ed): Nitrous Oxide/N_2O. New York, Elsevier, 1985, pp 281–304.
5. Malamed SF, Orr DL II, Hershfield S, et al: The recreational abuse of nitrous oxide by health professionals. Calif Dent Assoc J 1980;8:38–42.
6. Gillman MA: Nitrous oxide abuse in perspective. Clin Neuropharmacol 1992;15:297–306.
7. Clarke JH, Chiodo GT, Cowan FF: Chemical dependency among dentists: Prevalence and current treatment. Gen Dentistry 1988;36:227–229.
8. Rosenberg M: Drug abuse in oral and maxillofacial training programs. J Oral Maxillofac Surg 1986;44:458–462.
9. Ward CF, Ward GC, Saidman LJ: Drug abuse in anesthesia training programs. A survey: 1970 through 1980. JAMA 1983;250:922–925.
10. Talbot GD, Gallegos KV, Wilson PO, et al: The medical association of Georgia's impaired physician program. JAMA 1987; 257:2927–2930.
11. Rosenberg H, Orkin FK, Springstead J: Abuse of nitrous oxide. Anesth Analg 1979;58:104–106.
12. National Household Survey on Drug Abuse: Main Findings, 1991. (DHHS Publication No. [SMA] 93-1980.) Rockville, MD, Substance Abuse and Mental Health Services Administration, Office of Applied Studies, 1993.
13. Finck AD: Nitrous oxide analgesia. *In* Eger EI (ed): Nitrous Oxide/N_2O. New York, Elsevier, 1985, pp 41–55.
14. Sundin RH, Adriani J, Alam S, et al: Anxiolytic effects of low dosage nitrous oxide-oxygen mixtures administered continuously in apprehensive subjects. South Med J 1981;74:1489–1492.
15. Davy H: Researches, Chemical and Philosophical; Chiefly Concerning Nitrous Oxide, or Dephlogisticated Air, and Its Respiration. London, J Johnson, 1800.
16. Dohrn CS, Lichtor JL, Coalson DW, et al: Reinforcing effects of extended inhalation of nitrous oxide in humans. Drug Alcohol Depend 1993;31:265–280.
17. Yajnik S, Thapar P, Lichtor JL, et al: Effects of marijuana history on the subjective, psychomotor, and reinforcing effects of nitrous oxide in humans. Drug Alcohol Depend 1994;36:227–236.
18. Lassen HCA, Henriksen E, Neukirch F, et al: Treatment of tetanus: Severe bone-marrow depression after prolonged nitrous-oxide anaesthesia. Lancet 1956;1:527–530.
19. Amess JAL, Rees DM, Burman JF, et al: Megaloblastic haemopoiesis in patients receiving nitrous oxide. Lancet 1978;2:339–342.
20. Layzer RB, Fishman RA, Schafer JA: Neuropathy following abuse of nitrous oxide. Neurology (NY) 1978;28:504–506.
21. Sahenk Z, Mendell JR, Couri D, et al: Polyneuropathy from inhalation of N_2O cartridges through a whipped cream dispenser. Neurology (NY) 1978;28:485–487.
22. Layzer RB: Myeloneuropathy after prolonged exposure to nitrous oxide. Lancet 1978;2:1227–1230.
23. Gutmann L, Ferrell B, Crosby TW, et al: Nitrous oxide–induced myelopathy-neuropathy: Potential for chronic misuse by dentists. J Am Dent Assoc 1979;98:58–59.
24. Paulson GW: "Recreational" misuse of nitrous oxide. J Am Dent Assoc 1979;98:410–411.
25. Nevins MA: Neuropathy after nitrous oxide abuse. JAMA 1980;244:2264.
26. Gutmann L, Johnsen D: Nitrous oxide-induced myeloneuropathy: report of cases. J Am Dent Assoc 1981;103:239–241.
27. Blanco G, Peters HA: Myeloneuropathy and macrocytosis associated with nitrous oxide abuse. Arch Neurol 1983;40:416–418.
28. Sterman AB, Coyle PK: Subacute toxic delirium following nitrous oxide abuse. Arch Neurol 1983;40:446–447.
29. Heyer EJ, Simpson DM, Bodis-Wollner, I, et al: Nitrous oxide: Clinical and electrophysiologic investigation of neurologic complications. Neurology (NY) 1986;36:1618–1622.
30. Vishnubhakat SM, Beresford HR: Reversible myeloneuropathy of nitrous oxide abuse: Serial electrophysiological studies. Muscle Nerve 1991;14:22–26.
31. Stacy CB, Di Rocco A, Gould RJ: Methionine in the treatment of nitrous-oxide-induced neuropathy and myeloneuropathy. J Neurol 1992;239:401–403.
32. Brodsky JB, Cohen EN, Brown BW Jr, et al: Exposure to nitrous oxide and neurologic disease among dental professionals. Anesth Analg 1981;60:297–301.
33. Schilling RF: Is nitrous oxide a dangerous anesthetic for vitamin B_{12}–deficient subjects? JAMA 1986;255:1605–1606.
34. Holloway KL, Alberico AM: Postoperative myeloneuropathy: A preventable complication in patients with B_{12} deficiency. J Neurosurg 1990;72:732–736.
35. Flippo TS, Holder WD Jr: Neurologic degeneration associated with nitrous oxide anesthesia in patients with vitamin B_{12} deficiency. Arch Surg 1993;128:1391–1395.
36. Koblin DD, Waskell L, Watson JE, et al: Nitrous oxide inactivates methionine synthetase in human liver. Anesth Analg 1982;61:75–78.
37. Koblin DD, Tomerson BW, Waldman FM, et al: Effect of nitrous oxide on vitamin B_{12} metabolism in patients. Anesth Analg 1990;71:610–617.

38. Nunn JF, Chanarin I: Nitrous oxide inactivates methionine synthetase. *In* Eger EI (ed): Nitrous Oxide/N_2O. New York, Elsevier, 1985, pp 211–233.
39. Agamanolis DP, Chester EM, Victor M, et al: Neuropathology of experimental vitamin B_{12} deficiency in monkeys. Neurology (NY) 1976;26:905–914.
40. Dinn JJ, McCann S, Wilson P, et al: Animal model for subacute combined degeneration. Lancet 1978;2:1154.
41. Dinn JJ, Weir DG, McCann S, et al: Methyl group deficiency in nerve tissue: A hypothesis to explain the lesion of subacute combined degeneration. Ir J Med Sci 1980;149:1–4.
42. Scott JM, Dinn JJ, Wilson P, et al: Pathogenesis of subacute combined degeneration: a result of methyl group deficiency. Lancet 1981;2:334–337.
43. Duffield MS, Phillips JI, Veira-Makings E, et al: Demyelinisation in the spinal cord of vitamin B_{12} deficient fruit bats. Comp Biochem Physiol 1990;96C:291–297.
44. Weir DG, Keating S, Molloy A, et al: Methylation deficiency causes vitamin B_{12}-associated neuropathy in the pig. J Neurochem 1988;51:1949–1952.
45. Jacobson W, Gandy G, Sidman RL: Inhibition of transmethylation reaction in the central nervous system—an experimental model for subacute combined degeneration of the cord. J Physiol 1973;233:1–3.
46. Scott JM, Molloy AM, Kennedy DG, et al: Effects of the disruption of transmethylation in the central nervous system: An animal model. Acta Neurol Scand Suppl 1994;154:27–31.
47. McKeever M, Molloy A, Weir DG, et al: An abnormal methylation ratio induces hypomethylation in vitro in the brain of pig and man, but not in rat. Clin Sci 1995;88:73–79.

Chapter 4
COMPLICATIONS ASSOCIATED WITH WOUND HEALING

by

Charles N. Bertolami
Diana V. Messadi

Introduction

Tissue repair ordinarily occurs without intruding into the consciousness of the surgeon. Normal wound repair is the rule, not the exception. It is not surprising, therefore, that over many decades, little has been achieved in wound healing research that has led directly and unequivocally to improvements in either the quality or character of healing.

The few conditions uniquely associated with wound healing and leading to undesired results are: (1) wound contraction, (2) excessive repair (hypertrophic scarring, keloid formation), (3) deficient repair (wound breakdown, ulceration), and (4) wound infection.

In this chapter, a brief survey of normal wound healing and formation of the mature fibrous scar is presented. Derangements in wound healing are considered in detail, and various treatment options are presented. Advances in current research are discussed, even though many treatments remain purely theoretical at this point.

The Subjects Discussed in This Chapter Are:

- Normal soft tissue wound repair
  - Background
  - Early wound healing (inflammatory) phase
  - Remodeling phase
  - Late phase
- Wound contraction
- Hypertrophic scarring and keloid formation
- Deficient healing
- Factors affecting wound repair
  - Wound infection
  - Hypoxia
  - Radiation
  - Age
  - Drug therapy
  - Nutrition
- Growth factors and their role in wound healing

Normal Soft Tissue Wound Repair

Background

Wound healing, tissue repair, and *regeneration* are common, interchangeably used terms in clinical surgery. Wound biologists, however, ascribe a specific meaning to each term and draw clear distinctions between repair and regeneration.

A *wound* is defined as any anatomic or functional interruption in the continuity of a tissue that is accompanied by cellular damage and death. The causative agent may be physical, chemical, or biologic. Every such injury initiates a coordinated series of processes directed toward restoring injured tissues to their original condition. This process of tissue restitution constitutes healing.[1] Complete return to the preinjury state is not always possible.

The various stages constituting the healing process are parts of a continuum and are not readily separated from one another. These indistinct and overlapping events are generally schematized into the following phases: inflammatory, granulation (proliferative), and matrix remodeling.[2] Inasmuch as excellent reviews of soft tissue healing have been published,[3–6] the subject is considered only briefly here.

Wound healing encompasses two distinct categories of tissue restoration, regeneration and repair. These are radically different events, although they may take place concurrently. *Regeneration* yields a healed tissue that is structurally and functionally indistinguishable from the original. In contrast, the *repair* process achieves structural integrity through generation of a fibrous connective tissue scar. Scar tissue does not resemble the original preinjury tissue, structurally or functionally. Whether a tissue possesses the capacity to heal by regeneration or repair is genetically determined. Amphibians, for example, regenerate skin, bone, muscle, and nerve, allowing complete restitution of an amputated limb throughout life.

In contrast, human tissues are segregated into those that are capable of true regeneration and those that are not. In the case of skin, the epidermal component regenerates, whereas the dermal component repairs by scarring. The capacity of bone and liver to regenerate in humans is well known. However, these tissues require appropriate and specific conditions for their full regenerative potential to be realized. The ability of nerve and muscle to regenerate in the postnatal state has been lost in humans. It is in the realm of repair, not regeneration, that complications intrinsic to wound healing generally arise.

Early Wound Healing (Inflammatory) Phase

Injury initiates the reparative response. Extravasation of blood into the wound site leads to clot formation and to generation of a temporary fibrin matrix. This matrix acts as a provisional scaffolding that promotes ingrowth of new cells. In a sense, *healing* can be understood simply as the progressive remodeling and revivification of the provisional matrix produced immediately after tissue injury. After 3 to 4 days, the presence of inflammatory cells, fibroblasts, and neovascular endothelium, along with the structural and chemotactic secretory products released by these cells, compose a distinct entity known as *granulation tissue.* Granulation tissue is a fibrovascular connective tissue initiated with the formation of the fibrin clot and ending with establishment of the healed scar.

The inflammatory phase is a leukocyte-mediated response to injury directed toward eliminating both pathogens and necrotic tissue. This phase begins with the initial injury, when disruption of blood vessels permits extravasation of blood that, in turn, provokes platelet aggregation and blood coagulation. Contemporaneous with the inflammatory phase is the process of *neovascularization.* Soft tissue healing cannot occur without the ingrowth of new blood vessels. Accordingly, angiogenesis is a key event that necessitates endothelial phenotype alteration, chemotaxis, and mitosis. It requires a suitable extracellular matrix along which neovascular endothelial elements can migrate.

Accompanying these events is *reepithelialization,* which begins when tissue injury induces a loss of contact-inhibitory restraints. When contact between adjacent epithelial cells is lost, the resulting free-edge effect induces epithelial cells to dedifferentiate and begin migrating. This behavior continues until opposing migrating epithelial sheets make contact and attach. Reepithelialization begins within 24 hours after injury. This is a distinguishable difference between regenerative and repair processes, because resurfacing the wound with epithelium is already in progress for several days before discernible granulation tissue is evident.[7] Thereafter, reepithelialization and granulation tissue formation proceed simultaneously.

Although reepithelialization is generally described as beginning at a wound's free edge and proceeding by centripetal movement across the wound bed,[8] this description is true, strictly speaking, only for full-thickness wounds. In the case of partial-thickness wounds, disrupted epithelium of adnexal structures (such as hair follicles) is subject to precisely the same free-edge effects and thus begins to proliferate and migrate whenever adnexal epithelium is disturbed by injury (Fig. 4–1). The practical clinical consequence is that reepithelialization proceeds not only from the edge but also from the innumerable follicles and other adnexal structures distributed within the wound site. Importantly, the stimulus for cellular movement is unknown; however, various biologic response modifiers, so-called cytokines, like epidermal growth factor (EGF) and fibroblast growth factors (FGFs), are known to be mitogenic for epidermal cells and to influence epidermal cell migration.[9, 10] Such mediators may be involved in signaling the onset of epithelial cell division and movement.

From a purely clinical standpoint, the deepest portions of the organizing blood clot are efficiently remodeled into viable tissue. However, moisture loss through evaporation at the clot surface desiccates the superficial

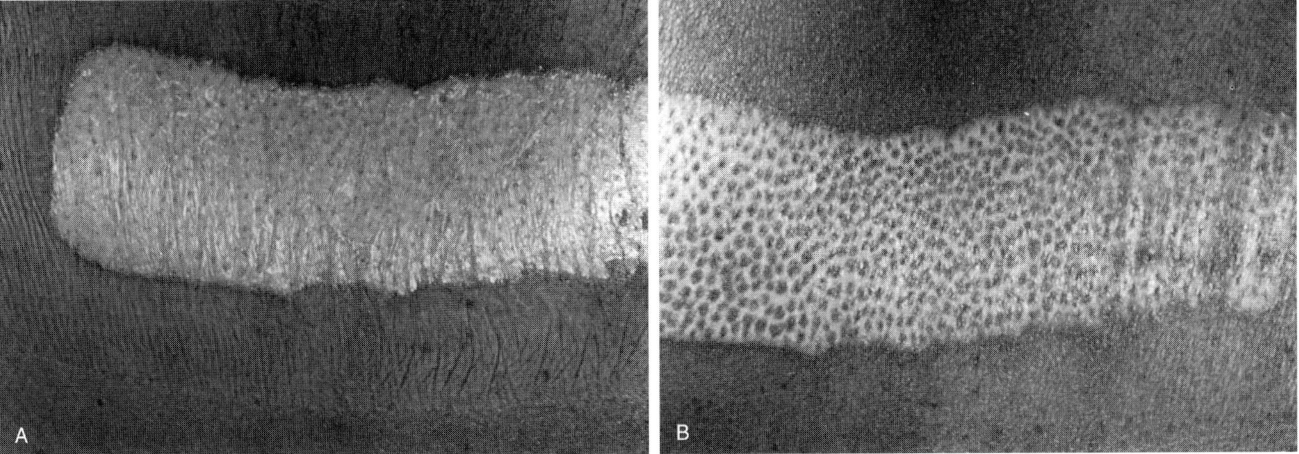

Figure 4–1. *A,* Split-thickness skin graft donor site at 10 days. *B,* Same donor site at 14 days. The darkly pigmented epithelial cells can be seen to migrate not only from the wound periphery, but also from adnexal elements scattered within the wound site. (Courtesy of Dr. Larry J. Peterson).

coagulum and impedes ingress of cells, vessels, and other viable elements. This causes the superficial portion of the clot to form a natural biologic dressing, the scab. Because dried clot is not conducive to cellular migration, epithelial cells migrate deep to the scab, insinuating themselves at the interface between viable (organizing) and nonviable clot. Therefore, as reepithelialization nears completion, the superficial desiccated clot detaches, revealing a wound site that has been newly resurfaced with epithelium.

Remodeling Phase

The process by which fibrin matrix is transformed into living tissue involves more than simple ingrowth of cells, vessels, and matrix. It also requires matrix *remodeling,* defined as a subtle but continuous disequilibrium between matrix production and breakdown. The remodeling process induces, incrementally and over time, gradual shifts in the cellular and molecular content of wound granulation tissue. In the case of healing by repair, remodeling continues until the dense collagen architecture of end-stage repair is attained. The various transitions a healing wound undergoes as repair proceeds are inevitably accompanied by the production and breakdown of large quantities of matrix, including constituents such as glycosaminoglycans, proteoglycans, fibronectin, and collagen.[6]

In the case of fibrous connective tissue repair, wound remodeling plays a key role. It is a failure of remodeling to generate a tissue architecture identical to that of the original, preinjury state that accounts for the inability of certain tissues to heal by regeneration. Nevertheless, the remodeling process continues long after the wound has apparently healed, continually altering the character and quality of the newly healed tissue. Remodeling of connective tissue matrix takes place during all phases of wound healing. It begins with the initial formation of granulation tissue and continues through development of the definitive scar. Remodeling reflects a wound's dynamic state of flux and the evolving mix of different matrix components required to meet functional demands at various points during healing. Details of the remodeling process for fibrous connective tissues have been described in depth elsewhere.[1]

Late Phase

In the case of normal healing, scar formation ordinarily represents the endpoint of connective tissue repair. In any consideration of complications secondary to wound healing, however, it must be recognized that undesirable outcomes do not result exclusively from abnormal repair. It is the simple incompetency of certain human tissues to regenerate that leads to disappointment and dissatisfaction when healing is complete. Thus, devastating injuries of the sort shown in Figure 4–2 are not solely the product of abnormal healing. Scar formation and wound contraction are not abnormalities. They are physical manifestations of the inability of connective tissue repair to perfectly recapitulate the ontogenetic events of early embryogenesis. The rate at which the scar endpoint is reached depends on how the economy of the wound site is managed with respect to matrix production and breakdown. Early on, anabolism predominates, and production of collagen and other matrix constituents exceeds catabolism. As healing progresses, overlying epithelium stratifies, and underlying connective tissue shows positivity for a variety of degradative enzymes, including metalloproteinases such as collagenase and various glycosidases. Over time, matrix catabolism permits connective tissue to remodel to form a thin, dense, white scar. In the event of a disequilibrium between synthesis and breakdown, abnormal healing may occur. Examples are considered subsequently, including both excesses in anabolism (or deficiencies in catabolism) leading to hypertrophic scarring and keloid formation and excesses in catabolism (or deficient anabolism) leading to

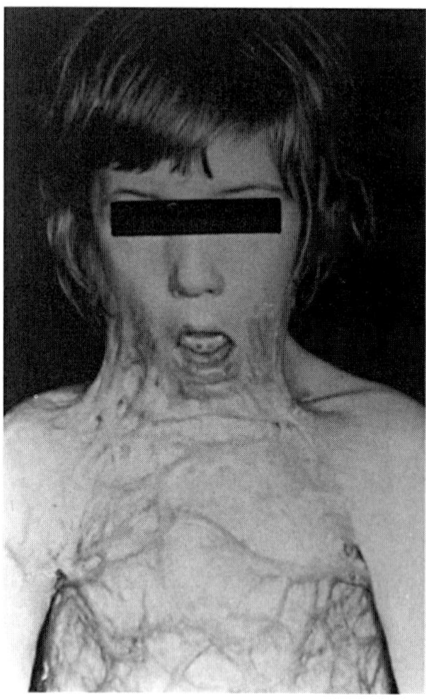
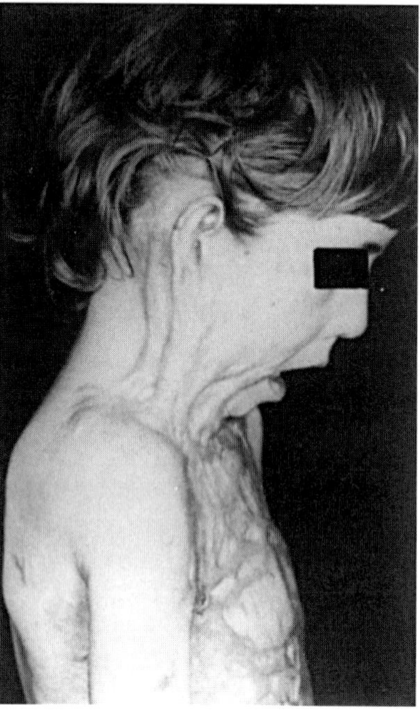

Figure 4–2. Dramatic scar formation and wound contraction subsequent to full-thickness skin loss of anterior chest, leading to anterior flexion deformity of the neck and distortion of facial features. (*From* Peacock EE, Van Winkle W: Surgery and Biology of Wound Repair. Philadelphia, WB Saunders, 1970, pp 171–251.)

deficient healing expressed as ulceration and tissue breakdown.

Wound Contraction

Wound contraction may be the single greatest factor in achieving closure of soft tissue wound defects, depending on the site and nature of the tissues injured. The character of the wound base and the mobility of the peripheral tissues are especially important variables.

Contraction is defined as a decrease in a wound's area by the drawing together of the margins, independent of the phenomenon of reepithelialization. In the absence of direct surgical intervention, contraction and reepithelialization are the two natural processes that account for complete wound closure, the former contributing substantially more in most cases than the latter.

Purely from the standpoint of survival, there is distinct evolutionary advantage to achieving wound closure as rapidly as possible, especially in a primitive, nontechnologic setting. When modern surgical management is available, however, the benefits of rapid wound closure are obviated by the invariable anatomic distortions produced by contractile forces. Such distortions are, to varying degrees, accompanied by functional loss.[11] This is most certainly the case in the oral and maxillofacial region, where wound contraction of the face, perioral, nasal, and periorbital regions generates significant compromise in the natural functions of these tissues. Even from a strictly oral perspective, contractile distortions subsequent to avulsive or burn injury may be associated with significant impairment of mastication, respiration, deglutition, and speech.

A classic scenario develops after a child has sustained an electrical burn of the oral commissures. The burn may be minor; however, subsequent wound contraction produces major distortion of the oral orifice and significant compromise in function. Similarly, burns (either chemical or thermal) as well as excision of pathologic lesions of the buccal mucosa, floor of the mouth, or base of the tongue may lead to major impairment as vigorous contraction ensues. The contractile process in loosely adherent oral mucosa is so active that a very small linear scar may result from a surprisingly large excisional or avulsive injury. Of course, this situation occurs only with significant wound contraction, generation of high tensile forces, and tissue distortion.

Clinical efforts at limiting contraction have often focused on physical methods such as splinting and application of skin grafts.[12–15] Burn, avulsive, and excisional injuries are frequently of such magnitude, however, that the amount of autogenous tissue available for reconstruction through free skin grafting may be insufficient.

Research efforts therefore have been directed at developing biocompatible nonautogenic substitutes for full-thickness grafts.[16–20] In general, such substitutes are bilaminar membranes composed of dermal and epidermal components. The intent is that such graft matrices are repopulated in the wound bed by the patient's own cells—both fibroblasts and epidermal cells. The system would produce a permanent skin or mucosal replacement composed of a functioning dermis/epidermis or mucosa/submucosa. Although such materials have now been shown to achieve relative success under specified experimental conditions (engendering as much as a 70% inhibition in contraction) (Figs. 4–3, 4–4, 4–5), they are not widely used. The reason may be related to the inconsistency of the results obtained.[21, 22]

Thus, the difficulties in preventing wound contraction do not have simple solutions. Physical splinting of wounds for protracted periods, perhaps as long as a

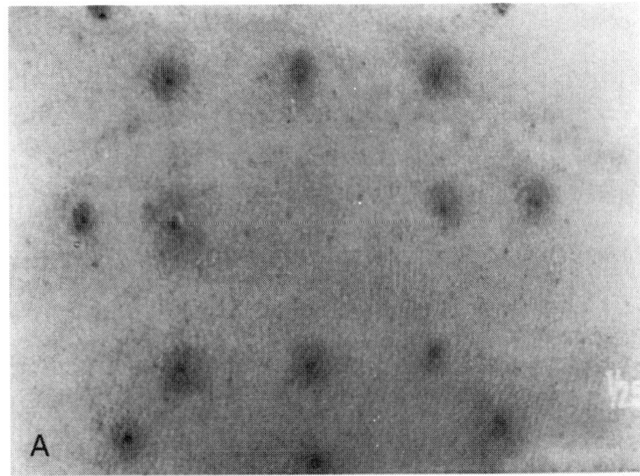

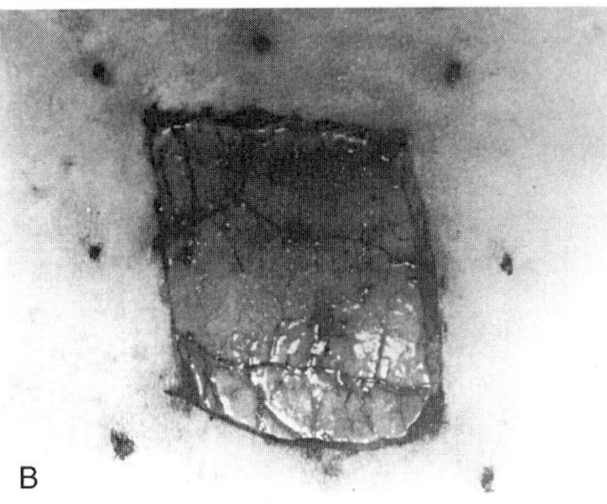

Figure 4–3. Experimental wound in animal for the purpose of studying the effect of grafting (using an artificial skin substitute) on wound contraction. *A,* Prior to excision, graft and control sites are tattooed with India ink at the four corners and at the midpoints between corners so that a 3.0 × 3.0-cm area is demarcated. In addition, an outer set of tattoos is placed 1 cm beyond the inner set. *B,* Full-thickness excision of skin is made to the level of the panniculus carnosus muscle layer by sharp dissection using the inner India ink tattoos as markers to ensure reproducible wound margins. (*From* Bertolami CN, Shetty V, Milavec JE, et al: Preparation and evaluation of a nonproprietary bilayer skin substitute. Plast Reconstr Surg 1991;87:1089–1098.)

year, may be successful. The practical difficulties of achieving splinting either in skin or mucosa for such periods, however, make these methods difficult to implement. In the case of burn injury, various elastic bandages have been devised both to impede contraction and to control hypertrophic scarring and keloid formation (discussed subsequently), but again, such approaches remain suboptimal.

There is no completely satisfactory approach to inhibiting wound contraction beyond very basic surgical principles. Perhaps the most important among these is to attain primary closure of cutaneous and mucosal wounds in the absence of actual tissue loss. The most common problem that may lead to a highly deforming contractile injury occurs in the setting of a large, gaping wound resulting from blunt trauma without any actual loss of tissue. Failure to recognize the absence of tissue loss may lead the clinician to conclude, erroneously, that healing must take place by secondary intention (Fig. 4–6). Thus, assiduous efforts at approximating tissue margins is not attempted. In fact, the highly irregular margins of the wound can be pieced together much like a large jigsaw puzzle. Recognizing the absence of tissue loss and proceeding with a very meticulous reassembly of injured tissues are the best means of preventing significant wound contraction.

When true avulsion or a large excisional wound is present, full-thickness skin grafting, splinting when possible, and carefully designed surgical closure strategies remain the only alternatives to minimize contraction.

Hypertrophic Scarring and Keloid Formation

Hypertrophic scarring and keloid formation represent serious derangements in orofacial healing that are defined by an abnormal accumulation of extracellular matrix (Figs. 4–2 and 4–7).[23] Such disturbances have been described as benign tumors arising in the reticular dermis in response to trauma. The wound healing process is arrested in the proliferative phase, resulting in massive tissue accumulation.[24, 25]

In the formation and remodeling of normal cutaneous scar, matrix production and degradation ordinarily balance each other; in hypertrophic scars and keloids, a disequilibrium between production and catabolism leads to matrix accumulation.[26–28] The cause of this disequilibrium is not known; however, the tendency to aberrant scar formation occurs with high frequency in African-American populations, in whom it is inherited as an autosomal dominant disorder with variable expression and incomplete penetrance.[29]

In comparison with caucasians, African-Americans experience up to a 15-fold higher incidence of postinjury keloid formation.[30] The occurrence of keloids in predominantly African-American and Hispanic populations is estimated at 4.5% to 16%,[31] and up to 16% in random samplings of black Africans.[32] Furthermore, keloids are five times more common in people of Japanese descent and three times more common in individuals of Chinese descent than among whites.

Hospital data suggest a preponderance of keloids and hypertrophic scars of the face.[33] However, this finding may be due to the fact that facial keloids are exposed and disfiguring, leading patients to seek surgical correction more often than when lesions are either hidden or have fewer functional consequences. The mandibular angle region is known to exhibit special predilection for keloid formation.[33] This tendency is of particular concern because fractures in this area are common, and open repair via an extraoral incision may be necessary. The long-term consequences of serious scar derangements in susceptible populations should not be overlooked or minimized when treatment decisions are made.

In numerous studies of hypertrophic scars and keloids, collagen accumulation has been an appropriate focus of inquiry. Significant derangements in other matrix components are also observed yet receive much less attention. For instance, glycosaminoglycan content

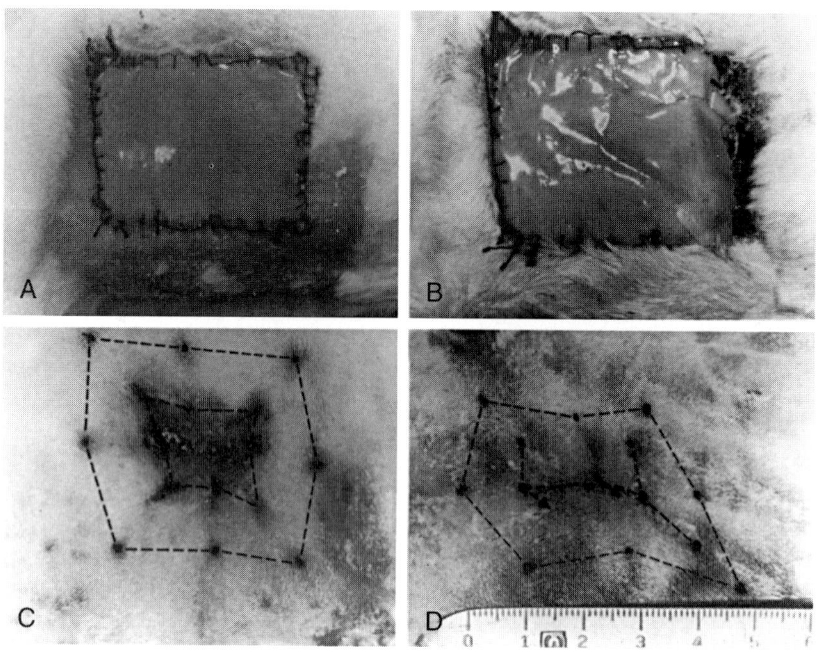

Figure 4–4. With the use of a bilayer artificial skin substitute, grafted cutaneous wounds are significantly inhibited in their rate and extent of wound contraction compared with ungrafted control wounds. As reepithelialization proceeds, the outer layer of the graft exfoliates, revealing altered scar formation. *A,* Appearance of bilayer graft at 14 days. Outer (Silastic) layer is still in place (original magnification ×1). *B,* By 21 days, Silastic has begun exfoliating along the periphery (original magnification ×1.2). *C,* Graft site at 56 days. Wound has completely reepithelialized. A set of dashed lines connecting the inner tattoos and another set connecting the outer tattoos make evident the extent of contraction retardation (original magnification ×1.7). *D,* Control wound on day 49. In contrast to grafted wound *(C),* control (ungrafted) wound has fully contracted. A set of dashed lines connecting the inner tattoos and another set connecting the outer tattoos demonstrate the full extent of contraction of the wound proper (inner lines) and the distorting effect of tensile forces produced in the skin by the contractile process 1 cm from the wound site (outer lines) (original magnification ×1.7). (*From* Bertolami CN, Shetty V, Milavec JE, et al: Preparation and evaluation of a nonproprietary bilayer skin substitute. Plast Reconstr Surg 1991;87:1089–1098.)

is altered both quantitatively and qualitatively in aberrant scars.[34] Hypertrophic scar tissue contains more sulfated glycosaminoglycans and more hyaluronan (both in absolute amount and as a percentage of total glycosaminoglycan) than either normal skin or normal scar.[35] Given their regulatory effects in developmental and reparative systems, glycosaminoglycans (hyaluronan in particular) are believed to participate in tissue fibrosis, matrix accumulation, remodeling, and scar persistence, and to do so to an extent disproportionate with the absolute magnitude of the derangement in glycosaminoglycan composition.[36–38]

Many efforts have been made to distinguish hypertrophic scars from keloids; however, few, if any, definitive criteria exist to distinguish between the two phenomena. This is not surprising, inasmuch as the

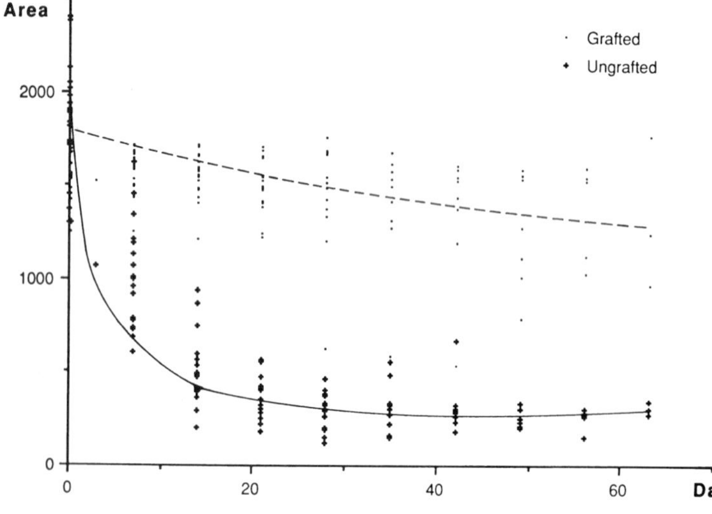

Figure 4–5. Comparison of wound contraction for experimental full-thickness skin donor sites in rabbits. The curves compare the effects of grafting with a bilayer skin substitute. Wound area (expressed in pixels) is shown as a function of postwound time (in days) and graft status (grafted versus ungrafted). (*From* Bertolami CN, Shetty V, Milavec JE, et al: Preparation and evaluation of a nonproprietary bilayer skin substitute. Plast Reconstr Surg 1991;87:1089–1098.)

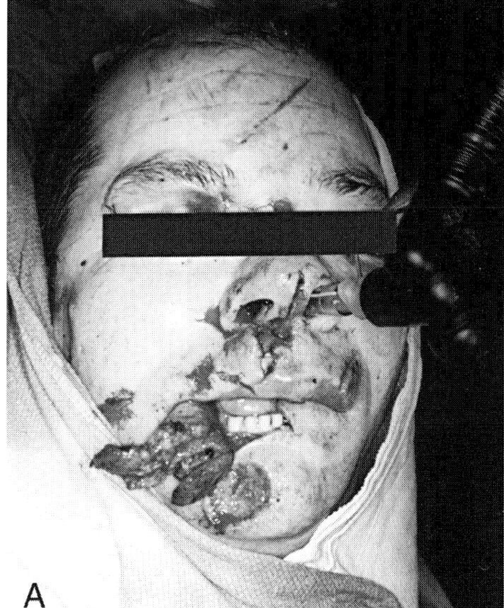

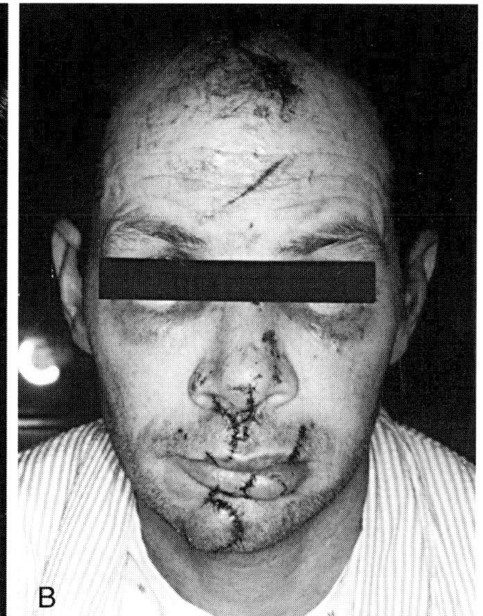

Figure 4–6. *A,* Motor vehicle accident has caused blunt trauma and significant tissue disruption. Although actual tissue avulsion might be suspected, meticulous closure of the wound site reveals that all tissue is physically present. *B,* Immediate postclosure result showing that there is no tissue loss.

histologic appearance of scars, whether normal or abnormal, is not nearly as great as clinical expression would suggest (Figs. 4–7 and 4–8). Keloids seem to differ from hypertrophic scars only in the relative amount of matrix produced. Scars showing the largest deposits of tissue are called *keloids,* whereas those that are larger than originally anticipated are termed *hypertrophic.* Peacock and Van Winkle[23] have advanced the view that scars that show moderate hypertrophic tendencies and then either regress or remain stable should be classified as hypertrophic; in contrast, deposits of collagen and other matrix constituents that continue to enlarge beyond the original size and shape of the wound are to be considered keloidal. From a purely clinical standpoint, the feature known as *overflow* may be useful. This term refers to the tendency of some scars to produce new collagen so rapidly that the resulting scar is pedunculated. Under such circumstances, the scar mass is many times the size of the scar base. Pedunculated scars are more likely to be identified clinically as keloids.

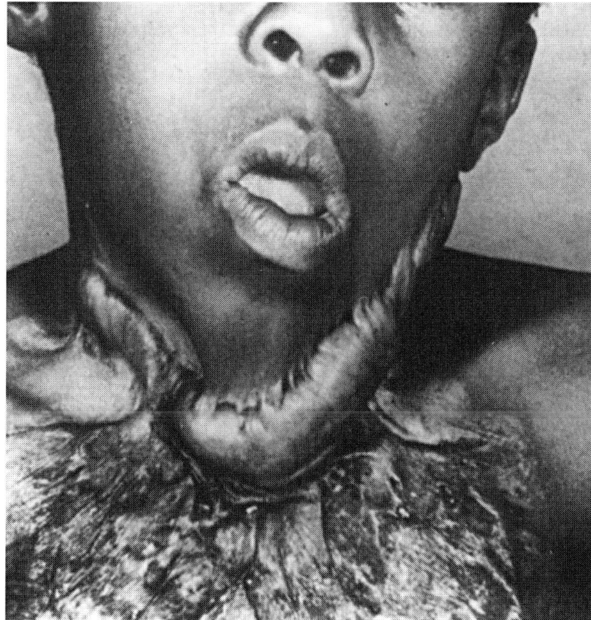

Figure 4–7. Combination of hypertrophic scar, wound contraction, and keloid formation resulting from thermal burn of the anterior neck and chest. (*From* Kischer CW, Shetlar MR, Chvapil M: Hypertrophic scars and keloids: A review and a new concept concerning their origin. Scanning Electr Microsc 1982;4:1699–1713.)

Surprisingly, for more than two decades, efforts at discriminating among abnormal scars (hypertrophic versus keloid) on the basis of biochemical, histologic, and molecular criteria have been unsuccessful. Except for the absolute amount of matrix present, clear differences in cell size, matrix solubility, and matrix architecture have not been demonstrated. When objective measures of the clinical properties of scar tissue are made by elastometry in vivo,[39] the essence of the problem is well seen (Fig. 4–9). Abnormal scars arrange themselves along a continuum from mildly abnormal to severely abnormal without clear distinctions. Scars in the extreme of the plot evince the best, perhaps archetypal, manifestation of abnormality; otherwise, the shades of transition between severe and mild derangement are subtle, continuous, and not readily recognized. Even the distinction between an overtly abnormal scar and a scar that is identified clinically as being normal is not always easy. Evidence has been advanced suggesting that molecular markers for normal versus abnormal scars may exist (Fig. 4–10).[40] These distinctions, although promising, cannot be interpreted as definitive at this time.

Abnormal scarring, when it occurs, may necessitate some form of treatment, provided that an improvement can be obtained. Many treatments have been proposed over the years, including ionizing radiation before and after surgical excision of scars, complete excision fol-

A. NORMAL SKIN

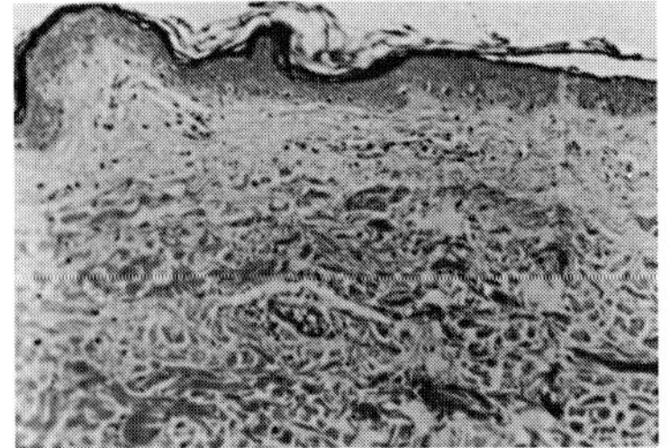

B. NORMAL SCAR

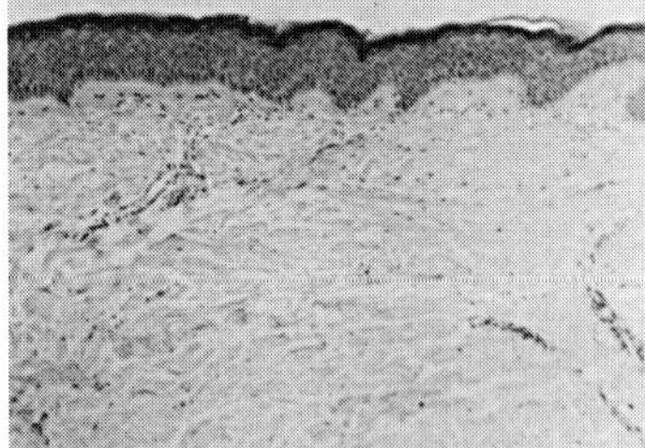

C. HYPERTROPHIC SCAR

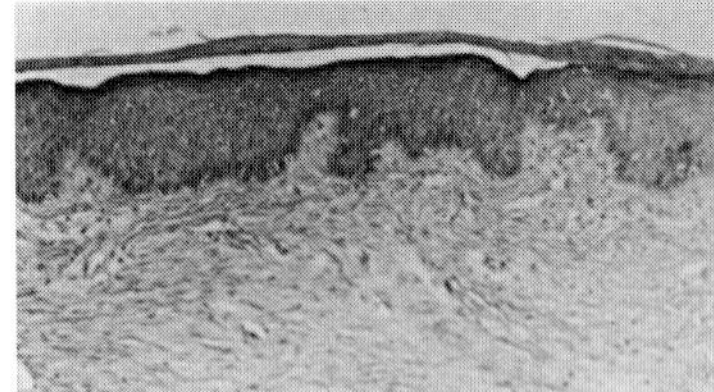

D. KELOID

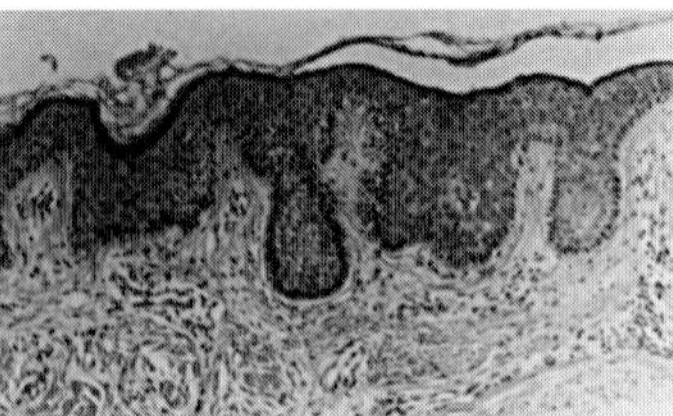

Figure 4–8. Histologic appearance of normal skin *(A)*, normal cutaneous scar *(B)*, hypertrophic scar *(C)*, and keloid *(D)*. Normal skin possesses a characteristic dermal architecture that is not adequately duplicated during the healing process. Fibrous connective tissue scar takes the form of dense bundles of collagen, readily visualized in these sections stained with hematoxylin and eosin. Despite the dramatic clinical appearance of hypertrophic scars and keloids, their histologic appearance is not easily distinguished from that of more normal scars (×100).

lowed by skin grafting, and partial excision with administration of steroids. Though each has been reported as successful at one time or another, none can be viewed as unequivocally effective. Certain manipulations that work in some patients at a given time may not be effective in the same or other patients at other times,[23] suggesting that the cause and character of hypertrophic scars and keloids are ambiguous or variable. Because severe hypertrophic scars and keloids do not consistently occur in either domestic or laboratory animals, research in the area has been limited to observations in human subjects. The data arising from such studies have necessarily been scattered, inconsistent, and, on the whole, inadequate. Even the matter of suitable controls is not easily addressed in the design of studies intended to develop therapies for hypertrophic scars and keloids.

Although basic science has not yielded clear approaches to preventing and treating hypertrophic scars and keloids, years of clinical observations by competent practitioners have pointed to certain principles that seem to help in minimizing and managing such disorders. One appears to be the relief of soft tissue tension at wound sites (including excisional sites). The release of wound tension by either grafting, undermining of soft tissue margins, or changing scar direction seems to help. Although the injection of corticosteroids makes sense from a purely theoretic standpoint and, correspondingly has been reported to be effective in many case reports, steroid injection cannot be viewed as a complete answer. Such injections are thought to soften scars and to decrease size, especially when accompanied by manual massage. Few adequately controlled studies unequivocally demonstrate a complete or partial resolution or a return to normal appearance and function after steroid injections.

Despite disappointment in the failure of basic science to provide clear direction for the future in relation to

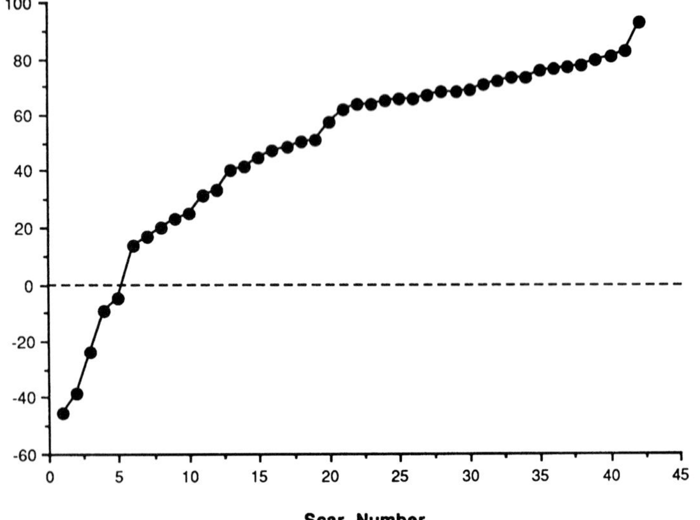

Figure 4–9. Plot of elastometric properties arranged in increasing order of elastometric index (EI) using the methodology of Bartell et al.[39] *EI*, shown along the *y* axis, offers a noninvasive way of measuring the biomechanical properties of scar tissue in vivo. It is computed using the formula $EI = [(x - y)](100)/x$, where y is percentage stretch of scar tissue and x is percentage stretch of the normal, mirror-image skin. The higher the EI, the less elastic the scar in comparison with normal skin. Thus, a scar with an EI of 60 would be interpreted as being 60% less elastic than normal skin. Although *normal, abnormal,* and *hypertrophic* are in common usage, assigning a comprehensive computed score reflects the reality that individual scars position themselves along a continuum, with innumerable gradations and transitions between normal and abnormal. In this plot, although there is clustering at the higher EI values, the continuity of data points over the range −45 to +90 clearly indicates a continuum, with gradual transitions between overtly normal and overtly abnormal scars.

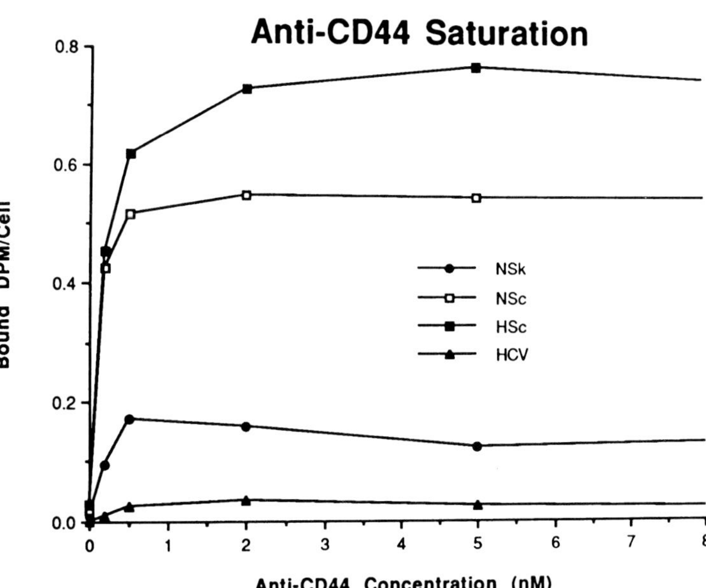

Figure 4–10. Human fibroblastic CD44 expression for cultures derived from normal skin *(NSk)*, normal scar *(NSc)*, and hypertrophic scar *(HSc)*. A negative control cell line derived from invasive human bladder cell carcinoma *(HCV)* is also shown. CD44 was revealed using mouse anti-CD44 IgG as a primary antibody and [^{35}S]-conjugated sheep anti-mouse antibody. Each data point represents the average of values from triplicate wells. Bound disintegrations per minute (DPM)/cell, shown along the *y* axis, reflects the amount of cell surface CD44. Fibroblasts derived from scar tissues are seen to be markedly higher in CD44 than those from normal skin. (*From* Messadi D, Bertolami CN: CD44 and hyaluronan expression in human cutaneous scar fibroblasts. Am J Pathol 1993;142:1041–1049.)

hypertrophic scarring and keloid formation, the tools available today to identify and, perhaps, alter genetic abnormalities at a systemic or local level are unprecedented.

Deficient Healing

When considering deficiency of healing, it is useful to categorize wounds into acute and chronic forms. Acute wounds heal in an orderly fashion and result in adequate repair, accompanied by both restoration of anatomic and functional integrity and by various degrees of scarring.

Chronic wounds, however, do not proceed through an orderly reparative process and fail to produce anatomic and functional integrity, leaving an underlying healing defect. Chronic wounds arise as a function of the character of the wound-healing process, host condition, and wound environment.[41] These wounds are considered models of deficient healing and are the product of predisposing conditions, including pressure (decubitus ulcers), diabetes mellitus, venous stasis, arterial insufficiency, vasculitis, and leprosy. Discussion is limited to diabetes-related wound healing problems because of their relevance to oral and maxillofacial surgeons.

Diabetes and Wound Healing

Diabetic patients are predisposed to a diversity of systemic disorders, including peripheral vascular disease, neuropathy, infection, and impaired healing.[42] Diabetic ulcers have always been defined in conjunction with the triad of neuropathy, ischemia, and infection. Vascular changes, such as impairment of blood flow, and neurologic abnormalities in diabetic patients are closely related. Infection plays a major role in the duration of such ulcers and is believed to be fostered by abnormalities in neutrophil function as a result of insulin deficiency.[43] The exact mechanism by which diabetes mellitus causes neuropathy and angiopathy remains unknown; however, several factors have been defined that contribute to a reduction in the healing potential of such patients after minor injuries. These factors are reduced hyperemic response to injury, a defect in the inflammatory response leading to impaired migration of neutrophils and macrophages, and abnormalities in the release and action of several growth factors and neuropeptides. The most common sites for deficient healing are the legs, either above or below the knee, and especially at places of repeated trauma such as toes, heel, and metatarsal heads on the plantar surface of the foot. In these regions, nonhealing diabetic ulcers are a wound healing challenge. The best treatment, of course, is prevention. The cause of an uncomplicated neuropathic ulcer in a diabetic patient is usually mechanical force. Accordingly, removing or moderating such forces can promote healing. The use of a total contact cast (TCC)—a below-the-knee plaster cast applied with minimal padding over bony prominences—can be an effective and safe way to treat such conditions. The therapy is altered in the presence of infection; however, antibiotic use in treating diabetic foot ulcers may not always be justified, because some diabetic patients with chronic wounds are at high risk for developing antimicrobial-resistant microorganisms. The best treatment for such infections, especially when osteomyelitis occurs, is prompt surgical débridement of all infected and necrotic tissues along with additional oral or intravenous antibiotics if necessary. Diabetic ulcers of the oral cavity are uncommon. If they occur, however, a similar strategy of treatment should be followed, i.e., relief of pressure, vigorous cleaning, and antibiotics.

Factors Affecting Wound Repair

A variety of factors contribute in subtle ways to the quality of healing; they are infection, hypoxia, radiation, age, drugs, nutrition, and various growth factors (cytokines).

Wound Infection

Bacterial infection is a major cause of impaired healing. Colonization of tissues already compromised by inflammation leads to further tissue damage. Clinically, tissue infection manifests as redness, heat, edema with tenderness, leukocytosis, fever, and pain. Bacteria and their toxins provoke the release of neutrophil proteases and O_2 radicals, causing cell lysis, destruction of the extracellular matrix, and impaired healing. Optimizing the wound environment for healing, together with maintaining hemodynamic stability, is necessary to prevent infection. Débridement of necrotic tissue, adequate postoperative care, nutrients, and vitamins are essential factors for proper healing.

In superficial wounds, several topical antimicrobial dressings, such as silver sulfadiazine, have been shown to be effective in decreasing the risk of infections. Reports have also shown that certain topical antimicrobials may exert a delaying effect on keratinocyte proliferation and subsequent healing.[44]

Hypoxia

Decreased oxygen contributes to impairment of wound repair. The decrease may be caused by constricting sutures, tissue edema, or residual necrotic tissue. Also, underlying systemic diseases such as anemia, malnutrition, and sepsis lower tissue PO_2, causing cell death and the release of proteases and glycosidases. This release contributes to tissue breakdown and impaired healing. Impaired circulation impedes the supply of oxygen and nutrients to the wound site. Reportedly, if tissue oxygen tension is greater than 80 mm Hg, wounds will heal; however, if wound PO_2 decreases to less than 30 mm Hg, the phagocytic defense system is altered, and bacteria proliferate.[44] Clinically, wounds with poor oxygen supply show decreases in epithelialization, collagen deposition, tensile strength, resistance to infection, and angiogenesis.

Radiation

The effects of radiation therapy are not always limited to neoplastic cells but can also extend to healthy tissues. Cells with a high turnover rate are the most radiosensitive. Radiation effect on tissues is dose dependent and may assume either an acute or a chronic form.[45] Acute changes manifest clinically as mucositis, erythema, desquamation, and decrease in bone marrow. Such changes accompany low to moderate doses of radiation and usually subside after a month. Chronic changes are irreversible and are evident in blood vessel walls and skin connective tissues. Collagen hyalinizes, and tissues become fibrotic and hypoxic because of obliterative vasculitis, increasing tissue susceptibility to infection. Also, patients who have been exposed to whole-body irradiation usually demonstrate impaired healing because of their inability to evoke a nonspecific cell-mediated response to bacterial diseases. Macrophages have been shown to be relatively radioresistant and survive for long periods in situ, but bone marrow progenitor cells that are known to provide more long-term protection are hindered by radiation from activation and repopulation.[46]

Age

The young heal more efficiently than the elderly, most likely because the aged patient experiences an overall decline in general health. The multifactorial nature of healing in the elderly makes it difficult to determine whether impaired healing is due to aging per se or to other factors, such as disease, nutrition, perfusion, and environment.[47]

Drug Therapy

Therapeutic drugs are known to affect healing. Some have highly focused therapeutic objectives and, therefore, can exert detrimental effects on the patient's overall health. Examples are antineoplastic, anticoagulant, and glucocorticosteroid agents. Others, such as growth hormone and vitamins A and C, are thought to stimulate healing. Retinoids may stimulate the healing of some wounds and inhibit that of others.[48] Exogenous antiinflammatory corticosteroids can impair healing by impeding the inflammatory response through inhibition of macrophage migration. They also affect the remodeling phase by reducing levels of protocollagen, proline hydroxylase, and collagen. Also, cortisone delays development of granulation tissue through its effects on fibroblast and capillary proliferation.[49] Antineoplastic drugs and chemotherapeutic drugs are known to inhibit wound repair; wounds of patients receiving chemotherapy may exhibit reduced tensile strength. Such agents specifically arrest the inflammatory phase, suppressing protein synthesis and inhibiting cell proliferation.

Nutrition

Malnutrition is most likely the single greatest contributor to poor wound healing, especially in the elderly. Nutrients enhance the immune response, stimulate hormone secretion, and diminish tissue oxidation.[50] Nutritional support therapy promotes immune competence, facilitates wound healing, and lowers the risk of infection. Predictably, the nutrients important for wound repair are protein, carbohydrates, fats, vitamins, and minerals.

Basically, nutritional deficiency impairs adequate wound repair by prolonging the exudative phase and inhibiting collagen synthesis. Protein promotes neovascularization, fibroblastic proliferation, collagen synthesis, matrix accumulation, and remodeling, as well as facilitating the formation of lymphatics and enhancing the competence of the immune response. Generally, when protein concentration falls below 2g/dL, significant impairment occurs in wound tensile strength. In contrast to expectation, however, a high-protein diet does not shorten the healing time.[51] Albumin appears to be especially important for wound repair. Its serum levels, together with those of prealbumin and transferrin, are indicators of the status of protein stores and are one predictor of the quality of wound healing. Albumin is known to protect intravascular oncotic pressure and to serve as an amino acid donor for extrahepatic tissue synthesis.[52] Dietary essential amino acids must be provided because the rate of synthesis, in a wounded patient, does not meet the metabolic requirements of anabolism. Arginine and glutamine have been reported to be important elements for adequate wound healing because they enhance immune function and increase resistance to infection.[53]

Carbohydrate (glucose) and free fatty acids provide energy to cells, contributing to cellular proliferation and phagocytic activity. Because cellular membranes are composed, in part, of fatty acids, their deficiency may contribute to abnormal tissue repair and regeneration. It is well known that the energy supplied by different carbohydrates and fats is vital to prevent gluconeogenesis, which, in turn, deprives tissues of essential amino acids important for different physiologic processes and maintenance of body weight.[54]

Vitamins are vital to the wound healing process. Their role is complex, and supplemental vitamins are always recommended to foster healing, especially in patients receiving long-term nutritional supplements.[55]

Growth Factors and Their Role in Wound Healing

The last decade has witnessed significant progress in the field of polypeptide growth factors and their receptors. Institutions all over the world are conducting research to investigate more closely the biologic activities, chemical structure, molecular mechanisms, and target receptors of these growth factors. Such agents, sometimes referred to as *biologic response modifiers,* are certain to play key regulatory roles in the process of wound healing. The discovery of growth factors is largely attributable to studies of the molecular biology of carcinogenesis. These studies have implicated oncogenes and peptide growth factors in the transformation and expression of cancer cells and also in the stimulation of certain changes in the tumor environment, among which are neovascularization and deposition of extracellular matrix. Subsequently, researchers recognized that growth factors participate in physiologic processes as well, including fetal growth and wound healing. As in growth and proliferation of malignant cells, wound healing encompasses complex cellular processes involving cell-cell and cell-matrix interactions. It is now clear that these cellular processes are initiated, controlled, and terminated by growth factors. By definition, growth factors are signaling peptides that exert various actions through specific cell surface receptors, resulting in a paracrine (adjacent cells) or autocrine (producer cells) stimulation or both. Such actions regulate several cellular mechanisms, such as proliferation, differentiation, and migration. The discovery that growth factors play a major role in the wound healing process held out hope that they could be used clinically to accelerate wound healing by application to wound sites and could promote healing of chronic wounds.[56] The growth factors that appear to contribute significantly to wound healing include platelet-derived growth factor (PDGF), transforming growth factor–β (TGF-β), epidermal growth factor (EGF), basic fibroblast growth factor (bFGF), insulin-like growth factor (IGF), and tumor necrosis factor–α (TNF-α).

Summary

Wound healing encompasses two related processes: tissue repair and tissue regeneration. Although commonly used interchangeably, these terms are not synonymous. Regeneration yields a healed tissue that is structurally and functionally indistinguishable from the original, whereas repair attains structural integrity by forming a fibrous connective tissue scar. Identifiable phases are observed during soft tissue healing, beginning with extravasation of blood into the wound site, clot formation, organization of the clot to form granulation tissue, and proceeding eventually to remodeling of granulation tissue to form definitive scar. In its earliest stages, repair of hard tissues resembles that of soft tissues; however, key differences emerge consonant with the need for hard tissues to undergo remineralization.

Subtle distinctions exist between what is desirable and what is undesirable in a healing wound. For instance, wound contraction, the single most important natural factor contributing to the closure of soft tissue defects, serves a necessary role from an evolutionary perspective. With the advent of technologic societies, however, disadvantages inherent in rapid wound closure outweigh the benefits. Hypertrophic scarring and keloid formation are relatively common (and clearly undesirable) abnormalities in healing associated with an excessive accumulation of extracellular matrix. Despite much research, little progress has been made in preventing and treating these disorders. Nevertheless, promising research technology is being applied to these problems to assist in discovering treatments. At the opposite extreme are nonhealing wounds. Most arise as a consequence of underlying predisposing conditions. Generally, adequate healing follows correction of the primary (and usually obvious) cause.

The identification of various growth factors has been an important step in understanding wound healing from a descriptive standpoint. The impact of their discovery on treatments for disordered repair is yet unknown. Those known to participate significantly in wound healing processes are platelet-derived growth factor (PDGF), transforming growth factor–β (TGF-β), epidermal growth factor (EGF), basic fibroblast growth factor (bFGF), insulin-like growth factor (IGF), and tumor necrosis factor–α (TNF-α).

References

1. Bertolami CN, Messadi DV: The role of proteoglycans in hard and soft tissue repair. Crit Rev Oral Biol Med 1994;5:311–337.

2. Goslen JB: Wound healing for the dermatologic surgeon. J Dermatolol Surg 1988;14:959–972.
3. Cohen K, Diegelman RF, Lindblat WJ: Wound Healing: Biochemical and Clinical Aspects. Philadelphia, WB Saunders, 1992.
4. Clark RAF: Overview and molecular considerations of wound repair. *In* Clark RAF, Hensen PM (eds): Molecular and Cellular Biology of Wound Repair. New York, Plenum Press, 1988, pp 3–33.
5. Zitelli J: Wound healing for the clinician. Adv Dermatol 1987; 2:243–268.
6. Clark RAF: Cutaneous tissue repair: Basic biologic considerations I. J Am Acad Dermatol 1985;13:701–725.
7. Stenn KS, DePalma L: Re-epithelialization. *In* Clark RAF, Henson PM (eds): Molecular and Cellular Biology of Wound Repair. New York, Plenum Press, 1988, pp 321–335.
8. Odland G, Ross R: Human wound repair I: Epidermal migration. J Cell Biol 1971;49:247–251.
9. Barrandon Y, Green H: Cell migration is essential for sustained growth of keratinocyte colonies: The roles of transforming growth factor–α and epidermal growth factor. Cell 1987;50:1131–1137.
10. O'Keefe EJ, Chin ML, Payne RE Jr: Stimulation of growth of keratinocytes by basic growth factor. J Invest Dermatol 1988; 90:767–769.
11. Peacock EE, Van Winkle W: Contraction. *In* Surgery and Biology of Wound Repair. Philadelphia, WB Saunders, 1970, pp 49–74.
12. Hill TG: The evolution of skin graft reconstruction [review]. J Dermatol Surg Oncol 1987;13:834–835.
13. Noordhoff MS: Control and prevention of hypertrophic scarring and contracture [review]. Clin Plast Surg 1974;1:49–68.
14. Willis BA, Larson DL, Abston S: Positioning and splinting the burned patient. Heart Lung 1973;2:696–700.
15. Cronin TD: The use of a molded splint to prevent contracture after split skin grafting on the neck. Plast Reconstr Surg 1961; 27:7–18.
16. Nalbandian RM, Henry RL, Balko KW, et al: Pluronic F-127 gel preparation as an artificial skin in the treatment of third-degree burns in pigs. J Biomed Mater Res 1987;21:1135–1148.
17. Sternberg I, Sternberg N, Seelenfreund MH, Levine MR: The use of artificial skin in the prevention of early wound healing. Ann Ophthalmol 1987;19:127–128.
18. Jaksic T, Burke JF: The use of "artificial skin" for burns [review]. Ann Rev Med 1987;38:107–117.
19. Yannas IV, Burke JF: Design of an artificial skin. I: Basic design principles. J Biomed Biomater Res 1980;14:65–81.
20. Yannas IV, Burke JF, Gordon PL, et al: Design of an artificial skin. II: Control of the chemical composition. J Biomed Biomater Res 1980;14:107–132.
21. Bertolami CN, Shetty V, Milavec JE, et al: Preparation and evaluation of a nonproprietary bilayer skin substitute. Plast Reconstr Surg 1991;87:1089–1098.
22. Bertolami CN, Ellis DG, Donoff RB: Healing of cutaneous and mucosal wounds grafted with collagen-glycosaminoglycan/Silastic bilayer membranes: A preliminary report. J Oral Maxillofac Surg 1988;46:971–978.
23. Peacock EE, Van Winkle W: Repair of skin wounds. *In* Surgery and Biology of Wound Repair. Philadelphia, WB Saunders, 1970, pp 171–237.
24. Garb J, Stone MJ: Keloids. Am J Surg 1942;58:315–335.
25. Bornstein P, Sage H: Structurally distinct collagen types. Ann Rev Biochem 1980;49:957–1003.
26. Kischer CW, Shetlar MR, Chvapil M: Hypertrophic scars and keloids: A review and a new concept concerning their origin. Scanning Electr Microsc 1982;4:1699–1713.
27. Babin RW, Ceilley RI: Combined modalities in the management of hypertrophic scars and keloids. J Otolaryngol 1979;8:457–460.
28. Linares HA, Larson DL: Proteoglycans and collagenase in hypertrophic scar formation. Plast Reconstr Surg 1978;62:589–593.
29. Bloom D: Heredity of keloids: Review of the literature and report of a family with multiple keloids in five generations. N Y State J Med 1956;56:511–519.
30. Ketchum LD, Cohen IK, Masters FW: Hypertrophic scars and keloids. Plast Reconstr Surg 1974;53:140–154.
31. Cosman B, Crikelair GF, Ju MC, et al: The surgical treatment of keloids. Plast Reconstr Surg 1961;27:335–358.
32. Oluwasanmi JO: Keloids in the African. Clin Plast Surg 1974; 1:179–195.
33. Murray JC: Scars and keloids. Dermatol Clin 1993;11:697–708.
34. Savage K, Swann DA: A comparison of glycosaminoglycan synthesis by human fibroblasts from normal skin, normal scar, and hypertrophic scar. J Invest Dermatol 1985;84:521–526.
35. Donoff RB, Swann DA, Schweidt SH: Glycosaminoglycans of normal and hypertrophic human scar tissue. Exp Mol Pathol 1984;40:13–20.
36. Polansky JR, Toole BP, Gross J: Brain hyaluronidase: Changes in activity during chick development. Science 1974;183:862–864.
37. Toole BP: Morphogenetic role of glycosaminoglycans (acid mucopolysaccharides) in brain and other tissues. *In* Barondes SH (ed): Neuronal Recognition. New York, Plenum Press, 1976, pp 275–329.
38. Bertolami CN, Donoff RB: Identification, characterization, and purification of mammalian skin wound hyaluronidase. J Invest Dermatol 1982;79:417–421.
39. Bartell TH, Monafo WW, Mustoe TA: A new instrument for serial measurements of elasticity in hypertrophic scar. J Burn Care Rehabil 1988;9:657–660.
40. Messadi DV, Bertolami CN: CD44 and hyaluronan expression in human cutaneous scar fibroblasts. Am J Pathol 1993;142:1041–1049.
41. Lazarus GS, Cooper DM, Knighton DR, et al: Definitions and guidelines for assessment of wounds and evaluation of healing. Arch Dermatol 1994;130:489.
42. Phillips TJ, Dover JS: Leg ulcers. J Am Acad Dermatol 1991; 25:965.
43. Falanga V: Chronic wounds: Pathophysiologic and experimental considerations. J Invest Dermatol 1993;100:721.
44. Smith DJ, Thomson PD, Garner WL, et al: Burn wounds: Infection and healing. Am J Surg 1994;167:46S.
45. Shetty V, Bertolami CN: The physiology of wound healing. *In* Peterson LJ (ed): Principles of Oral and Maxillofacial Surgery, vol 1. Philadelphia, JB Lippincott, 1992, p 3.
46. Conklin JJ, Walker RI, Hirsch EF: Current concepts in the management of radiation injuries and associated trauma. Surg Gynecol Obstet 1983;156:809.
47. Jones PL, Millman A: Wound healing and the aged patient. Nurs Clin North Am 1990;25:263–277.
48. Frosch PJ, Czarnetzki BM: Effect of retinoids on wound healing in diabetic rats. Arch Dermatol Res 1989;281:424.
49. Min DI, Monaco AP: Complications associated with immunosuppressive therapy and their management. Pharmacotherapy 1991;11:119S.
50. Telfer NR, Moy RL: Drug and nutrient aspects of wound healing. Dermatol Clin 1993;11:729–737.
51. Levenson SM, Demetriou AA: Metabolic factors. *In* Cohen IK, Diegelman RF, Lindblad WJ (eds): Wound Healing: Biochemical and Clinical Aspects. Philadelphia, WB Saunders, 1992, pp 248–260.
52. Young ME: Malnutrition and wound healing. Heart Lung 1988; 17:60.
53. Daly JM, Reynolds J, Sigal RK: Effect of dietary protein and aminoacids on immune function. Crit Care Med 1990;18(suppl 2):S86.
54. Windsor JA, Hill GL: Weight loss with physiologic impairment: A basic indicator of surgical risk. Ann Surg 1988;207:290.
55. Bassler KH: Significance of vitamins in parenteral nutrition. Infusionstherapie 1990;17:19.
56. Steenfos HH: Growth factors and wound healing. Scand J Plast Reconstr Hand Surg 1994;28:95.

Section 2
Surgical Complications

Chapter 5
COMPLICATIONS OF THIRD MOLAR SURGERY

by

M. A. Pogrel

Introduction

Third molar (wisdom tooth) surgery remains the procedure most commonly carried out by oral and maxillofacial surgeons. Indeed, in some areas of the United States, it is the most commonly performed of any medical procedure, according to records held by third party insurance carriers. It is estimated that third molar removal may furnish around 65% of the gross income of the average oral and maxillofacial surgeon. It is therefore a commonly performed and, in most cases, relatively benign procedure that has generally been judged to have a good risk-to-benefit ratio. Complications do occur from this procedure, however, and they should be taken into account when a patient is being counseled regarding the removal of third molars.

THE SUBJECTS DISCUSSED IN THIS CHAPTER ARE:

- Natural history of wisdom teeth
- Complications of local anesthetics
- Sensory nerve damage
- Infection
- Periodontal complications
- Maxillary sinus involvement
- Fracture of the mandible
- Displacement of teeth and other foreign bodies
- Hemorrhage
- Pain and swelling
- Temporomandibular joint complications

Natural History of Wisdom Teeth

There is general agreement that symptomatic third molars that will not erupt normally should be removed. The natural history of wisdom teeth, however, is unclear, as was shown at the National Institutes of Health (NIH) consensus meeting in 1979, at which a request was made for prospective studies of third molars.[1] When third molars are to be removed, the complication rate is lower if the procedure is carried out at a younger age, and it has been suggested that one should evaluate patients for third molar removal by the time skeletal growth is complete (16 to 18 years of age).[2] Anecdotal reports document problems that can arise from retention of nonfunctional third molars,[3, 4] although other reports document the unpredictable nature of these teeth, which can change direction even at a comparatively late age.[5, 6] With the exception of preliminary reports,[7] however, information is still lacking on the long-term sequelae of retained third molars, so that an accurate risk-to-benefit ratio can be calculated. A 4-year follow-up of 20-year-old patients showed many wisdom teeth may still erupt normally.[8] The application of decision analysis to evaluate the need for extraction of asymptomatic third molars has been suggested.[9]

Third molar removal remains the most common single surgical procedure performed by oral and maxillofacial surgeons.[10] There is, however, associated morbidity even in routine cases, including lost working time. Iatrogenic injury and complications also occur with third molar removal. In particular, because many third molars are asymptomatic at the time of their removal, one needs to be cognizant of the risk-to-benefit ratio of such surgery. One should be aware of the risks and complications associated with the procedure[11] and of the techniques for minimizing these complications and treating them if they occur.

Complications of Local Anesthetics

The majority of patients undergoing third molar removal receive local anesthetics, either alone or in combinations with agents to produce sedation or general anesthesia. Rarely, local anesthesia alone can cause complications, which on occasion may be difficult to separate from complications resulting from the surgical procedure itself.

Hematoma formation is usually associated only with regional block injections. Although it can occur with the inferior alveolar nerve block if the inferior alveolar vessels bleed, hematoma formation is more usually reported from the posterior superior alveolar nerve block. When the needle enters the pterygoid venous plexus, a low-pressure venous ooze occurs, which can result in considerable swelling and bruising. There is no specific treatment, the application of pressure and ice being all that is available.

Infections from local anesthetic injections are fortunately extremely rare, provided that a sterile technique is adhered to at all times. Infection resulting from inferior alveolar nerve block appears in the medial pterygoid space and therefore may become a matter of importance, as mentioned later.

Local anesthetic injections may also be responsible for nerve damage. This complication can be extremely difficult to distinguish from nerve damage resulting from the surgical procedure itself, and direct evidence for this phenomenon can come only from patients given nerve blocks for restorative procedures. Estimates of the incidence of nerve damage from inferior alveolar nerve blocks range from 1 in 400,000 to 1 in 750,000 injections but may be much higher.[12, 13] The possible theoretical mechanisms involved include a direct injury from the needle,[14] epineurial hematoma formation,[15] and local toxicity from the anesthetic agent.[16, 17] Hematoma formation within the epineurium appears to be the most likely cause of nerve damage.[13] The rate of spontaneous recovery following nerve damage from a local anesthetic injection may be less than that after surgically created nerve damage; if spontaneous recovery has not occurred within 3 weeks, its chance of occurring at all is about one in three.[14] The role of nerve decompression and other microsurgical procedures has not been delineated in these cases.[18–20] A particular cause of nerve injury may be associated with the use of a needle that has developed a barb as a result of contacting bone as part of a normal inferior alveolar nerve block procedure. It is suggested that following inferior alveolar nerve block, the needle should not be reused unless it can be passed over a piece of sterile gauze without catching on it in any way.[21] Hard contact with bone should also be avoided with a local anesthetic needle.

Sensory Nerve Damage

Nerve damage, which occurs almost exclusively during removal of lower third molars, has been reported in the inferior alveolar nerve and lingual nerve and, less frequently, the long buccal nerve. A review of the literature shows that nerve damage occurs following 0.6% to 5% of third molar removals.[22–26] Most patients recover without treatment, as shown in a definitive review by Alling,[26] wherein over 96% of patients with inferior alveolar nerve injuries and 87% of those with lingual nerve injuries recovered spontaneously.[26] The higher incidence of inferior alveolar nerve recovery is probably due to the fact that the nerve is retained within a bony canal and the damaged nerve endings are better approximated spontaneously. Though there is general agreement that most spontaneous recovery occurs within 9 months and that after 2 years there is very little likelihood of further spontaneous recovery, well-documented reports describe recovery occurring several years after injury,[27, 28] so this possibility cannot be dismissed.

Damage to the inferior alveolar nerve occurs primarily because of the anatomic relationship between the third molar tooth and the nerve. This relationship can be partially determined from preoperative radiographs (Fig. 5–1).[29] The inferior alveolar nerve canal can normally be visualized on a panoramic radiograph. It is of consistent width and has a radiopaque cortical outline

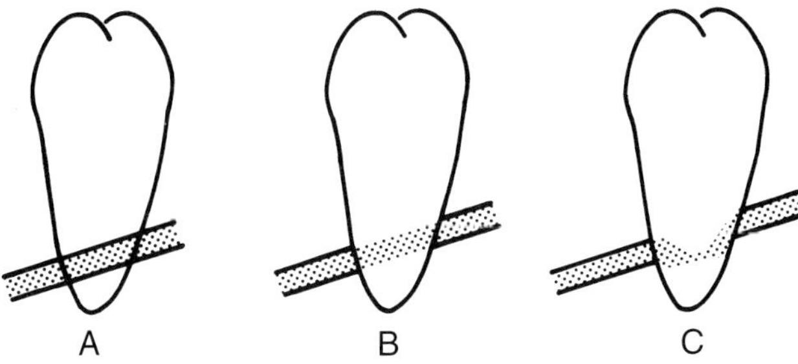

Figure 5–1. The radiographic relationship of the inferior alveolar nerve and the lower third molar. *A*, Cortical outline of the canal is intact. This probably represents superimposition only. *B*, There is loss of the cortical outline of the nerve canal. The nerve may be grooving the tooth. *C*, There is loss of cortical outline as well as narrowing and deviation of the nerve canal, denoting an intimate relationship of the nerve with the tooth and possible perforation of the tooth roots by the nerve.

visible superiorly and inferiorly. If the outline of the nerve is seen crossing the roots of the third molar and the nerve canal retains its size and cortical outline, the tooth is probably not intimately related to the nerve (Fig. 5–2). If, however, the nerve loses its cortical outline, it may well be grooving the tooth. If, in addition to losing its cortical outline, the nerve canal is narrowed or displaced, there is a very intimate relationship between the tooth and the nerve, which may even perforate the tooth roots; in these circumstances, there is a high incidence of nerve damage (Fig. 5–3). Statistically, a number of factors have been shown to be associated with a higher instance of inferior alveolar nerve damage following wisdom tooth removal.[22] They are:

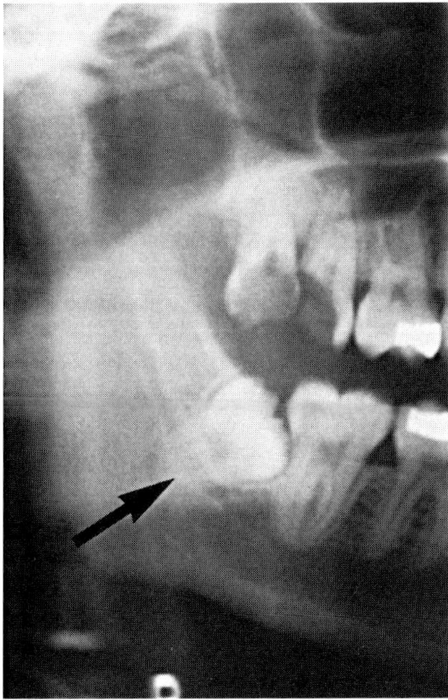

Figure 5–2. Radiograph of inferior alveolar nerve crossing the roots of a third molar (*arrow*), showing no loss of cortical outline, narrowing, or deviation. Relationship is probably one of superimposition only.

1. Full bony impactions.
2. Horizontal impactions.
3. Use of burs for removal.
4. Apices extending into or below the level of the neurovascular bundle.
5. Clinical observation of the bundle during surgery.
6. Excessive hemorrhage into the socket during surgery (presumably, this can cause pressure on the nerve, the resulting clot organization and fibrosis may cause additional nerve damage).
7. The age of the patient.

Within certain limits, the incidence of inferior alveolar nerve damage appears to increase with the age of the patient.[2, 30–32] In patients over the age of 25, incidence of nerve damage certainly appears to be higher, but the incidence in older age groups is unclear, because the majority of people in older age groups also have more difficult impactions. The relationship may become one of the difficulty of the impaction rather than the age of the patient.

Once the assessment of the likelihood of inferior alveolar nerve damage has been made, the tooth should be removed in such a way as to minimize the risk. This will often involve sectioning of the tooth. It is generally believed, however, that differences in surgical technique have relatively little influence on the overall incidence of inferior alveolar nerve damage.

Injuries to the lingual nerve have been more difficult to explain. Although they occur less commonly than inferior alveolar nerve injuries (in about 1% of lower third molar removals),[11, 30, 32] they are often more distressing to the patient, because they often include abnormal taste sensation, and spontaneous recovery is less likely.[26] Anatomic dissections have demonstrated variation in the position of the lingual nerve and have shown that in some cases, the lingual nerve may run over the retromolar pad.[33, 34] Such a nerve may be traumatized by flap-raising and retraction techniques, by follicle removal, and by suturing procedures. Developmental perforation of the lingual plate of the mandible by the roots of the third molar tooth[35] or other pathology (e.g., a cyst) in the approximate area where the lingual nerve is closely adapted to the periosteum may also explain some cases of lingual nerve damage.

Variations in the surgical technique for lower third molar removal appear capable of decreasing the incidence of lingual nerve damage, unlike that of inferior alveolar nerve damage. Flaps can be made from a more buccal approach to avoid a lingual nerve lying on the retromolar pad (Fig. 5–4). The lingual bone-splitting technique may be contraindicated, as it is known to be associated with a higher incidence of lingual nerve damage.[36–38] Aggressive curettage and follicle removal should be avoided on the lingual side of the socket; although there is a theoretical possibility of residual cyst formation due to retained follicle, this complication is extremely rare and is relatively easy to deal with if it does occur. Bone removal should be carried out predominantly from a buccal approach, and the tooth sectioned if necessary to facilitate its removal in a buccal direction. Perforation of the lingual plate by

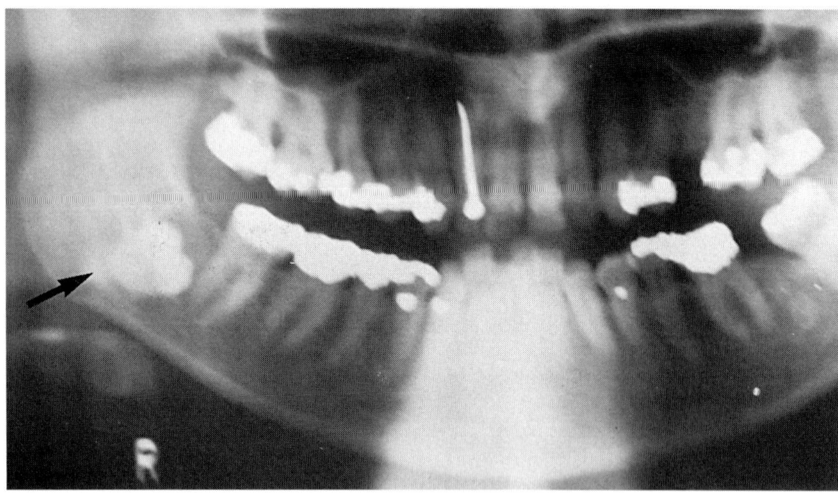

Figure 5–3. Radiograph showing loss of cortical outline and deviation of the inferior alveolar nerve canal as it crosses the third molar roots (*arrow*), denoting an intimate association.

the bur should be avoided. If suturing is to be carried out postoperatively, sutures should be placed superficially in the lingual flap to avoid possible nerve trauma. The question of raising a lingual flap and using a lingual retractor is more controversial. Placement of a lingual retractor is associated with a 13% temporary paresthesia rate[39] but no permanent nerve damage, the rate of permanent lingual nerve damage is around 2.0% if no retractor is used. It may be preferable, therefore, to carefully elevate a lingual flap and place a retractor,[40, 41] and special instruments have been designed for this purpose.[42]

If nerve damage does occur, its extent should be documented, preferably by photographs, so that any improvement can be accurately recorded. The sensory branches of the trigeminal nerve transmit sensations of pain, pressure, temperature, touch, and proprioception. In addition, the chorda tympani nerve (the pretrematic branch of the facial nerve that accompanies the lingual nerve) carries taste sensation from the anterior two thirds of the tongue. Because these sensations are relayed by different diameters of nerve fiber, differential loss and recovery of these components can, and do, occur. It is for this reason that monitoring of all components of sensation is generally recommended. Loss of all sensory components carries a worse prognosis and is more likely to indicate a discontinuity defect. The technique of nerve testing is covered in Chapter 6.

In most cases of nerve damage, recovery occurs over 6 to 8 weeks, and the remainder usually within 6 to 9 months. There is still some possibility of recovery up to 18 months, but after 2 years, further spontaneous recovery is rare. After 6 months, total recovery is rare.[43] Regular follow-up must therefore be carried out for this period. A suggested regimen consists of evaluations (1) every 2 weeks for 2 months; (2) every 6 weeks for 6 months; (3) every 6 months for up to 2 years; and then (4) annually for an indefinite period. The indications for microneurosurgery are discussed in Chapter 6.

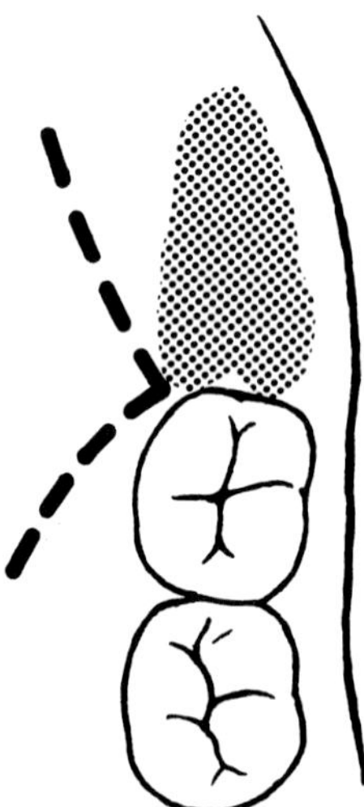

Figure 5–4. Suitable buccally placed incision (*dotted line*) for removal of a lower third molar. Incision goes down the external oblique ridge to the distobuccal angle of the second molar and down into the buccal sulcus.

Infection

Infection is common in association with third molars both before and after their surgical removal. Preoperative infections usually arise from a preexisting pericoronitis, and postoperatively, a localized osteitis can become infected. Infections appear to be more common after removal of partial or full bony impactions.[32] The strategic position of the third molar at the junction of a number of different fascial spaces mandates any infection in this area must be taken seriously, because of the ability of such an infection to spread along the fascial planes and compromise the airway (Fig. 5–5). Infections in the buccal space and buccinator space are usually localized on the lateral side of the mandible. Submasseteric infections occupy the potential space between the lateral border of the mandible and the masseter muscle. This is not a fascial-lined space; infection in this area is in direct contact with the masseter

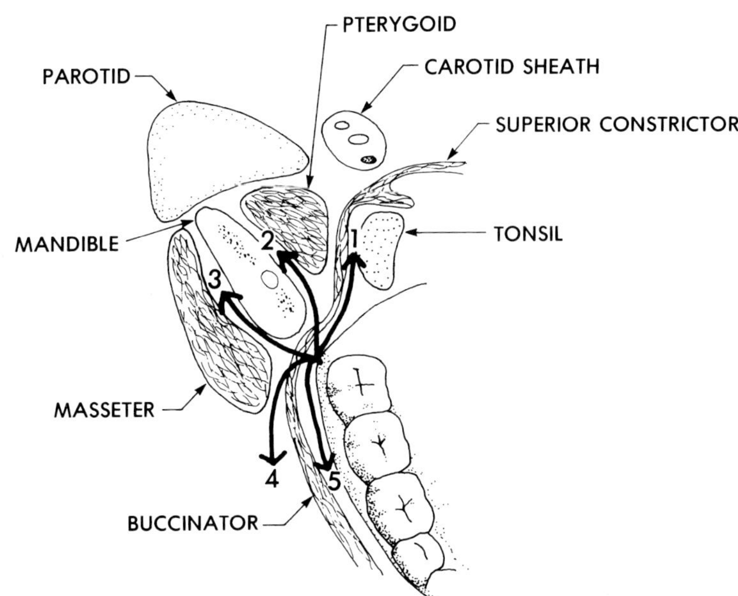

Figure 5–5. Coronal cut through the ascending ramus of the mandible just cephalic to the mandibular teeth. *1*, parapharyngeal space; *2*, internal pterygoid space; *3*, submasseteric space; *4*, buccinator space; *5*, buccal space.

muscle and usually induces intense spasm in the muscle, resulting in a profound trismus.

Internal pterygoid space infections occupy the fascia-lined space between the internal pterygoid muscle and the medial aspect of the mandible. Infections in this area cause a less profound trismus but can result in airway embarrassment. They can also result from inferior alveolar nerve block.

The submandibular space consists of a splitting of the investing fascia of the neck to enclose the submandibular salivary gland and is in continuity with the internal pterygoid and parapharyngeal spaces. Infections in this region can cause airway embarrassment and, when bilateral with associated cellulitis, is termed *Ludwigs angina.*

Parapharyngeal space infections occur between the pharyngeal mucosa and superior constrictor muscle. Infections in this region are potentially life-threatening and require urgent attention.

The main principles of treatment remain surgical with dependent drainage of pus augmented by antibiotic therapy. The infective organisms are normal oral flora, and penicillin remains the antibiotic of first choice. With the increasing recognition of the role of anaerobic oral bacteria in these infections,[44, 45] clindamycin can be substituted for penicillin in severe infections or metronidazole added to the penicillin. Studies show an average of four bacterial species in any oral infection, with anaerobic species outnumbering aerobic species, although streptococci remain the largest single group of organisms.[45]

A study of British oral and maxillofacial surgeons[46] showed penicillin still to be the antibiotic of choice for oral infections, but a substantial minority (22%) chose a broad-spectrum penicillin. Metronidazole was added routinely by 10% of surgeons.

A specific localized form of osteitis occurring at extraction sites is termed *dry socket*. Studies have shown that this phenomenon occurs in about 3% of extractions,[47, 48] and its incidence may be increasing,[48] though this apparent trend may be related to the greater likelihood of the patient's reporting the phenomenon. It is more common in relation to lower teeth and to the use of local anesthesia, and it is directly related to the difficulty of tooth removal.[47] The etiology appears to be a breakdown of a normal blood clot due to fibrinolytic action from the alveolar bone and, possibly, the saliva in association with local oral flora.[49, 50] The usual symptom is pain in the absence of lymph adenopathy and other signs of systemic infection. It is more common when the tooth is removed because of preexisting periapical infection or pericoronitis.[47] The incidence of dry socket can be decreased by prescribing systemic prophylactic antibiotics, packing sockets prophylactically with antibiotics and steroid paste, or, possibly, using antifibrinolytic agents prophylactically.[51–53] In normal circumstances, however, these measures are not used, because dry socket has a low incidence and low morbidity. Treatment normally consists of irrigation of the socket followed by packing with iodoform gauze or any of a number of proprietary medications. Antibiotics are rarely necessary unless there are systemic symptoms. Cultures from dry sockets have shown normal oral flora only, although metronidazole given prophylactically does decrease the incidence of the complication, perhaps indicating a role for anaerobic bacteria.[53] Other antibiotics given prophylactically may also decrease the incidence of dry socket.[54]

The role of prophylactic antibiotics in third molar surgery, to decrease the incidence of infection, remains controversial.[55, 56] Studies have shown that prophylactic antibiotics are unnecessary and may even make the management of subsequent infections more difficult.[57–60] In the only three controlled studies to have been carried out on third molars, two showed antibiotics to be without value,[59, 61] and the third showed them to be of possible value in deep impactions only.[62] Other studies, however, have shown a lower incidence of pain following third molar removal when antibiotics are prescribed,[63] and it is known that despite the evidence, prophylactic antibiotics are widely prescribed for third molar removal.[64, 65] There does, however, seem to be a move toward prescribing antibiotics for shorter periods; 24 hours of antibiotics may be all that is necessary.[66] Penicillin remains the antibiotic of choice, though metronidazole has been shown to be as effective as penicillin, demonstrating the mixed aerobic-anaerobic nature of many oral infections.[67] A short course of high-dose amoxicillin has also been shown to be effective for treatment of acute dentoalveolar infections.[68]

Periodontal Complications

Pericoronitis is a localized periodontal condition occurring around many erupting teeth. In the case of lower third molars in particular, it can become a recurrent condition if the teeth remain incompletely erupted. Most cases of pericoronitis are mild and respond to local measures, including irrigation, débridement, and chlorhexidine mouth washes.[69] On occasion, however, antibiotics are required. The bacteria species most commonly incriminated are *Peptostreptococcus, Fusobacterium*, and *Bacteroides*.[70–72] Penicillin or metronidazole is usually equally effective in these circumstances.[67] When pericoronitis is mild and the lower third molar is expected to erupt normally, local measures alone may suffice, though on occasion, a operculectomy may be performed or the opposing upper third molar may be extracted. In most instances, however, when the lower third molar is not expected to erupt normally, it should be removed.

Removal of third molars is often carried out to preserve periodontal health or, in some situations, to treat existing periodontitis.[73] With a partially impacted lower third molar, there is already a periodontal pocket on the mesial aspect of the third molar as well as an osseous defect in the bone on the distal root of the second molar. This situation can, under certain circumstances, progress to rapid periodontal destruction. Postoperative measurements show lower bone levels and deeper pocket depth than desirable. Some studies have grouped patients into treatment groups according to age. It is suggested that patients 19 years and younger, between 20 and 35 years, older than 35 years may have different periodontal healing potentials following lower third molar removal.[74] In most young patients, bone height after third molar removal appears similar to the preoperative level.[75–77] In fact, some studies even show a gain in bone level following surgery.[78] If the bone level distal to the second molar is compromised before third molar removal, it normally remains below the normal level postoperatively. There seems to be general agreement that the postoperative periodontal condition around the second molar is better if the third molar is removed when the patient is young.[75–81] The greatest bone defects occur in older patients, in whom the third molars have already resorbed part of the second molar. Periodontal pocket depth appears to be the same postoperatively as preoperatively,[75, 80, 82] and in older patients, pocket depth may even increase following removal of the third molar. In younger patients, however, there appears to be no adverse effect on pocket depth. In younger patients, reduction in pocket depth can occur for up to 4 years following surgery,[79] though this benefit may not occur in older patients.[77, 79]

Maxillary Sinus Involvement

The maxillary sinus is normally intimately related with the roots of the upper molar and premolar teeth. The risk of a communication occurring between the oral cavity and sinus following removal of an upper molar tooth should be discussed with any patient preoperatively. It is likely that many small openings remain undiagnosed, but provided that a healthy blood clot forms in the socket, closure occurs spontaneously with no untoward complications. Even when a communication is noted postoperatively, antibiotics and nasal decongestants coupled with good oral hygiene often allow spontaneous closure to occur over 6 to 8 weeks. If spontaneous closure does not occur, surgical closure, which normally consists of advancement of a buccal flap after freeing of the periosteum is required.[83] The mucosa is normally cut back on the palatal side so that suturing is carried out over bone rather than over the opening. Vertical mattress sutures are used to ensure a good soft tissue closure, and antibiotics and nasal decongestants are normally required (Fig. 5–6). The antibiotic chosen should be effective against nasal organisms as well as oral, and either a betalactamase-resistant penicillin or a first-generation cephalosporin is appropriate.

Teeth, roots, and other foreign bodies can occasionally be displaced into the sinus.[84, 85] Although they are sometimes seen as a chance asymptomatic finding on routine panoramic radiographs, such foreign bodies are generally removed because of the possible complication of sinus infection or polyp formation. Suction can be applied to the opening immediately after the foreign body has been displaced into the sinus. If this

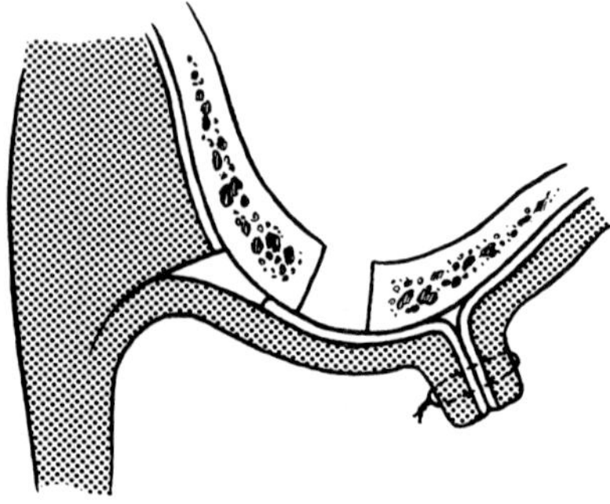

Figure 5–6. Closure of an oroantral fistula by raising of a buccal advancement flap, incision of buccal periosteum, cutting back of palatal side, and closure with vertical mattress sutures. Note suture line lies over palatal bone and not over the opening.

maneuver is unsuccessful, the sinus can be irrigated via the oral opening, and suction reapplied to try to remove the foreign body. If this second maneuver is unsuccessful, however, the procedure should be aborted, and the patient started on antibiotics and nasal decongestants. The foreign body should be removed via a Caldwell-Luc antrostomy as a secondary procedure coupled with surgical closure of the oral antral opening and a temporary intranasal antrostomy to aid surgical drainage of the sinus.

Fracture of the Mandible

Mandibular fracture is a recognized complication of lower third molar removal and should be listed as such on a routine consent form. There are, however, a number of predisposing conditions, such as mandibular atrophy, osteoporosis, and the presence of associated pathology such as a cyst or tumor. If a fracture occurs, it should be treated like any similar fracture. A number of medicolegal cases have revolved around the fact that the practitioner treated an iatrogenic fracture of the mandible differently from how it would have been treated if it had occurred as a result of any other traumatic episode, and complications arose.

Displacement of Teeth and Other Foreign Bodies

Upper third molars can be displaced distally into the infratemporal space if excessive distal elevation is used without an object behind the tuberosity to guide the tooth down into the oral cavity. A periosteal elevator or even the operator's finger is suitable for minimizing the incidence of this complication. If the tooth is displaced in this way, it should be retrieved immediately if at all possible. On occasion, however, venous oozing from the pterygoid venous plexus may make retrieval difficult; in these circumstances, packing of the area with iodoform gauze may be preferable, with removal of the tooth or root performed as a secondary procedure 7 to 10 days later.[86]

When a lower third molar is displaced into the lingual space, it normally passes inferior to the mylohyoid muscle onto the cervical fascia of the neck (Fig. 5–7). This complication normally results from excessive posterior and lingual elevation in the presence of a very thin or perforated lingual plate. The operator's thumb should be placed under the lower border of the mandible, and an attempt should be made to "milk" the tooth back along the lingual surface of the mandible. It may be necessary to incise the attachment of the mylohyoid muscle on the mylohyoid ridge in order to allow the tooth to return to the oral cavity, and care should be taken to avoid damage to the lingual nerve at this site. On occasion, the tooth cannot be recovered in this manner and must be recovered from an extraoral approach. Because the fascial planes have been invaded by the tooth, antibiotics are mandatory following this procedure.

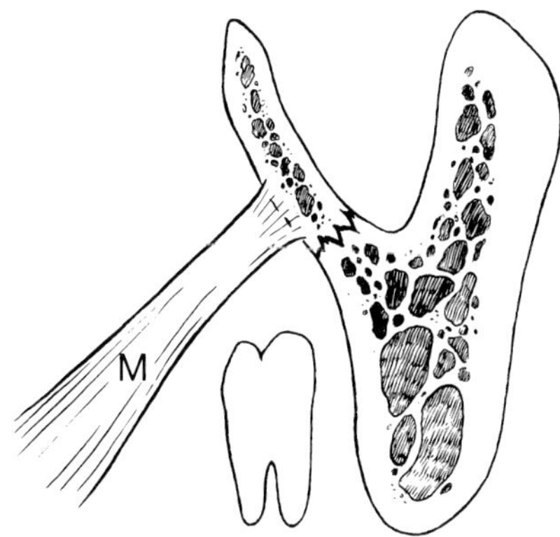

Figure 5–7. Tooth displaced into the lingual pouch. Note usual site of fracture of thin lingual plate and position of the tooth below the mylohyoid muscle (*M*).

Hemorrhage

Most patients with a bleeding diathesis are diagnosed early in life, and their medical history is available to the surgeon. Nevertheless, cases are still occasionally diagnosed for the first time following dental extraction. The majority of patients who bleed after extractions do not have any underlying hematologic disorder, and they generally have had extractions previously without complication, suggesting a purely local factor in the hemorrhage. It has been shown that preoperative screening of patients with no relevant history for coagulation disorders is not an effective means of identifying patients who may bleed postoperatively.[87] There exists a small group of patients who bleed after dental extractions on each occasion but do not bleed after extraoral trauma and do not show any abnormality on hematologic testing.[88] It has been suggested that oral fibrinolysis, probably of salivary origin, may be responsible for lysis of the blood clots and consequent hemorrhage in such patients.[89, 90] Fibrin-stabilizing factors, such as epsilon-aminocaproic acid and transexamic acid, may be helpful in these cases.[91]

Pain and Swelling

Discomfort, swelling, and edema are normally considered inevitable consequences of third molar removal, but as part of general improvement in patient care, all reasonable steps should be taken to minimize them. Excessive operative time and flap retraction increase the swelling associated with surgery.[11] Ice is generally recommended to reduce swelling, but its effectiveness is questionable,[92] and in the only controlled study, cold packs were found to be without value.[93] Steroids undoubtedly decrease swelling and are preferably given intravenously before the procedure. Though several studies have shown the efficacy of steroids in the reduction of postoperative swelling following wisdom tooth removal, there is no consensus of opinion as to the most appropriate steroid to use or the appropriate dosage.[94, 95] Conceptually, it would appear preferable to utilize a steroid with maximum antiinflammatory reaction and minimum glucocorticoid and mineralocorticoid activity. A fluorinated steroid such as betamethasone[96] or dexamethasone[97] would appear to be preferable. Studies utilizing a variety of antihistamines and proteolytic enzymes have obtained conflicting results for minimizing postoperative pain and swelling, so these agents are not generally employed for these purposes.[98, 99] Metronidazole[100] and penicillin[101] have been shown to reduce postoperative pain and swelling, though the relationship to any bacteria is unproven.[63, 101] A dressing rather than closure of the socket may decrease pain,[102] but the simplest and most effective measure may be copious irrigation of the socket.[103, 104] Postoperative saline rinses are usually prescribed, but their value is unproven in aiding healing, and patients cannot consistently mix an isotonic solution.[105] The postoperative use of a long-acting local anesthetic such as bupivacaine can decrease patient discomfort as well as the amount of systemic analgesia required.[106, 107]

Temporomandibular Joint Complications

Internal derangements of the temporomandibular joint (TMJ) appear to increase with the degree of sophistication of the society being examined. Females present for treatment more often than males. Epidemiologic studies, however, have shown that up to 60% of the population may suffer from some degree of temporomandibular joint dysfunction at some time, and the sex distribution is equal.[108] Fortunately, most cases are mild and require no treatment. With third molar removal being such a common procedure and temporomandibular joint dysfunction being so common as well, there inevitably are cases in which there is a temporal relationship between the two, but not necessary an etiologic relationship. Undoubtedly, however, removal of wisdom teeth may cause or exacerbate a preexisting TMJ problem. This complication is best prevented by allowing the patient to bite on a prop and rest every few minutes if the procedure is prolonged. If TMJ problems do occur following third molar removal or other oral surgical procedures, they must be treated in the normal way utilizing predominantly nonsurgical modalities, such as rest, heat, muscle relaxants, and, possibly, splint therapy.

Conclusions

Avoiding complications with third molar surgery involves three basic principles common to all surgical procedures:

1. A correctly designed treatment plan derived from clinical judgment and radiographic and ancillary investigations.
2. Informed patient consent including alternative treatment plans and possible risks and complications; this is best obtained in written form, and an explanatory videotape or interactive laser disc may be helpful.
3. Use of correct surgical techniques as well as diagnosis and treatment of complications in a timely fashion.

One should not hesitate to obtain a consultation or referral if indicated.

References

1. National Institute of Dental Research and Office of Medical Applications, National Institutes of Health: Removal of Third Molars. NIH Consensus Development Conference Summary 1979; 2.
2. Osborn TP, Frederickson G, Small IA, et al: A prospective study of complications related to mandibular third molar surgery. J Oral Maxillofac Surg 1985; 43:767.
3. Hinds EC, Frey KF: Hazards of retained third molars in older persons: Report of 15 cases. J Am Dent Assoc 1980; 101:246.
4. Stanley HR, Diehl DL: Ameloblastoma potential of follicular cysts. Oral Surg 1965; 20:260.
5. Oliver RG: An enigmatic wisdom tooth. Br Dent J 1983; 154:128.
6. Allen CD: An enigmatic wisdom tooth. Br Dent J 1983; 155:4.
7. Stanley HR, Alattar M, Collett WK, et al: Pathological sequelae of "neglected" impacted third molars. J Oral Pathol 1988; 17:113.
8. Von Wowern N, Nelson HO: The fate of impacted lower molars after the age of 20. Int J Oral Maxillofac Surg 1989; 18:277.
9. Tulloch JF, Antczak AA, Wilkes JW: The application of decision analysis to evaluate the need for extraction of asymptomatic third molars. J Oral Maxillofac Surg 1987; 45:855.
10. Friedman JW: Containing the cost of third molar extractions. Public Health Rev 1983; 98:376.
11. Van Gool AV, Ten Bosch JJ, Boering G: Clinical consequences of complaints and complications after removal of the mandibular third molar. Int J Oral Surg 1977; 6:29.
12. Ehrenfeld M, Cornelius CP, Altenmuller E, et al: Nervinjektionsschaden wach leitungsanasthesie im spatium pterygomandbulare. Dtsch Zahnarztl 1992; 47:36.
13. Pogrel MA, Bryant J, Regezi J: Nerve damage associated with inferior alveolar nerve blocks. J Am Dent Assoc 1995; 126:1150.
14. Harn SD, Durham TM: Incidence of lingual nerve trauma and postinjection complications in conventional mandibular block anesthesia. J Am Dent Assoc 1990; 121:519.
15. Rayan GM, Pitha JV, Wisdom P, et al: Histologic and electrophysiologic charges following subepineurial hematoma induction in rat sciatic nerve. Clin Orthop 1988; 229:257.
16. McCaughey W: Adverse effects of local anesthesia. Drug Safety 1992; 7:178.
17. Nickel AA: Regional anesthesia. Oral Maxillofac Clin North Am 1993; 5:17.
18. Hudson AR: Injection nerve injuries. Clin Plast Surg 1984; 11:27.
19. Clark WK: Surgery for injection injuries of peripheral nerves. Surg Clin North Am 1972; 52:1325.
20. Yaffe B, Pri-Chen S, Lin E, et al: Peripheral nerve injury: An experimental pilot study of treatment modalities. J Reconstr Microsurg 1986; 3:33.
21. Stacy GC, Hajjar G: Barbed needle and inexplicable paresthesias and trismus after dental regional anesthesia. Oral Surg Oral Med Oral Pathol 1994; 77:585.
22. Kipp DP, Goldstein BH, Weiss WW: Dysesthesia after mandibular third molar surgery: A retrospective study and analysis of 1,377 surgical procedures. J Am Dent Assoc 1980; 100:185.
23. Wofford DT, Miller RI: Prospective study of dysesthesia following odontectomy of impacted mandibular third molars. J Oral Maxillofac Surg 1987; 45:15.
24. Merrill RG: Prevention, treatment and prognosis of nerve injury related to the difficult impaction. Dent Clin North Am 1979; 23:471.
25. Goldberg MH, Nemarich AN, Marco WP: Complications after mandibular third molar surgery: A statistical analysis of 500 consecutive procedures in private practice. J Am Dent Assoc 1985; 111:277.
26. Alling CC: Dysesthesia of the lingual and inferior alveolar nerves following third molar surgery. J Oral Maxillofac Surg 1986; 44:454.

27. Girard KR: Considerations in the management of damage to the mandibular nerve. J Am Dent Assoc 1979; 98:65.
28. Alling CC: Editorial comment. J Oral Maxillofac Surg 1987; 45:204, 286.
29. Howe GL, Poyton HG: Prevention of damage to the inferior dental nerve during extraction of mandibular third molars. Br Dent J 1960; 109:355.
30. Bruce RA, Frederickson GC, Small GS: Age of patients and morbidity associated with mandibular third molar surgery. J Am Dent Assoc 1980; 101:240.
31. Fielding AF, Douglass AF, Whitley RD: Reasons for early removal of impacted third molars. Clin Prev Dent 1981; 3:19.
32. Rud J: The split-bone technique for removal of impacted mandibular third molars. J Oral Surg 1970; 28:416.
33. Kiesselbach JE, Chamberlain JG: Clinical and anatomic observations on the relationship of the lingual nerve to the mandibular third molar region. J Oral Maxillofac Surg 1984; 42:565.
34. Pogrel MA: The relationship of the lingual nerve to the mandibular third molar region. J Oral Maxillofac Surg 1995; 53:1178.
35. Killey HC, Kay LW: The Impacted Wisdom Tooth. Edinburgh, E & S Livingstone, 1965.
36. Rud J: Reevaluation of the lingual split-bone technique for removal of impacted mandibular third molars. J Oral Maxillofac Surg 1984; 42:114.
37. Rood JP: Lingual split technique. Br Dent J 1983; 154:402.
38. Mason DA: Lingual nerve damage following third molar surgery. Int J Oral Maxillofac Surg 1988; 17:290.
39. Rood JP: Permanent damage to inferior alveolar and lingual nerves during the removal of impacted mandibular third molars: Comparison of two methods of bone removal [see comments]. Br Dent J 1992; 172:108.
40. Blackburn CW, Bramley PA: Lingual nerve damage associated with the removal of lower third molars. Br Dent J 1989; 167:103.
41. Mason D: To retract or not retract. Br Dent J 1989; 168:94.
42. Browne WG: Lingual flap retractor for surgery in third molar area. Br Dent J Oral Surg 1982; 20:151.
43. Robinson PP: Observations on the recovery of sensation following inferior alveolar nerve injuries. Br J Oral Maxillofac Surg 1988; 26:177.
44. Labriola JD, Mascardo J, Alpert B: The microbiological flora of orofacial abscesses. J Oral Maxillofac Surg 1983; 41:711.
45. Quayle AA, Russell C, Hearn B: Organisms isolated from severe odontogenic soft tissue infections. Br J Oral Maxillofac Surg 1987; 25:34.
46. Gill Y, Scully C: The microbiology and management of acute dentoalveolar abscess: View of British oral and maxillofacial surgeons. Br J Oral Maxillofac Surg 1988; 26:452.
47. Heasman PA, Jacobs DJ: A clinical investigation into the incidence of dry socket. Br J Oral Maxillofac Surg 1984; 22:115.
48. Field EA, Speechley JA, Rotter E, et al: Dry socket incidence compared after a 12 year interval. Br J Oral Maxillofac Surg 1985; 23:419.
49. Birn H: Etiology and pathogenesis of fibrinolytic alveolitis (dry socket). Int J Oral Surg 1973; 2:211.
50. Gersel-Pedersen N: Fibrinolytic activity of blood and saliva before and after oral surgery. Int J Oral Surg 1981; 10:114.
51. Julius LL, Hungerford RW, Nelson WJ, et al: Prevention of dry socket with local application of Tera-Cortil in Gelfoam. J Oral Maxillofac Surg 1982; 40:285.
52. Gersel-Pedersen N: Transexamic acid in alveolar sockets in prevention of alveolitis sicca dolorosa. Int J Oral Surg 1969; 8:421.
53. Rood JP, Murgatroyd J: Metronidazole in the prevention of "dry socket." Br J Oral Surg 1979; 17:62.
54. Laird WRE, Stenhouse D, MacFarlane T: Control of postoperative infection. Br Dent J 1972; 133:106.
55. Pieluch JF, Arzadon J, Lieblich SE: Prophylactic antibiotics for third molar surgery: A supportive opinion. J Oral Maxillofac Surg 1995; 53:53.
56. Zeitler DL: Prophylactic antibiotics for third molar surgery: A dissenting opinion. J Oral Maxillofac Surg 1995; 53:61.
57. Paterson JA, Cardon VA, Strategos GT: An examination of antibiotic prophylaxis in oral and maxillofacial surgery. J Oral Surg 1970; 28:753.
58. MacGreger AJ: Anti-prophylactic antibiotics. J Oral Surg 1976; 34:1063.
59. Curran JB, Kennett S, Young AR: An assessment of the use of prophylactic antibiotics in third molar surgery. Int J Oral Surg 1974; 3:1.
60. Laskin DM: Prophylactic antibiotics: A problem or a panacea? J Oral Surg 1976; 34:585.
61. Happonen RP, Backstrom AC, Ylipaavalniemi P: Prophylactic use of phenoxymethyl penicillin and tinidazole in mandibular third molar surgery: A comparative placebo controlled clinical trial. Br J Oral Maxillofac Surg 1990; 28:12.
62. Macgregor AJ, Addy A: Value of penicillin in the prevention of pain, swelling and trismus following the removal of ectopic mandibular third molars. Int J Oral Surg 1980; 9:166.
63. Hellem S, Nordenram A: Prevention of postoperative symptoms by general antibiotic treatment and local bandage in removal of mandibular third molars. Int J Oral Surg 1973; 2:273.
64. Killey HC, Seward GR, Kay LW: Outline of Oral Surgery. Bristol, Wright, 1975.
65. Guralnick W: Third molar surgery. Br Dent J 1984; 156:389.
66. Conover MA, Kaban LB, Mulliken JB: Antibiotic prophylaxis for major maxillofacial surgery. J Oral Maxillofac Surg 1985; 43:865.
67. Ingham HR, Hood FJC, Bradnum P, et al: Metronizadole compared with penicillin in the treatment of acute dental infections. Br J Oral Surg 1977; 14:264.
68. Lewis MAO, McGowan DA, MacFarlane TW: Short course high dose amoxycillin in the treatment of acute dentoalveolar abscess. Br Dent J 1986; 161:299.
69. Peterson LJ: Rationale for removing impacted teeth. Am Dent Assoc 1992; 123:198.
70. Heimdahl A, Nord CE: Treatment of orofacial infections of odontogenic origin. Scand J Infect Dis 1985; 45:101.
71. Van Winkelhoff AJ, Caries AW, deGraaff J: *Bacteroides endodontalis* and other black-pigmented Bacteroides species in odontogenic abscesses. Infect Immun 1985; 49:494.
72. Mombelli A, Busser D, Lang NP, et al: Suspected periodontopathogens in erupting third molar sites of periodontally healthy individuals. J Clin Periodontol 1990; 17:48.
73. Leone SA, Edenfield MJ, Cohen ME: Correlation of acute pericoronitis and the position of the mandibular third molar. Oral Surg Oral Med Oral Pathol 1986; 62:245.
74. Amler MH: The age factor in human extraction wound healing. J Oral Surg 1977; 35:193.
75. Osborne WH, Snyder AJ, Tempel TR: Attachment levels and crevicular depths at the disc of mandibular second molars following removal of adjacent third molars. J Periodontol 1982; 53:93.
76. Meister FJ, Nery EB, Angell DM, et al: Periodontal assessment following surgical removal of mandibular third molars. Gen Dent 1986; 34:120.
77. Marmary Y, Brayer L, Tzukert A, et al: Alveolar bone repair following extraction of impacted mandibular third molars. Oral Surg Oral Med Oral Path 1985; 60:324.
78. Kugelberg CF, Ahlstrom U, Ericson S, et al: Periodontal healing after impacted lower third molar surgery. Int J Oral Surg 1985; 14:29.
79. Kugelberg CF: Periodontal healing two and four years after impacted lower third molar surgery. Int J Oral Maxillofac Surg 1990; 19:341.
80. Grondahl HG, Lekholm U: Influence of mandibular third molars on related supporting tissues. Int J Oral Surg 1973; 2:137.
81. Ash MMJ, Costich ER, Hayward JR: A study of periodontal hazards of third molars. J Periodontol 1962; 333:209.
82. Chin Quee TA, Gosselin D, Millar EP, et al: Surgical removal of the fully impacted mandibular third molar. J Periodontol 1985; 56:625.
83. Fickling BW: Oral surgery involving the maxillary sinus. Br Dent J 1957; 103:191.
84. Lee FMS: The displaced root in the maxillary sinus. Oral Surg 1970; 29:491.
85. Killey HC, Kay LW: Possible sequelae when a tooth or root is dislodged into the maxillary sinus. Br Dent J 1964; 116:73.
86. Gulbrandsen SR, Jackson IT, Turlington EG: Recovery of a maxillary third molar from the infratemporal space via a hemicoronal approach. J Oral Maxillofac Surg 1987; 45:279.
87. Suchman AL, Mushlin IA: How well does activated partial thromboplastin time predict postoperative hemorrhage? JAMA 1986; 256:750.

88. Gillbe GV, Fellingham FP: Repeated postextraction hemorrhage. Br Dent J 1968; 125:385.
89. Bjorlin G: Local fibrinolysis in the oral cavity. Scand J Hematol 1984; 33:411.
90. Nilsson IM: Local fibrinolysis as a mechanism for hemorrhage. Thromb Diath Haemorrh 1975; 34:623.
91. Wedgewood D: The fibrinolytic system with special reference to its relevance to oral surgery. Br J Oral Surg 1970; 8:82.
92. Zimmerman DC: Preplanning, surgical and postoperative considerations in the removal of the difficult impaction. Dent Clin North Am 1979; 23:451.
93. Forsgren H, Heimdaal A, Johansson B, et al: Effect of application of cold dressings on the postoperative course in oral surgery. Int J Oral Surg 1985; 14:223.
94. Holland CS: The influence of methylprednisolone on post-operative swelling following oral surgery. Br J Oral Maxillofac Surg 1987; 25:293.
95. Bierne OR, Hollander B: The effect of methylprednisone on pain, trismus and swelling after removal of third molars. Oral Surg 1986; 61:134.
96. Skjelbred P, Lokken P: Post-operative pain and inflammatory reaction reduced by injection of a corticosteroid. A controlled trial in bilateral oral surgery. Eur J Clin Pharmacol 1982; 21:391.
97. El Hag M, Coghlan K, Christmas P, et al: The inflammatory effect of dexamethasone and therapeutic ultrasound in oral surgery. Br J Oral Maxillofac Surg 1985; 23:17.
98. Cameron IW: An investigation into some of the factors concerned in the surgical removal of the impacted lower wisdom tooth including a double blind trial of Chymoral. Br J Oral Surg 1980; 18:112.
99. Seymour RA, Walton JG: Pain control after third molar surgery. Int J Oral Surg 1984; 13:457.
100. Kaziro GS: Metronidazole (Flagyl) and *Arnica montana* in the prevention of post-surgical complications. A comparative placebo controlled clinical trial. Br J Oral Maxillofac Surg 1984; 22:42.
101. Macgregor AJ, Hart P: Effect of bacteria and other factors on pain and swelling after removal of ectopic mandibular third molars. J Oral Surg 1969; 27:174.
102. Holland CS, Hindle MO: The influence of closure or dressing of third molar sockets on postoperative swelling and pain. Br J Oral Maxillofac Surg 1984; 22:65.
103. Sweet JB, Butler DP, Drager JL: Effects of lavage techniques with third molar surgery. Oral Surg 1976; 41:152.
104. Butler DP, Sweet JB: Effect of lavage on the incidence of localized osteitis in mandibular third molar extraction sites. Oral Surg 1977; 44:14.
105. Verser SJ, Alexander RE: Use of saline as a postoperative rinse. Oral Surg Oral Med Oral Pathol 1994; 77:438.
106. Laskin JL, Wallace WR, Deleo B: Use of bupivacaine hydrochloride in oral surgery: A clinical study. J Oral Surg 1977; 35:25.
107. Tuffin JR, Cunliffe DR, Shaw SR: Does local anesthesia injected at the time of third molar removal under general anesthesia reduce significantly postoperative analgesic requirements? A double blind controlled trial. Br J Oral Maxillofac Surg 1989; 27:27.
108. Rieder CE, Martinoff JT, Wilcox SA: The prevalence of mandibular dysfunction. J Prosth Dent 1983; 50:81.

Chapter 6
EVALUATION AND MANAGEMENT OF NEUROLOGIC COMPLICATIONS

by

Roger A. Meyer

Introduction

Injuries to peripheral branches of the fifth (trigeminal) and seventh (facial) cranial nerves are ever-present risks during surgical procedures performed in the oral cavity and associated maxillofacial region. The resulting loss of sensory or motor function in an area of the body that is highly visible and in which important bodily functions are located can be distressing or even devastating to those patients in whom spontaneous return of nerve function does not occur.

Contrary to previous opinion,[1–3] nerve injuries do not always heal spontaneously.[4–6] Fortunately, advances in microsurgical technique that have evolved during the past 30 years have made possible the surgical repair of selected maxillofacial peripheral nerve injuries when done in a timely fashion by a skilled surgeon.[7–15]

THE SUBJECTS DISCUSSED IN THIS CHAPTER ARE:

- Neuroanatomy of the trigeminal and facial nerve
- Classification of nerve injuries
- Trigeminal nerve injuries
  - Etiology and incidence
  - Evaluation
  - Indications for and timing of surgery
  - Surgical techniques
  - Results of surgery
  - Prognosis
- Facial nerve injuries
  - Surgical anatomy
  - Evaluation
  - Treatment and prognosis

Neuroanatomy

Knowledge of the internal structure of a nerve is helpful in understanding the pathophysiologic mechanisms of nerve injuries and in evaluating various methods of their surgical repair. There is no anatomic or physiologic distinction between a motor and a sensory nerve. Indeed, a sensory nerve is often the donor when an autogenous nerve graft is required in the surgical repair of an injured facial nerve.[16]

The anatomic structure of a nerve is similar in many ways to the structure of a telephone cable (Fig. 6–1). The axon, which transmits electrical impulses, is the basic functional unit of the nerve. Following an injury, the axon may undergo a process of degeneration distal to the area of injury and an exaggerated metabolic response proximal to the injury (so-called wallerian degeneration).[17, 18] Axons are individually covered by a layer of connective tissue, the *endoneurium*, and they are grouped together into fascicles or funiculi, which are in turn surrounded by *perineurium*. Nerves may contain one, a few, or many fascicles. The intrabony portion of the facial nerve contains one fascicle[19], for example, whereas the inferior alveolar nerve may consist of as many as 18 to 21 fascicles.[20] The outer surface of the nerve consists of *epineurium*, which also extends between fascicles as the *intraneural epineurium*. The major blood supply of the nerve is contained in vessels (the vasa nervorum) within the epineurium. The cross-sectional diameter of a nerve may contain 22% to 88% epineurium. The more epineurium contained in the nerve's diameter, the better able the nerve is to withstand compressive forces (e.g., prolonged retraction) and resist injury.[21] Unfortunately, the inferior alveolar and lingual nerves contain very little intraneural epineurium.[22]

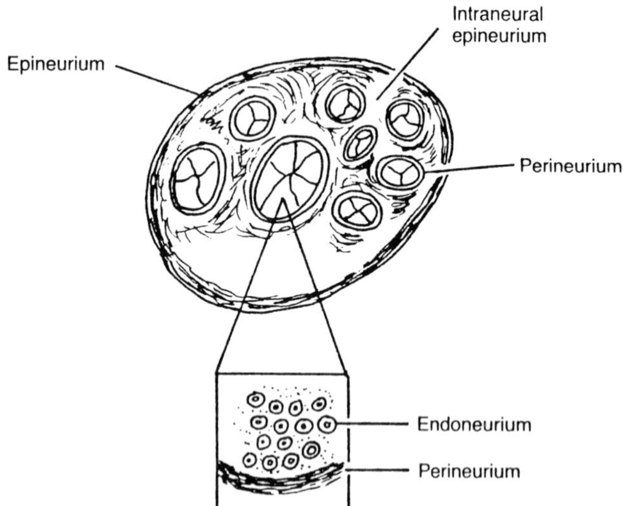

Figure 6–1. Internal anatomy of a nerve. Endoneurium surrounds each *axon*, the basic functional unit of the nerve. Axons are grouped together into *fascicles* (funiculi), which are covered by perineurium. The outer surface of the nerve is composed of epineurium, which extends between fascicles as the intraneural epineurium. (*From* Meyer RA: Applications of microneurosurgery to the repair of trigeminal nerve injuries. Oral Maxillofac Surg Clin North Am 1992;4:405–416.)

Classification of Nerve Injuries

Classification of nerve injuries assists the clinician in making a diagnosis, developing a rational plan of management, determining the need for and timing of surgical intervention, and estimating the prognosis of an injury. Systems of nerve injury classification developed by Seddon[6, 23] and by Sunderland[24, 25] are most useful to clinicians.

Seddon[6, 23] has described three types of nerve injury: neurapraxia, axonotmesis, and neurotmesis. *Neurapraxia* is a mild, temporary injury often caused by compression or retraction. There is no axonal degeneration distal to the area of injury. There is a temporary conduction block (sensory loss, motor weakness). Spontaneous recovery usually occurs within 4 weeks or less, and surgical intervention is not necessary.

Axonotmesis is a more significant injury. There is disruption or loss of continuity of some axons, which undergo wallerian degeneration distal to the site of injury. The general structure of the nerve remains intact, however. There is prolonged conduction failure, and initial signs or symptoms of recovery of nerve function do not appear for 1 to 3 months after injury. Eventual recovery is often less than normal (paresis, hypoesthesia). Sensory nerve injuries may develop persistent painful sensations (dysesthesias).

Neurotmesis is complete severance or internal physiologic disruption of all layers of the nerve. Wallerian degeneration of all axons occurs distal to the injury. There is a total permanent conduction block of all impulses (paralysis, anesthesia). The discontinuity gap between proximal and distal nerve stumps becomes filled with scar tissue, and proximal axonal sprouts are prevented from recannulating distal endoneurial tubules. No recovery is expected without surgical intervention.

Sunderland's classification[24, 25] is based on detailed descriptions of the pathophysiology and anatomy of the injured nerve. A comparison of Sunderland's and Seddon's classifications of nerve injuries is given in Table 6–1. Seddon's neurapraxia is comparable to a Sunderland class I injury; axonotmesis to classes II, III, and IV; and neurotmesis to class V. A sixth class of injury, in which there is a mixed combination of normal nerve tissue and varying degrees of injury (classes I–V) within the same nerve trunk, has been added by Mackinnon and Dellon.[26] Such complex injuries present the greatest challenge to the surgeon who must treat them.

Trigeminal Nerve Injuries

Lost or altered sensation *(paresthesia)* or painful symptoms *(dysesthesias)* that result from injuries to the maxillary or mandibular divisions of the trigeminal nerve may be permanent and unacceptable to afflicted patients.[27] Unpleasant sensations such as numbness, tingling, burning, itching, crawling, constant or inter-

Table 6–1. Seddon[6, 23] Classification of Nerve Injuries*

	Neurapraxia	Axonotmesis	Neurotmesis
Sunderland classification[24, 25]	I	II, III, IV	V
Nerve sheath	Intact	Intact	Interrupted
Axons	Intact	Interrupted	Interrupted
Wallerian degeneration	None	Yes, partial	Yes, complete
Conduction failure	Transitory	Prolonged	Permanent
Spontaneous recovery	Complete	Partial	Poor to none
Time of recovery	Within 4 weeks	Months	Begun by 3 months, if any

*Superscript numbers refer to chapter references.

mittent pain described as sharp or throbbing, and hypersensitivity can involve the chin, lips, cheeks, gingiva, tongue, or face. Loss of or changes in taste sensation are common with lingual nerve injury. Normal functions—speaking, chewing food, drinking fluids, swallowing, shaving, smoking, kissing, and washing—are unpleasant, difficult, or intolerable. Accidental cheek, lip, or tongue biting becomes a common problem. In susceptible patients, serious interference with the important functions of the oral and maxillofacial regions may cause significant depression, loss of self-worth, or interference with activities of daily living. Such untoward effects, especially if they are permanent and unexpected sequelae of elective surgery, may result in a distressed patient.

Etiology and Incidence

The various surgical procedures associated with a series of 308 nerve injuries I have treated,[15] in descending order of frequency, are as follows:

- Impacted tooth removal
- Osteotomy (bilateral sagittal split ramus)
- Fracture (mandible, zygoma)
- Root canal filling and/or apicoectomy
- Dental implants
- Calcium hydroxyapatite augmentation
- Genioplasty (osteotomy or implant)
- Tumor or cyst resection
- Salivary gland excision
- Mandibular vestibuloplasty
- Gunshot wound or laceration
- Local anesthetic injection

All but six of the patients in this series had an injury of the inferior alveolar, mental, lingual, or infraorbital nerve. Injury causing sensory deficits of the long buccal, mylohyoid, palatal, or superior alveolar nerves, although common, is seldom perceived by the patient.[13]

The incidence of nerve injuries associated with standard surgical procedures provides important information that may help a patient make a decision about elective surgery. Statistics vary according to the particular study consulted (Table 6–2).[28–48] For example, according to the report of a workshop on the management of patients with third molar teeth conducted by the American Association of Oral and Maxillofacial Surgeons in 1993, the removal of impacted mandibular third molars is associated with inferior alveolar nerve injury in 1.0% to 7.1% of patients, whereas the incidence of injury to the lingual nerve is estimated at 0.02% to 0.06%.[29] The difference between a temporary and a permanent sensory deficit and the possible lasting sensory sequelae (see earlier discussion) should be emphasized.

Evaluation

Documentation of sensory nerve injuries is essential in determining the type (classification) of injury, the objective nature of the sensory deficit, the potential for spontaneous recovery, and the indications for and optimal timing of surgical intervention.

The first step is to ascertain the patient's main complaint, whether it be loss of sensation, pain or other abnormal sensation, or functional impairment.[49, 50] A checklist completed by the patient, such as the example shown in Table 6–3, is helpful to the clinician in assessing perceived functional difficulties.

In taking the patient's history, the clinician must determine the type of trauma or surgical procedure associated with the injury, the date of the incident, and the progress of symptoms or functional complaints. Return of sensation within the first 4 weeks indicates neurapraxia and an excellent prognosis. Later onset of symptoms of recovery (1 to 3 months) has a less certain prognosis, usually associated with axonotmesis. Total lack of signs or symptoms of recovery of sensory function for 12 weeks or longer generally indicates neurotmesis and a poor prognosis for significant spontaneous recovery.[14]

The purpose of the nerve injury examination is to complete a series of testing maneuvers to outline the area of sensory deficit, quantify the magnitude and character of the deficit, and record it for comparison in an *objective* manner with the results of subsequent evaluations. Any clinician, with or without microneurosurgical skills, should be able to complete the examination. Information gained from the nerve injury examination will enable a non-microsurgeon to make an appropriate decision regarding referral for further evaluation and possible microsurgical repair of a nerve injury. Excellent protocols for neurosensory evaluation suitable for research[50] or practical clinical applications[49] are suggested to the reader interested in detailed discussions beyond the scope of this chapter.

Table 6–2. Incidence of Sensory Nerve Injuries After Various Surgical Procedures

Procedure*	Incidence of Sensory Deficit (%)	
	Temporary Deficit	*Permanent Deficit*
Third molar removal[28–39]	0.4–11.5†	0.1–1.05†
Sagittal split ramus osteotomy (SSRO)[40]	100	9–45‡
SSRO with rigid fixation[41–43]	100	20.1 52‡
Mandibular vestibuloplasty and ridge augmentation[44–47]	100	2–54
Vertical ramus osteotomy[40, 41, 48]	0.1	0.1

*Superscript numerals refer to chapter references.
†Lingual and inferior alveolar nerves combined.
‡Most permanent deficits after SSROs were minor variations from normal in response to standardized neurosensory testing.

The clinician should begin the examination by looking for evidence of recent injury or surgery or *neurotrophic* changes (edema, erythema, ulcerations, hypohydrosis, loss of hair, hypokeratosis) and signs of hyperactivity of the sympathetic nervous system (blanching, flushing, changes in skin temperature, sweating) in the skin distribution area of the injured nerve (Fig. 6–2). Palpation directly over accessible portions of the injured nerve (lingual aspect of mandible adjacent to second and third molars, buccal vestibule over the mental foramen, skin over the infraorbital foramen), or percussion of the teeth may produce a Tinel-like sign.[51] Localized tingling, burning, or other painful symptoms without radiation may indicate nerve severance with a proximal stump neuroma. Localized symptoms that radiate to areas distal to the suspected location of the nerve injury may be present with a neuroma in continuity and viable nerve tissue distal to the injury or a severed nerve with phantom pain. Pulp testing of the mandibular teeth is a reproducible method of assessing the sensory function of the inferior alveolar nerve. Radiographs may demonstrate distortion or disruption of the inferior alveolar canal, displaced bone or tooth fragments, or foreign material (wire, fixation screw, missile fragments, alloplastic material, dental implant, root canal filling) impinging on a nerve canal or foramen (Fig. 6–3).

Neurosensory testing is designed to evaluate as objectively as possible the patient's responses to a series of standardized maneuvers.[52] Von Frey monofilaments are used for contact detection (static light touch) and brush directional strokes. The Two-Point Anesthesiometer (Research Design, Inc., Houston, TX) tests the patient's ability to differentiate contact with one or two points. Normal distances for two-point discrimination

Table 6–3. Checklist for Determining Functional Impairment Associated with Sensory Nerve Injuries

Rating*	Patient Complaint or Symptom
_____	1. Lip, cheek or tongue biting?
_____	2. Burning lips or mouth with hot food/fluids?
_____	3. Drooling of saliva or dribbling food on chin?
_____	4. Difficulty chewing or drinking?
_____	5. Decreased, altered or absent taste?
_____	6. Difficulty speaking or being understood?
_____	7. Difficulty smiling, frowning, laughing?
_____	8. Difficulty with toothbrushing, flossing, dental care?
_____	9. Difficulty with yawning, swallowing?
_____	10. Lowered sense of self-worth, general health, work performance

*0, no interference with normal function; 1, minimal (smallest interference with normal function); 2, moderate (interference with function 50% of the time); 3, severe (interference with function almost all the time).

After Zuniga JR, Essick GK: A contemporary approach to the clinical evaluation of trigeminal nerve injuries. Oral Maxillofac Surg Clin North Am 1992;4:353.

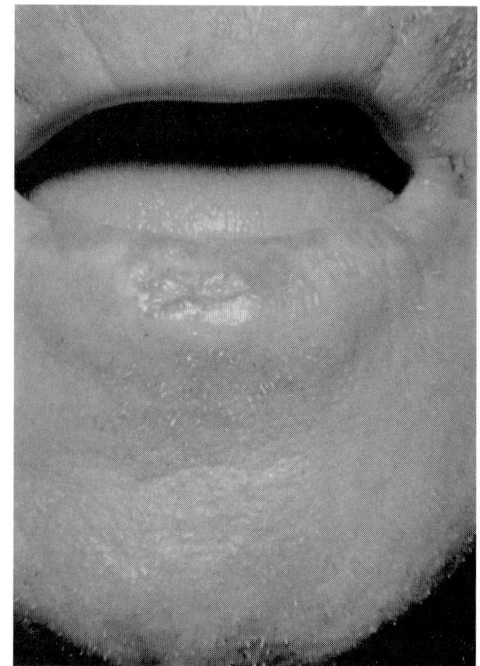

Figure 6–2. Neurotrophic changes in lower lip of patient with bilateral inferior alveolar neurotmesis 1 year after mandibular fractures; appearance of lip raised suspicion of squamous cell carcinoma.

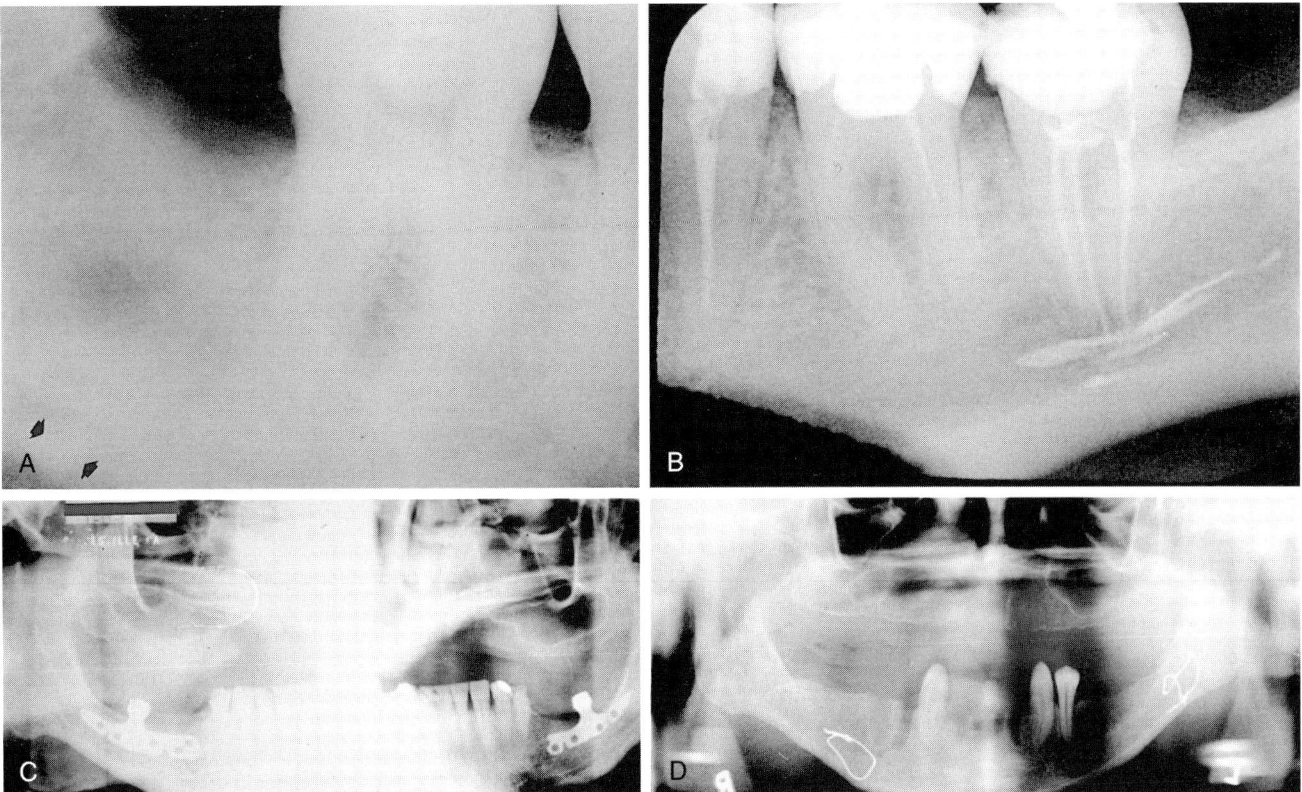

Figure 6–3. Radiographs of patients with sensory complaints reveal *(A)* displaced tooth root *(arrows)*, *(B)* extravasated root canal filling material, *(C)* dental implant impinging upon the inferior alveolar canal, and *(D)* fixation wires overlying inferior alveolar canals.

of the tongue, lips, and chin vary from 5 to 15 mm.[49] Pinprick detection (painful stimulus) is determined using a hand-held 22- or 23-gauge needle. Thermal discrimination is assessed with a cotton swab saturated with ethyl chloride spray and immediately applied lightly to the skin. Responses to directional stroke identification and two-point discrimination measure the function of larger-diameter (5 to 12 μ) myelinated nerve fibers, the so-called rapidly adapting mechanoreceptors. These fibers are the last to regain their function in the recovery phase of a nerve injury. Contact detection or static light touch assesses the conductivity of impulses in smaller-diameter (4 to 8 μ), slowly adapting myelinated fibers. Noxious stimuli (pinprick, thermal discrimination, pulp testing of teeth) determine the integrity of small-diameter (0.05 to 1.0 μ), poorly myelinated fibers. Perception of painful stimuli is usually the first function to return in a recovering sensory nerve. For each test, the patient's eyes are closed, and the response, lack of response, or onset of painful symptoms is compared with the normal, contralateral side and recorded. Photographs or diagrams[53] of the affected area are helpful in documentation and for comparison with results of subsequent testing (Fig. 6–4).

Somatosensory evoked potentials of the trigeminal nerve[54–56] and sophisticated methods of measuring touch-pressure,[57] vibration, and thermal sensation[58] have value in the research laboratory and in generating normal data for future comparison in clinical studies. At present, however, these modalities are either too cumbersome, expensive, or unpredictably variable in their results to have practical applications in the clinical setting.

Local anesthetic nerve blocks are indicated in evaluating painful nerve injuries.[59] Failure to relieve pain in the presence of an otherwise effective nerve block suggests a central—sympathetic or psychological—rather than peripheral cause of dysesthesia.[60]

Results of testing are compared with findings at sequential examinations, which are repeated at 4-week intervals until sensory function has returned to normal or there is an indication for surgical intervention. Detailed algorithms are available to guide the clinician in the evaluation and treatment of the various trigeminal nerve injuries,[61] and the reader is referred to them for further in-depth study.

Indications for and Timing of Surgery

Following injury to a nerve, the pathophysiologic events (wallerian degeneration)[18] that occur dictate the optimal time for successful nerve repair surgery. Phagocytosis of necrotic axonal debris distal to the injury and initial sprouting of axons from the proximal nerve stump occur within 1 to 2 months. Then the distal endoneurial tubules (basal lamina and Schwann cells),[62] if not recannulated by new axons, begin to atrophy sequentially and are obliterated by scar tissue. End-organ receptors in the skin or mucosa degenerate

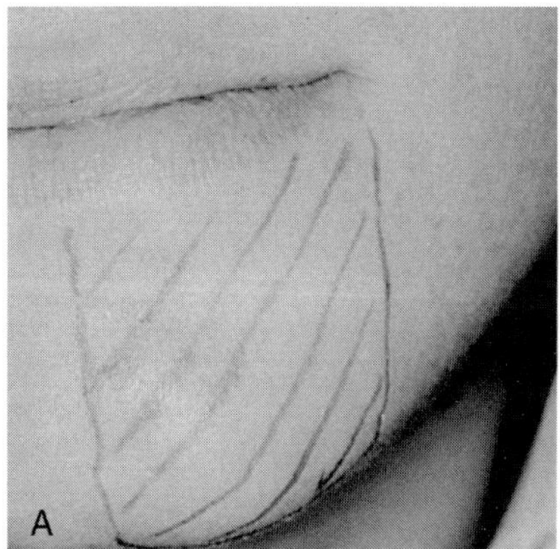

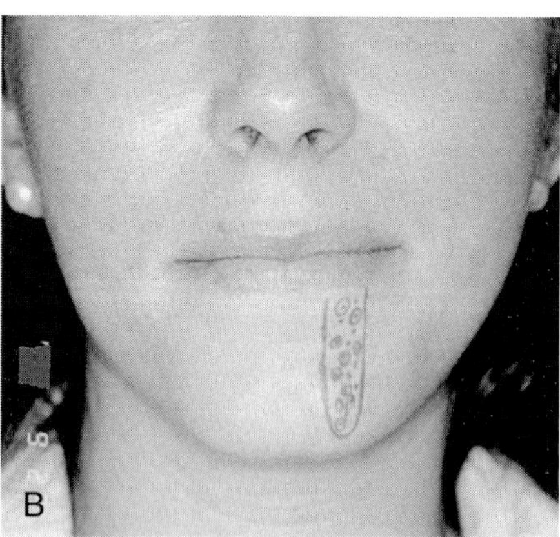

Figure 6–4. *A,* Area of total anesthesia in patient 1 week after bilateral mandibular sagittal split ramus osteotomies. *B,* Same patient 8 weeks after surgery. Note the decrease in the area of altered sensation. Responses to both pinprick *(dots)* and static light touch *(circles)* had returned.

and lose their ability to receive new axons also.[63] Once this process is complete, axons can no longer be guided to end-organ receptors, and all potential for recovery is lost. It is difficult to determine in humans exactly when surgical repair of nerve injuries becomes impossible. Sunderland[64, 65] has estimated, however, that 75% to 90% of the distal nerve will have atrophied and become irreparable if axonal invasion (neuralization) has not occurred by *1 year.*

Girard[1] has speculated that the inferior alveolar nerve could continue to have potential for recovery from injury for as much as 2 years. Anecdotal reports of late recovery of sensation after inferior alveolar or lingual nerve injury[2, 3] have not provided the objective documentation needed to assess their validity.[66] Blackburn and Bramley,[30] in a study of 1,117 patients whose lower third molars were removed, found an 11% incidence of lingual nerve dysfunction, with 0.5% of cases permanent. No patient experienced full recovery of lingual sensation later than 36 weeks after surgery. Kipp and associates[33] determined, in an analysis of mandibular third molar removals in 1,377 patients, that no sensory abnormality of the inferior alveolar nerve that persisted beyond 6 months resolved completely.[33] I have followed 23 patients with initial total anesthesia secondary to injury of the inferior alveolar or lingual nerve, all of whom refused surgical treatment but agreed to be followed for sequential neurosensory evaluation for at least 2 years.[67, 68] *None* of those patients, who remained totally anesthetic to objective clinical testing and had no subjective symptoms of early recovery (tingling, itching, crawling sensations, etc.) at *12 weeks* after injury, went on to experience significant spontaneous recovery of sensory function. In a prospective study of 1,107 cases of dentoalveolar surgery, patients who sustained only minor inferior alveolar or lingual nerve injury experienced complete spontaneous recovery by the third or fourth postoperative month.[37]

Donoff and Colin[60] have observed generally less persistent sensory dysfunction in inferior alveolar nerve injuries than in lingual nerve injuries. Anatomic factors as well as timing may have an impact on the spontaneous healing of nerve injuries. For example, the inferior alveolar nerve resides in a bony canal,[69] which may serve as a guide for regenerating axons and a barrier to ingrowth of scar tissue across the area of injury from the periphery. The lingual nerve, on the other hand, coursing through soft tissues medial to the mandible, enjoys no such protection.[70] These considerations of anatomy and pathophysiology have prompted experienced microneurosurgeons to explore promptly all sensory nerve injuries exhibiting total anesthesia that persist beyond 3 months.[7, 14, 71] Further delay in the presence of lack of spontaneous recovery reduces the likelihood of successful surgical intervention.

Surgical Techniques

Nerve injuries are described clinically as "open" or "closed." Open injuries are observed directly by the surgeon at the time they occur. Closed injuries may or may not be suspected, and they are not visualized at the time of their occurrence.

Open Injuries

Open injuries are best managed by tension-free, *immediate primary* repair.[62, 72] Examples are intentional sacrifice of the inferior alveolar or lingual nerve during excision of a tumor and immediate repair by autogenous nerve grafting,[73, 74] and unintentional severance of the inferior alveolar nerve during a sagittal split mandibular ramus osteotomy with immediate suturing of the nerve.[75] The patient may not be a candidate for immediate primary repair if (1) the physical status is compromised, (2) the wound is contaminated (e.g., missile injury) and there is risk of infection, or (3) a surgeon with microsurgical skills is not immediately available. Treatment can be delayed until conditions are optimal.

Delayed primary repair (up to 1 week after injury) or *early secondary repair* (after appearance of scar tissue in the wound at 1 to 3 weeks) provides restoration of function as good as that following immediate primary repair.[76] Although retracted nerve stumps, scar tissue, and neuroma formation add to technical difficulty of secondary repair, thickening of the epineurium may make suturing easier.[62] In crushing, stretching, or chemical burn injuries (e.g., toxic root canal filling materials), it may be prudent to intentionally delay repair

Table 6–4. Indications for and Contraindications to Microneurosurgery

Indications
Observed nerve severance
Total anesthesia beyond 3 months
Dysesthesia beyond 4 months
Severe hypoesthesia without improvement beyond 4 months
Contraindications
Central neuropathic pain
Dysesthesia not abolished by local anesthetic nerve block
Improving sensation
Sensory deficit acceptable to the patient
Metabolic neuropathy
Medically compromised patient
"Excessive" delay after injury

in order to be able to better identify the demarcation between normal and injured nerve tissues.[62]

Closed Injuries

Closed injuries are followed expectantly with repeated examinations every 4 weeks. Injuries that produce significant unacceptable loss of sensation, painful or unpleasant sensation, or interference with normal function should receive exploration and microsurgical repair according to the guidelines listed in Table 6–4, which also lists situations in which surgical intervention may be contraindicated. Although "excessive delay" (greater than 1 year) between the time of a nerve injury and its surgical repair is a relative contraindication,[77, 78] exploration beyond that time occasionally reveals viable distal nerve tissue whose repair may restore significant sensory function.[79]

Microneurosurgery

The technical requirements and surgical principles applicable to repair of injuries of the peripheral branches of the trigeminal nerve are controlled general anesthesia, visualization and magnification of the surgical field, good hemostasis, removal of pathologic tissue or foreign material, proper alignment and coaptation of proximal and distal nerve stumps, and suturing without tension.[13, 14, 62, 72, 80, 81]

Microsurgical operations upon the injured nerve are performed using general endotracheal anesthesia in the operating room. The patient must remain motionless during the lengthy surgical procedure, and sterile conditions reduce the incidence of infection. Head elevation, control of blood pressure, and injection of local anesthetic containing epinephrine minimize capillary oozing.

The inferior alveolar nerve is exposed by either a transoral (Fig. 6–5) or a submandibular (Fig. 6–6) approach, depending on the location and circumstances (intentional or unintentional) of the injury and the experience and preference of the surgeon.[10] The mental nerve is approached by a buccal sulcus incision (Fig. 6–7),[14] whereas the lingual nerve is operated through an incision around the lingual aspects of the premolar and molars that extends posteriorly along the superior border of the ascending mandibular ramus (Fig. 6–8).[82] The infraorbital nerve is visualized through intraoral (maxillary labiobuccal vestibule) or external (subciliary, transconjunctival) incisions (Fig. 6–9).[83] An external approach provides better access to the inferior orbital canal, whereas exposure of the nerve distal to the infra-

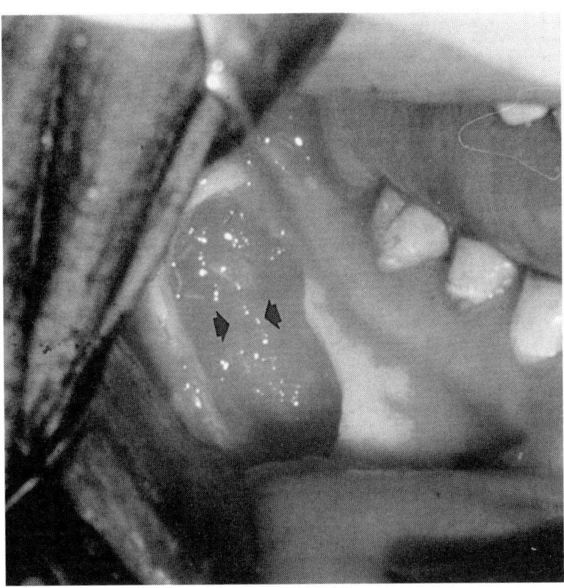

Figure 6–5. Transoral exposure of the inferior alveolar nerve *(arrows)* by removal of overlying buccal cortical mandibular bone. (*From* Meyer RA: Applications of microneurosurgery to the repair of trigeminal nerve injuries. Oral Maxillofac Surg Clin North Am 1992;4:405–416.)

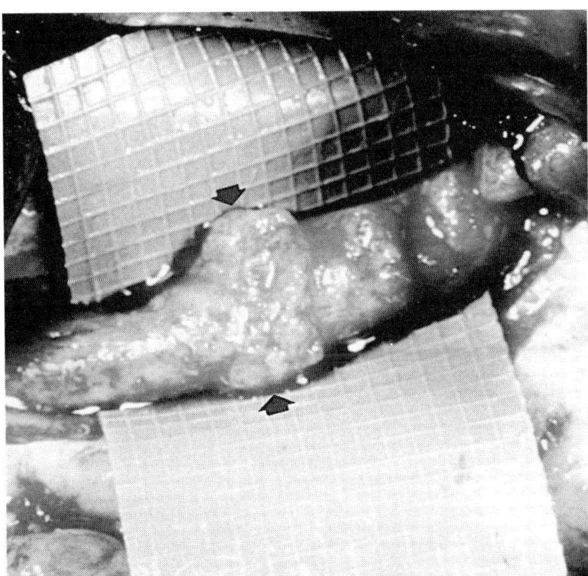

Figure 6–6. Submandibular approach to the inferior alveolar nerve. Note neuroma-in-continuity *(arrows)*. In the posterior portion of the inferior alveolar canal, access to the nerve through a submandibular incision is often better than that possible by an intraoral approach.

orbital foramen is difficult through a transconjunctival incision.

Visualization is enhanced by appropriate retraction of surrounding tissues and stabilization of nerve ends by an assistant surgeon. Magnification of the nerve (generally 1.0 to 2.5 cm in diameter) is provided by surgical loupes and by the operating microscope. Custom-made loupes of 2 to 5 power are useful in isolating and dissecting the nerve from surrounding tissues, in débridement, and in placing sutures intraorally, where access for the microscope may be compromised. Microscopic magnification facilitates dissection within the nerve and placement of sutures.

Once the nerve is exposed, impinging scar tissue, bone, or foreign material is removed (external decompression) (Fig. 6–10). The epineurium may be opened and interfascicular scarring relieved (internal neurolysis) (Fig. 6–11). Careful technique and control of bleeding are important, or neurolysis may cause increase in the scar tissue it seeks to remove.[84, 85] Internal inspection of the nerve, however, is also necessary to detect neuromas or discontinuity of individual fascicles. When neuromas are excised, the existing pathology or its removal may create a discontinuity defect. If so, the proximal and distal nerve ends are assessed, and serial 1-mm sections are removed, as indicated, until viable fascicles are visualized or identified on frozen sections.[86] The nerve stumps are fully mobilized and advanced, if possible, to close any gap. Preexisting gaps of 1 to 1.5 cm can often be closed in the lingual nerve (Fig. 6–12), but seldom in the infraorbital, mental, or inferior alveolar nerves. The coapted nerve ends are secured with tension-free sutures (neurorrhaphy) of fine (8-0, 10-0), nonreactive material.[87–89] Sutures are generally placed through the epineurium only.[14] Because the inferior alveolar, mental, lingual, and infraor-

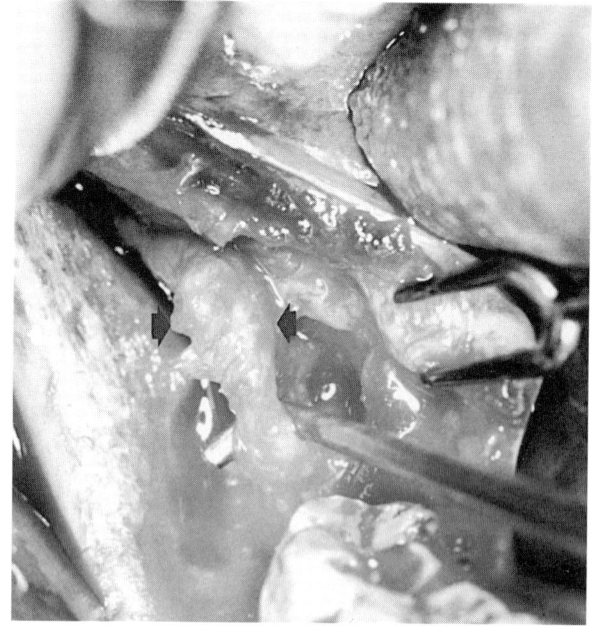

Figure 6–8. Exposure of lingual nerve *(arrows)* lying adjacent to site of previously removed mandibular third molar.

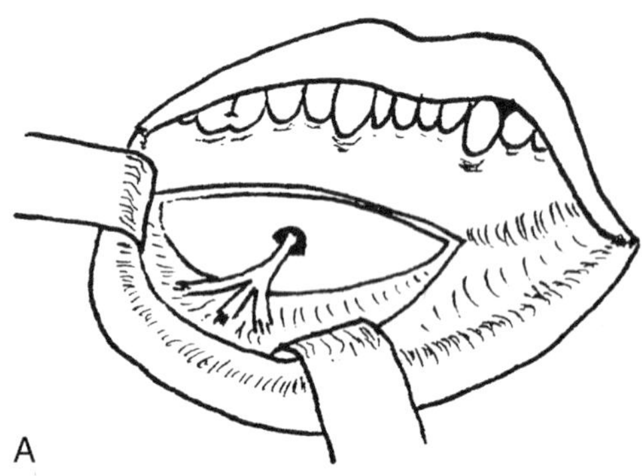

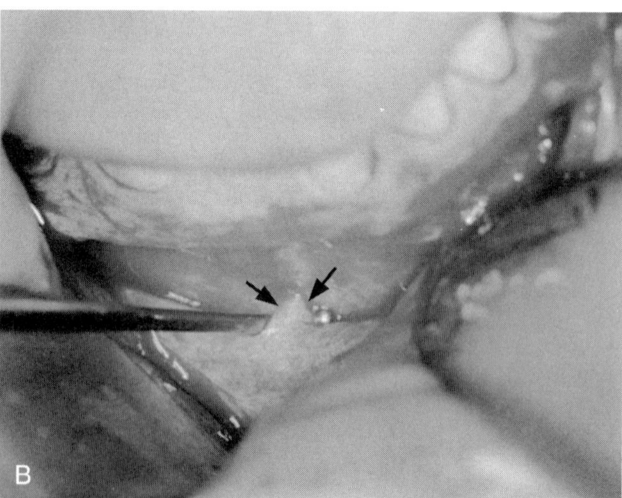

Figure 6–7. *A,* The right mental nerve is exposed by an incision in the mandibular labiobuccal sulcus. After it exits the mental foramen, the nerve normally divides into three branches as it enters the labial soft tissue. *B,* The mental nerve is surrounded by dense scar tissue *(arrows).*

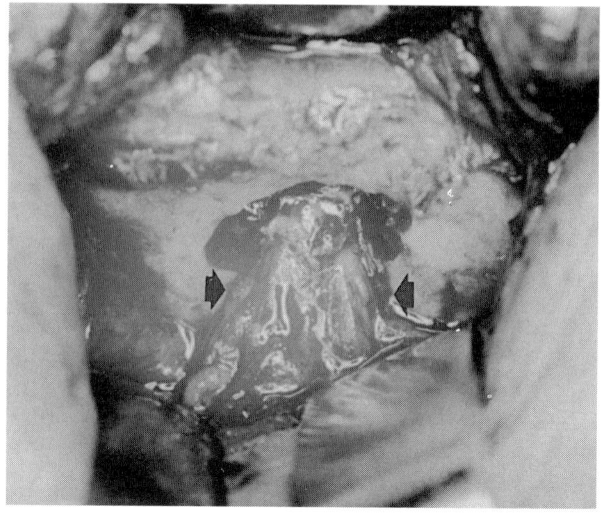

Figure 6–9. Subciliary approach to infraorbital nerve *(arrows).* Nerve is surrounded by scar tissue in area of previous inferior orbital rim fracture.

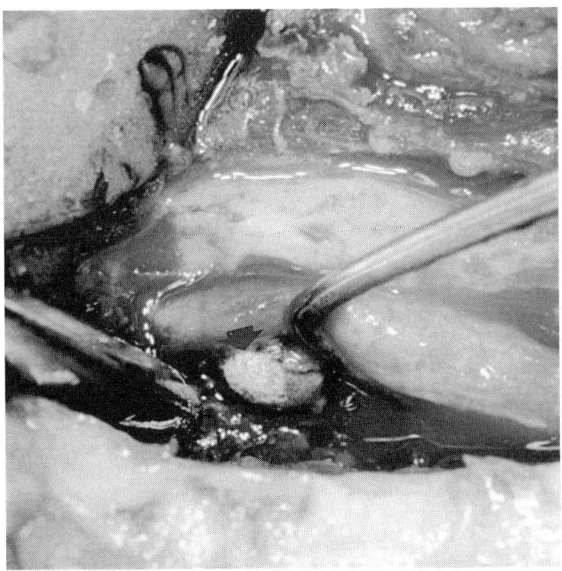

Figure 6–10. External decompression procedure: The inferior alveolar nerve is exposed for relocation away from an impinging osseointegrated dental implant *(arrow).*

bital nerves are purely sensory and polyfascicular, perineural suturing provides no special advantages.[90]

Tension across the suture line of greater than 25 g produces a "stretching effect" that is detrimental to successful nerve regeneration.[81, 91] An autogenous *nerve graft* interposed between the nerve stumps eliminates tension and facilitates healing potential equal to that of a tension-free neurorrhaphy.[26, 80] The great auricular (neck) and sural (lower extremity) nerves are common donors (Fig. 6–13).[92–95] The medial antebrachial cutaneous nerve (forearm) is also advocated.[72, 96]

Nerve sharing offers several approaches to special clinical challenges in microneurosurgery. For example, a sural nerve graft can be used to unite the greater auricular nerve with the visible distal stump of the inferior alveolar[97] or mental[98] nerve when the injured nerve's proximal stump is excessively atrophied or inaccessible. Haschemi[99] achieved primary repair of an unexpected loss of a 1-cm segment of the inferior alveolar nerve during excision of a large dentigerous cyst by rotating a pedicle graft from a portion of the ipsilateral lingual nerve. An autogenous crossover graft can be used to unite the distal stump of irreparable infraorbital nerve with the contralateral infraorbital nerve.[83]

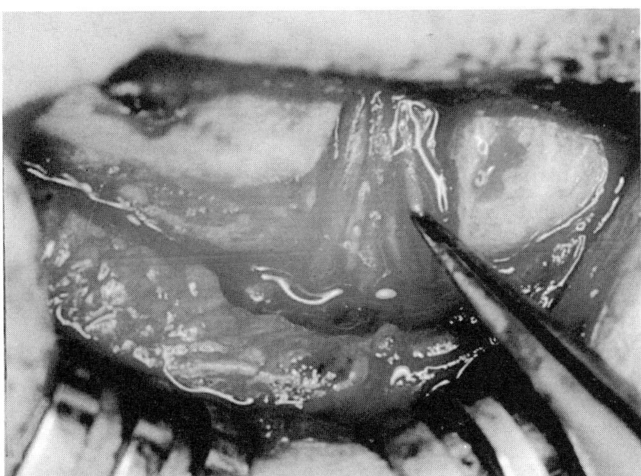

Figure 6–11. Internal neurolysis procedure has been done to remove scar tissue and separate multiple fascicles in an infraorbital nerve injured by an inferior orbital rim fracture.

Planned *repositioning* of the inferior alveolar or mental nerves is helpful in preventing injury when operations (dental implants, fixation screws, alloplastic augmentation) might otherwise place the nerve in jeopardy (Fig. 6–14).[46, 100–102]

Short-span (1 to 3 cm) nerve gaps may be repaired without autogenous nerve grafting by the technique of *guided nerve regeneration.*[103] Axonal growth is directed across the discontinuity by a tube made of alloplastic materials (polytetrafluoroethylene,[104] polyglycolic acid,[105] collagen with laminin gel)[106, 107] or autogenous tissue (vein graft),[108, 109] which prevents ingrowth of scar tissue (Fig. 6–15).

Results of Surgery

The immediate postoperative effect of microneurosurgery is anesthesia of the distribution of the operated nerve. Estimates of the rate of growth of regenerating axons have been given as 0.5 to 3.0 mm per day[110] after necrotic axonal material has been cleared by phagocytosis from the distal endoneurial tubules. For example, the distance from an injury of the inferior alveolar nerve in the third molar region of the mandible to the lower lip midline is about 90 mm. Therefore, one might expect the first symptoms of sensory recovery, correlating with reconnection of regenerating axons with sensory receptor endplates in the lip, at between 1.5 and 6 months, with a mean of about 3 months. Typically, this onset is followed by spontaneous and evoked sensation (abnormal, unpleasant, or painful) for several more months, while the new axons slowly reform their myelin sheath and impulse conduction speed is less than normal (Fig. 6–16). As maturation of axons progresses (increase in diameter and myelination) and conduction speed increases, abnormal sensations decrease in intensity and frequency and anesthesia to stimuli is replaced by progressively lessened hypoesthesia until the process is completed by about 1 year.[64] Patients better tolerate the long and often bothersome period of recovery if they are informed about it beforehand.[14]

Early reports of microsurgical repair of mandibular nerve injuries claimed highly successful results. In one series of lingual nerve injuries, "complete return of sensation" was reported for 13 of 18 patients operated within 9 months, although 5 patients operated beyond 8 months experienced only partial recovery.[79] In another report of 23 patients, "full recovery" of sensory function was experienced by all patients whose microsurgical repair of the inferior alveolar nerve was done within 12 months of injury, but in only 57% of those patients whose operations were done after more than

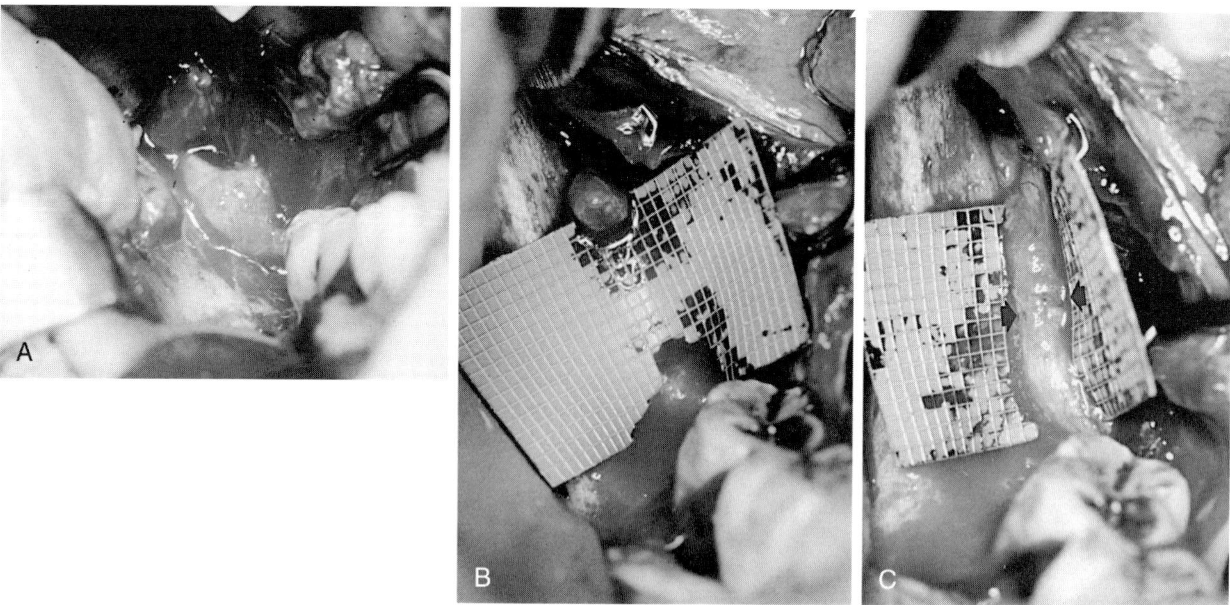

Figure 6–12. *A*, Neuroma-in-continuity of the lingual nerve. *B*, Neuroma excised and nerve stumps prepared for suturing. *C*, Proximal and distal nerve stumps mobilized, advanced to approximation without tension, and repaired with 8-0 nylon epineural sutures *(arrows)*. (*From* Meyer RA: Applications of microneurosurgery to the repair of trigeminal nerve injuries. Oral Maxillofac Surg Clin North Am 1992;4:405–416.)

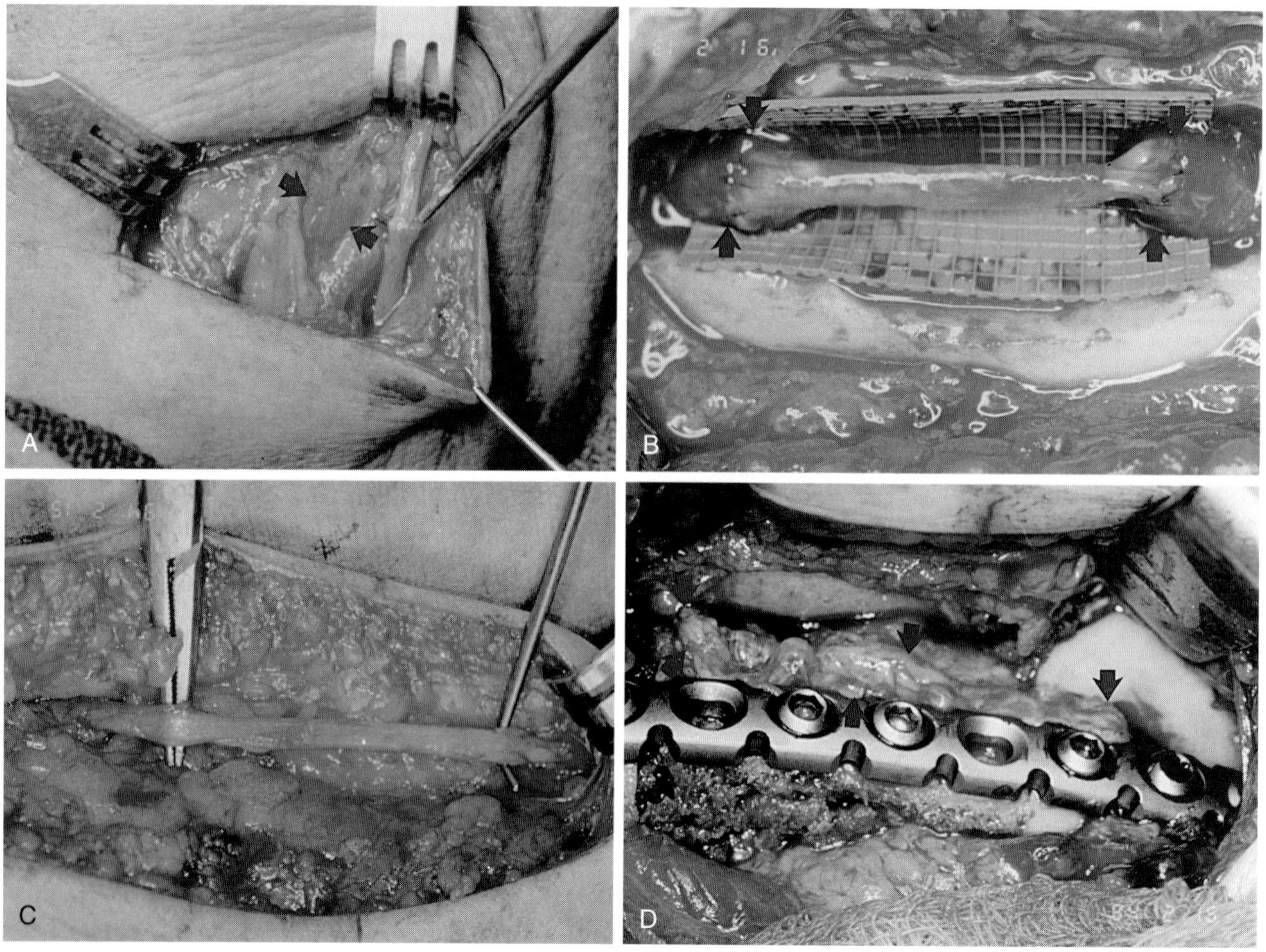

Figure 6–13. Autogenous nerve grafting. *A*, Great auricular nerve (cradled in nerve hook) located posterior to external jugular vein *(arrows)*. *B*, Graft of 2.0 cm has been placed *(arrows)* to reconstruct the inferior alveolar nerve. *C*, Sural nerve exposed superior to lateral malleolus. *D*, Graft of sufficient length can be taken to reconstruct any nerve defect in the maxillofacial region. Sural nerve *(arrows)* has been used to reconstruct 9-cm defect in inferior alveolar nerve following resection of mandible for ameloblastoma and replacement with autogenous bone graft.

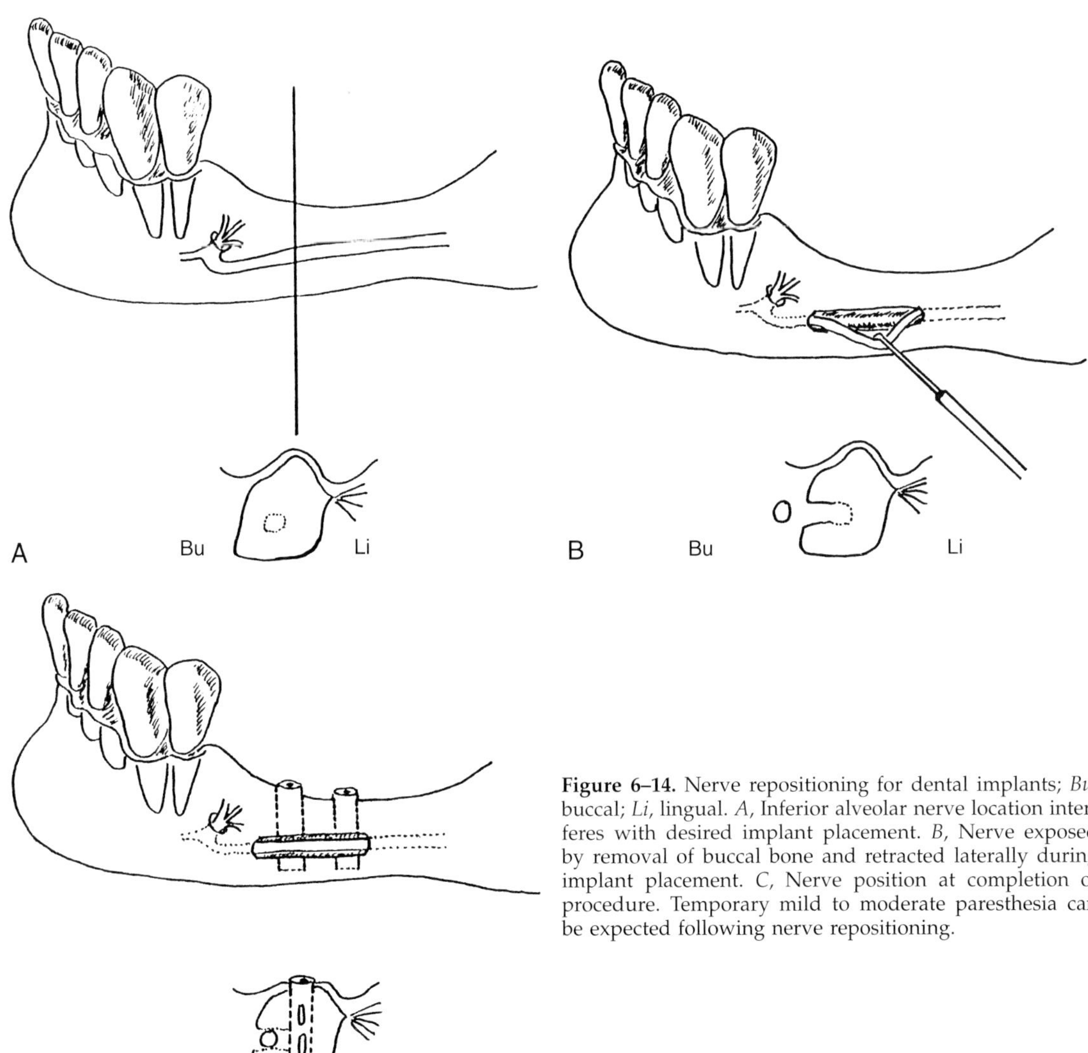

Figure 6–14. Nerve repositioning for dental implants; *Bu*, buccal; *Li*, lingual. *A*, Inferior alveolar nerve location interferes with desired implant placement. *B*, Nerve exposed by removal of buccal bone and retracted laterally during implant placement. *C*, Nerve position at completion of procedure. Temporary mild to moderate paresthesia can be expected following nerve repositioning.

1 year.[78] Six of 7 patients had complete return of sensation, and 1 patient had partial sensory recovery following repair of infraorbital nerve injuries at up to 12 months after injury.[77] Unfortunately, the methods of evaluating neurosensory function were not described in these reports.

In a study of seven patients who required microsurgical repair of severed lingual nerves, documentation by neurosensory testing revealed significant improvement in tongue sensation 1 year or longer after the surgery. Patients' assessment of gustatory function did not, however, correlate well with objective results of testing of taste sensation.[111] Donoff and Colin[60] analyzed results of repair of 30 lingual and 14 inferior alveolar nerve injuries. Restoration of sensory function was more likely (77%) than relief of pain (42%) in the lingual nerve injuries. All but one of the inferior alveolar nerve injuries were primarily painful, and 77% improved after surgery. The timing of surgery did not correlate well with pain relief, but early surgical intervention (by 6 months) had a positive association with improved sensation.

In a series of 308 nerve injury patients (339 nerves) I treated,[15] 80% to 90% of those operated for anesthesia within 6 months of injury gained improved sensation, but only 10% of those operated beyond 1 year were judged to be better (Fig. 6–17). All patients were evaluated by standard neurosensory tests before and after microneurosurgery and were followed for at least 1 year postoperatively.[15] A retrospective, multi-institutional study of the surgical repair of inferior alveolar and lingual nerve injuries in 521 patients reported an overall success rate of 76.2%. There was no significant difference in success of restoring lost sensation in either nerve (85.4% for inferior alveolar nerves, 87.0% for lingual nerves). Relief of pain, however, was more likely to occur following lingual nerve repair (67.5%), than after inferior alveolar nerve repair (55.6%).[9]

Patients with painful nerve injuries are different from patients whose principal complaint is lost sensation. Painful nerve injury patients generally do poorly if their injuries are repaired more than 12 months after injury.[67] In fact, there is a rapid decline in success rate after 9 months (Fig. 6–18). Gregg's[112] analysis of pa-

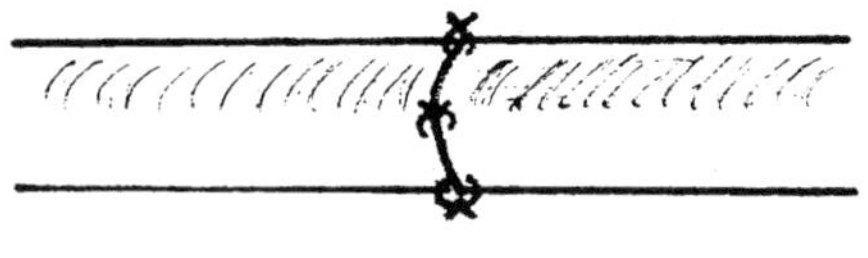

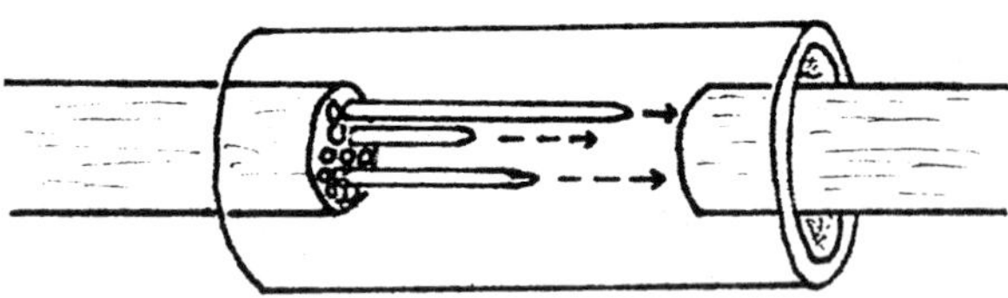

Figure 6–15. *A,* An alloplastic or autogenous "guide" can be used to bridge short-span gap (1.0 to 3.0 cm) between nerve stumps. *B,* Autogenous graft taken from the external jugular vein has been sutured to the proximal and distal ends of a discontinuity defect of the inferior alveolar nerve *(arrows)* resulting from a gunshot wound four months previously.

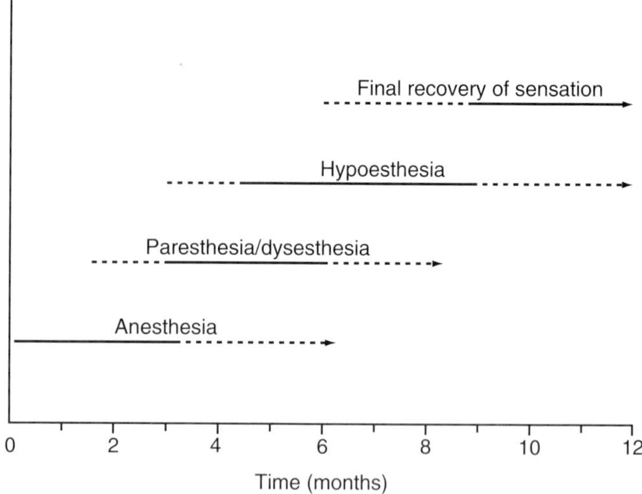

Figure 6–16. Process of recovery over time following microsurgical repair of sensory nerve injuries.

tients with painful trigeminal nerve injuries identified four subtypes: Pain relief was poor following microsurgical repair for *anesthesia dolorosa* (only 14.6% of patients improved) and *sympathetically mediated pain* (20.7%), whereas patients with *hyperalgesia* (60.5%) and *hyperpathia* (56.3%) gained far more improvement after surgery. The pathophysiology of such injuries is complex and may involve input from peripheral neuromas, somatic and autonomic collateralization, and central deafferentation.[93, 113, 114, 115] Psychological factors such as neuroticism and depression may contribute to difficulty in assessing and managing the painful nerve injury patient.[115] Results of local anesthetic blocks of the injured peripheral nerve correlate well with prospects for pain relief from microsurgical repair of trigeminal nerve injuries.[67, 112]

The general consensus gained from reviewing results of microsurgery of the peripheral branches of the trigeminal nerve is that nerve continuity can be reestablished, responses to neurosensory testing are improved, and painful sensations are reduced or relieved with timely and technically skilled surgery.[116]

Patients often continue to complain of subjective feelings of "numbness" despite normal or nearly normal responses to neurosensory testing.[14, 116] New connections created at the repaired area of the nerve, varying velocities of impulse transmission, and arrival of impulses at different locations within the central nervous

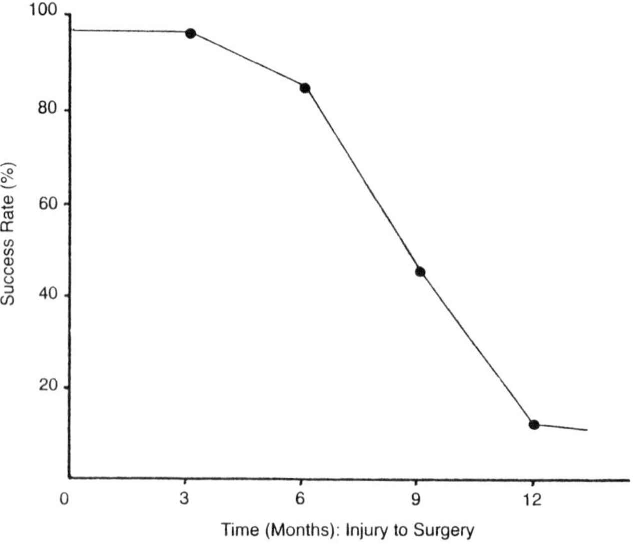

Figure 6–17. Comparison of favorable outcome (improved or recovered) of microsurgical repair of injuries causing loss of sensation of the inferior alveolar, lingual, mental, or supraorbital nerves with the time from injury to surgery. Best results (80% to 90%) occur when repair is done within 6 months of injury for correction of anesthesia. (*From* Meyer RA: Applications of microneurosurgery to the repair of trigeminal nerve injuries. Oral Maxillofac Surg Clin North Am 1992;4:405–416.)

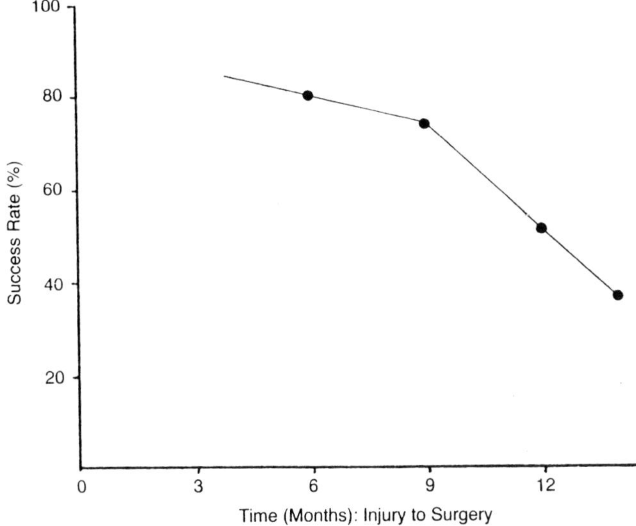

Figure 6–18. Comparison of success rate for microsurgical repair of painful injuries of the inferior alveolar, lingual, mental, or infraorbital nerve with the time from injury to surgery. Best results (reduced or relieved pain) are achieved when surgical repair is performed within 9 months of injury. (*From* Meyer RA: Applications of microneurosurgery to the repair of trigeminal nerve injuries. Oral Maxillofac Surg Clin North Am 1992;4:405–416.)

system create a "scrambling" effect, consisting of distorted recognition of position sense as well as difficulty with localization of stimulus (synesthesia) and assessment of quality and intensity of stimulus.[117] Resolution requires a learning process, which is assisted by a regimen of sensory exercises *(sensory reeducation)*,[118] originally devised for hand-injured patients,[119] that should be initiated as soon as the patient begins to perceive any sensation. Alternating massage or stimulation of the contralateral normal side and the affected area is done with various textures (finger, cotton swab, bobby pin). These maneuvers can also be accomplished during normal activities such as toothbrushing, washing, shaving, and applying makeup or lipstick. Hypersensitive areas should not be avoided, although their stimulation may be unpleasant at first. Sensory exercises should be repeated several times daily and continued for 6 to 12 months. Repetition helps the central nervous system to learn new, more acceptable responses to stimuli arriving by connections newly created by the nerve repair.

Painful or other abnormal sensations and impaired function may persist despite technically excellent surgical repair or improvement in responses to neurosensory testing.[120] Serious interference with the performance of everyday activities, relationships, and employment may develop. Management with medications (antidepressants, anticonvulsants, antineuralgics, local anesthetics), psychological counseling, psychotherapy or behavior modification programs, physical therapy, transcutaneous electrical nerve stimulation (TENS), acupuncture, or a global approach by a multidisciplinary pain clinic may be helpful for these unfortunate patients.[121–123]

Prognosis

The potential for spontaneous recovery of a nerve injury is most closely related to the type of injury that created the conditions from which the nerve must attempt recovery. Types of injuries are severance (partial or complete), avulsion, stretching, pressure (compression, crush), and burns (chemical, thermal). Tyndall and colleagues[124] studied crushing and severance (with passive approximation) injuries of the infraorbital nerve. Spontaneous regeneration of axons and return of sensory function were more nearly complete after crushing injury. Spontaneous recovery is probably least likely with a stretching, avulsion, or burn injury, because a segment of nerve undergoes ischemic necrosis or is lost or coagulated by heat or toxic chemicals, respectively, leaving that segment as a scarred barrier to advancing axons (Table 6–5).

Factors important in recovery after microsurgical repair of a nerve injury are the age of the patient, the technical quality of the operation, and the time lapse between the injury and its surgical repair.[14, 62, 72, 80] Young patients have fewer systemic illnesses (vascular disease, diabetes mellitus) that interfere with normal tissue healing than the elderly. Nerves that are approximated surgically with a high degree of accuracy, minimal tissue trauma, and lack of tension have the best chance to heal favorably. The time from injury to repair is critical, because the distal nerve becomes progressively replaced with scar tissue and loses its ability to receive advancing axons from the proximal nerve stump. The clinical studies previously discussed have repeatedly emphasized the importance of timely surgical intervention and serve to validate Seddon's[6] comment made in 1947: "If a purely expectant policy is pursued, the most favorable time for operative intervention will always be missed."

Facial Nerve Injuries

Weakness *(paresis)* or total flaccidity *(paralysis)* of facial muscles is a feared functional and aesthetic complication of operations performed near peripheral branches of the facial nerve. Altered motor function of the lips, cheeks, forehead, and eyelids produces significant problems for the affected patient.[125] Loss of protection for the cornea of the eye can lead to pain, infection, and reduced visual acuity. Loss of motor control of the lips and cheeks makes the drinking of fluids and mastication of food difficult or clumsy. Fa-

Table 6–5. Nerve Injuries: Spontaneous Healing Potential

Type of Injury	Prognosis
Pressure (compression, crush)	Best
Severance	↓
Stretch	↓
Avulsion or burns	Worst

cial expression becomes asymmetric (if the injury is unilateral) and is socially embarrassing for the sensitive patient (Fig. 6–19).

Surgical situations in which the facial nerve is known to be at risk for injury include facial trauma (lacerations and fractures),[126, 127] orthognathic surgery,[128, 129] temporomandibular joint (TMJ) arthrotomy[130–135] and arthroscopy,[136, 137] parotid gland surgery,[138, 139] and facial aesthetic surgery.[140, 141] The incidence of such injuries, according to various reports, ranges from 1% to as high as 55% for TMJ surgery.[130] Most injuries, however, produce only temporary motor dysfunction that resolves within 6 months.[134] Exact data are difficult to establish, but the overall risk of permanent motor deficit from facial nerve injury during surgical procedures (excluding those in which the nerve must be intentionally sacrificed) is probably much less than 1%. Nonetheless, presentation of such risk should be included in an informed consent discussion with the patient before elective surgery.

When a significant facial nerve injury does occur, the surgeon must be able to make an accurate assessment, establish a prognosis, and develop a rational plan of nonsurgical management or timely surgical intervention in order to maximize the patient's chance for a favorable outcome. Many of the principles of diagnosis and treatment of trigeminal nerve injuries discussed previously are directly applicable to the facial nerve and are not repeated in this discussion.

Surgical Anatomy

The extracranial portion of the facial nerve is particularly at risk for injury, because variability of its several branches[142] makes its exact location difficult to predict in individual patients. Many common surgical procedures are necessarily performed in close proximity to these branches.

The facial nerve leaves the cranium through the stylomastoid foramen. It courses inferolaterally forward through the retromandibular region, and bifurcates into *temporofacial* and *cervicofacial* divisions just posterior to the subcondylar portion of the mandible, usually within the substance of the parotid gland. Identification of the nerve is facilitated during parotid gland dissection by injecting a dye such as methylene blue into the Stensen duct before commencing surgery; the gland tissues are stained blue, but the nerve remains a glistening, translucent white structure. The main nerve trunk bifurcation has been variously reported to be 15.6 mm (range, 12 to 20 mm) inferior to the posterior aspect of the tragus of the ear (PAT)[135] or 23 mm (range, 15 to 28 mm) inferior to the lowest concavity of the bony external auditory canal (EAC).[143] The temporofacial division continues anterosuperiorly and is found at a mean distance of 22.5 mm (range, 16 to 29 mm) anterior to the PAT[136] or 20 mm (range, 8 to 35 mm) anterior to the anterior margin of the bony EAC[143] (Fig. 6–20). At this location, the facial nerve lies within the temporal fascia superficial to the periosteum of the zygomatic arch. The temporofacial division gives rise to the buccal, zygomatic, and temporal (frontal) branches, which supply muscles of the cheek and upper lip, eyelids, and forehead, respectively. These branches are at risk when dissections are carried too far inferiorly, contacting the temporofacial division, or anterosuperiorly (such as with a "hockey-stick" extension of the incision for TMJ arthrotomy), involving primarily the temporal branch. Although trocar puncture sites for introduction of an arthroscope into the TMJ are often placed in close contact with branches of the temporofacial division, branches of the nerve are

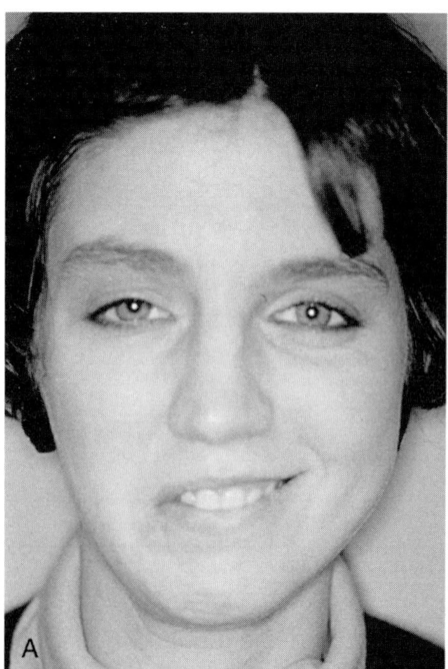

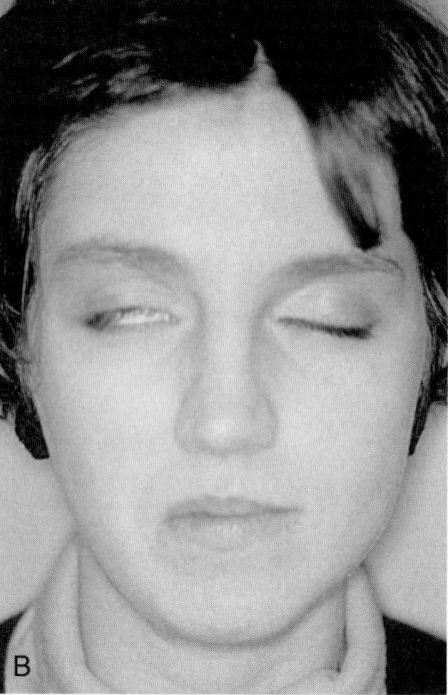

Figure 6–19. *A* and *B*, Persistent unilateral facial weakness 2 years after right facial nerve injury during a sagittal split osteotomy of the mandibular ramus. Uncontrollable bleeding posterior to the right mandibular angle required extensive dissection for control.

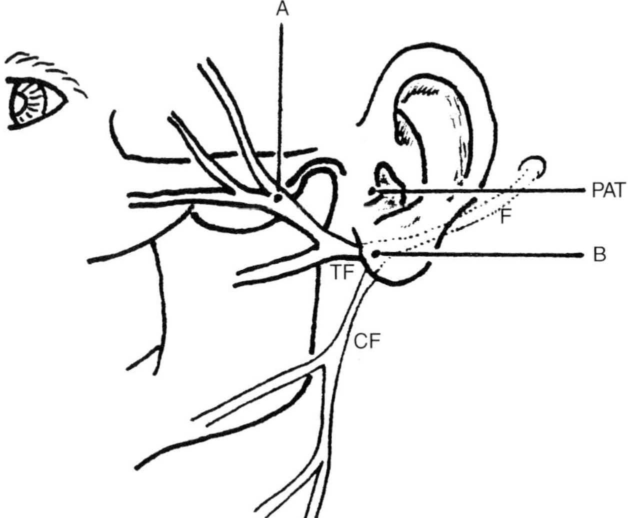

Figure 6–20. The extracranial facial nerve and its relationship to the posterior aspect of the tragus of the ear *(PAT)*. Distance from *PAT* to point *A* averages 22.5 mm; distance from PAT to point B averages 23 mm. The anteroposterior location of an incision to expose the temporomandibular joint and the inferior extent of that incision are limited by the location of the facial nerve. *F*, nerve trunk, facial nerve; *CF*, cervicofacial division; *TF*, temporofacial division.

most likely displaced rather than impaled by the trocar.[136]

The cervicofacial division proceeds forward, just lateral to the angle of the mandible, and divides into mandibular and cervical branches, which continue forward and inferiorly deep to the platysma muscle to supply the lower lip and cervical muscles, respectively. The mandibular branch may or may not dip below the angle of the mandible, but it generally is found just superior to a lymph node that overlies the facial artery and vein as they cross the inferior border of the mandible. Rather than a single nerve, the mandibular branch may consist of several discrete nerves that individually supply the depressor anguli oris, depressor labii inferioris, and mentalis muscles.[144] Incisions placed well below the inferior border (submandibular) or posterior to the angle (retromandibular) of the mandible should avoid direct contact with the mandibular branch. For an intraoral approach to the angle and ramus of the mandible, maintaining the integrity of the surrounding periosteum and pterygomasseteric sling should protect against direct injury of the facial nerve. Indirect injury from retraction of tissues, hematoma formation, extravasation of injected local anesthetic solutions, or compression by repositioned osteotomy or fracture segments are less easily avoided, but the resulting facial paresis is usually temporary.[129]

Evaluation

The patient who exhibits facial nerve dysfunction following surgery requires prompt evaluation. Local anesthetics injected during the operation to reduce bleeding or minimize early postoperative pain may, however, complicate the situation and necessitate delay in initiating assessment for several hours, until their effects have dissipated.

Examination of the patient reveals which facial areas have lost motor function. It is important to differentiate weakness (paresis) from total flaccidity (paralysis). The location of the injury can be surmised by inference from the associated surgical procedure and by observing whether a single branch, a major division, or the entire nerve is affected. The Facial Nerve Function Index (FNFI), devised by Peckitt and associates,[145, 146] is a method of measuring asymmetric facial movement. It is also useful for monitoring progress of returning facial nerve function after surgery.

Important documentation of the status of a facial nerve injury, its prognosis, and the best course of management is gained from electrodiagnostic testing (EDT), which evaluates peripheral nerve conduction and muscle electrical activity. EDT is used to determine whether (1) the affected nerve is completely or partially transected, (2) the injury is reversible, and (3) surgical intervention is indicated.[11] The Maximal Stimulability Test (MST) is applied to the affected nerve and measures the stimulus intensity required to elicit a muscle response.[147] Because of delayed onset of wallerian degeneration in the distal nerve, falsely normal MST results may persist for 72 to 96 hours after the injury.[148] Therefore, the MST is first given at 3 days after injury and repeated at 2- to 3-day intervals until full function returns or completely disappears. *Electromyography* (EMG)[149] is useful in distinguishing normal from denervated muscle and in determining the degree of muscle degeneration that has occurred following nerve injury. The presence of voluntary muscle action potentials is a strong indicator that the nerve has not been completely transected. Because a denervation pattern (i.e., fibrillation) does not appear for 14 to 21 days after injury, EMG results may be equivocal during that time.[11]

Facial nerve injuries are classified according to Seddon[6, 23] or Sunderland[24, 25] (see earlier), as previously discussed, but such classification may require serial evaluations during a transition period in closed injuries to assess recovery of function, if any. Neurapraxia resolves promptly with return of facial mobility in a few weeks. Axonotmesis exhibits prolonged weakness with gradual return of function after several months. Total and prolonged paralysis of affected facial musculature with little or no return of function is the usual fate of untreated neurotmesis.

Treatment and Prognosis

Open injuries of the facial nerve should be repaired as soon as possible.[11] As with trigeminal nerve injuries, immediate primary repair at the time of intentional or unintentional transection (neurotmesis) probably gives the best result, although delayed primary repair or early secondary repair are acceptable when delay is necessary for various reasons (contaminated wound, compromised medical status, extensive tissue destruction).[76] Because of progressive distal nerve degeneration and muscle atrophy, 12 months is often considered the time limit for successful facial nerve repair.[11] Good results have been reported, however, as late as 2 or 3 years after injury.[150]

The method of choice for surgical repair of the transected facial nerve is direct end-to-end coaption and suturing.[11] If there is loss of nerve that produces a gap between the proximal and distal stumps, autogenous nerve grafting is necessary. The hypoglossal nerve has been a very effective autogenous graft for facial nerve reconstruction.[151] The sural nerve is an alternative donor.[16] Crossover nerve grafting[151] from the contralateral side of the face may be the only option when the distal nerve stump alone is available, as in massive tissue loss from trauma (e.g., missile injury) or malignant tumor resection. A major disadvantage of the crossover nerve graft is the resulting uncoordinated movement (dyskinesia) of reinnervated muscles with loss of appropriate spontaneous facial expression.[11]

Factors influencing the results of extracranial facial nerve repair are the level of the injury, the prevailing biologic condition of the wound, and the technique of repair.[152] The more distal the injury, the better the functional result, because more axons are available from the proximal stump for reinnervation.[11] The amount of tissue damage or loss, scar tissue formation, vascular supply in the area of the repair, patient age, and general health have direct effects on wound (and nerve) healing.[62] As with trigeminal nerve injuries, the preparation of the nerve stumps, their coaptation without tension, and placement of a minimum number of small-diameter sutures to reduce reactive scar tissue are critical technical requirements of nerve repair.[11] Careful attention to prevention of disturbance of the nerve repair area during recovery from anesthesia and in the first few postoperative days is also important to successful nerve regeneration. Avoidance of talking and intake of solid food in the first 48 hours followed by minimal facial movement for the next 5 days is emphasized.[11]

Supportive postoperative care is important. Depending on which branch or branches of the facial nerve are involved, a tarsorrhaphy or eye patch and methylcellulose drops are provided when eyelid closure is inadequate to protect the cornea from injury. Application of heat to the face, massage of facial muscles, and attempted facial exercises are helpful in activating intact nerve fibers and maintaining muscle tone. Nerve stimulation does not increase axonal growth, but it may retard atrophy of facial muscles.[153] Electrodiagnostic studies are done serially until there is evidence of reinnervation. Once this has occurred, intensive physical therapy (facial muscle exercises, reeducation of facial muscles, and biofeedback) is begun to stimulate and facilitate coordinated movements of the facial muscles. Patients should be followed for at least 3 years, because facial muscle function continues to improve for at least that long.

Closed injuries are evaluated and observed expectantly, supported by electrodiagnostic testing. *Delayed onset* and incomplete loss of function (paresis) have the best prognosis for spontaneous recovery. Delayed onset of paresis that progresses to complete paralysis may still have a good prognosis for spontaneous partial or complete recovery of function.[154] Onset of edema in the nerve and surrounding tissues, rather than anatomic disruption of the nerve, may account for the delay in loss of function. If the injured nerve is not trapped in a closed (i.e., bony) space, this process may be reversible.

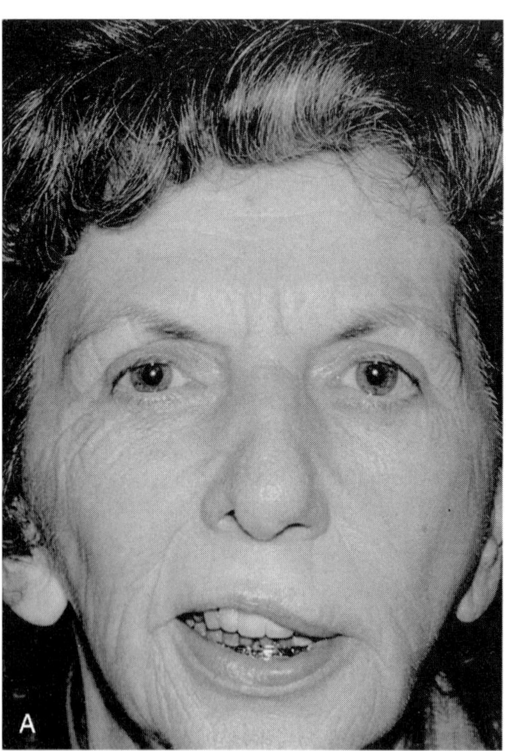

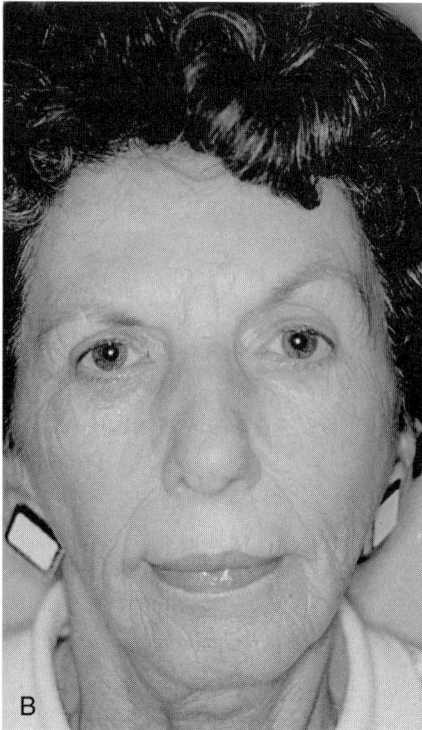

Figure 6–21. *A*, Patient with left forehead and upper lip weakness secondary to temporal branch of facial nerve injury after multiple temporomandibular joint procedures. *B*, Upper lip paresis resolved. Forehead lift procedure improved elevation of left eyebrow.

Steroids may be beneficial in such cases, although their efficacy had not been established. Immediate and complete facial paralysis carries the worst prognosis. The implication is, of course, that a complete transection of the nerve has taken place. This situation may be immediately known in an open surgical procedure but only inferred initially in a closed injury.

Of reassurance to the anxious clinician is information regarding closed injuries of the facial nerve associated with orthognathic[128, 155–161] and TMJ[130–134] surgery. Most such injuries were reported to have improved or resolved spontaneously within 8 months. Nonetheless, an aggressive approach should be taken. Patients are given appropriate supportive care, as discussed previously for postoperative facial nerve repair. Serial examination and electrodiagnostic testing are done. As soon as there is evidence of nerve discontinuity or muscle degeneration, surgical exploration is indicated. Although spontaneous recovery of facial muscle function has been reported after resection of the facial nerve during tumor surgery,[162] such return is unpredictable. Communication between the peripheral branches of the trigeminal and facial nerves may be involved.[163] The optimal time for nerve repair should not be lost to a vain hope of unlikely spontaneous recovery.

Patients seen with long-standing (i.e., more than 12 months) injuries may have distal nerve degeneration and muscle atrophy that preclude nerve repair procedures. Such patients might be candidates for muscle transfers, fascial slings, or facial elevation procedures (Fig. 6–21).[164, 165]

Conclusion

At present, the standard of care for the nerve-injured patient comprises recognition and evaluation of the neurologic deficit, supportive care, recommendations for microsurgical treatment if indicated, and appropriate timing of such treatment. The use of standardized neurologic testing should enable clinicians now and in the future to more thoroughly evaluate and categorize sensory or motor deficits in the nerve-injured patient and to compare and assess the results of microsurgical intervention.

Further refinements in technique, development of improved instrumentation, and the growth of microsurgical skills and experience in concert with ever-expanding knowledge of neurophysiology will extend the surgeon's capability to deal with the challenge of peripheral trigeminal and facial nerve injuries in the future.[166]

References

1. Girard KR: Considerations in the management of damage to the mandibular nerve. J Am Dent Assoc 1979;98:65.
2. Hayward JR: The triumphant trigeminal nerve [letter]. J Oral Maxillofac Surg 1986;44:2.
3. Lytle JJ: Etiology and indications for the management of impacted teeth. Oral Maxillofac Surg Clin North Am 1993;5:63.
4. Meyer RA: Indications for microneurosurgery [letter]. J Oral Maxillofac Surg 1986;44:758.
5. Meyer RA: Microneurosurgery: Current status in the repair of peripheral trigeminal nerve injuries. American Association of Oral and Maxillofacial Surgeons Annual Meeting, Boston, Oct 3, 1988 (Audiotapes W276-12 A & B, Garden Grove, CA, Info-Medix).
6. Seddon HJ: Nerve lesions complicating certain closed bone injuries. JAMA 1947;135:691.
7. Colin W, Conoff RB: Restoring sensation after trigeminal nerve injury: A review of current management. J Am Dent Assoc 1992;123:80.
8. Donoff RB, Guralnick WC: The application of microneurosurgery to oral-neurologic problems. J Oral Maxillofac Surg 1982;40:156.
9. La Banc JP, Gregg JM: Trigeminal nerve injuries: Basic problems, historical perspectives, early successes, and remaining challenges. Oral Maxillofac Surg Clin North Am 1992;4:277.
10. La Banc JP, Van Boven RW: Surgical management of inferior alveolar nerve injuries. Oral Maxillofac Surg Clin North Am 1992;4:425.
11. Lee KK, Terzis JK: Management of acute extratemporal nerve palsy. Clin Plast Surg 1984;11:203.
12. Merrill RG: Oral-neurosurgical procedures for nerve injuries. Transactions of the Third International Conference on Oral Surgery. London, E & S Livingstone, 1970, pp 131–140.
13. Merrill RG: Prevention, treatment and prognosis for nerve injury related to the difficult impaction. Dent Clin North Am 1979;23:471.
14. Meyer RA: Applications of microneurosurgery to the repair of trigeminal nerve injuries. Oral Maxillofac Surg Clin North Am 1992;4:405.
15. Meyer RA: Nerve injuries: Current concepts of management. Surgical Clinic, American Association of Oral and Maxillofacial Surgeons, Toronto, Canada, Sept 12, 1995.
16. Scaramella LF: On the repair of the injured facial nerve. Ear Nose Throat J 1979;58:45.
17. Sunderland S: Nerves and Nerve Injuries, ed. 2. Edinburgh, Churchill Livingstone, 1978, pp 31–60.
18. Young JZ: The functional repair of nervous tissue. Physiol Rev 1942;22:318.
19. Sunderland S: Some anatomical and pathophysiological data relative to facial nerve injury repair. *In* Fisch U (ed): Facial Nerve Surgery. Birmingham, AL, Aesculapius Publishing, 1977.
20. Svane TJ, Wolford LM, Milam SB, et al: Fascicular characteristics of the human inferior alveolar nerve. J Oral Maxillofac Surg 1986;44:431.
21. Lundborg G: The nerve trunk. *In* Lundborg G (ed): Nerve Injury and Repair. New York, Churchill Livingstone, 1988, p 65.
22. La Banc JP: Reconstructive microneurosurgery of the trigeminal nerve. *In* Bell WH (ed): Modern Practice in Orthognathic and Reconstructive Surgery, vol 2. Philadelphia, WB Saunders, 1992, p 1083.
23. Seddon HJ: Three types of nerve injury. Brain 1943;66:237.
24. Sunderland S: A classification of peripheral nerve injuries produced by loss of function. Brain 1951;74:491.
25. Sunderland S (ed): Nerve Injuries and Their Repair: A Critical Appraisal. New York, Churchill Livingstone, 1991, p 221.
26. Mackinnon SE, Dellon AL (eds): Surgery of the Peripheral Nerve. New York, Thieme, 1988, p 91.
27. Hegtvedt AK: Adaptation to mental nerve anesthesia [letter]. J Oral Maxillofac Surg 1990;48:1352.
28. Alling CC: Dysesthesia of the lingual and inferior alveolar nerves following third molar surgery. J Oral Maxillofac Surg 1986;44:454.
29. American Association of Oral and Maxillofacial Surgeons: Report of a workshop on the management of patients with third molar teeth. J Oral Maxillofac Surg 1994;52:1102.
30. Blackburn CW, Bramley PA: Lingual nerve damage associated with the removal of lower third molars. Br Dent J 1985;167:103.
31. Hochwald OP, Davis WH, Martinoff J: Modified distolingual splitting technique for removal of impacted mandibular third molars: Incidence of postoperative sequelae. Oral Surg 1983;56:9.
32. Howe GL, Poyton HG: Prevention of damage to the inferior dental nerve during the extraction of mandibular third molars. Br Dent J 1960;109:355.
33. Kipp DP, Goldstein BH, Weis WW Jr: Dysesthesia after mandib-

ular third molar surgery: A retrospective study and analysis of 1,377 surgical procedures. J Am Dent Assoc 1980;100:185.
34. Mason PA: Lingual nerve damage following lower third molar surgery. Int J Oral Maxillofac Surg 1988;17:290.
35. Middlehurst RJ, Barker GR, Rood JP: Postoperative morbidity with mandibular third molar surgery: A comparison of two techniques. J Oral Maxillofac Surg 1988;46:474.
36. Rud J: The split bone technique for removal of impacted mandibular third molars. J Oral Surg 1970;28:416.
37. Schultze-Mosgau S, Reich RH: Assessment of inferior alveolar and lingual nerve disturbances after dentoalveolar surgery and of recovery of sensitivity. Int J Oral Maxillofac Surg 1993;22:214.
38. Sisk AL, Hammer WB, Shelton DW, et al: Complications following removal of impacted third molars. J Oral Maxillofac Surg 1986;44:855.
39. Wofford DT, Miller RI: Prospective study of dysesthesia following odontectomy of impacted mandibular third molars. J Oral Maxillofac Surg 1987;45:855.
40. Zaytoun HS, Phillips C, Terry BC: Long term neurosensory deficits following transoral vertical ramus and sagittal split osteotomies for mandibular prognathism. J Oral Maxillofac Surg 1986;44:193.
41. Karas ND, Boyd SB, Sinn DP: Recovery of neurosensory function following orthognathic surgery. J Oral Maxillofac Surg 1990;48:124.
42. Nishioka GJ, Zysset MK, Van Sickels JE: Neurosensory disturbance with rigid fixation of the bilateral sagittal split osteotomy. J Oral Maxillofac Surg 1987;45:20.
43. Pansegrau KJ, Fridrich KL, Holton TJ: Neurosensory changes following bilateral sagittal split osteotomies. J Oral Maxillofac Surg 1993;51(suppl 3):145.
44. Bailey PH, Bays RA: Evaluation of long-term sensory changes following mandibular augmentation procedures. J Oral Maxillofac Surg 1984;42:722.
45. Campbell RL, Shamaskin RG, Harkins SW: Assessment of recovery from injury to inferior alveolar and mental nerves. Oral Surg 1989;64:519.
46. Haers PE, Sailer HF: Neurosensory function after lateralization of the inferior alveolar nerve and simultaneous insertion of implants. Oral Maxillofac Surg Clin North Am 1994;4:707.
47. Steinhauser E: Vestibuloplasty—skin grafts. J Oral Surg 1971;29:777.
48. Tornes K, Gilhuus-Moe OT: The surgical technique of vertical subcondylar osteotomy for correction of mandibular prognathism: A 10 year survey. Acta Odontol Scand 1987;45:203.
49. Ghali GE, Epker BN: Clinical neurosensory testing: Practical applications. J Oral Maxillofac Surg 1989;47:1074.
50. Zuniga JR, Essick GK: A contemporary approach to the clinical evaluation of trigeminal nerve injuries. Oral Maxillofac Surg Clin North Am 1992;4:353.
51. Henderson WR: Clinical assessment of peripheral nerve injuries: Tinel's test. Lancet 1948;2:801.
52. La Banc JP, Query-Herrera G: Quantitative static light touch and nociceptive examination: A prerequisite for microneurosurgery. J Oral Maxillofac Surg 1986;44:M10.
53. Robinson RC, Williams CW: Documentation method for inferior alveolar and lingual nerve paresthesias. Oral Surg 1986;62:128.
54. Barker GR, Bennett AJ, Wastell DG: Applications of trigeminal somatosensory evoked potentials (TSEPs) in oral and maxillofacial surgery. Br J Oral Maxillofac Surg 1987;25:308.
55. Godfrey RM, Mitchell KW: Somatosensory evoked potentials to electrical stimulation of the mental nerve. Br J Oral Maxillofac Surg 1987;25:300.
56. Pogrel MA: Trigeminal evoked potentials and electrophysiological assessment of the trigeminal nerve. Oral Maxillofac Surg Clin North Am 1992;4:535.
57. Dyck PJ, Schulty PW, O'Brien PC: Quantitation of touch-pressure sensation. Arch Neurol 1972;26:465.
58. Dyck PJ, Zimmerman IR, O'Brien PC, et al: Introduction of automated systems to evaluate touch-pressure, vibration, and thermal cutaneous sensation in man. Ann Neurol 1978;4:502.
59. Campbell RL: The role of nerve blocks in the diagnosis of traumatic neuralgia. Oral Maxillofac Clin North Am 1992;4:369.
60. Donoff RB, Colin W: Neurologic complications of oral and maxillofacial surgery. Oral Maxillofac Surg Clin North Am 1990;2:453.
61. Alling CC III, Schwartz E, Gregg JM, et al: Algorithm for diagnostic assessment and surgical treatment of traumatic trigeminal neuropathies and neuralgias. Oral Maxillofac Surg Clin North Am 1992;4:555.
62. Dellon AL: Wound healing in nerve. Clin Plast Surg 1990;17:545.
63. Dellon AL, Witebsky FG, Terrill RE: The denervated Meissner corpuscle: A sequential histologic study following nerve division in the rhesus monkey. Plast Reconstr Surg 1975;56:182.
64. Sunderland S: Nerves and Nerve Injuries, ed. 2. Edinburgh, Churchill Livingstone, 1978, p 366.
65. Sunderland S, Bradley DC: Denervation atrophy of the distal stump of a severed nerve. J Comp Neurol 1950;93:401.
66. Meyer RA: Complications of exodontia. *In* Waite DE (ed): Textbook of Practical Oral and Maxillofacial Surgery, ed. 3. Philadelphia, Lea & Febiger, 1987, pp 158–161.
67. Meyer RA: *Discussion of* Gregg JM: Studies of traumatic neuralgias in the maxillofacial region: Symptom complexes and response to microsurgery. J Oral Maxillofac Surg 1990;48:141.
68. Meyer RA: Protection of the lingual nerve during placement of rigid fixation after sagittal ramus osteotomy [letter]. J Oral Maxillofac Surg 1990;48:1135.
69. Carter RB, Keen EN: The intramandibular course of the inferior alveolar nerve. J Anat 1971;108:433.
70. Kiesselbach JE, Chamberlain JG: Clinical and anatomic observations on the relationship of the lingual nerve to the mandibular third molar region. J Oral Maxillofac Surg 1984;42:565.
71. Zuniga JR, La Banc JP: Advances in micro-surgical nerve repair. J Oral Maxillofac Surg 1993;51(suppl 1):62.
72. Dellon AL: Management of peripheral nerve injuries: Basic principles of microneurosurgical repair. Oral Maxillofac Surg Clin North Am 1992;4:393.
73. La Banc JP: Inferior alveolar nerve repair after treatment of benign cysts and tumors of the mandible. Oral Maxillofac Surg Clin North Am 1993;3:209.
74. Noma H, Kakizawa T, Yamane G, et al: Repair of the mandibular nerve by autogenous grafting after partial resection of the mandible. J Oral Maxillofac Surg 1986;44:31.
75. Wessberg GA, Epker BN: Transoral inferior alveolar neurorrhaphy via a sagittally split mandible. J Max-Fac Surg 1982;10:173.
76. Jabaley ME: Current concepts of nerve repair. Clin Plast Surg 1981;8:33.
77. Mozsary PG, Middleton RA: Microsurgical reconstruction of the infraorbital nerves. J Oral Maxillofac Surg 1983;41:697.
78. Mozsary PG, Syers CS: Microsurgical correction of the injured inferior alveolar nerve. J Oral Maxillofac Surg 1985;43:353.
79. Mozsary PG, Middleton RA: Microsurgical reconstruction of the lingual nerve. J Oral Maxillofac Surg 1984;42:415.
80. Mackinnon SE: Surgical management of the peripheral nerve gap. Clin Plast Surg 1989;16:587.
81. Millesi H: Interfascicular grafts for repair of peripheral nerves of the upper extremity. Orthop Clin North Am 1977;8:405.
82. Gregg JM: Surgical management of lingual nerve injuries. Oral Maxillofac Surg Clin North Am 1992;4:417.
83. Epker BN, Gregg JM: Surgical management of maxillary nerve injuries. Oral Maxillofac Surg Clin North Am 1992;4:439.
84. Gentili F, Hudson AR, Kline DG, et al: Morphological and physiological alteration following internal neurolysis of normal rat sciatic nerve. *In* Gorio A, Millesi H, Mingrino S, et al (eds): Posttraumatic Peripheral Nerve Repair. New York, Raven Press, 1981, pp 183–196.
85. Rydevik B, Lundborg G, Nordborg C: Intraneural tissue reaction induced by internal neurolysis. Scand J Plast Reconstr Surg 1976;10:3.
86. Wessberg GA, Wolford LM, Epker BN: Experiences with microsurgical reconstruction of the inferior alveolar nerve. J Oral Maxillofac Surg 1982;40:651.
87. Lee S, de Macedo AR, Hweidi SA, et al: Efficacy of polyglycolic acid (Dexon) microsutures in peripheral nerve anostomoses in the rat 2: Perineural suture. Microsurgery 1984;5:123.
88. Matras H, Dinges HP, Manioli B, et al: Non-sutured nerve transplantation. J Max-Fac Surg 1973;1:37.
89. Yamazaki Y, Noma H: Comparison of suture methods and materials in experimental inferior alveolar nerve grafting. J Oral Maxillofac Surg 1983;41:34.
90. Orgel MG: Epineurial versus perineurial repair of peripheral nerves. Clin Plast Surg 1984;11:101.

91. Terzis J, Faibisoff B, Williams HB: The nerve gap: Suture under tension vs graft. Plast Reconstr Surg 1975;56:166.
92. Eppley BL, Snyders RV Jr: Microanatomic analysis of the trigeminal nerve and potential nerve graft donor sites. J Oral Maxillofac Surg 1991;49:612.
93. Schultz JD, Dodson TB, Meyer RA: Donor site morbidity of greater auricular nerve graft harvesting. J Oral Maxillofac Surg 1992;50:803.
94. Wolford LM: Autogenous nerve graft repairs of the trigeminal nerve. Oral Maxillofac Surg Clin North Am 1992;4:447.
95. Woods DD, La Banc JP: Complications and morbidity associated with trigeminal nerve repairs. Oral Maxillofacial Surg Clin North Am 1992;4:473.
96. McCormick SU, Buchbinder D, McCormick SA, et al: Microanatomic analysis of the medial antebrachial nerve as a potential donor nerve in maxillofacial grafting. J Oral Maxillofac Surg 1994;52:1022.
97. La Banc JP, Epker BN, Jones DL, et al: Nerve sharing by an interpositional sural nerve graft between the great auricular and inferior alveolar nerve to restore lower lip sensation. J Oral Maxillofac Surg 1987;45:621.
98. Kaban LB, Upton J: Cross mental nerve graft for restoration of lip sensation after inferior alveolar nerve damage: case report. J Oral Maxillofac Surg 1986;44:649.
99. Haschemi A: Partial anastomosis between the lingual and mandibular nerves for restoration of sensibility in the mental nerve area after injury to the mandibular nerve. J Max-Fac Surg 1981;9:225.
100. Dario LJ, English R Jr: Achieving implant reconstruction through bilateral mandibular nerve repositioning. J Am Dent Assoc 1994;125:305.
101. Jensen O, Nock D: Inferior alveolar nerve repositioning in conjunction with placement of osseointegrated implants: A case report. Oral Surg 1987;63:263.
102. Meyer RA: Nerve injuries associated with dental implants. *In* Fagan MJ Jr (ed): Implant Prosthodontics. Chicago, Yearbook Medical, 1990, pp 313–330.
103. Seckel BR, Ryan SE, Gague RG, et al: Target-specific nerve regeneration through a nerve guide in the rat. Plast Reconstr Surg 1986;78:793.
104. Ruskin JD, Markin R, Davis LF: Evaluation of polytetrafluoroethylene (Gore-Tex) tubes for use as synthetic nerve grafts. American Association of Oral and Maxillofacial Surgeons, Poster Session, Annual Scientific Session, Anaheim, CA, Sept 18, 1987.
105. Mackinnon SE, Dellon AL: Clinical nerve reconstruction with a bioabsorbable polyglycolic acid tube. Plast Reconstr Surg 1990;85:419.
106. Colin W, Donoff RB: Nerve regeneration through collagen tubes. J Dent Res 1984;63:987.
107. Eppley BL, Delfino JJ: Collagen tube repair of the mandibular nerve: A preliminary investigation in the rat. J Oral Maxillofac Surg 1988;46:41.
108. Chiu DTW, Strauch B: A prospective clinical evaluation of autogenous vein grafts used as a nerve conduit for distal sensory nerve defects of 3 cm or less. Plast Reconstr Surg 1990;86:928.
109. Walton RL, Brown RE, Matroy WE Jr, et al: Autogenous vein graft repair of digital nerve defects in the finger: A retrospective clinical study. Plast Reconstr Surg 1989;84:944.
110. Wessberg GA, Wolford LM, Epker BN: Simultaneous inferior alveolar nerve graft and osseous reconstruction of the mandible. J Oral Maxillofac Surg 1982;40:384.
111. Hillerup S, Hjorting-Hansen E, Reumert T: Repair of the lingual nerve after iatrogenic injury: A follow-up study of return of sensation and taste. J Oral Maxillofac Surg 1994;52:1028.
112. Gregg JM: Studies of traumatic neuralgia in the maxillofacial region: Symptom complexes and responses to microsurgery. J Oral Maxillofac Surg 1990;48:135.
113. Gregg JM: Studies of traumatic neuralgia in the maxillofacial region: Surgical pathology and neural mechanisms. J Oral Maxillofac Surg 1990;48:228.
114. Peszowski MJ, Larsson A: Extraosseous and intraosseous oral traumatic neuromas and their association with tooth extraction. J Oral Maxillofac Surg 1990;48:463.
115. Walter JM, Gregg JM: Analysis of postsurgical neurologic alteration in the trigeminal nerve. J Oral Surg 1979;37:410.
116. Zuniga JR: Multimodal scaling of sensory recovery after microsurgical repair. J Oral Maxillofac Surg 1990;48(suppl 1):85.
117. La Banc JP: Classification of nerve injuries. Oral Maxillofac Surg Clin North Am 1992;4:285.
118. Dellon AL: Functional sensation and its reeducation. *In* Terzis JK (ed): Microreconstruction of Nerve Injuries. Philadelphia, WB Saunders, 1987, p 181.
119. Wynn Parry CB, Salter M: Sensory reeducation after median nerve lesions. Hand 1976;8:250.
120. Zuniga JR: Perceived expectation, outcome and satisfaction of microsurgical nerve repair. J Oral Maxillofac Surg 1991; 49:(suppl 1)77.
121. Gregg JM: Nonsurgical management of traumatic trigeminal neuralgias and sensory neuropathies. Oral Maxillofac Surg Clin North Am 1992;4:375.
122. Turner JA, Chapman CR: Psychological interventions for chronic pain: A critical review I: Relaxation and biofeedback. Pain 1982;12:1.
123. Turner JA, Chapman CR: Psychological interventions for chronic pain: A critical review II: Operant conditioning, hypnosis and cognitive-behavioral therapy. Pain 1982;12:121.
124. Tyndall DA, Gregg JM, Hanker JS: Evaluation of peripheral nerve regeneration following crushing or transection injuries. J Oral Maxillofac Surg 1984;42:314.
125. Smith JW: Advances in facial nerve repair. Surg Clin North Am 1972;52:1287.
126. Brussati R, Paini P: Facial nerve injury secondary to lateral displacement of the mandibular ramus. Plast Reconstr Surg 1978;62:728.
127. Goin DW: Facial nerve paralysis secondary to mandibular fracture. Laryngoscope 1980;90:1777.
128. Behrman S: Complications of sagittal osteotomy of the mandibular ramus. J Oral Surg 1972;30:554.
129. Jones JK, Van Sickels JE: Facial nerve injuries associated with orthognathic surgery: A review of incidence and management. J Oral Maxillofac Surg 1991;49:740.
130. Dingman RO, Dingman DL, Lawrence RA: Surgical correction of lesions of the temporomandibular joint. Plast Reconstr Surg 1975;55:335.
131. Dolwick MF, Kretzschmar DP: Morbidity associated with the preauricular and perimeatal approaches to the temporomandibular joint. J Oral Maxillofac Surg 1982;40:699.
132. Hall MB, Brown RW, Lebowitz MS: Facial nerve injury during surgery of the temporomandibular joint: A comparison of two dissection techniques. J Oral Maxillofac Surg 1985;43:20.
133. House LR, Morgan DH, Hall WP: Clinical evaluation of temporomandibular joint arthroplasties with insertion of articular eminence prosthesis on ninety patients. Laryngoscope 1977;87:1182.
134. Keith DA: Surgery of the Temporomandibular Joint: Success, Failure and Complications of Temporomandibular Joint Surgery. Boston, Blackwell Scientific, 1988, pp 272–282.
135. Weinberg S, Kryshtalsky B: Facial nerve function following temporomandibular joint surgery using the preauricular approach. J Oral Maxillofac Surg 1992;50:1048.
136. Greene MW, Hackney FL, Van Sickels JE: Arthroscopy of the temporomandibular joint: An anatomic perspective. J Oral Maxillofac Surg 1989;47:386.
137. Westesson PL, Erickson L, Leiberg J: The risk of damage to facial nerve, superficial temporal vessels, disk and articular surfaces during arthroscopic examination of the temporomandibular joint. Oral Surg 1986;62:124.
138. Byars LT: Preservation of the facial nerve in parotid surgery. Ann Surg 1952;136:412.
139. Lathrop FD: Management of the facial nerves during operation of the parotid gland. Ann Otolaryngol 1967;72:780.
140. Baker DC, Conley J: Avoiding facial nerve injuries in rhytidectomy. Plast Reconstr Surg 1979;64:781.
141. Rudolph R: Depth of the facial nerve in face lift dissections. Plast Reconstr Surg 1990;85:537.
142. Davis RA, Anson BJ, Budinger JM, et al: Surgical anatomy of the facial nerve and parotid gland based upon a study of 350 cervico-facial halves. Surg Gynecol Obstet 1956;102:385.
143. Al-Kayat A, Bramley P: A modified preauricular approach to the temporomandibular joint and malar arch. Br J Oral Surg 1980;17:91.

144. Nelson DW, Gingrass RP: Anatomy of the mandibular branches of the facial nerve. Plast Reconstr Surg 1979;64:479.
145. Fields MJ, Peckitt NS: Facial Nerve Function Index: A clinical measurement of facial activity in patients with facial nerve palsies. Oral Surg 1990;69:681.
146. Peckitt NS, Walker RV, Barker GR: The facial nerve function coefficient: Analysis of 100 normal subjects. J Oral Maxillofac Surg 1992;50:338.
147. May M, Harvey JE, Marovitz WF, et al: The prognostic accuracy of the maximal stimulability test compared with that of the nerve excitability test in Bell's palsy. Laryngoscope 1971;81:931.
148. Crumley RL: Recent advances in facial nerve surgery. Head Neck Surg 1982;4:233.
149. Blumental E, May M: Electrodiagnosis. *In* May M (ed): The Facial Nerve. New York, Thieme, 1986, pp 241–263.
150. Conley J: Longstanding facial paralysis rehabilitation. Laryngoscope 1974;84:2155.
151. Conley J, Baker D: Hypoglossal-facial anastomosis for reinnervation of the paralyzed face. Plast Reconstr Surg 1979;63:63.
152. Conley J: Facial nerve palsy: Physiopathology and therapeutic approach. *In* Moldaver J and Conley J (eds): The Facial Palsies. Springfield, IL, Charles C Thomas, 1980, pp 205–235.
153. Post CF: Value of galvanic muscle stimulation immediately after paralysis in reanimation of the paralyzed face. *In* Rubin LR (ed): Reanimation of the Paralyzed Face: New Approaches. St Louis, CV Mosby, 1977.
154. May M, West RJ: Iatrogenic injury—prevention and management. *In* May M (ed): The Facial Nerve. New York, Thieme, 1986, pp 549–560.
155. Dendy RA: Facial nerve paralysis following sagittal split mandibular osteotomy: A case report. Br J Oral Surg 1973;11:101.
156. Eygedi P, Houwing M, Juten E: The oblique subcondylar osteotomy: Report of results of 100 cases. J Oral Surg 1981;39:871.
157. Guralnick WC, Kelly JP: Palsy of the facial nerve after intraoral oblique osteotomies of the mandible. J Oral Surg 1979;37:743.
158. Karabouta-Voulgaropoulav I, Martis CS: Facial paresis following sagittal split osteotomy: Report of two cases. Oral Surg 1984;57:600.
159. Kline SN: Electrical testing for injuries of the seventh nerve. J Oral Surg 1975;33:215.
160. Martis CS: Complication of sagittal split ramus osteotomy. J Oral Maxillofac Surg 1984;42:10.
161. Piecuch JF, Lewis RA: Facial nerve injury as a complication of sagittal split ramus osteotomy. J Oral Maxillofac Surg 1982;40:309.
162. Norris CW, Proud GO: Spontaneous return of facial motion following seventh cranial nerve resection. Laryngoscope 1981;91:211.
163. Baumel JJ: Trigeminal-facial nerve communications: Their function in facial muscle innervation and reinnervation. Arch Otolaryngol 1974;99:34.
164. Harrison DH: Current trends in the treatment of established unilateral facial palsy. Ann R Coll Surg Engl 1990;72:94.
165. May M, Drucker C: Temporalis muscle for facial reanimation. A 13-year experience with 224 procedures. Arch Otolaryngol Head Neck Surg 1993;119:378.
166. Zuniga JR, Hegtvedt AK, Alling CC III: Future applications in the management of trigeminal nerve injuries. Oral Maxillofac Surg Clin North Am 1992;4:543.

Chapter 7
COMPLICATIONS OF TEMPOROMANDIBULAR JOINT SURGERY

by

M. Franklin Dolwick
Jeffrey W. Armstrong

Introduction

Potential complications associated with temporomandibular joint (TMJ) surgery and arthroscopy are discussed in this chapter. Complications that occur in the perioperative period are hemorrhage, infection, damage to the fifth and seventh cranial nerves, auriculotemporal nerve syndrome, otologic injury, perforation into the middle cranial fossa, parotid injury, and anesthesia related events. Complications specific to arthroscopy include extravasation of irrigation fluid, iatrogenic damage to intraarticular structures, breakage of instruments within the joint space, and thermal damage secondary to the use of the electrocautery or laser. Long-term complications include occlusal changes, restricted range of motion, implant failure, and persistent pain. Prevention and management of these complications are discussed. The importance of proper patient selection, the criteria for success of TMJ surgery, and the value of precise careful technique are reviewed.

THE SUBJECTS DISCUSSED IN THIS CHAPTER ARE:

- Avoidance of complications
  - Proper patient selection
  - Criteria of surgical success
- Perioperative complications
  - Vascular injury and hemorrhage
  - Neurologic injury
  - Peripheral nerve injury
  - Infection
  - Otologic complications
  - Trauma to the parotid gland: Sialocele or fistula formation
- Complications specific to arthroscopy
  - Extravasation of irrigating fluid
  - Iatrogenic intraauricular injury
  - Instrument failure or breakage
  - Laser complications
  - Complications of electrocautery
- Long-term complications
  - Malocclusion
  - Ankylosis
  - Implant failure
  - Persistent pain in the multiply-operated patient

Avoidance of Complications

TMJ surgical procedures, whether arthroscopy or arthrotomy, carry the risk of potential complications as do all surgical procedures. The purpose of the chapter is to review the potential complications and their management with a discussion of how to best avoid their occurrence.

Proper Patient Selection

Before a review of the specific complications in detail, the most important criteria for successful TMJ surgery, patient selection, needs to be discussed. The most common reasons for failure of TMJ surgery are inadequate patient selection and misdiagnosis. The patient needs to be able to accurately describe his or her symptoms and localize the pain to the preauricular area. It must be emphasized that the criterion for surgery is not simply refractory pain but pain that is localized to the TMJ. The more localized the symptoms are to the TMJ, the better the surgical prognosis.[1] Clinical indications for TMJ surgery are relative, and the following general indications have been recommended[2]:

- The TMJ is the source of pain and/or dysfunction that results in a significant impairment to the patient in his or her daily activities.
- The TMJ pain is refractory to appropriate nonsurgical therapies.
- The pain is localized to the TMJ.
- There is pain on loading of the TMJ.
- There is pain on movement of the TMJ.
- There are mechanical interferences in TMJ function.

Criteria of Surgical Success

Currently, a wide spectrum of surgical procedures, ranging from arthrocentesis to complex open joint procedures, are used in the treatment of internal derangement of the TMJ. The success of TMJ surgery depends on appropriate case selection. Also, the patient must be an acceptable surgical candidate from a general health standpoint. Criteria for declaring success of a TMJ procedure should include the following[3]:

- An increased range of function
- Ability to chew and eat a normal diet with few restrictions
- No alteration of occlusion
- Significant reduction or elimination of joint pain.

It is critical that the patient's goals and expectations are realistic and are in line with those of the surgeons, for a successful outcome to be achieved. Ninety percent of operated patients benefit from TMJ surgery, but both the patient and the surgeon must realize that TMJ surgery may worsen the patient's problem. Therefore, the decision to operate must be made carefully.[4]

Perioperative Complications

Vascular Injury and Hemorrhage

Arthroscopy

With the density of vascular structures surrounding the TMJ, there is a definite possibility for hemorrhage during arthroscopy. Because of the extensive collateral blood supply in the head and neck region, adverse sequelae are rarely associated with vascular injury compared with orthopedic procedures. In orthopedics, surgery is performed in joints, where there are single terminal arteries, in which an injury can result in a compromised extremity.

Operative arthroscopy requires multiple punctures. A vessel can be penetrated, punctured, or torn with the insertion of the sharp trocar. Use of a rotational movement upon insertion of the trocar may prevent this event.

The superficial temporal artery may be punctured at any time during the procedure. Palpation of the artery and identification of landmarks prior to insertion of the trochar can prevent damage to the artery.[5] Westesson and colleagues[6] and Holmlund and associates[7] showed that the puncture site closely approximates the superficial temporal artery and vein. If the artery is encountered, the resultant pulsatile flow usually responds to pressure and suturing of the puncture site. If this maneuver fails to control bleeding, open exploration with identification and ligation of the vessel is indicated. There is no accurate way to determine the exact location of the superficial temporal vein prior to joint puncture. If the vein is injured, the resultant bleeding usually is controlled with pressure and suturing of the skin puncture site.[8]

Intracapsular bleeding can be encountered during an anterior release in the region of the lateral pterygoid muscle or during débridement in the area of the posterior attachment. Use of electrocautery, laser ablation, and injection of local anesthetic with vasoconstrictor are options to be considered in controlling the bleeding. After hemorrhage is controlled, copious irrigation with suction evacuation of blood clots is indicated. Medial advancement of the arthroscope through the capsule wall can damage the pterygoid venous plexus or the internal carotid artery.

Pseudoaneurysm and formation of an arteriovenous (AV) fistula of the superficial temporal vessels has been reported.[9, 10] Clinical signs and symptoms of an AV fistula are a palpable thrill and a audible bruit. Arteriography is indicated and will demonstrate the AV fistula. Surgical exploration with isolation and ligation should be undertaken. A pseudoaneurysm results from incomplete transection of the artery with bleeding continuing into the surrounding tissues until a hematoma large enough to counter arterial pressure is formed. The hematoma liquefies in the center, and an endothelium-lined pulsatile cavity continuous with the vessel is formed. A carotid angiogram should be obtained, and surgery to ligate the vessel and excision of the aneurysm is accomplished if indicated. Embolization of the AV fistula is another treatment option. If embolization is to be performed, the patient needs to be made aware of the potential complications, i.e., pain, trismus, skin necrosis, temporary or permanent cranial nerve palsies, stroke, blindness, and death. A permanent complication rate of 1% has been reported.[9]

With any TMJ arthroscopy procedure, the patient may develop a hemarthrosis. No significant adverse outcomes related to hemarthrosis have been reported. A pressure dressing is usually applied for the first 24 hours postoperatively to minimize risk of hematoma formation and oozing.

Arthrotomy

During open TMJ surgery, as with arthroscopy, meticulous attention to hemostasis is critical throughout the procedure to prevent postoperative hematoma formation and to allow the dissection to progress smoothly.

The vessels at risk during TMJ surgery are the superficial temporal artery and vein, the maxillary artery, and the middle meningeal artery. With use of the standard preauricular approach with appropriate dissection as described by Dolwick and Sanders,[11] the superficial temporal vessels are located in the anterior flap and bluntly retracted out of the surgical field. If the vessels are encountered, ligation may be necessary to ensure hemostasis and avoid postoperative hematoma, which can increase the risks of infection and development of adhesions.

At the level of the lateral capsule, a vein is usually encountered, which also must be cauterized or ligated to ensure hemostasis.

The middle meningeal artery may be encountered if aggressive bone removal is performed during eminectomy, so meticulous attention to the surgical procedure and location of the instruments is required.

The maxillary artery crosses medial to the condyle and has been found to be on the average 20 mm below the superior aspect of the condyle.[8] Variations occur, so great care is mandatory for operating in the extreme medial and inferior aspects of the joint.

Hemorrhage from the maxillary artery can be very problematic and difficult to control. Usually, the bleeding is controlled with pressure or with use of vascular clips. Husted[12] has reported bleeding in two cases, that necessitated ligation of the external carotid artery. Peoples and associates[13] reported hemorrhage from the maxillary artery that was controlled via selective embolization because of the possibility of persistent bleeding from collateral vessels distal to the bleeding site. Possible complications of selective embolization were discussed previously.

Neurologic Injury

Middle Cranial Fossa Perforation During Arthroscopy

Owing to the thinness of the temporal bone making up the roof of the articular fossa, extreme care must be taken to avoid its perforation. Green and coworkers[8] found the average thickness to be 0.9 mm. Inadvertent puncture of the roof of the glenoid fossa during arthroscopy has been reported by McCain,[14] for which an immediate neurosurgery consultation was obtained. The proposed surgical procedure was accomplished, and no neurologic sequela was reported. Perforation into the middle cranial fossa may result in a tear of the dura and a cerebrospinal fluid (CSF) leak. In most cerebrospinal fluid leaks, the dura seals and the leak ceases spontaneously. If CSF continues to collect in the wound or continues to drain through the incision, a pressure dressing is applied, and the head is kept elevated. If the leak persists longer than 48 hours, the neurosurgeon is consulted again. Surgical repair of the middle cranial fossa, however, is rarely necessary. A persistent leak may be treated with a lumbar subarachnoid drain, and a CT scan obtained to document the site of the leak.

The anatomic landmarks identified prior to entering the superior joint space have been well described. Careful identification of the landmarks and minimal use of force prior to feeling the "loss of resistance" upon entering the superior joint space are important to prevent perforation into the middle cranial fossa. Case selection is also important in preventing middle cranial fossa puncture. Patients who are obese with unpalpable landmarks or have a history of open procedures with diminished superior joint spaces represent high-risk cases that should be avoided by the inexperienced arthroscopist.

Middle Cranial Fossa Perforation Secondary to Foreign Body Reaction

Extensive bony destruction and perforation of the roof of the glenoid fossa secondary to foreign body reaction has been well documented.[15] The temporal bone perforations are rarely located in the area of articulation and, in the majority of cases, do not need to be repaired. If repair is indicated, use of cranial bone, autogenous auricular cartilage, and allogenic cartilage have been considered.[16, 17] In the presence of a dural tear with a resultant CSF leak, the surgical site is packed off, the head is elevated, and an intraoperative neurosurgical consultation is obtained. When there is a small dural perforation and when surgical access is complicated by the location, the use of fibrin adhesive has been recommended.[18, 19] Absorbable gelatin sponge (Gelfoam) is placed over the site of the dural tear, and the fibrin adhesive is applied and allowed to gel. The surgical procedure is then completed, with a lumbar subarachnoid drain placed prior to awakening of the patient. Postoperative management includes keeping the patient's head elevated. The subarachnoid drain is removed as recommended by the neurosurgeon, usually in 2 to 3 days.

Middle Cranial Fossa Involvement due to Pneumatization of the Articular Eminence of the Temporal Bone (PAT)

Unless pneumatization of the articular eminence is large, the presence of pneumatization is not a contraindication to performing an eminoplasty or eminectomy in the treatment of chronic recurrent mandibular dislocation. Thorough radiographic evaluation of the articular eminence is always indicated prior to surgery. Use of panoramic radiographs to screen for PAT is the method of choice for the best visualization, image clarity, and cost (Fig. 7–1). Common characteristics of PAT are as follows:

- Asymptomatic radiolucent defect in the zygomatic process of the temporal bone with similar appearance of the mastoid air cells
- Extension of this defect anteriorly as far as the articular eminence but not extending beyond the zygomaticotemporal suture
- No enlargement or cortical destruction of the zygoma

Incidence of PAT has been reported to be 1% to 2.6%; there is no sex predilection, and the mean age is 32.5 years with a range of 15 to 74 years.[20, 21] PAT is distinguished from other pathologic entities, such as hemangioma, by the lack of clinical signs and symptoms.[21] When a PAT is large, elimination of the defect can be difficult, and an alternative method of surgical treatment should be considered. During surgery, care is taken to avoid sudden penetration through the defect with resultant perforation into the middle cranial fossa. Clinically, these defects have no soft tissue lining. After completion of the eminoplasty or eminectomy, the surgeon needs to rule out the possibility of dural tear by having anesthesia personnel perform a vascular maneuver and observe for a CSF leak. An intraoperative neurosurgery consultation is indicated if a dural tear and CSF leak are noted. Small perforations can be treated with fibrin tissue adhesive as described previously or according to the neurosurgeon's preference. The bony defect may have to be obliterated to avoid interference with disk function and jaw movement. An autogenous graft utilizing the previously removed eminence and autogenous auricular cartilage or allogenic cartilage has been described.[22]

Peripheral Nerve Injury

Facial Nerve Injuries

The proximity of the temporal branches of the facial nerve to the surgical field increases the risk of damage during arthroscopy or open surgery. The temporal branches lie in a dense fusion of periosteum, temporal fascia, and superficial fascia at the level of the zygomatic arch. Al-Kayat and Bramley[23] found the nerve to lie on an average of 2.0 cm from the anterior concavity of the external auditory canal, with a range of 0.8 to 3.5 cm. A preauricular incision as described by Dolwick and Sanders[11] is the most common approach to minimize the risk of nerve damage. The reported incidence of facial nerve transient neurapraxia after open surgery ranges from 1% to 25%; it is generally limited to the temporal branch and usually resolves in 3 to 6 months.

Cadaveric studies by Greene and colleagues[8] and Westesson and associates[8] have addressed the risk of facial nerve damage during arthroscopy. They found the puncture site to be as close as 3 mm to the temporal branch of the facial nerve, although no damage to the nerve was reported. Retrospective studies of arthroscopic complications show the rate of facial nerve injury to be less than 1%.[24, 25]

To avoid damage to the temporal branch of the facial nerve during arthroscopy, the surgeon needs to utilize predetermined measurements, as described by McCain,[26] and to further minimize the risk by using a rotational motion in placing the trocar and cannula systems, sliding past the nerve rather than impaling it. Unless the sharp trocar actually transects the nerve, the prognosis for a full recovery should remain excellent. Facial nerve damage following TMJ surgery usually results in eyebrow lag with occasional decrease in or-

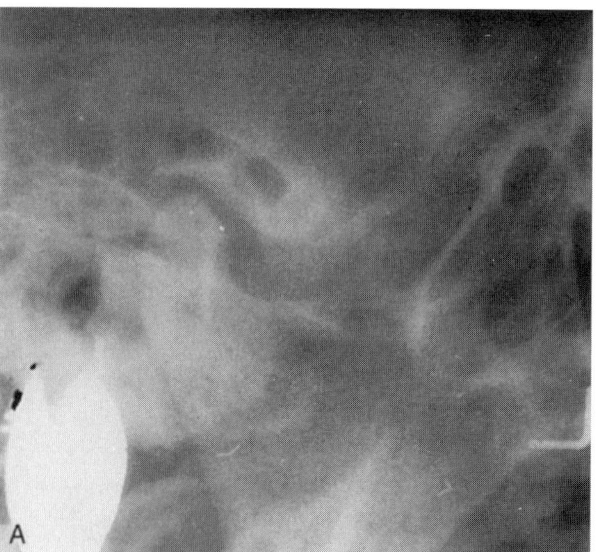

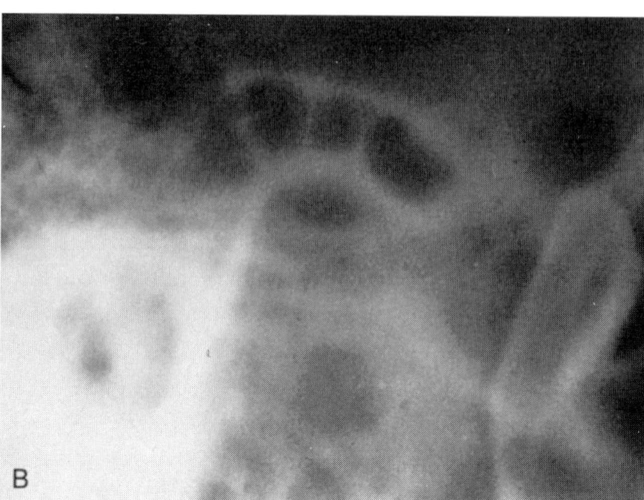

Figure 7–1. *A* and *B*, Radiographs showing pneumatization of articular eminence.

bicularis oculi function, preventing complete closure of the eyelid. For patients with a residual brow or forehead weakness, a period of observation is warranted. Postoperative management for a case of eyelid involvement includes use of artificial tears and ocular lubricant and taping of eye at night to prevent excessive corneal desiccation and abrasion. Ophthalmologic consultation is indicated. Physical therapy with electrical stimulation may be helpful in maintaining muscle tone as function returns. For more extensive injury involving other branches of the facial nerve or complete paralysis, evaluation with nerve excitability testing is performed. With a facial nerve neuropraxia, the percutaneous threshold is normal, and full recovery is likely. If there is evidence that the nerve has been severed or irreversibly crushed, surgical exploration with nerve repair should be considered.[27]

Many surgeons utilize a long-acting local anesthetic at the conclusion of the arthroscopic procedure for postoperative pain management. Extravasation of the local anesthesia may result in a facial nerve weakness that can mimic a true neurologic injury. Also, extravasation of irrigating fluid with resultant edema can be responsible for this occurrence. Thus, it is extremely important to inform the patient preoperatively of these possible effects.

Trigeminal Nerve Injuries

Infraorbital Nerve

The postoperative complication of infraorbital nerve paresthesia has been infrequently reported.[28] Typically it is associated with extravasation of irrigation fluid into the medial tissues because of extended operating time. In the few observed occurrences, it appears to resolve rapidly without sequela.

Lingual Nerve

Injury to the lingual nerve is rarely mentioned as a problem in open TMJ surgery. Neuropraxia of the lingual nerve may result from the mandibular angle clamp utilized to distract the mandibular condyle inferiorly and anteriorly. With arthroscopy, medial extravasation of fluid may result in paresthesia of the ipsilateral lingual nerve. Also, compression of the tongue during mandibular manipulation may be responsible for a limited deficit. It is important to distinguish the local compression injury from a more proximal nerve compression secondary to the extravasation of fluid. Carter and Testa[29] report no instances of permanent lingual nerve injury.

Inferior Alveolar Nerve

Injury to the inferior alveolar nerve has been more commonly reported. There are two mechanisms for this injury. As with other nerve injuries reported, medial extravasation of irrigating fluid can result in compression of this nerve. Resolution is usually rapid. The other mechanism of injury is secondary to the use of a clamp placed at the angle of the mandible to assist in distraction of the condyle. Heffez and Blaustein[30] reported a compression injury to the inferior alveolar nerve as a result of this technique. The prognosis for recovery from this type of injury is much less predictable. Care must be utilized in placement of this clamp. It should be placed posteriorly and inferiorly to avoid compression and penetration of the buccal or lingual cortex over the inferior alveolar nerve canal. Sanders[31] describes a technique that avoids the use of the mandibular clamp. The surgical assistant manipulates and distracts the mandible transorally through a sterile drape, maintaining the sterile surgical field.

Auriculotemporal Nerve Injuries

The auriculotemporal nerve travels immediately adjacent to the superficial temporal vessels and thus is subjected to the potential risk of injury. Carter and Testa[29] reported that auriculotemporal nerve injuries were the most commonly reported complications with arthroscopy, representing 59% of all neurologic injuries. Lateral puncture can impinge on the nerve and surrounding vessels. Injury can result from direct severance, compression, and contusion. Local hematoma formation resulting from puncture of an adjacent vessel can result in nerve compression, as can extravasation of irrigating fluids. Paresthesia as a result of damage to this nerve is quite common following arthrotomy.[32] There were no reports of long-term problems associated with this injury; it is temporary and usually resolves within 6 months. With the high incidence of occurrence and relative long duration, of this complication, inclusion of its possibility in the preoperative discussion with the patient is indicated.

Auriculotemporal Nerve Syndrome (Frey Syndrome)

Frey syndrome is manifested by gustatory "sweating" and flushing with warmth in the temporal and preauricular areas. It is the result of auriculotemporal nerve damage with reinnervation of the eccrine sweat glands by parasympathetic salivary fibers. The clinical presentation is variable, and its severity can be evaluated with the Minor starch iodine test,[33] which is conducted as follows:

1. The test should be performed in a climate-controlled clinic.
2. A solution of 3 g iodine, 20 g castor oil, and 200 mL absolute alcohol is applied by brush to both preauricular regions of the face.
3. As the solution dries, the region is lightly dusted with starch powder.
4. The patient is instructed to chew a piece of fresh lemon for 4 minutes to elicit a salivary response.
5. Sweat dissolves the starch powder and reacts with the iodine to produce dark blue spots.

Kryshtalsky and Weinberg[33] reported a 15% incidence of Frey syndrome in a group of 20 TMJ surgery patients. Options for treating Frey syndrome include topical application of anticholinergic compounds such as glycopyrrolate, transection of the auriculotemporal nerve, and implantation of freeze-dried dura or fascia lata under the skin in the involved areas.[34]

Infection

To minimize the risks of postoperative infection, careful selection of patients is important. If an infection is present in adjacent structures, such as regional cellulitis secondary to insect bite or acne, acute parotitis, or otitis media or externa, cancellation of the surgical procedure is indicated. The existence of an active infection at a remote site has been shown to increase the risks of postoperative infection twofold to fourfold.[35] It is important that all patients be evaluated and treated for any urinary tract, respiratory tract, or soft tissue infection prior to surgery.

Other factors have also been shown to have an effect on infection rates. Hospital admission 24 hours to 1 week prior to surgery for patients undergoing clean elective procedures showed a twofold increase in postoperative infections,[35] presumably secondary to nosocomial sources of contamination. Hair removal, although a matter of surgeon preference, has profound implications if performed more than 6 hours prior to surgery, at which time the probability of infection increases tenfold. When hair removal is planned, it should be done immediately before the procedure. In TMJ surgery, the microbial flora of the skin is a source of wound contamination. Skin preparation may remove bacteria from the epidermis, but it is impossible to fully eliminate those residing in the underlying hair follicles and sebaceous glands because of poor penetration of disinfecting agents into an oily environment. Thus, the overall number of bacteria are reduced, but the skin can rarely be made sterile.

Prophylactic antibiotics to prevent postoperative infection are routinely used. However, controversy over the value of prophylaxis in head and neck surgery not involving the oral cavity still exists. In clean surgical wounds, the anticipated infection rate ranges from 1% to 5%.[35] Incidence of postoperative infection with TMJ surgery has been reported within this range.[24, 29] King[36] denounced the use of antibiotic prophylaxis in head and neck surgery because of additional expense, questionable usefulness, and incidence of allergic reactions. Ketchum and associates[37] advocated the use of prophylactic antibiotics. Because of the small number of their patients undergoing head and neck procedures, however, statistical analysis of these data was not performed. Eppley and Delfino,[35] in their prospective study on TMJ surgery, found no significant difference in the incidence of infection with or without the use of antibiotic prophylaxis. The organisms most commonly isolated were *Staphylococcus aureus* and *Staphylococcus epidermidis.* In retrospective studies by Carter and Testa[29] and McCain and colleagues,[24] the frequency of postoperative infection in patients undergoing TMJ arthroscopy was less than 1%. Otitis media has been reported[31] and is discussed later along with other otologic complications.

The current trend for prophylactic antibiotics in open TMJ surgery and arthroscopy is to use a cephalosporin intravenously in the perioperative period. A dose is given immediately preoperatively, followed by a single dose in the recovery room. If an autogenous graft or total joint reconstruction is planned, antibiotic coverage is extended for 10 to 14 days.[38]

In the event of postoperative infection, indicated treatment consists of instituting chemotherapy empirically for the potential pathogen, obtaining a specimen for culture and sensitivity testing, wound débridement, and irrigation. Resolution of infection without long-term sequelae has been the reported outcome.[35, 39–41]

Otologic Complications

The close proximity of the ear to the TMJ increases the risk for potential damage during surgical procedures. With the greater use of diagnostic and surgical arthroscopy, the numbers and types of reported otologic complications have increased.

Sanders[31] in 1986 reported a single occurrence of otitis media in a very large series of arthroscopies. Van Sickels and Nishioka[42] in 1987 reported a perforation of the tympanic membrane with ossicular disruption resulting in a moderate hearing loss and tinnitus in the affected ear. The error was discovered when middle ear structures were noted through the arthroscope. Applebaum and associates[43] in 1988 reported a severe sensorineural hearing loss in two cases and a conductive component in another. Two of the patients had previously undergone open surgical procedures; it was thought that the resultant scar tissue with distortion of landmarks made entry into the joint more difficult and may have predisposed the patients to these complications. Laughner and colleagues[44] in 1989 reported one case of hearing loss after arthroscopy and one case after open surgery with resulting total deafness. Excessive mobilization and distraction of the mandible, producing tension on the sphenomandibular ligament and disrupting the malleus via its attachment to the anterior malleolar ligament, were thought to be responsible.

In avoiding these possible arthroscopic complications, strict attention to the following considerations are most important[5, 42]:

- Maintenance of proper horizontal patient head position
- Attention to anatomic landmarks
- Maintenance of anterior inclination of the trocar
- Use of a blunt trocar to penetrate the lateral capsule and enter the superior joint space
- Attention to the average puncture depths from the skin surface to the lateral aspect of the joint at 25 mm; perforation of the medial capsule can occur at 50 ± 5 mm
- Visualization of canicular systems directed posteriorly for instrumentation by means of triangulation as they penetrate and enter the joint space
- Awareness of complicating factors; e.g., obesity of the patient and joint stiffness make palpation of the landmarks very difficult
- Otoscopic examination is mandatory preoperatively

and postoperatively to document any abnormalities of the external auditory canal (EAC) or tympanic membrane. Consultation with an otolaryngologist and audiologist should be accomplished if any abnormalities of the EAC or tympanic membrane or alteration in auditory acuity is noted. Specific otologic complications are now discussed.

Laceration or Hematoma of the External Auditory Canal

Laceration injuries occur at the junction of the cartilaginous EAC with the bony portion of the canal because of the anteromedial inclination of the canal.[5] If a laceration occurs, it is important to control hemorrhage with bipolar cautery. Antibiotic-hydrocortisone suspension otic drops for 10 to 14 days postoperatively are used to prevent infection and aid healing. Any developing granulation tissue is removed using silver nitrate or bipolar cautery. An aural-TMJ fistula may develop as a long-term complication of EAC laceration.

Aural-TMJ Fistula

Occurrence of an aural-TMJ fistula is very rare, and only a few cases have been reported.[45, 46] The fistula, which is a permanently epithelialized communication between the ear and the TMJ, may result from either open TMJ surgery or arthroscopy. In the treatment of bony ankylosis, there is a risk of posterior displacement of the tympanic plate into the EAC, which may lead to stenosis of the EAC and resultant hearing impairment. Also, with the need for aggressive bony recontouring, the risk of forming an aural-TMJ fistula increases. If the communication is small, it usually heals without a residual defect. If the communication is large, however, or if a chronic infection is present, a permanent tract or fistula may form and require surgical management. The fistula interferes with the normal quality of the synovial tissue, so crepitus and loud joint noises may be present.

Otoscopic examination usually reveals a polypoid mass protruding into the EAC, and synovial fluid may be expressed on joint movement. Local measures utilized to treat the fistula have consisted of cauterization with silver nitrate or local excision with packing of the EAC. If the fistula persists, a CT scan is obtained to delineate the course of the fistula. Closure is achieved by means of a temporalis flap.[45] The temporalis flap provides necessary bulk of tissue to cover the fistula, is easily developed, and obviates a secondary donor, site thus decreasing morbidity and preventing recurrence. The goals of surgical intervention are to create a barrier between the EAC and TMJ, to reestablish a normal environment within the intraarticular space, and to prevent an ascending infection from the EAC.

Perforation of the Tympanic Membrane

Perforation of the tympanic membrane occurs when the arthrocsope or an instrument used to pack off the EAC is inadvertently passed medially through the membrane. Small perforations in the anterior or inferior portion of the tympanic membrane result in minimal hearing loss and heal uneventfully. Injuries to the tympanic membrane in the posterior region may result in disruption of the middle ear ossicles and may cause a significant hearing loss.[42] If a perforation is noted, referral to an otolaryngologist is indicated.

Otitis Externa

Accumulation of irrigation fluid in the EAC or abrasion of the epithelial surface may destroy the natural barriers to infection, allowing bacterial proliferation and penetration and predisposing the patient to otitis externa postoperatively.[14]

Clinical signs and symptoms of otitis externa include ear pain that can be extreme, tenderness upon movement of the tragus and auricle, a feeling of aural fullness, and itching. Otoscopic examination reveals a edematous EAC with erythema and discharge.

Treatment consists of relieving pain and discomfort with analgesics, thorough cleansing of the EAC with repeated weekly débridements until resolution, and instilling an antibiotic-hydrocortisone suspension for 10 to 14 days. If the infective process does not respond to this treatment, obtaining a specimen for culture of the EAC and referral to an otolaryngologist are indicated.[47]

Otitis Media

Otitis media has been reported as a postoperative complication that can lead to a residual hearing loss.[31] It may develop as a result of direct injury to the middle ear structures, perforation of the tympanic membrane, or eustachian tube dysfunction secondary to postoperative edema.

The patient presents complaining of ear pain and fever. There may be a purulent discharge if a perforation is present in the tympanic membrane. Otoscopic examination reveals a full or bulging, opaque tympanic membrane with limited mobility to pneumatic otoscopy. Erythema of the tympanic membrane is an inconsistent finding.

Treatment consists of systemic antibiotic therapy, i.e., amoxicillin 500 mg every 8 hours orally for 10 days.[28] Additional supportive therapy such as analgesics, antipyretics, and an antihistamine-decongestant may be of some benefit.[48] If the middle ear fluid persists after 10 days of antibiotic therapy, referral to an otolaryngologist is indicated.

Trauma to the Parotid Gland: Sialocele or Fistula Formation

Injury to the superficial lobe of the parotid gland is possible because of the gland's close proximity to the TMJ. There is mention of this risk in the literature, although no reported cases were found. Primary management of a parotid gland injury is straightforward and should be similar to that of a traumatic injury in this region.[49] It is very important to obtain good approximation and closure of the parotid capsule prior to continuing the anatomic closure of the subcutaneous tissues and skin. A pressure dressing is placed for 24 to 48 hours following primary repair.

Postoperatively, saliva can accumulate subcutaneously. If there is a significant accumulation, needle aspiration and the use of an antisialagogue should be considered. A nondependent location is selected for the needle aspiration to prevent fistula formation. A pressure dressing is then placed for 24 to 48 hours following aspiration.

When the parotid gland is inadvertently injured and a primary repair is not accomplished, a sialocele, a true cyst, or a salivary fistula may form. The treatment of a sialocele consists of needle aspiration and placement of a pressure dressing as previously described. If the accumulation continues, exploration with primary repair should be accomplished. With the persistence of an untreated sialocele, cyst formation may occur, necessitating surgical excision. The development of a salivary fistula is treated by surgical excision with primary closure and application of a pressure dressing. Any inadvertent injury to the parotid duct needs to be ruled out prior to treating the fistula. Unobstructed salivary flow through the parotid duct should be documented. Meticulous attention to surgical detail and a thorough knowledge of the regional anatomy should prevent inadvertent injury to the superficial lobe of the parotid gland and postoperative complications.

Dysrhythmias

The development of a dysrhythmia is usually reported as an anesthetic-related complication. A local anesthetic solution containing epinephrine is routinely the choice of surgeons performing arthroscopic procedures to distend the superior joint space. Epinephrine can be rapidly absorbed, however, resulting in a dysrhythmia. Premature ventricular contractions have been noted to occur and have been successfully treated with lidocaine.[28]

Sinus dysrhythmias have also been noted with the repeated forced manipulation of the mandible during surgical procedures. Sinus bradycardia has been observed and is thought to arise from simultaneous carotid body massage. When sinus bradycardia is encountered, cessation of manipulation usually resolves the bradycardia.

Gomez and Gilder[50] described an occurrence of profound bradycardia during arthroscopy thought to be secondary to the trigeminovagal reflex. Increased pressure in the joint is thought to stimulate the trigeminal sensory innervation. This then activates the afferent arc of the reflex that in turn activates the efferent pathway via the vagus nerve, resulting in profound bradycardia. Another possibility is the stimulation of the periosteal innervation of the zygomatic arch. The bradycardia can be treated with atropine or glycopyrrolate. The surgeon needs to be aware that a dysrhythmia can occur and thereby ensure that the patient is appropriately monitored and has intravenous access.

Complications Specific to Arthroscopy

Extravasation of Irrigating Fluid

Interstitial extravasation of irrigating fluid into the temporal, parotid, and masseteric regions may occur and can be a limiting factor in the length of the procedure.[5] Attention to the placement of the inflow and outflow cannulae and confirmation of unobstructed outflow are important in the prevention of this problem. The depth of the trocar upon insertion into the superior joint space must be carefully monitored to avoid perforation of the medial capsule. McCain[5] reported the average depth to the midportion of the joint to be 25 mm from the skin and the depth to the medial capsule to be 50 ± 5 mm from the skin. Continuous monitoring of the inflow-outflow circuit is necessary. If obstruction of the outflow part goes unnoticed and excessive pressure is required to irrigate, excessive pressure within the joint can lead to extravasation and distention of the soft tissues. Strict attention to detail during the procedure should help the surgeon recognize the imbalance between inflow and outflow irrigant volumes.

No long-term irreversible sequelae secondary to the extravasation of irrigating fluid are reported in the literature. It appears to be an infrequent occurrence with spontaneous resolution in 24 to 48 hours. Indresano[51] reported three cases of extravasation in 50 operations with spontaneous resolution; however, one case was associated with a transient temporal and zygomatic branch paralysis. Goss and Bosanquet[52] reported excessive extravasation in three cases of 50 arthroscopies, with complete resolution seen at 1 week postoperatively.

Difficult and lengthy triangulation procedures, in which large volumes of irrigation fluid are used, may increase the risk of excessive extravasation into the tissue planes medial to the TMJ. The subsequent distention may lead to edema of the medial masticator space and lateral pharyngeal space, producing an acute upper airway obstruction if there is rapid extubation at the completion of the procedure. To avoid the possibility of this complication, the surgeon should inspect the pharynx for asymmetry. The neck must also be examined for swelling and tracheal deviation prior to extubation.[53] If a significant amount of edema exists, the patient should not be extubated but rather should be monitored in the recovery room until symmetry returns. Lateral pharyngeal edema usually resolves in 2 to 4 hours. Extubation of the patient can then be carried out in the standard fashion. Upper airway obstruction secondary to extravasation has been reported by Hendler and Levin[53] to be complicated by the development of postoperative pulmonary edema. To avoid the possibility of extravasation leading to upper airway obstruction, the surgeon must constantly monitor for free flow of irrigation fluid with minimal irrigation pressure, avoid medial capsule puncture, monitor for imbalance between inflow and outflow volumes, and be expedient in technique.

Iatrogenic Intraarticular Injury

Intraarticular injury, such as scuffing or laceration of the articular fibrocartilage of the fossa, eminence, or condyle and perforation of the disk during arthroscopy, has been reported. Westesson and associates[6] found evidence of iatrogenic injury on the articular surfaces in more than half of the cadaver joints undergoing arthroscopic examination. McCain[5] reported a single incidence of disk perforation during arthroscopy. There have been no other reports of the clinical significance of iatrogenic injury. However, Bjornland and colleagues[54] report irreversible postoperative changes after arthroscopy in their animal model, suggesting that there might be long-term detrimental effects of iatrogenic arthroscopic injury. They recommend human prospective follow-up studies to correlate their findings.

Iatrogenic injury can be prevented by use of a blunt trocar as well as careful puncture with controlled force and attention to the tactile sensation of a "loss of resistance" signifying entrance into the superior joint space. Needles used for joint insufflation or as outflow ports need to be precisely placed to avoid heavy bone contact. No sharp instruments should be used in the joint unless first visualized with triangulation.

Instrument Failure or Breakage

Instruments used for arthroscopic TMJ surgery are extremely fine and delicate; thus, the potential for breakage is always present. Every effort must be made to avoid this problem, as follows:

- Use devices standardized and manufactured specifically for TMJ arthroscopy.
- The structural integrity of the instruments must be verified prior to insertion into the joint.
- Avoid the excessive use of force and bending of the instrument.
- Use ferromagnetic instruments.
- Have duplicate instruments and a magnetic retriever available.
- Make sure each instrument is closed prior to its removal.

The operator must be prepared in the event that an instrument does fail or break during arthroscopy. A well-thought-out approach for instrument retrieval is essential. The following protocol has been suggested for retrieval of a broken instrument[55, 56]:

1. Stop the procedure and maintain the position of the arthroscope and working cannulas.
2. Keep the instruments in view.
3. Inform operating room and anesthesia staff to ensure a coordinated effort and to avoid confusion.
4. Check the inflow bag to ensure that adequate irrigation fluid is available, so the joint will always be filled during instrument retrieval.
5. Record and measure the depth of the instrument.
6. Adjust inflow in the arthroscopic portal to force the object toward the working cannula.
7. Take a radiograph if the piece can not be found arthroscopically.
8. Remove the fragment.

If instrument removal can not be achieved arthroscopically, immediate open surgery is indicated to retrieve the object.[38] Patients undergoing TMJ arthroscopy must be informed of the potential risk of instrument breakage, and their consent for open arthrotomy should be obtained.

Laser Complications

A dramatic increase in the use of lasers during TMJ arthroscopic surgery is taking place. Introduction of the holmium:yttrium-aluminum-garnet (Ho:YAG) laser, with a wavelength of 2,100 nm, offers many features that have made it a very useful arthroscopic instrument. The laser energy can be transmitted through readily available fiberoptics, standard irrigating solutions can be used, tissue penetration is lower with more precise control, and minimal heat is generated compared with motorized shavers, suction punch instruments, and electrocautery.[39]

The main advantage of the Ho:YAG laser is that it generates significantly less heat and the resultant tissue damage is much less compared with electrocautery. The initial zone of injury is 0.4 to 0.6 mm with the Ho:YAG laser, which decreases with time; this zone is 0.7 to 1.8 mm with electrocautery and increases with time, causing more undesirable tissue damage.[39, 57]

The surgeon must be familiar with and must implement the principles of laser safety. Adequate working knowledge of lasers with laboratory experience is necessary prior to its use in patients. The laser is used with the working tip in motion in a pulsed mode. Continuous firing of the laser in a static position, which can result in undesired destruction of tissues in the joint and penetration into surrounding structures, should be avoided. Metallic instruments in the arthroscopic field can reflect the laser energy, resulting in undesirable tissue damage. The arthroscope must be kept away from the laser beam, because direct contact of the laser beam with the optical end of the scope will destroy the fiberoptics.

With the advent of laser arthroscopy and the many features that make the Ho:YAG laser in particular a very useful arthroscopic instrument, this technique must not be used indiscriminately or by an inexperienced operator. Complications can range from considerable local tissue destruction to deep penetration and perforation into the middle cranial fossa, resulting in death of the patient.

Complications of Electrocautery

The use of high-flow irrigation is required for electrocautery in arthroscopic surgical procedures, to control the generated heat. The zone of adjacent tissue injury has been reported to be 0.7 to 1.8 mm, and the zone increases with time. A nonconductive irrigant is advocated for use with electrocautery. Sterile water has been recommended as an irrigant,[28] but the hypoosmolar solution has been shown to cause dramatic changes in synovial surface cells and superficial chondrocytes and does not support proteoglycan synthesis.[58] Ringer's lactate is the irrigating fluid recommended by others because it supports cartilage metabolism and because no adverse effects have been reported. Tarro[39] reports its use in over 300 cases with no adverse effects.

During electrocautery, the tip as well as the length of the electrode needs to be monitored closely to prevent current arcing backward into the working canula, resulting in a soft tissue and skin thermal injury. The resultant concentric cutaneous burn may cause a cutaneous depression and a residual area of hyperpigmentation requiring secondary scar revision. Also, irreversible thermal damage to a motor nerve can occur if the cannula is adjacent to it, resulting in facial paralysis. In their retrospective review, Carter and Testa,[29] found a high correlation between nonresolving seventh nerve injury and the use of electrocautery. The correlation was much stronger than that seen with arthroscopic lysis and lavage.

The use of electrocautery in arthroscopic surgical procedures requires advanced surgical training and a knowledge of the possible complications secondary to thermal injury.

Long-Term Complications

Malocclusion

Occlusal changes seen after conservative TMJ surgery usually consisted of a limited posterior open bite, secondary to edema, that resolves within a few weeks. Minor occlusal discrepancies that fail to resolve may be treated with minimal occlusal adjustment.

Patients who have undergone a meniscectomy, patients who present with extreme degeneration of the condyle following extensive débridement with removal of alloplastic implants, and patients who have undergone aggressive arthroplasty for bony ankylosis can have significant occlusal changes. The development of an anterior open bite can result from these changes in posterior vertical height and may become a factor in continued symptoms. Correction of postoperative malocclusions may be very challenging and requires the services of surgeons, orthodontists, and prosthodontists experienced in treating such patients (Fig. 7–2). The TMJ symptoms first must be controlled. A stabilization splint is constructed, the occlusion is monitored for any continued change, and splint adjustments are made as necessary to allow for the continued change in occlusion. When there has been no change in the occlusion for at least 6 months, definitive treatment for the malocclusion can now be considered. Treatment options include orthodontics and orthognathic surgery.

Ankylosis

Fibrous ankylosis can form between the disk and the articular eminence following surgical arthroscopy and arthrotomy if meticulous hemostasis is not obtained and a hemarthrosis develops. Patient noncompliance with a postoperative physical therapy regimen can also result in fibrous ankylosis. True bony ankylosis can occur following diskectomy without proper postoperative physical therapy and is seen with increasing incidence after multiple surgical procedures secondary to inadequate bone removal or incomplete separation of bone surfaces.[59–61]

Clinically, the patient with fibrous ankylosis presents with a limited opening—less than 20 mm—and the absence of translation in the affected joint. The limited opening is usually less than 10 mm with bony ankylosis. If ankylosis is suspected, a computed tomography (CT) examination is indicated to delineate the location and extent of heterotopic bone formation. A CT examination with axial, coronal, and sagittal cuts enables the joints to be viewed from all perspectives, allowing precise planning of the procedure to ensure adequate resection and reducing the chances of reccurrence.

The goals of surgical treatment for fibrous and bony ankylosis are to restore range of motion and function, to avoid the development of a malocclusion, and to prevent recurrence of ankylosis. Surgical treatment of fibrous ankylosis depends on the extent and severity of adhesions. Treatment can range from aggressive physical therapy to passive stretching under anesthesia to arthroscopic lysis or arthrotomy for extensive intraarticular fibrosis.

Severe limitation in opening can make palpation of arthroscopic landmarks difficult, increasing the risks of surgical complications.

Ankylosis with intraarticular bony fusion and heterotopic bone formation is treated with a gap arthroplasty to create a 4- to 5-mm joint space and placement of an interpositioned material to prevent recurrent ankylosis. Aggressive bone recontouring can increase the risk of developing an aural-TMJ fistula, if the tympanic plate is posteriorly displaced into the external auditory canal (EAC). The bony segment requires reduction to prevent stenosis of the EAC, which may cause hearing impairment and or fistula formation. Numerous materials have been used since the concept was first advocated by Verneud in 1860. Alloplastic materials are no longer used, and there is not a consensus among surgeons as to the autogenous material of choice. Autogenous tissue grafts in use include temporalis muscle/fascia, dermis, and cartilage.

Recurrent ankylosis can occur secondary to inadequate bone removal or incomplete separation of bone surfaces. It usually occurs on the medial aspect of the joint where access is very difficult, resulting in an insufficient gap. It is therefore difficult to visualize placement of the interpositional graft and to ensure that all bony surfaces are covered. Preventive strategies, including the use of nonsteroidal antiinflammatory drugs (NSAIDs) have been reported in the orthopedic literature.[62, 63] NSAIDs may inhibit the differentiation and irrigation of heterotopic ossification. Indomethacin, 25 mg three times daily for 6 weeks postoperatively, is advocated.[64] In patients who have difficulty with gastrointestinal side effects, antacid use or rectal administration of the NSAID can be helpful.[65]

The postoperative range of motion depends on the

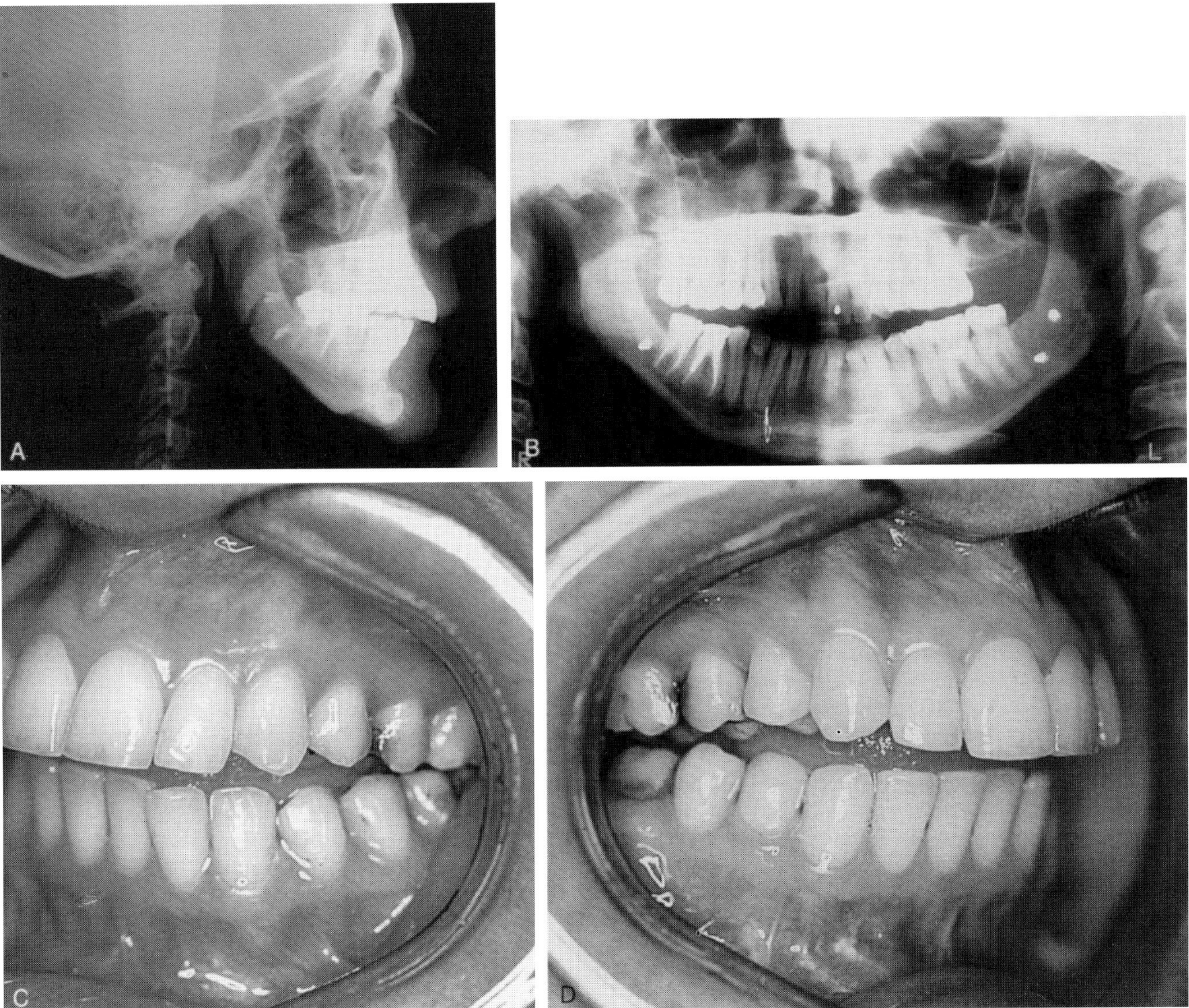

Figure 7–2. This 30-year-old female underwent a bilateral sagittal split osteotomy and genioplasty followed by bilateral TMJ surgery. Bilateral condylar resorption developed postoperatively, with resultant open-bite malocclusion. *A*, Lateral cephalograph. *B*, Panoramic radiograph. *C* and *D*, Photographs showing occlusion.

extent of ankylosis, the extent of muscle fibrosis and atrophy, and the patient's compliance with the prescribed physical therapy regimen. Postoperative physical therapy is vital to the success of treatment of ankylosis. Therapy is directed at maintaining the range of motion obtained surgically. Active range-of-motion exercise are begun in the immediate postoperative period or after the release of intermaxillary fixation, avoiding overly aggressive stretching, which can cause intraarticular hemorrhage and recurrent ankylosis. Close postoperative supervision by the surgeon is paramount to ensure patient compliance and commitment to the physical therapy regimen. It must be stressed that the range-of-motion exercises are as important to overall success as the surgery itself. Patient failure to comply with the range-of-motion exercises results in recurrent limitation of movement.

Ankylosis presents a formidable challenge to the surgeon. Careful clinical examination with appropriate imaging to delineate the extent and location of the bony fusion is necessary to formulate an appropriate treatment plan. The complexity and extent of the surgical procedure should reflect the severity of ankylosis. The patient's cooperation and maintenance of the postoperative exercise regimen are most important to ensure a successful outcome.

Implant Failure

All alloplastic implants fail with time.[17] When the implant is subjected to the forces of articulation, particulation occurs, and a foreign body giant cell reaction ensues, causing degeneration or resorption of the surrounding bone and soft tissue. The subjective symptoms of implant failure include increasing joint pain with limited function, the feeling of swelling or tightness in the area of the joint, and fullness in the ears in spite of a negative otologic examination. Clinically, there is a decrease in range of motion, crepitus, and occlusal changes usually presenting as an anterior open bite. With Proplast-Teflon interpositional implants, severe bone loss may occur without clinical signs or symptoms, the only evidence, in an asymptomatic patient, being found on imaging of the joint. Panoramic radiographs are a good screening film to detect condylar change; however, the temporal aspect of the joint is not always clearly visualized on such studies. The superimposition of bone over the giant cell granulomatous destruction necessitates the use of CT scanning or magnetic resonance imaging (MRI) to adequately visualize the soft tissue changes. CT scanning is preferred for determining the extent of destruction of the temporal bone and condyle (Fig. 7–3). MRI allows visualization of both the implant and the surrounding soft tissues. For nonmetallic implants, MRI is the most efficient method to detect signs of a foreign body giant cell response, implant deterioration, and destruction of the surrounding bone and soft tissues.[66]

Patients with alloplastic implants should be contacted, should undergo a clinical examination, and should have a CT or MRI evaluation.[67] The surgeon must not wait for clinical signs and symptoms to manifest. Ultimately, it is the patient's decision to have the implant removed. The risks and complications should be presented along with treatment options. If there are no clinical signs or symptoms of implant failure and the patient refuses removal, periodic reevaluation and imaging should be considered. With the current trend in health care reform and cost containment, however, it hardly seems justified to spend $800 to $1200 every 6 months to image an implant that will ultimately fail.[17]

Current recommendations for the management of patients with failing implants are as follows[17]:

- All implants should be removed with thorough débridement of the surrounding soft tissues in the joint. Débridement utilizing an operative microscope has been advocated. Because of the difficulty of complete débridement of all traces of the foreign body giant cell reaction and particles of the implant, no disk replacement is recommended. Migration of particles into autogenous replacements can lead to failure. Recurrent foreign body giant cell reaction can occur, so patients need to undergo long-term periodic reevaluation and imaging.
- Temporal bone perforation can be a result of the foreign body giant cell reaction. However, most perforations occur away from the area of articulation, are small, and need not be repaired. If a perforation is large and repair is indicated, cranial bone, autogenous cartilage, and allogenic cartilage have been utilized. If a dural tear with a resultant CSF leak is noted, an immediate neurosurgical consultation is indicated. Fibrin tissue adhesive can be used for the repair, as previously described.
- Reconstruction of the joint may not be indicated if the patient's range of motion is acceptable and occlusal changes are not significant. Use of elastic traction and physical therapy can decrease the adverse occlusal changes caused by the loss of posterior vertical dimension. If occlusal changes are significant, a stabilization splint is indicated to determine the progression and magnitude of change prior to the performance of osteotomies to correct occlusal discrepancies. It is imperative that the patient be informed of the possibility of recurrent granuloma formation with the risk of continued occlusal changes. The recurrent granuloma can develop as late as 2 years after removal of the implant.

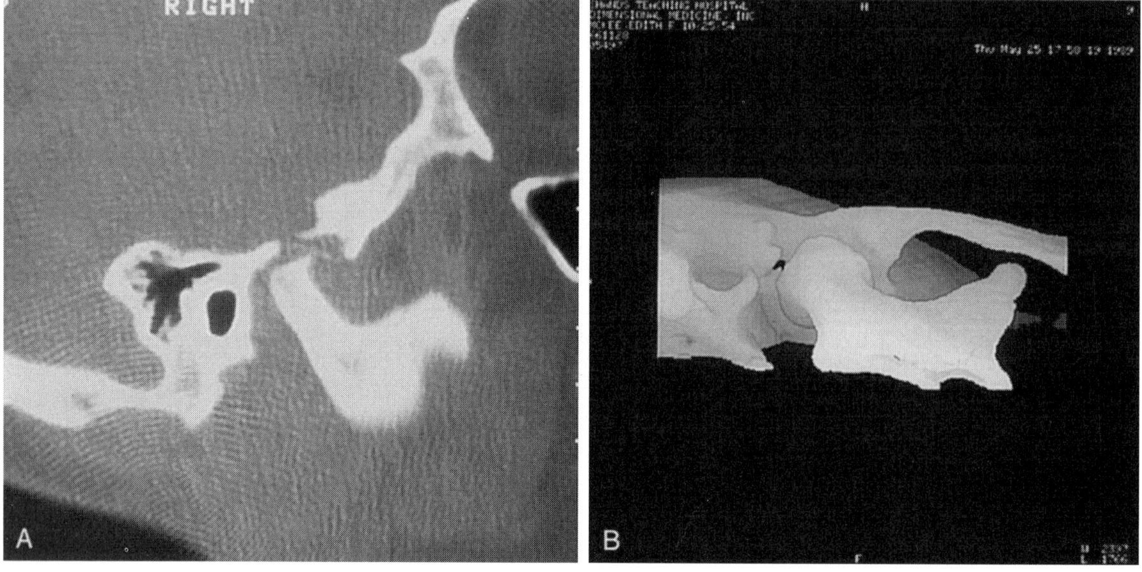

Figure 7–3. This 35-year-old female developed a foreign body reaction to the Proplast-Teflon implant. *A*, CT scan demonstrating perforation of the fossa. *B*, Three-dimensional CT scan demonstrating perforation of the fossa.

Persistent Pain in the Multiply-Operated Patient

Surgical treatment of TMJ internal derangement has proved effective for reducing pain and dysfunction in about 80% of patients regardless of operative technique.[2] Even if a successful surgical procedure has been performed, the patient's pain and dysfunction may not be significantly improved, therefore, the decision to perform surgery must be carefully made.

The most common reasons for failure of surgical management to resolve a patient's TMJ pain and dysfunction are improper patient selection and misdiagnosis. On the basis of the patient's history and clinical examination, the surgeon must be convinced that the patient's symptoms arise within the TMJ and that the pain and dysfunction are localized to the TMJ. It must be remembered that imaging can identify specific anatomic abnormalities; however, the lack of correlation of these findings with pain preclude their use as a primary consideration for surgery.[1]

The literature is virtually devoid of any long-term recommendations for the management of the multiply-operated patients, here again reinforcing the need for careful patient selection and treatment planning. The tendency is to recommend another surgical procedure to these patients, because the original diagnosis was not correct or an inappropriate surgical procedure was performed and resulted in the persistence of the pain and dysfunction. However, the percentage of success is dramatically reduced with each subsequent surgical procedure.

Usually, the patient who has undergone previous surgery and experiences persistent symptoms presents with a complex history. Evaluation by an integrated team approach of which the surgeon is a member is recommended.[68] Consultation with a pain specialist in conjunction with a physical therapist and clinical psychologist can be very beneficial in enabling the patient to deal with, and manage, chronic pain and dysfunction.

To properly assess this type of patient, the sequence of events leading to the present situation need to be reviewed along with previous imaging records, treatment notes, and operative reports. Direct contact with previous providers for their perspective about the prior treatment and its outcome may be very beneficial. Also, the status of any pending litigation should be known, because the patient's symptoms may change with the success or failure of the proceedings.

Proceeding with an integrated nonsurgical program is recommended before consideration of any further surgical intervention. Nonsurgical management is directed at unloading the joints, reducing inflammation, relieving muscle spasms, teaching behavior management and pain coping skills, offering treatment of depression and sleep disturbances, of pain with the various pain control modalities, and of any coexisting pain problems.

The integrated approach to and assessment of patients with a history of multiple surgical procedures are especially prudent, and the indications for additional TMJ surgery should be made much more rigid. Most such patients look to surgery as a "quick fix" for their pain and dysfunction. The consideration for additional surgery should be made after careful deliberation by the team. Surgical management is unique in each case, and the type and extent of the procedure depend on the existing symptoms, functional impairment, and condition of the joint structures. However, despite a successful surgical procedure, the patient's pain may not be significantly improved immediately, and continued nonsurgical management may be necessary for long-term successful relief of pain and dysfunction.

Summary

The potential complications discussed in this chapter range from perioperative complications common to both TMJ arthroscopy and arthrotomy, to specific complications associated with arthroscopy, to long-term complications. The strategies for their prevention and management are discussed. These complications are infrequent and can be prevented with meticulous attention to surgical anatomy and technique.

Careful patient selection is paramount, because the most common reasons for failure of TMJ surgery are improper patient selection and misdiagnosis. It must be emphasized that the criterion for surgery is not simply refractory pain, but pain localized to the TMJ.

When TMJ surgery is considered, the possible complications, their management, and their implications for the overall success of the proposed procedure should be reviewed with the patient. Good patient-doctor rapport can prevent a complication from becoming a major hindrance to a successful outcome.

The literature is virtually devoid of any long-term recommendations for the management of the multiply-operated patients who present with persistent pain and dysfunction. Evaluation and treatment using an integrated team approach, involving a pain specialist, a clinical psychologist, and a physical therapist as well as the surgeon, is recommended. This nonsurgical approach can be very beneficial, enabling the patient to deal with and manage chronic pain and dysfunction. The consideration for additional surgery should be made after careful deliberation by the team. It must be remembered that a successful surgical procedure may not significantly reduce the patient's pain.

References

1. Dolwick M, Nitzan D: The role of disc-repositioning surgery for internal derangements of the temporomandibular joint. Oral Maxillofac Surg Clin North Am 1994;6:271.
2. Dolwick M, Dimitroulis G: Is there a role for temporomandibular surgery? Br J Oral Maxillofac Surg 1994;32:307.
3. Ad Hoc Study Group in TMJ Meniscus Surgery: 1984 Criteria for TMJ Meniscus Surgery. American Association of Oral and Maxillofacial Surgeons, 1984.
4. Dolwick M, Ochs M: Surgical management of TMJ internal derangement. *In* Zarb G (ed): TMJ and Masticatory Muscle Disorders, Copenhagen, Munksgaard, 1994, p 449.

5. McCain J: Complications of TMJ Arthroscopy. J Oral Maxillofac Surg 1988;46:256.
6. Westesson P, Eriksson L, Liedbert J: The risk of damage to facial nerve, superficial temporal vessles, disk and articular surfaces during arthroscopic examination of the temporomandibular joint. Oral Surg 1986;62:124.
7. Holmlund A, Hellsing G: Arthroscopy of the TMJ: An autopsy study. Int J Oral Surg 1985;14:169.
8. Greene M, Hackney F, Van Sickels J: Arthroscopy of the tempromandibular joint: An anatomic perspective. J Oral Maxillofac Surg 1989;47:386.
9. Kornbrot A, Shaw A, Toohey M: Pseudoaneurysm as a complication of arthroscopy: A case report. J Oral Maxillofac Surg 1991;49:1226.
10. Moses J, Topper D: Arteriovenous fistula: An unusual complication associated with arthroscopic TMJ surgery. J Oral Maxillofac Surg 1990;48:1220.
11. Dolwick M, Sanders B: TMJ internal derangement and arthrosis. *In* Surgical Atlas. St Louis, CV Mosby, 1985, p 142.
12. Husted E: Surgical diseases of the TMJ. Acta Odontol Scand 1956;14:119.
13. Peoples J, Euzenio G, Dion J: Management of internal maxillary artery hemorrhage from TMJ surgery via selective embolization. J Oral Maxillofac Surg 1988;46:1005.
14. McCain J: Arthroscopy of the human temporomandibular joint. J Oral Maxillofac Surg 1988;46:648.
15. Yih W, Merrill R: Pathology of alloplastic interpositional implants in the temporomandibular joint. Oral Maxillofac Surg Clin North Am 1989;1:415.
16. Hartog J, Slavin A, Kline S: Reconstruction of the TMJ with cryopreserved cartilage and freezed dried dura: A preliminary report. J Oral Maxillofac Surg 1990;48:919.
17. Ryan D: Alloplastic disc replacement. Oral Maxillofac Surg Clin North Am 1994;6:307.
18. Lerner R, Binur N: Current research review, current status of surgical adhesive. J Surg Res 1990;48:165.
19. Tayapogsak P, O'Brien D, Monteiro C: Autogenous fibrin adhesive in mandibular reconstruction with particulate cancellous bone and marrow. J Oral Maxillofac Surg 1994;52:161.
20. Kaugers G, Mercuri L, Laskin D: Pneumatization of the articular eminence of the temporal bone: Prevalence, development and surgical treatment. J Am Dent Assoc 1986;113:55.
21. Tyndall D, Matteson R: Radiographic appearance and population distribution of the pneumatized articular eminence of the temporal bone. J Oral Maxillofac Surg 1985;43:493.
22. Kulikowski B, Schow S, Kraut R: Surgical management of a pneumatized articular eminence of the temporal bone. J Oral Surg 1982;40:311.
23. Al-Kayat A, Bramley P: A modified pre-auricular approach to the temporomandibular joint and malar arch. Br J Oral Surg 1979;17:91.
24. McCain J, Sanders B, Koslin M, et al: TMJ arthroscopy: A 6-year multicenter retrospective study of 4,831 joints. J Oral Maxillofac Surg 1992;50:926.
25. Greene M, Van Sickles J: Survey of TMJ arthroscopy in oral and maxillofacial surgery residency programs. J Oral Maxillofac Surg 1989;47:574.
26. McCain J: An Illustrated Guide to TMJ Arthroscopy. Andover, MA, Dyonics Corporation, 1987.
27. Weinberg S, Kryshtalsky J: Facial nerve function following TMJ surgery using the preauricular approach. J Oral Maxillofac Surg 1992;50:1048.
28. Carter J, Schwaber M: Temporomandibular joint arthroscopy: Complications and their management. Oral Maxillofac Surg Clinics North Am 1989;1:185.
29. Carter J, Testa L: Complications of TMJ arthroscopy: A review of 2,225 cases: Review of the 1988 Annual Scientific Sessions abstracts. J Oral Maxillofac Surg 1988;46:M14.
30. Heffez L, Blaustein D: Diagnostic arthroscopy of the temporomandibular joint. I: Normal arthroscopic findings. Oral Surg 1987;64:653.
31. Sanders B: Arthroscopic surgery of the temporomandibular joint: Treatment of internal derangement with persistent closed lock. Oral Surg 1986;62:361.
32. Dolwick M, Kretzschmar D: Morbidity associated with the preauricular and perimeatal approaches to the temporomandibular joint. Oral Surg 1982;40:699.
33. Kryshtalsky J, Weinberg S: An Assessment for auriculotemporal syndrome following temporomandibular joint surgery through the preauricular approach. J Oral Maxillofac Surg 1989;47:3.
34. Berrois R, Quinn P: Frey's syndrome: Complication after orthognathic surgery. Intl J Adult Orthod-Orthog Surg 1986;1:219.
35. Eppley B, Delfino J: Use of prophylactic antibiotics in temporomandibular joint surgery. J Oral Maxillofacial Surg 1985; 43:675.
36. King G: The case against antibiotic prophylaxis in major head and neck surgery. Laryngoscope 1961;71:647.
37. Ketchum A, Block J, Crawford D, et al: The role of prophylactic antibiotic therapy in control of staphylococcal infections following cancer surgery. Surg Gynecol Obstet 1962;114:345.
38. Vallerand W, Dolwick M: Complications of temporomandibular joint surgery. Oral Maxillofac Surg Clin North Am 1990;2:481.
39. Tarro A: TMJ Arthroscopy: A Diagnostic and Surgical Atlas. Philadelphia, JB Lippincott, 1993, p 143.
40. Hall H: The role of discetomy for treating internal derangement of the temporomandibular joint. Oral Maxillofac Surg Clin North Am 1994;6:287.
41. McCain J, Zabiegalski N, Levine R: Joint infection as a complication of temporomandibular joint arthroscopy: A case report. J Oral Maxillofac Surg 1993;51:1389.
42. Van Sickles J, Nishioka G, Hegewald M, et al: Middle ear injury resulting from temporomandibular joint arthroscopy. J Oral Maxillofac Surg 1987;45:962.
43. Applebaum E, Berg L, Kumar A, et al: Otologic complications following temporomandibular joint arthroscopy. Ann Otol Rhinol Laryngol 1988;97:675.
44. Laughner B, Larkin H, Mahan P: Discomalleolar and anterior malleolar ligaments: Possible causes of middle ear damage during temporomandibular joint surgery. Oral Surg 1989;68:14.
45. Sinn D, Theramen W, Culbertson M, et al: Surgical correction of an aural-TMJ fistula with a temporalis flap. J Oral Maxillofac Surg 1994;52:197.
46. Cecine A, Ng P: Polyp of the external ear canal arising from the TMJ: A case report. J Otolaryngol 1991;20:168.
47. Myerhoff W, Caruso V: Trauma and infections of the external ear. *In* Paparella M, Shumrick DA, Gluckman JL, Mayerhoff WL (eds): Otolaryngology, ed 3. Philadelphia, WB Saunders, 1991, p 1227.
48. Bluestone C, Meyerhoff W: Diseases and Disorders of the Eustachian Tube–Middle Ear. *In* Paparella M, Shumrick DA, Gluckman JL, Mayerhoff WL (eds): Otolaryngology, ed 3. Philadelphia, WB Saunders, 1991, p 1289.
49. Epker B, Burnette J: Trauma to the parotid gland and duct: Primary treatment and management of complications. J Oral Surg 1970;28:657.
50. Gomez T, Gilder J: Reflex bradycardia during TMJ arthroscopy: A case report. J Oral Maxillofac Surg 1991;49:543.
51. Indresano A: Arthroscopic surgery of the temporomandibular joint: Report of 64 patients with long-term follow-up. J Oral Maxillofac Surg 1989;47:439.
52. Goss A, Bosanquet A: Temporomandibular joint arthroscopy. J Oral Maxillofac Surg 1986;44:614.
53. Hendler B, Levin L: Postobstructive pulmonary edema as a sequela of TMJ arthroscopy: A case report. J Oral Maxillofac Surg 1993;51:315.
54. Bjornland T, Rorvik M, Haanoes J, et al: Degenerative changes in the temporomandibular joint after diagnostic arthroscopy. Int J Oral Maxillofac Surg 1994;23:41.
55. McCain J, De La Rua H: Foreign body retrieval: A complication of TMJ arthroscopy. J Oral Maxillofac Surg 1989;47:1221.
56. Tarro A: Instrument breakage associated with arthroscopy of the temporomandibular joint: Report of a case. J Oral Maxillofac Surg 1989;47:1226.
57. Hendler B, Gateno J, Mooar P, et al: Holmium:Yag laser arthroscopy of the temporomandibular joint. J Oral Maxillofac Surg 1992;50:931.
58. Thomas M, Lane C, Koslin M: Electrocautery and fluid mediums. *In* Bronstein S (ed): Arthroscopy of the TMJ. Philadelphia, WB Saunders, 1991, p 204.
59. Rotskoff K: Management of hypomobility and hypermobility

disorders of the TMJ. *In* Peterson LJ (ed): Principles of Oral and Maxillofacial Surgery. Philadelphia, JB Lippincott, 1992, p 1989.

60. Norman J: Ankylosis of the TMJ. Aust Dent J 1978;56.
61. Linquist C, Soderholm A-L, Hallikainen D, et al: Erosin and heterotopic bone formation after alloplastic TMJ reconstruction. J Oral Maxillofac Surg 1992;50:942.
62. Warren S: Heterotopic ossification after total hip replacement. Orthop Re 1990;19:603.
63. Sodermann B, Persson P, Nilsson O: Prevention of heterotopic ossification by non-steroid anti-inflammatory drugs after total hip arthroplasty. Clin Orthop 1988;237:158.
64. Cella J, Salvati E, Sculo T: Indocin for the prevention of heterotopic ossification following total hip arthroplasty. J Arthroplasty 1988;3:229.
65. Knahr K, Salzer M, Eyb R, et al: Heterotopic ossification with hip endoprosthesis in various models of thrombosis prophylaxis. J Arthroplasty 1988;3:1.
66. Smith R, Goldwasser M, Sabol S: Erosion of a Teflon-Proplast implant into the middle cranial fossa. J Oral Maxillofac Surg 1993;51:1268.
67. US Food and Drug Administration: FDA Safety Alert. Rockville, MD, US Food and Drug Administration, Sept 1991.
68. Roser S, Sanders B, Merrill R, et al: Management of the failed surgical patient. *In* Peterson L (ed): Principles of Oral Max Surgery. Philadelphia, JB Lippincott, 1992, p 2043.

Chapter 8
DONOR SITE MORBIDITY

Diagnosis, Treatment, and Prevention

by

Thomas B. Dodson

Introduction

Oral and maxillofacial surgeons commonly harvest autologous hard and soft tissues for reconstructive procedures. The literature consists primarily of technique papers describing a variety of donor sites and harvesting operations, although some reports address donor site morbidity anecdotally along with other subjects. In recent years, more emphasis has been placed on systematically reviewing the issue of donor site morbidity. This chapter reviews the common hard and soft tissue donor sites used in oral and maxillofacial surgery, emphasizing the diagnosis, treatment, and prevention of donor site morbidity. For the purposes of this chapter, donor site morbidity has been categorized as early or late, according to when the complications develop. *Early complications* are defined as those that develop during the perioperative period or self-limiting complications; *late complications* occur several weeks to months postoperatively or are persistent early complications.

The Subjects Discussed in This Chapter Are:

- Donor site morbidity with free autologous bone grafts
  - Iliac crest
  - Chest
  - Calvaria
  - Mandible
  - Tibia
- Donor site morbidity with vascularized autologous bone grafts
  - Radial forearm
  - Fibula
- Donor site morbidity with soft tissue grafts
  - Split-thickness skin grafts
  - Mucosa
- Donor site morbidity with nerve grafts
  - Sural nerve
  - Greater auricular nerve
  - Medial antebrachial cutaneous nerve

Donor Site Morbidity with Free Autologous Bone Grafts

Free autologous bone is the material of choice for reconstructing skeletal defects in the host with a healthy recipient site. Autogenous bone grafts become vascularized in a short time, and healing is accompanied by a better quality and quantity of bone formation than are seen with allogeneic grafts. In addition, autogenous grafts do not elicit an immune response, and there is no question of transmission of communicable diseases such as hepatitis and AIDS. When autologous bone is used, however, the patient is subject to donor site problems such as pain, functional limitations, infection, hemorrhage, and deformities. In addition, there may be an inadequate quantity of bone, especially in the pediatric or geriatric patient.

Iliac Crest

Early Morbidity

The iliac crest is a common source of particulate marrow, corticocancellous chips, and corticocancellous blocks. Morbidity depends on the amount and type of graft harvested and the donor site (anterior or posterior iliac crest). Documented early donor site morbidity commonly includes pain and gait disturbances. Less common complications are excessive blood loss, ileus, wound breakdown, infection, and hematoma or seroma formation.

Pain and Gait Disturbance

Patients commonly complain of pain and gait disturbances after an iliac crest bone graft has been harvested. Between 6% and 100% of patients complain of postoperative donor site pain that ranges from moderate to severe.[1–6] More pain is associated with the removal of bone grafts involving both cortical plates.[7]

Gait disturbances are attributable to muscle dissection and stripping of the iliacus, gluteus, and tensor fascia lata muscles to expose the underlying bone.[5, 8–15] In contrast, patients report little pain or gait disturbance when particulate marrow alone is harvested. Kreibich and associates[16] recommend using a percutaneous approach if <10 mL of particulate marrow is needed.

Donor site location and anterior or posterior iliac crest affect the incidence and severity of pain and gait disturbance. Bloomquist and Feldman[12] anecdotally reported that pain was less with graft removal from the posterior than from the anterior iliac crest. This finding was confirmed in a randomized clinical trial comparing anterior and posterior iliac crest donor sites. In this latter study, Marx and Morales[5] found that patients in whom bone was harvested via a posterior approach walked sooner than patients who had an anterolateral approach (1.7 days versus 3.6 days; $P < .005$). Patients who had had a posterior approach, however, reported having greater difficulty climbing stairs or rising from a sitting position.[12]

Generally, pain is self-limiting and lasts 3 to 60 days.[1, 2, 7, 13, 17] The duration of gait disturbance ranges from less than 4 days to 4 months, with no gait disturbances reported at 1-year follow-up.[1, 3, 5, 10, 11] Younger patients commonly have both a shorter duration of pain and less gait disturbance than older patients.[8, 15]

Infection and Delayed Wound Healing

The rate of donor site infection ranges from 0 to 4%. Infections are minor and can be treated with local wound care.[1–3, 8] Rate of delayed wound healing averages 1.3% (range, 0 to 5%) (Fig. 8–1).[8, 11, 13] Placing the incision directly over the bony prominence of the iliac crest increases the risk of delayed wound healing.[13] To avoid this complication, the incision should be placed either medial or lateral to the iliac crest. The skin can then be shifted over the crest, avoiding postoperative pressure. This technique also reduces the muscle dissection needed. The incision should be at least 2 cm medial to the crest to avoid spontaneous shifting of the wound to over the crest when the patient stands.[1, 18]

Blood Loss and Hematoma or Seroma Formation

Blood loss is minimal when harvesting cancellous bone grafts and increases with the size of the full-thickness corticocancellous graft. Intraoperative blood loss from the donor site ranges from 75 to 800 mL per operation.[1, 5, 12, 13, 17, 19] In one study, there was a statistically significant difference in the mean intraoperative blood loss between the posterior and anterior approaches (306 mL and 474 mL, respectively; $P < .001$).[5] The volume of postoperative drainage of blood from the wound ranges from 150 mL to 256 mL.[9, 13] To reduce intraoperative blood loss, it is recommended (1) to remove cancellous bone expeditiously and (2) to use bone wax.[1] Because of the significant amount of post-

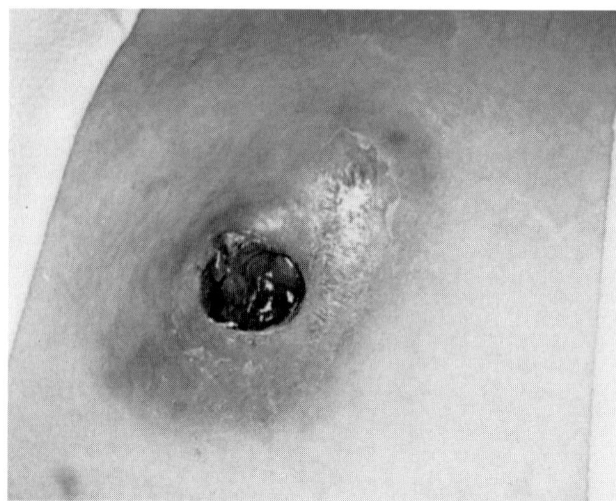

Figure 8–1. Right iliac crest of a supine patient illustrating wound breakdown after harvesting of bone graft. (*From* Dodson TB, Kaban LB: Donor site morbidity: Diagnosis, treatment, and prevention. Oral Maxillofac Surg Clin North Am 1990;2:489.)

operative oozing from the site, a suction drain may be placed in the donor wound for at least 24 hours, or until the output is less than 25 mL in an 8-hour period. Significant hemorrhage is uncommon, because most intraoperative bleeding is localized to the wound and readily controlled. There is, however, a case report of retroperitoneal bleeding that resulted in patient death.[20] Vessels at risk during harvesting of an anterior iliac crest bone graft are the deep circumflex iliac artery and the gluteal artery. Signs and symptoms of significant retroperitoneal bleeding are hypotension, hemodynamic instability, decreasing hematocrit, and lower abdominal mass. Recommended diagnostic tests include CT scanning and ultrasonography.

The rate of hematoma formation ranges from 0 to 6%.[1-3, 5, 21] Most hematomas are minor; however, one case report documents a patient who developed a retroperitoneal hematoma following an anterior approach to the ilium.[22] Seromas occur with a reported frequency of 0 to 50%.[1, 3, 5, 8, 10, 13, 14, 17, 23] Both complications are less common when the donor site is drained. When compared with the anterior approach, hematoma or seroma formation is less frequent after harvesting posterior iliac crest.[5]

Adynamic Ileus

Adynamic ileus is a rare complication of iliac crest harvest. It was mentioned as a potential complication in two studies, but no case was reported.[13, 17] There is a report of ileus occurring as a complication of this procedure in two elderly women.[24]

Orthopedic Complications

Orthopedic complications include fracture of the iliac spine or acetabulum, iliac crest subluxation, and pelvic instability. The risk of these complications increases with the size of the graft. Fractures of the anterior iliac crest spine occur uncommonly (2% to 13.3%) in the early postoperative period.[5, 10, 25, 26] Acetabular fracture and iliac crest subluxation are rare, particularly if exposure is adequate and the force used to free and deliver the graft is not excessive.[18, 27] Pelvic instability is a complication of posterior iliac crest harvest.[28, 29] Injury of the sacroiliac crest joint and weakening of the posterior sacroiliac crest ligaments may lead to stress at the pubic rami and subsequent pelvic fractures.

Late Morbidity

Late complications of iliac bone harvest are uncommon. They include persistent pain and gait disturbance, contour defects and unaesthetic scars, paresthesia, hernia, and pseudoaneurysm formation.

Whereas pain and gait disturbances are rare after 6 months, contour defects are common, especially when the crest has been removed to harvest a large full-thickness corticocancellous block (Fig. 8–2).[13, 21, 30] The crest is replaced as a free graft, and the contour abnormality results from remodeling and resorption during healing. Sagittal splitting of the iliac crest to gain access is associated with an excessively wide contour.

Two modifications of the harvesting technique help to avoid contour abnormalities. If a small to medium-sized piece of bone is needed, the iliac crest may be left intact, and the graft harvested as a plug from below the crest. When a large block of bone is needed, it is possible to elevate the crest as a flap attached to muscle (Figs. 8–3 and 8–4). With these two techniques, the iliac crest maintains its blood supply. Therefore, resorption, with a resultant contour defect, does not occur. A wide or hypertrophic scar is not uncommon and may result from wound breakdown, infection, or poor incision placement.[13, 14] For example, the classic incision used to access the posterior iliac crest follows the line of the underlying bone and is associated with a higher risk for neuroma formation, paresthesia, and a widened scar. A suggested alternative incision follows a line from the fourth lumbar vertebra to the greater trochanter. In a study comparing the two incisions, patients receiving the alternative approach reported less pain, fewer neurosensory changes, and a more aesthetic scar.[31] Another common complication is the presence of suture tracks when the skin sutures are not removed early.[13]

The frequency of persistent paresthesia of the lateral femoral cutaneous nerve ranges from 0 to 17%.[1, 3, 11, 17] Also, there are reports of injury to the femoral, ilioinguinal, cluneal, sciatic, and subcostal and iliohypogastric lateral cutaneous nerves.[5, 12, 26, 32] The most common mechanism of injury is excessive soft tissue traction. A painful paresthesia known as meralgia is a neurologic disorder characterized by altered sensation with a burning or tingling feeling or stabbing pain. Fortunately, it is rare, ranging in frequency from 0 to

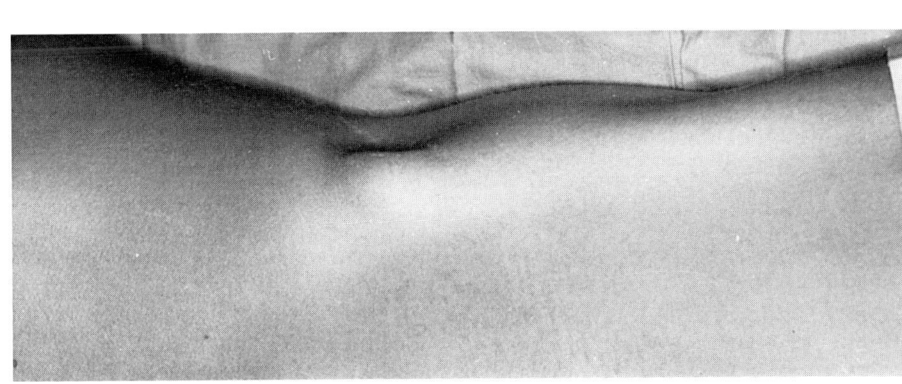

Figure 8–2. Contour deformity after harvesting of bone graft from left iliac crest. Patient is supine. (*From* Dodson TB, Kaban LB: Donor site morbidity: Diagnosis, treatment, and prevention. Oral Maxillofac Surg Clin North Am 1990;2:489.)

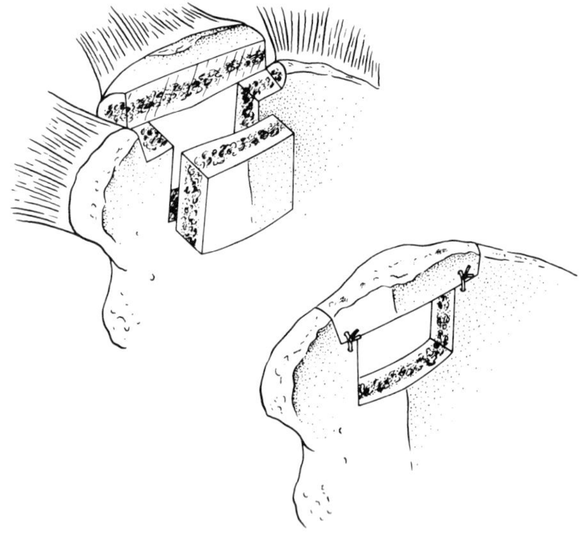

Figure 8–3. Technique for harvesting full-thickness iliac crest bone graft. Note that crest is pedicled to soft tissue medially and fits tightly into place on a bone ledge created by osteotomy. (*From* Dodson TB, Kaban LB: Donor site morbidity: Diagnosis, treatment, and prevention. Oral Maxillofac Surg Clin North Am 1990;2:489.)

1.8%.[13, 23, 27] To avoid injury to the nerve, 1 cm of bone should be left intact proximal to the anterior iliac spine. Excessive retraction should be avoided.

Rare complications are hernia, arteriovenous fistula, and ureteral injury.[33, 34] Harvesting large full-thickness bone grafts with a poor approximation of dissected muscle may result in a hernia. Hernias are rare, with a reported frequency of 0 to 0.8%, and appear from 5 months to 11 years after the operation.[17, 21, 27, 35–37] To prevent herniation, excessive muscle dissection should be avoided, and the detached muscles reattached carefully.

Chest

Early Morbidity

The chest is an excellent source of bone and cartilage in the form of rib or costochondral graft. Harvesting is technically easy with little morbidity. The graft may be harvested with or without cartilage and may be used in full thickness, split longitudinally, or milled into corticocancellous chips. Complications depend on the number of ribs or amount of cartilage harvested and, to some extent, on the incision site. Early complications include pleural tears with the development of pneumothorax or hemothorax, pain and associated respiratory difficulties such as atelectasis and pneumonia, infection, and delayed wound healing.

Pleural Injury

Pleural injury (pleural tear or pneumothorax) is associated with harvesting multiple ribs and with the use of a small incision for aesthetic reasons. In addition, the frequency of pleural tears increases with the removal of large segments of cartilage. The frequency of well-documented pleural injuries averages 4.4%.[7, 13, 30, 38–42] In one paper, a complication rate of 20% to 30% was reported.[15] These were poorly documented cases, however, and such a high complication rate has not been seen in other studies.

After the rib or costochondral graft is removed, the surgeon should examine the wound carefully for a pleural tear. The donor site is filled with normal saline, and a maximal positive-pressure breath is delivered by the anesthesiologist. The appearance of air bubbles in the wound suggests a pleural tear. A postoperative chest radiograph is mandatory, because intraoperative examination may not demonstrate a small pleural opening or pneumothorax. Matthews[40] reported three cases of pneumothorax identified postoperatively despite careful intraoperative examination of the donor site with a well expanded lung.[40] Although there may be no intraoperative evidence of pleural injury, the sharp ends of the cut rib may puncture the pleura if the patient coughs vigorously during extubation or during the early postoperative period. Straight cuts of the rib reduce the incidence of pleural injury.

Pain, Atelectasis, and Pneumonia

Postoperative donor site pain is a universal complaint, with a mean duration of 2 weeks (range 1 to 8 weeks).[6, 13] Pain may result in splinting with a decreased tidal volume, atelectasis, and pneumonia. The overall frequency of postoperative pneumonia is 2.9% (range, 0 to 12.2%).[13, 37, 38, 42] Respiratory difficulty is decreased if two or fewer ribs are harvested.[41] An intercostal nerve block or an epidural drip with bupivacaine is useful to decrease chest pain and improve respiratory effort. Effective postoperative physiotherapy reduces the risk of postoperative pneumonia following rib harvest.

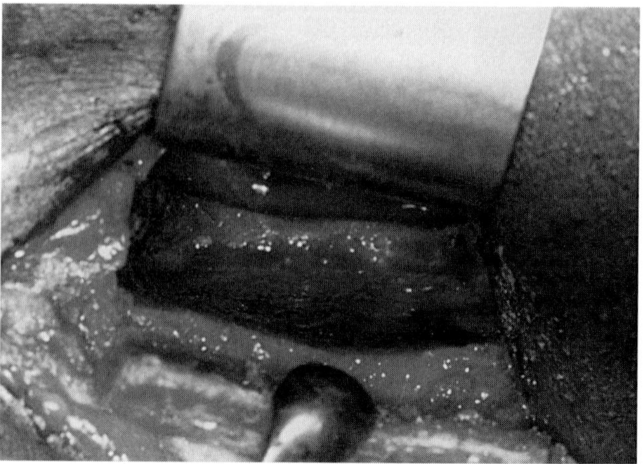

Figure 8–4. Alternative technique for harvesting corticocancellous bone graft from the iliac crest. Donor site is right anterior iliac crest and the crest is pedicled to soft tissue laterally.

Wound Infection

The frequency of postoperative wound infections ranges from 0 to 2.4%.[13, 37, 38, 42] The reported frequency of delayed wound healing ranges from 0 to 2.4%.[12, 13, 38]

Late Morbidity

Late complications of rib harvesting include pleuritic pain, a hypertrophic scar, and a contour defect. The frequency of persistent pleuritic pain after 2 years ranges from 0 to 6.8%.[13, 42] This pain probably is secondary to scar formation between the parietal and the visceral pleura. Laurie and colleagues[13] reported the mean length and width of the incision as 7.5 cm and 0.3 cm, respectively. More than half the patients (26 of 44) had suture tracks present. Such tracks can be avoided by using dermal sutures with early removal of skin sutures or by using buried subcuticular closure. Korlof and coworkers[30] reported that five of 46 patients had a wide, conspicuous scar (Fig. 8–5). To obtain the best aesthetic result, the incision should be in the inframammary fold in adults and 2.5 cm from the edge of the nipple-areolar complex in children. Although some surgeons still use a lateral thoracotomy incision to harvest ribs, such a placement may result in an unsightly scar.[38] Adequate amounts of bone or cartilage can be obtained via the inframammary approach. The lateral thoracotomy approach offers no advantages and should be avoided.

Visible contour defects generally are associated with harvest of cartilage. The defect can be well camouflaged, particularly in female patients, if the incision is placed in the inframammary fold and the rib is harvested under the breast.

Calvaria

Early Morbidity

The skull is an excellent source of corticocancellous bone with little donor site morbidity. In children the skull can provide an abundant source of grafting material.[43] In maxillofacial surgery, the operating field often includes the donor site, and harvesting time is short with little blood loss. The mean time for harvesting a cranial bone graft is 35 minutes (range, 30 to 45 minutes) with blood loss ranging from 20 to 200 mL.[44–46] In addition, there is greater retention of residual graft volume compared with iliac bone grafts.[43] Early complications of calvarial bone grafting are perforation of the inner table with dural injury, formation of a seroma or hematoma, and infection. Patients report little postoperative pain.[45, 47, 48]

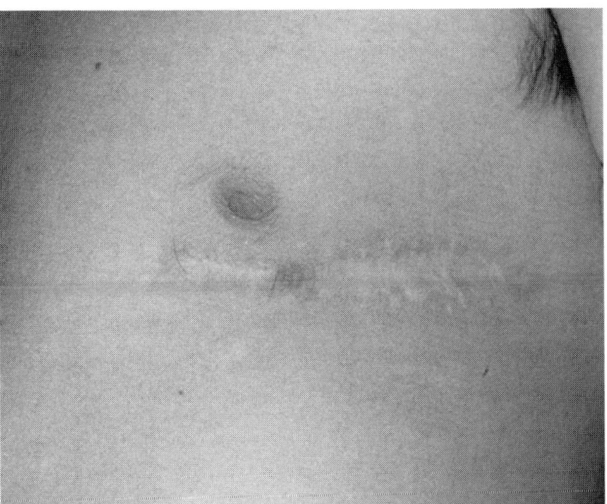

Figure 8–5. A wide, conspicuous scar with suture tracks after harvesting of rib graft. (*From* Dodson TB, Kaban LB: Donor site morbidity: Diagnosis, treatment, and prevention. Oral Maxillofac Surg Clin North Am 1990;2:489.)

Perforation of the Inner Cortical Plate

A potentially serious complication of calvarial bone graft harvesting is inadvertent perforation of the inner cortical plate with dural injury. This complication is associated with harvesting of full-thickness cortical bone or with technical errors during harvest of partial-thickness grafts. Complications of inner cortical plate perforation include subdural hematoma, dural exposure or tear, cerebrospinal fluid leak, sagittal sinus penetration, and central nervous system infection. The reported frequency of inner table perforation ranges from 0 to 13%, and that of dural exposure or tear from 0 to 4.9%.[23, 43–45, 48–52] Powell and Riley[46] reported one instance of sagittal sinus entry in a series of 62 patients. A second case report of sagittal sinus laceration has also been published.[53] To prevent entering the sagittal sinus during harvest of cranial bone, it is recommended to stay at least 2 cm from the midline and not to cross the midline.[52, 54] Central nervous system infections, subdural hematomas, intracerebral hematomas, arachnoid bleeding, and cerebrospinal fluid leaks are uncommon,[43, 50, 55] but they may have devastating consequences. Therefore, some authors have recommended harvesting the cranial bone graft from the side of the nondominant hemisphere of the brain.[23, 54, 55]

Several recommendations may help to decrease the risk of an inadvertent neurologic injury. Lateral skull films or CT scans provide some information regarding skull thickness. A less objective, but recommended approach is to tap the skull with the same instrument in each procedure to gain experience in relating the tone to the thickness of the skull.[54] Another author recommends use of a sharp osteotome and patience.[50] The bone should not be forcefully elevated with the osteotome. Otherwise, the inner cortex may fracture with dural exposure. In children younger than age 5 years, the dura is firmly attached to the inner cortical bone, which increases the risk of a dural tear. Careful dissection is necessary in this age group to avoid a dural tear.

Dural exposure is generally not serious, but coverage of the exposed dura with bone graft is recommended.[23] If there is a dural laceration, the craniotomy needs to be extended to expose the limits of the tear. The underlying cerebral cortex is carefully examined for injury. In the event of cerebral cortex injury, an immediate neurosurgical consultation should be obtained. In the absence of cerebral cortex injury, bleeding of the torn dura is controlled with bipolar cautery, and a meticulous dural repair is performed either directly or with a pericranial patch. The repaired dura is covered with bone graft.[23] Postoperatively, the patient is kept under neurologic observation for 24 hours. Antibiotic coverage with a broad-spectrum antibiotic for 5 days is recommended.[51]

Age is an important consideration for harvest of cranial bone grafts from children. In children less than 3 years old, the skull is thin, and the presence of a diploic space is unreliable. Consequently, split cranial bone grafts should not be planned. After age 3, a preoperative CT scan is suggested to ensure the presence of a diploic space. After the thickness of the parietal region is 6.0 mm, which occurs about age 9 years, it becomes appropriate to consider harvesting split-thickness grafts.[56]

Infection, Hematoma, Seroma, and Delayed Wound Healing

Hematoma or seroma formation and subsequent infection are uncommon, minor postoperative complications associated with failure to provide wound drainage.[23, 43–45, 49, 51, 52, 54, 57, 58] Delayed wound healing is associated with hematoma or seroma formation and infection. Jackson and associates[57] reported two cases of delayed wound healing in a series of 247 free cranial bone grafts.

Late Morbidity

The reported late complication of calvarial bone graft harvesting is a contour deformity of the cranium. The severity ranges from no residual defect to subtle but palpable depressions.[47, 57–59] Some patients complain of the scalp depression, and Jackson and associates[57] recommended filling such a defect with cranial bone dust or skull shaving grafts to obtain a more aesthetic result. Alternatively, the bony edges of the skull defect can be smoothed to a feather edge to make the defect less apparent.[23, 50] In male patients, care should be taken to place the incision far enough posterior that it will not be exposed later if the hairline recedes. Alopecia secondary to damaged hair follicles is a potential, although unreported, complication. Its likelihood can be reduced by incising the skin parallel to the hair follicles.

Mandible

The mandibular symphysis is an excellent source of bone graft material when small amounts of corticocancellous bone may be required to graft alveolar clefts, to reconstruct the alveolus before placing osseointegrated implants, or to augment facial bones.[23, 60–63] The advantages of using the mandibular symphysis as a donor site include ease of access (the donor and recipient sites in the same operative field), shorter operating time and length of hospital stay, decreased morbidity, and avoidance of a cutaneous scar. The bone, additionally, is of membranous origin. Potential complications are injury to teeth or the mental nerve, periodontal defects, infection, wound breakdown, and aesthetic problems due to the presence of a chin defect, the development of a ptotic or "witch's" chin, or alteration of lip function or appearance.[60, 61]

Early complications following harvesting a chin graft are uncommon. There are no reports of mental nerve or tooth injury in the literature. The reported rate of wound breakdown ranges from 4% to 5%. Late complications are also uncommon. Lip function and appearance return to normal within a few months of the procedure. The bony defect shows healing by 6 months postoperatively. It is commonly advocated, although probably not necessary, to fill the bony chin defect with an allograft. Accurate reattachment of the mentalis muscle prevents the development of the ptotic chin.[60, 61]

Tibia

The search for donor sites for small amounts of bone has extended beyond the mandible. On the basis of the experience of orthopedic surgeons, maxillofacial surgeons have begun harvesting corticocancellous grafts from the proximal tibia. The proximal tibia provides a limited amount of corticocancellous bone graft material (<45 mL).[64] The advantages of using the proximal tibia include ready donor site accessibility, harvest in the office setting, minimal postoperative pain and functional limitations, low risk of delayed wound healing due to infection or hematoma or seroma formation, and minimal risk for nerve injury or the development of unaesthetic scars. Potential complications are delayed wound healing, gait disturbance or fracture, and persistent pain (Fig. 8–6).

Two large patient series (total n = 710) reported in the orthopedic literature review harvesting of proximal tibia bone grafts.[65, 66] In these studies, the reported early complications included two cases of delayed wound

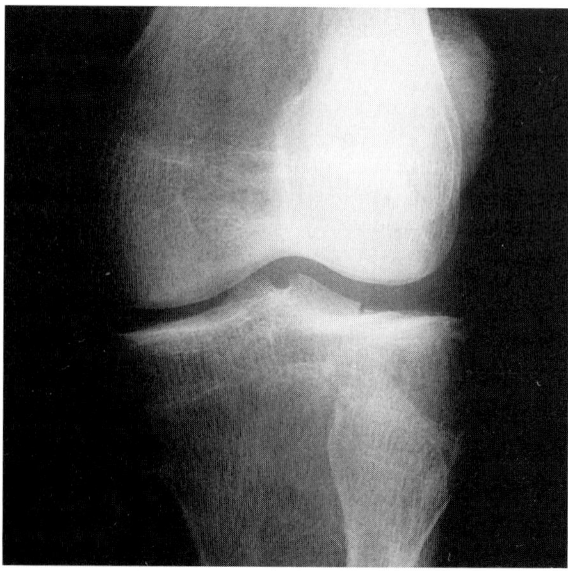

Figure 8–6. Comminuted, slightly depressed fracture of the lateral plateau of the left tibia following tibial bone graft. (Courtesy of Dr. Rebeka G. Silva, San Francisco, CA.)

healing due to infection (n = 1) and hematoma formation (n = 1). In two smaller studies (total n = 23), there were no reported cases of delayed wound healing.[23, 64] Stress fractures of the tibia occurred at a rate of 5.6%. These fractures were treated nonsurgically and healed without complications.[65, 66] Twelve patients (total n = 710) developed pathologic fractures postoperatively. There was no report of symptomatic nerve injury. One study noted a short-term (<3 weeks) duration of gait disturbance.[64] The patients used canes to assist walking. In one study of patients with multiple injuries, thrombophlebitis developed in 3.8%, and pulmonary embolus occurred in 2.8%.[66] These complications were not reported in any other study and may reflect the patient population treated and not the expected complications of harvesting tibial bone in otherwise healthy people.

Long-term complications are uncommon. Persistent donor site pain ranges from 0 to 5.4%.[64–66] There were no reports of long-term neurosensory change or unaesthetic donor site appearance. Of interest, in one report, the tibial donor site was misdiagnosed as tumor because the radiologist noted a radiolucency in the proximal tibia on a routine radiograph (Fig. 8–7).[67] Consequently, it is important to inform the patient of, as well as to document well, the donor site location.

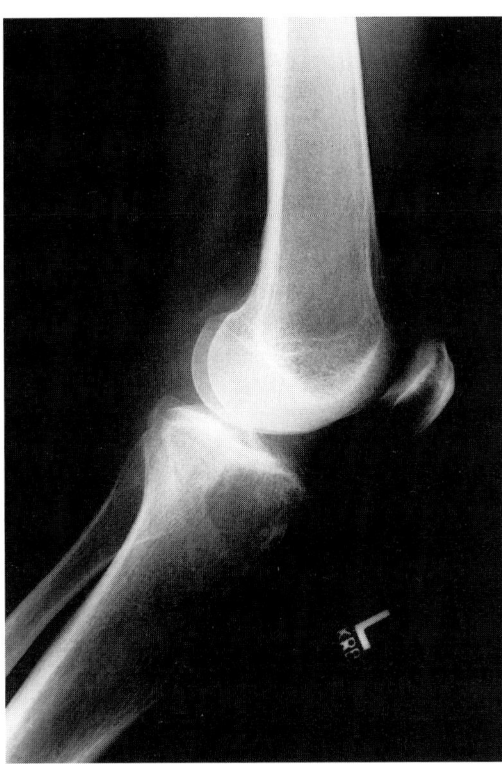

Figure 8–7. Lateral view of the knee following harvesting a bone graft from the tibia. The graft harvest has created a radiolucent defect in the proximal tibia that could be mistaken for a lesion. (Courtesy of Dr. Rebeka G. Silva, San Francisco, CA.)

Donor Site Morbidity with Vascularized Autologous Bone Grafts

Over the last 15 years, the use of vascularized bone grafts to reconstruct maxillofacial defects has become common. In theory, the vascularized bone graft is ideal. The graft has its own blood supply. It is osteoconductive and osteoinductive, and has osteoprogenitor elements in the donor bone. The graft heals primarily with minimal bony necrosis.[68] For the recipient bed compromised by fibrosis, radiation injury, or infection, the vascularized bone graft is becoming the reconstructive modality of choice.

The major problem with vascularized bone grafts, especially for mandibular reconstruction, is that they generally are unsuitable for conventional (non–implant-supported) prosthetic reconstruction. The operation may be defined as a technical success with a healed bone graft with restoration of mandibular continuity. Owing to inadequate shape or size of the bone graft, however, the operation may be a resounding failure for functional prosthetic reconstruction. The use of osseointegrated implants placed in vascularized bone grafts has resulted in both satisfactory reconstruction of the mandibular defect and functional prosthetic reconstruction.[69] Given the increased use of vascularized bone grafts, the oral and maxillofacial surgeon is more likely to evaluate a patient with a vascularized bone graft for osseointegrated implant placement. Consequently, the surgeon should be aware of the potential donor site complications. Multiple donor sites have been described, but this chapter focuses on two common donor sites for vascularized grafts, the radial forearm and the fibula.

Radial Forearm

Early Complications

The radial forearm flap has multiple features, making it an attractive donor site for maxillofacial reconstruction. The forearm is a versatile source for grafts. Vascularized bone (radius) can be harvested. The overlying skin and fascia may be harvested for intraoral and extraoral soft tissue replacement. A composite flap consisting of the radius and skin and fascia may be harvested to replace hard and soft tissues simultaneously. The skin is thin, with limited amounts of adipose tissue, and has little hair. These features facilitate its use to replace intraoral soft tissue by reducing bulk and permit draping over complex shapes. To facilitate the execution of the operation, the graft has a long vascular stem, the radial artery has a wide lumen, and multiple veins are available for anastomosis. In addition, flap re-innervation is possible.[51, 70] Potential complications include delayed wound healing, orthopedic complications, poor aesthetic result, and nerve injury.

Delayed Wound Healing

Delayed wound healing due to wound breakdown at the forearm donor site is a serious complication particularly associated with harvest of fasciocutaneous or composite vascularized grafts. Wound breakdown leads to tendon exposure (brachioradialis and flexor carpi radialis tendons) and may result in scarring and limitation of wrist motion.[51, 71, 72] Rate of wound breakdown ranges from 6.7% to 53%.[51, 72–76] Forearm weakness due to injury of the flexor pollicis longus muscle is generally a temporary complication with the patients reported to recover by 3 months postoperatively. The weakness is more likely to occur in bone harvest than in a fasciocutaneous flap.[72, 75, 77]

After a fasciocutaneous or composite flap is harvested, the surgeon has three options for covering the donor site: primary closure alone, primary closure using a flap from the ulnar aspect of the forearm, or free skin graft.[51, 70, 71, 73] Because of the high frequency of donor site wound breakdown, it is suggested to allow the oral wound to heal by secondary intention and thereby to avoid harvesting radial forearm skin for oral soft tissue coverage.[76] It is also recommended to use the nondominant arm as the donor and to undergo postoperative physiotherapy to maximize wrist mobility and reduce donor site morbidity.

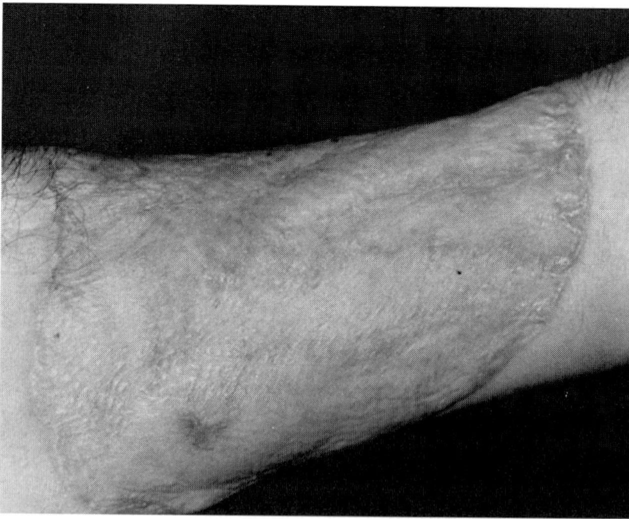

Figure 8–8. Typical donor site 6 months after harvest of a fasciocutaneous forearm flap. The original wound was covered by a split-thickness free skin graft. Note the unaesthetic result due to the poor color match of the donor skin and the residual soft tissue defect.

Orthopedic Complications

A complication of harvesting the radius is fracture of the donor bone. The frequency of fracture ranges from 0 to 43%.[51, 72, 74–79] Limitation in wrist or elbow mobility (in unfractured donor sites) has also been reported. Although the stiffness generally resolves, it may be persistent.[75]

An uncommon but potentially disastrous complication of harvesting the radial forearm flap is the development of hand ischemia.[80, 81] In most patients, the major blood supply to the hand is via the ulnar artery. If the major blood supply to the hand is via the radial artery, the hand will manifest signs of ischemia after harvest of the forearm flap. The radial artery can be reconstructed, if necessary, using an interpositional vein graft from the saphenous or cephalic vein.

Late Complications

The common, almost universal, long-term complication of radial forearm flap harvests is an unaesthetic donor site.[70, 79, 81] The donor site commonly has a wide scar when closed primarily. When it is covered by a skin graft, the color match is poor, and there is a visible, palpable tissue defect due to loss of tissue bulk (Fig. 8–8).

Although nerve injury is not commonly reported, some patients do complain of nerve injury producing dysesthesia in the distribution of the superficial branch of the radial nerve.[51, 72, 77, 79] One article reported two patients (n = 75) who developed painful neuromas at the donor site.[51] In older papers, however, paresthesia and cold-induced symptoms are more common.[75]

Fibula

Early Complications

The vascularized fibula bone graft provides a greater bulk of bone for reconstructing the mandible than the radial forearm flap.[82] The indication for using a vascularized fibula is the reconstruction of bone in a compromised recipient site where additional soft tissue may or may not be required.[82, 83] The nutrient vessel supplying the bone graft is a branch of the peroneal artery. Potential complications of using the fibula are primarily orthopedic in nature. Problems with wound healing are rare unless a composite flap is harvested.

Orthopedic Complications

Reported early complications after harvest of a vascularized fibula are fracture, compartment syndrome, transient motor nerve weakness, and gait disturbance. The overall early complication rates vary from 0 to 6.3%.[83–85] In a series of 132 patients, 1 patient had ipsilateral tibia fracture, 1 patient developed compartment syndrome, and 5 patients had transient peroneal nerve paralysis.[85] After graft harvest, the patients were not permitted to walk for several days. On average, patients began walking about 9 days postoperatively (range, 5 to 14 days).[82] Generally, when the donor site was closed primarily, a good aesthetic result was obtained and the patient began walking sooner. If a free skin graft was used to cover the wound, there was a delay in walking.

Delayed Wound Healing

Harvesting a composite flap increases the risk for donor site complications compared with harvesting bone alone. There is also a greater risk for delayed wound healing due to skin edge necrosis or the development of leg edema.[82] As with the radial forearm flap, if a composite flap is harvested and covered with a free skin graft, the donor site is not cosmetic and there can be incomplete graft take with tendon exposure.

Late Complications

Late complications of fibula grafts, primarily orthopedic, are extremity weakness, stiffness in the knee, tendon contracture, joint inflammation, loss of toe function, and growth deformities. Diffuse pain complaints, although uncommon, have been reported. The overall long-term complication rate ranges from 0 to 50%.[83, 85, 86] In a small series of 10 patients with an average of 7 years of follow-up, 5 patients had persistent donor site problems following harvest of the fibula.[6] The orthopedic complications included bursitis (n = 1), weakness (n = 2), weakness and a stiff knee (n = 1). All patients, however, could stand and function well despite their complaints.[86] In another report reviewing 16 cases, 1 patient lost dorsiflexion of the great toe.[83] In a third report (n = 132), 3 patients developed tendon contracture (flexor hallucis longus).[85] To alleviate some long-term orthopedic complications, extended postoperative physiotherapy should be prescribed to strengthen areas of weakness.[86] In growing patients, deformities can develop following harvest of the fibula. Reported growth deformities are tibial bowing and a valgus deformity of the ankle.[87, 88]

Summary

Morbidity is but one component in the decision-making process to select a donor site for bone harvesting. Other important factors are the amount and type of bone required, the location of the recipient site (e.g., forehead, zygoma, maxilla, mandible), and the type of skeletal defect (e.g., contour deficiency, osteotomy gap, continuity defect).

The iliac crest is a versatile common source for bone. Large quantities of particulate marrow, corticocancellous chips, and partial- or full-thickness corticocancellous blocks are available. The grafts can be used to repair osteotomy gaps, defects resulting from cyst enucleation, alveolar clefts, and continuity defects. Although pain and gait disturbances are common early complications of iliac crest harvest, these complaints are usually short lived and may be managed with analgesics and physiotherapy. Late morbidity is uncommon and can be avoided by careful graft procurement.

The chest is an excellent source for cartilage, costochondral grafts, and corticocancellous chips. Ribs provide excellent donor bone for augmentation of the atrophic mandible and for reconstruction of the mandibular ramus and condyle. Usually, ribs are not satisfactory for contour augmentation because of the high rate of graft resorption.

Calvarial bone is an excellent source of corticocancellous chips or blocks and cortical bone for contour augmentation. The overall morbidity is low, especially for harvest of a partial-thickness graft. A neurosurgeon should be present to assist with harvest of a full-thickness cranial bone graft. The chief indication for cranial bone is for contour augmentation, although this type of bone also is excellent for osteotomy gaps. Cranial bone is dense, and there may be less resorption than with either rib or iliac crest. The long-term results of contour augmentation are therefore more predictable.

When smaller grafts of cortical or corticocancellous bone are needed, mandible or tibial bone grafts may be particularly useful for reconstruction of alveolar bone for purposes of placing osseointegrated implants or repairing an alveolar cleft. The major advantage of using these donor sites is ready accessibility with minimal donor site complications.

Autogenous, free bone grafts are the material of choice for maxillofacial reconstruction in most clinical situations. There is a role, however, for vascularized bone grafts with or without attached soft tissue. In theory, vascularized bone graft is the material of choice, because the graft carries its own blood supply and heals primarily. Because of technical difficulty, generally poor shapes for replacing facial skeletal structures, and significant donor site morbidity, vascularized bone grafts are not the first choice for maxillofacial reconstruction in a host with an uncompromised recipient bed. Compared with autogenous bone, the benefits of harvesting vascularized bone do not exceed the risks. If, however, the recipient site is compromised because of previous radiation, injury, infection, or failed previous bone grafts, the vascularized bone graft offers a genuine alternative to the free bone graft.

The donor site morbidity after harvest of vascularized bone is common and not trivial. Whatever site, radial forearm or fibula, the common complications are wound breakdown with exposure of underlying tendons and potential compromised function of the involved extremity, fracture of the donor bone, universal complaints regarding the unaesthetic appearance of the donor site, and symptomatic nerve injury. In the growing patient, deformities of the lower leg have been reported following harvest of the fibula.

Donor Site Morbidity with Soft Tissue Grafts

Oral and maxillofacial surgeons commonly harvest free skin and mucosal grafts for soft tissue defect repair, scar release, and vestibuloplasty. Common areas of harvest are the buttocks, lateral thigh, upper arm, and forearm. Buccal and palatal mucosa are the most common sources for full-thickness mucosal grafts. The early complications of harvesting split-thickness skin grafts are pain, infection, delayed wound healing, and excessive blood loss.

Split-Thickness Skin Grafts

Early Morbidity

Pain

Donor site pain of varying severity is a universal complaint after the harvesting of split-thickness skin grafts.[4, 89–91] The intensity of the pain depends on graft size and the type of dressing. Semipermeable occlusive dressing decreases pain at the donor site, whereas air-

or heat-dry dressings are associated with greater pain.[4, 91, 92]

Infection and Delayed Wound Healing

The frequency of donor site infection ranges from 0 to 4.8% and is unrelated to the dressing used.[4, 91–95] There is one report of an epidemic of donor site infections that were associated with the use of improperly sterilized fine mesh gauze.[93]

In an attempt to prevent infection and promote wound healing, several types of donor site dressings have been proposed. Dressings can be divided into two types, closed and open. The closed or occlusive dressings are associated with less pain but may delay the identification of infection. The open technique, which consists of air- or heat-drying the donor site, has a lower infection rate as indicated by anecdotal reports but is associated with more pain. As clinicians, we must carefully weigh the risks and benefits of our choice of dressings. Anecdotally, a higher infection rate is associated with occlusive semipermeable dressings, but this claim is not substantiated by comparative studies.[4, 92, 95] Given that infection is rare regardless of the dressing type and that pain is a universal complaint, the author recommends careful application of semipermeable occlusive dressings and diligent postoperative follow-up to detect wound infections early.

Despite dressing type, the average time to healing of a donor site ranges from 9.7 to 12 days (total range, 7 to 20 days).[4] In a series of 210 patients, only 2 had delayed wound healing.[4] If a full-thickness skin graft is taken unintentionally, the likelihood of delayed wound healing increases. Therefore, if a full-thickness graft is harvested inadvertently, it should be replaced and another graft harvested. There is one report of a split-thickness skin graft that failed to heal, in a patient with anhidrotic ectodermal dysplasia, because of the lack of skin adnexa.[96]

Blood Loss

Blood loss is related to the size of the graft and generally does not produce patient management problems. The average estimated blood loss for a 4 × 8–inch split-thickness skin graft is 46 mL.[90] Blood loss increases with the size of the graft. In a series of 113 burn cases in which the entire scalp was harvested as split-thickness skin grafts, the estimated blood loss was between 400 and 600 mL, and one patient became hypotensive because of excessive blood loss from the donor site.[97] Blood loss can be reduced by the topical application of epinephrine to the donor site prior to placement of dressings.

Late Morbidity

Generally, patients are pleased with the eventual appearance of the donor site. Late complications include pain, paresthesia, and aesthetic concerns such as hypertrophic scars or keloid formation, abnormal skin pigmentation or condition, and alopecia.

Long-term pain and paresthesia are variable in frequency. In a small follow-up study, Bell[89] reported that almost half the patients (10 of 21) had some degree of pain or paresthesia at the donor site three years postoperatively. In a 5-year follow-up study by Hjorting-Hansen and coworkers,[98] however, 1 of 84 patients (1.2%) complained of pain.

Whereas unsightly scar or keloid formation is uncommon (1.2% at 5 years), alteration in skin color and condition is common (Fig. 8–9). The frequency of abnormal pigmentation ranges from 49% to 76%.[98, 99] After forearm grafts, Zoltie[99] reported that 6 of 13 patients had "lumpy" surface texture.

Although other chapters evaluate problems with wound healing, a brief comment may be appropriate here regarding the status of the clinical management of hypertrophic scars and keloids. Several excellent review articles have been recently published.[100–106] All of the articles have a common theme: The treatment of hypertrophic scars and keloids is uniformly unsatisfactory, because the clinical results are variable and unpredictable. Although the clinical risk factors for hypertrophic scars and keloid formation (e.g., race, age, family history, location) are known, the underlying cellular mechanisms that produce hypertrophic scars or keloid formation are poorly understood.

The clinical treatment of hypertrophic scars and keloids includes surgical treatment using excision with scalpel, laser, electrocautery, or cryotherapy in combination with direct primary closure, closure with local flaps, skin grafting, or healing by secondary intention.[100, 101, 107] Medical therapy includes lesional injection with steroids or interferon, radiation therapy, topical application of silicone, or occlusion and hydration.[108–117] Finally, combinations of both surgical and medical therapy have been applied.[114, 118–122] Because so many treatment options have been used with varying success, clearly, no treatment appears especially effective. Until a better understanding of the biologic basis of abnormal scar formation is achieved, there is little expectation of major clinical breakthroughs in this area.

Extensive clinical research has been done in the treatment of hypertrophic scars and keloids. Most studies, however, are of little use owing to general failures of study design and execution. First, most researchers used a case series study design, commonly a consecutive series of treated patients, without attempting to control for confounding variables or to compare the treatment results with some standard. Another major challenge to the researchers was, and continues to be, the lack of an unambiguous clinical definition for *hypertrophic scar* or *keloid*. Consequently, there exists the constant problem of lesion misclassification, such as classifying a normal scar as a hypertrophic scar. Finally, lesional changes are difficult to measure. Most studies report treatment results in semiquantitative terms such as "improved," "worse," or "no change." These problems make it difficult to interpret treatment results, compare treatments among studies, or generalize the applicability of results to clinicians' patients. Consequently, most studies offer little incremental value for

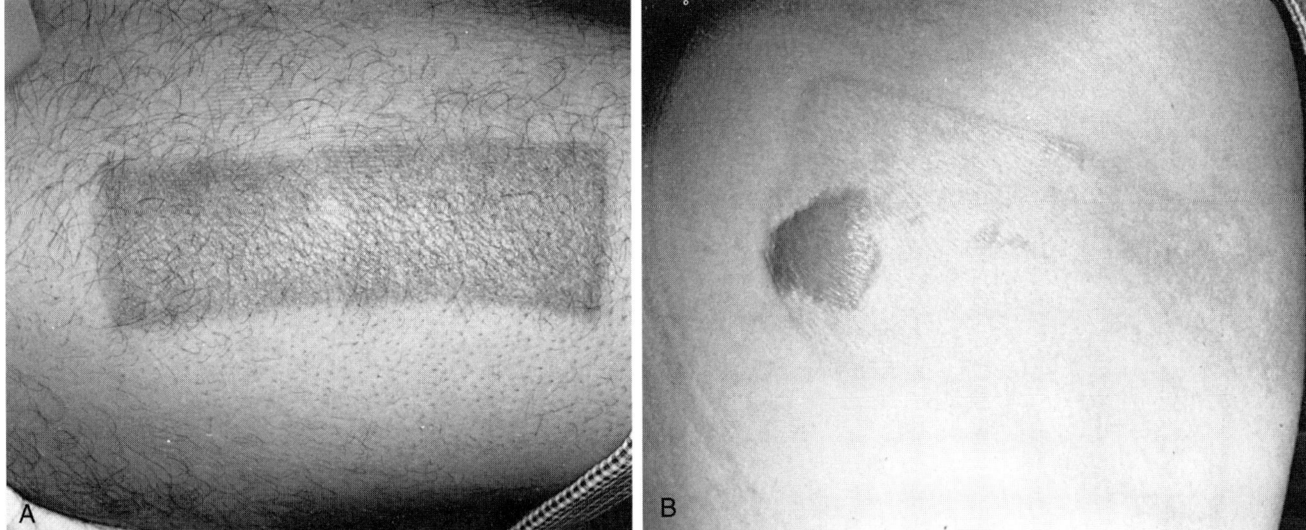

Figure 8–9. Complications of harvesting of split-thickness skin grafts. *A,* Abnormal skin pigmentation of lateral thigh. Patient is supine. *B,* Hypertrophic scar on right buttock. Patient is standing. (*From* Dodson TB, Kaban LB: Donor site morbidity: Diagnosis, treatment, and prevention. Oral Maxillofac Surg Clin North Am 1990;2:489.)

patient management or for a better understanding of the biologic and clinical behavior of these lesions.

A 1990 study applied sound clinical research principles to the problem of treating keloids.[112] Consequently, the study is valuable to both the clinician and the basic science researcher. The investigators used a randomized clinical trial study design to evaluate the role of intralesional interferon injections in treating keloids. The study was double-blinded and placebo-controlled. The sample consisted of ten patients with two keloids matched for size and location. One lesion was treated with the active agent (interferon, 0.1 mg or 0.01 mg) and the other lesion was treated with placebo (5% glucose solution). The outcome variables were lesion size and histologic changes. In the patients who completed the study, the active treatment resulted in a mean lesional height reduction of 30.4% compared with 1.1% in the placebo-treated lesions. Histologic examination found that the active treatment lesions displayed alterations in both the epidermis and dermis.

Because alterations of skin color and texture are common, choosing the donor site is imperative so it can be well camouflaged. Clothing commonly hides upper thigh sites, whereas a forearm donor site is visible during supination. The inner aspect of the upper arm provides an inconspicuous donor area. Finally, the scalp is a suitable donor site, because the area used can be covered with hair. One must take care, however, to use very thin grafts and to avoid removing skin adnexa during harvesting, because there are reported cases of alopecia associated with scalp donor sites.[94, 97] During the first year after harvesting, the donor site should be shielded from sun exposure to decrease the chance of abnormal pigmentation.

Mucosa

The two common donor sites for oral mucosal grafts are the buccal mucosa and palatal mucosa. The results at the two graft sites are similar, but the palate heals slowly.[19, 123–127] No complications such as palatal paresthesia, pain, or infection have been reported.

Palatal donor sites heal by secondary intention, and the discomfort is proportional to the size of the donor site. The time necessary for reepithelialization ranges from 3.5 to 6.5 weeks. Strip grafts of the palatal mucosa heal in 3.5 to 4 weeks, whereas sites of full palatal grafts heal in 6 to 6.5 weeks.[123, 124] In contrast, buccal mucosal donor sites can be closed primarily and heal in 7 to 12 days.[126]

The only late complication reported for palatal mucosal harvest is ulceration of the regenerated area. This complication is associated with full-thickness grafts, and the frequency ranges from 8.3% to 22%.[19, 123, 124] Clinically, the healed mucosa is normal in color but may appear thin and atrophic.[123, 124] Thus, regenerated palatal tissue may be less tolerant of slight faults in denture construction, although it is not clear whether this ulceration is associated with the donor site per se or with faulty denture construction. The ulcers occur in denture-bearing areas and resolve after alteration of the denture.

Summary

For small wounds, oral mucosal tissue is satisfactory. There may not be any strong indication for choosing palatal over buccal mucosa, except for grafting of gingival defects. For larger wounds, such as mandibular or maxillary vestibuloplasties, the split-thickness skin graft is the graft of choice. Meticulous postoperative wound care may reduce the frequency of donor site infections almost to zero. Pain can be lessened by using semipermeable occlusive dressings. Careful selection of a well-camouflaged donor site may decrease aesthetic problems secondary to pigmentation changes.

Donor Site Morbidity with Nerve Grafts

Oral and maxillofacial surgeons may require donor nerve tissue to reconstruct the inferior alveolar or lingual nerve. Potential donor nerves include the lateral and medial cutaneous nerves of the forearm, the sensory branch of the radial nerve of the hand, the lateral femoral cutaneous nerve of the thigh, the sural nerve, and the greater auricular nerve.[128–132] The sural and greater auricular nerves have been used commonly to repair inferior alveolar or lingual nerve defects.[128, 130] Potential complications of nerve harvesting are paresthesia with a residual functional disability and an unaesthetic donor site scar.

Sural Nerve

The sural nerve is an excellent source of nerve tissue because it is readily accessible, has several large fascicles, provides 30 to 40 cm of graft material, and can be obtained with minimal donor site morbidity, which consists of nerve injury with associated paresthesia and scar formation.[129]

The resulting sensory deficit covers the lateral border of the foot, the posterolateral part of the ankle, and the lateral edge of the sole. Although the deficit is permanent, the area of the deficit appears to shrink with time. No functional disability is associated with the deficit. In earlier studies, there were no reports of patient dissatisfaction with the donor site scar or the sensory deficit.[129, 133]

A later study by Woods and LaBanc[134] shed less favorable light on the results of sural nerve harvest, especially regarding complaints of nerve injury and scar appearance. In a systematic review of patients undergoing sural nerve harvest, 11 of 20 patients responded to a questionnaire assessing postoperative donor site morbidity. All of the patients who responded had complaints of donor nerve injury. All respondents had altered sensation involving the distribution of the sural nerve. Fifty percent of respondents reported nerve pain at an average of 35 on the Visual Analog Scale (0 = no pain, 100 = worst pain ever).

Generally, the scar is well camouflaged because it is hidden by the prominence of the lateral malleolus and by clothing. In the study by Woods and LaBanc,[134] however, 50% of the patients reported that their scar was unaesthetic.

A potential but unreported hazard of sural nerve harvest is injury to the lesser saphenous vein.

After harvest of the nerve, the foot is wrapped and elevated. Ambulation is discouraged for as long as 2 weeks, a stricture that may be inconvenient for some patients.

Greater Auricular Nerve

Systematic reports on the use of the greater auricular nerve (GAN) as a donor nerve are rare.[132] The advantages of this nerve for mandibular or lingual nerve reconstruction are its size and proximity to the operative field. The reported morbidity associated with the donor site is sensory alteration.[130] After harvest, there is a transient sensory deficit involving the ear and the skin overlying the parotid gland. Full sensation returns within 6 months. A more critical review revealed that patients commonly have long-term symptomatic neurosensory complaints at the donor site.[132] In a review of 29 patients, 13 patients (46%) reported symptomatic donor site nerve injury. For 6 patients, the complaints resolved within 6 months. In the remaining 7 patients, the symptoms had not resolved by the end of the study. Three patients developed symptomatic neuromas at the donor site. To prevent symptomatic neuroma formation, it has been advocated either to ligate the proximal stump and bury it underneath fascia or to oversew the proximal stump.[132, 134] There are no reports of delayed wound healing.[130, 132] The dissection of the donor nerve may be completed in the same wound as that for the primary operation. When a separate incision is used to harvest the GAN, there is a small risk that a hypertrophic scar may develop.[132]

Medial Antebrachial Cutaneous Nerve

According to a cadaver study, the medial antebrachial cutaneous nerve (MACN) may be suitable for grafting the inferior alveolar or lingual nerve.[135] The potential advantages of this donor nerve are minimal donor site neurosensory deficit and a less visible scar. In a review of 14 patients in whom the MACN was harvested for repair of digital nerves, there were no reports of long-term dysesthesia; however, hypesthesia was present in all patients.[131] One patient developed a hypertrophic scar on the forearm.

Summary

On the basis of limited reports on the use of sural or greater auricular nerve donor sites, there are few strong indications for choosing one donor site over the other. Equivalent results are reported, the sensory disturbances are mild with no functional impairment, and aesthetic concerns are minimal. The only advantage that the greater auricular nerve may offer is that only one operative site is needed, because it is possible to harvest the nerve through the incision used to access the mandible.

Overall, the donor site morbidity associated with nerve harvest may be considered mild and therefore not clinically important. When nerves are harvested for reconstruction following a major ablative procedure, the donor site morbidity with greater auricular nerve grafts may indeed be minor in comparison with the original operation or subsequent reconstructive procedures. When nerves are harvested to reconstruct a lingual or inferior alveolar nerve injured by elective dentoalveolar or orthognathic surgery, any donor site morbidity, no matter how minor, assumes greater significance. Consequently, the clinician must be aware of the potential donor site complications so as to better inform the patient of the risks and benefits of reconstructive nerve surgery using nerve grafts. Because the greater auricular and sural nerves are the common choices for donor nerves, it has been recommended to give preoperative nerve blocks at the potential donor site.[134] After experiencing and comparing the blocks, the patient is better able to choose the donor site.

References

1. Tayapongsak P, Wimsat JA, LaBanc JP, et al: Morbidity from anterior ilium bone harvest: A comparative study of lateral versus medial surgical approach. Oral Surg Oral Med Oral Pathol 1994;78:296.
2. Taher AA: Reconstruction of gunshot wounds of the mandible. 128 cases treated by autogenous iliac crest bone grafts. J Craniomaxillofac Surg 1990;18:310.
3. Canady JW, Zeitler DP, Thompson SA, et al: Suitability of the iliac crest as a site for harvest of autogenous bone grafts. Cleft Palate Craniofac J 1993;30:579.
4. Brady SC, Snelling CFT, Chow G: Comparison of donor site dressings. Ann Plast Surg 1980;5:238.
5. Marx RE, Morales MJ: Morbidity from bone harvest in major jaw reconstruction: A randomized trial comparing the lateral anterior and posterior approach to the ilium. J Oral Maxillofac Surg 1988;48:196.
6. Whitaker LA, Munro IR, Jackson IT, et al: Problems in craniofacial surgery. J Maxillofac Surg 1976;4:131.
7. Salyer KE, Taylor DP: Bone grafts in craniofacial surgery. Clin Plast Surg 1987;14:27.
8. Keller EE, Triplett WW: Iliac bone grafting: Review of 160 consecutive cases. J Oral Maxillofac Surg 1987;45:11.
9. Keathley CJ, Alexander JM: Postoperative morbidity of iliac crest donor sites in preprosthetic surgery patients [abstract]. American Association of Oral and Maxillofacial Surgeons, 64th Annual Meeting, Atlanta, Ga, Oct. 1982.
10. Hall M, Smith GR: The medial approach for obtaining iliac bone. J Oral Surg 1981;39:462.
11. Grillon GL, Gunther SF, Connole PW: A new technique for obtaining iliac bone graft. J Oral Maxillofac Surg 1984;42:172.
12. Bloomquist DS, Feldman GR: The posterior ilium as a donor site for maxillo-facial bone grafting. J Maxillofac Surg 1980;8:60.
13. Laurie SWS, Kaban LB, Mulliken JB, et al: Donor site morbidity after harvesting rib and iliac bone. Plast Reconstr Surg 1984;73:933.
14. Stoll P, Schilli W: Long-term follow-up of donor and recipient sites after autologous bone grafts for reconstruction of the facial skeleton. J Oral Surg 1981;39:767.
15. Whitaker LA, Munro IR, Salyer KE, et al: Combined report of problems and complications of 793 craniofacial operations. Plast Reconstr Surg 1979;64:198.
16. Kreibich DN, Scott IR, Wells JM, et al: Donor site morbidity at the iliac crest: Comparison of percutaneous and open methods. J Bone Joint Surg Br 1994;76:847.
17. Beirne OR: Comparison of complications after bone removal from lateral and medial plates of the anterior ilium for mandibular augmentation. Int J Oral Maxillofac Surg 1986;15:269.
18. Kaban LB, Longaker MT: Ancillary surgical procedures. *In* Kaban LB (ed): Pediatric Oral and Maxillofacial Surgery. Philadelphia, WB Saunders, 1989, p 52.
19. Goldberg JS, Byers SS, Distefano J: Follow-up study of palatal graft donor sites in 24 patients. J Oral Surg 1978;36:608.
20. Brazaitis MP, Mirvis SE, Greenberg J, Ord RA: Severe retroperitoneal hemorrhage complicating anterior iliac bone graft acquisition. J Oral Maxillofac Surg 1994;52:314.
21. Wolfe SA, Kawamoto HK: Taking the iliac-bone graft. J Bone Joint Surg Am 1978;60:411.
22. Ziccardi VB, Lalikos JF, Solercanois GC: Retroperitoneal hematoma as a complication of anterior iliac crest harvest. J Oral Maxillofac Surg 1992;50:1113.
23. Kline RMJ, Wolfe SA: Complications associated with the harvesting of cranial bone grafts. Plast Reconstr Surg 1995;95:5.
24. James JD, Geist ET, Gross BD: Adynamic ileus as a complication of iliac bone removal: Report of two cases. J Oral Surg 1981;39:289.
25. Blakemore ME: Fractures at cancellous bone graft donor sites. Injury 1983;14:519.
26. Guha SC, Poole MD: Stress fractures of the iliac bone with subfascial femoral neuropathy: Unusual complications at a bone graft donor site. Br J Plast Surg 1983;36:305.
27. Cockin J: Autologous bone grafting: Complications at the donor site. J Bone Joint Surg Br 1971;53:153.
28. Coventry MB, Tapper EM: Pelvic instability. J Bone Joint Surg Am 1972;54:83.
29. Lichtblau S: Dislocation of the sacro-iliac joint: A complication of bone-grafting. J Bone Joint Surg Am 1962;44:193.
30. Korlof B, Nylen B, Rietz K: Bone grafting of skull defects: A report of 55 cases. Plast Reconstr Surg 1963;52:378.
31. Hunt DM, Morley TR, Webb PF: A revised skin incision for operations on the posterior iliac crest and sacro-iliac joint. J Bone Joint Surg Br 1984;66:146.
32. Smith SE, DeLee JC, Ramamurthy S: Ilioinguinal neuralgia following iliac bone grafting. J Bone Joint Surg Am 1984;66:1306.
33. Escalas F, De Wald RL: Combined traumatic arterio-venous fistula and ureteral injury: A complication of iliac bone-grafting. J Bone Joint Surg Am 1977;59:270.
34. Catinella FP, De Laria GA, De Wald RL: False aneurysm of the superior gluteal artery: A complication of iliac crest bone grafting. Spine 1990;15:1360.
35. Cowley SP: Hernia through donor sites for iliac-bone grafts. J Bone Joint Surg Am 1983;65:1023.
36. Kinninmonth AWG, Patel P: Herniation through a donor site for iliac bone graft. J R Coll Surg Edinb 1987;32:246.
37. Reid RL: Hernia through an iliac bone-graft donor site. J Bone Joint Surg Am 1968;50:757.
38. James DR, Irvine GH: Autogenous rib grafts in maxillofacial surgery. J Maxillofac Surg 1983;11:201.
39. Lindqvist C, Pihakari A, Tasanen A, Goran H: Autogenous costochondral grafts in temporomandibular joint arthroplasty. J Oral Maxillofac Surg 1986;14:143.
40. Matthews DN: Experiences in major craniofacial surgery. Plast Reconstr Surg 1977;59:163.
41. Munro IR, Guyuron B: Split-rib cranioplasty. Ann Plast Surg 1981;7:341.
42. Skouteris CA, Sotereanos GC: Donor site morbidity following harvesting of rib grafts. J Oral Maxillofac Surg 1989;47:808.
43. Jackson IT, Helden G, Mark R: Skull bone grafts in maxillofacial and craniofacial surgery. J Oral Maxillofac Surg 1986;44:949.
44. Blankstein KC, Turvey TA: A review of 144 cranial bone grafts. J Oral Maxillofac Surg 1989;47(suppl 1):98.
45. Harsha BC, Turvey TA, Powers SK: Use of autogenous cranial bone grafts in maxillofacial surgery: A preliminary report. J Oral Maxillofac Surg 1986;44:11.
46. Powell NB, Riley RW: Cranial bone grafting in facial aesthetic and reconstructive contouring. Arch Otolaryngol Head Neck Surg 1987;113:713.
47. Petroff MA, Burgess LPA, Anonsen CK, et al: Cranial bone grafts for post-traumatic facial defects. Laryngoscope 1987;97:1249.
48. Tessier P: Autogenous bone grafts taken from the calvarium for facial and cranial applications. Clin Plast Surg 1982;9:531.
49. Wolfe SA, Berkowitz S: The use of cranial bone grafts in the closure of alveolar and anterior palatal clefts. Plast Reconstr Surg 1983;72:659.
50. Frodel JL Jr, Marentette LJ, Quatela VC, et al: Calvarial bone graft harvest. Techniques, considerations, and morbidity. Arch Otolaryngol Head Neck Surg 1993;119:17.
51. Juretic M, Car M, Zambelli M: The radial forearm free flap: Our experience in solving donor site problems. J Craniomaxillofac Surg 1992;20:184.
52. Kellman RM: Safe and dependable harvesting of large outer-table calvarial bone grafts. Arch Otolaryngol Head Neck Surg 1994;120:856.
53. Cannella DM, Hopkins LN: Superior sagittal sinus laceration complicating an autogenous calvarial bone graft harvest: Report of a case. J Oral Maxillofac Surg 1990;48:741.
54. Ilankovan V, Jackson IT: Experience in the use of calvarial bone grafts in orbital reconstruction. Br J Oral Maxillofac Surg 1992;30:92.
55. Young VL, Schuster RH, Harris LW: Intracerebral hematoma

complicating split calvarial bone-graft harvesting. Plast Reconstr Surg 1990;86:763.
56. Koenig WJ, Donovan JM, Pensler JM: Cranial bone grafting in children. Plast Reconstr Surg 1995;95:1.
57. Jackson IT, Adham M, Bite U: Update on cranial bone grafts in craniofacial surgery. Ann Plast Surg 1987;18:37.
58. Larsen PE, Markowitz NR: Morbidity associated with calvarial bone graft harvest. J Oral Maxillofac Surg 1989;47(suppl 1):110.
59. Spear SL, Wiegering CE: Temporal fossa bone grafts: A new technique in craniofacial surgery. Plast Reconstr Surg 1987;79:531.
60. Sindet-Pedersen S, Enemark H: Mandibular bone grafts for reconstruction of alveolar clefts. J Oral Maxillofac Surg 1988;46:533.
61. Sindet-Pedersen S, Enemark H: Reconstruction of alveolar clefts with mandibular or iliac crest bone grafts: A comparative study. J Oral Maxillofac Surg 1990;48:554.
62. Dario LJ, English R Jr: Chin bone harvesting for autogenous grafting in the maxillary sinus: A clinical report. Practical Periodontics and Aesthetic Dentistry 1994;6:87.
63. Jensen J, Riche-Fischel O, Sindet-Pedersen S: Autogenous mandibular bone grafts for malar augmentation. J Oral Maxillofac Surg 1995;53:88.
64. Catone GA, Reimer BL, McNeir D, et al: Tibial autogenous cancellous bone as an alternative donor site in maxillofacial surgery: A preliminary report. J Oral Maxillofac Surg 1992;50:1258.
65. O'Keefe RM, Reimer BL, Butterfield SL: Harvesting of autogenous cancellous bone graft from the proximal tibial metaphysis. J Orthoped Trauma 1991;5:469.
66. Belcher DC, Janes J: Tibial donor site morbidity: 500 consecutive cases with long term follow-up. J Bone Joint Surg Am 1975;57:1032.
67. Daffner RH: Case report 592: Bone graft donor site of tibia. Skeletal Radiol 1990;19:73.
68. Yarenchuk MJ: Vascularized bone grafts for maxillofacial reconstruction. Clin Plast Surg 1989;16:29.
69. Sclaroff A, Haughey B, Gay WD, et al: Immediate mandibular reconstruction and placement of dental implants: At the time of ablative surgery. Oral Surg Oral Med Oral Pathol 1994;78:711.
70. Vaughan ED: The radial forearm flap in orofacial reconstruction. Int J Oral Maxillofac Surg 1994;23:194.
71. Gaukroger MC, Langdon JD, Whear NM, et al: Repair of the radial forearm flap donor site with a full-thickness graft. Int J Oral Maxillofac Surg 1994;23:205.
72. Evans HB, Lampe HB: The radial forearm flap in head and neck reconstructions. J Otolaryngol 1987;16:382.
73. Urken ML, Futran N, Moscoso JF, et al: A modified design of the buried radial forearm free flap for use in oral cavity and pharyngeal reconstruction. Arch Otolaryngol Head Neck Surg 1994;120:1233.
74. Muldowney JB, Cohen JI, Porto DP, et al: Oral cavity reconstruction using the free radial forearm flap. Arch Otolaryngol Head Neck Surg 1987;113:1219.
75. Timmons MJ, Missotten FEM, Poole MP, et al: Complications of radial forearm flap donor site. Br J Plast Surg 1986;39:176.
76. Martin IC, Brown AE: Free vascularized fascial flap in oral cavity reconstruction. Head Neck 1994;16:45.
77. Boorman JG, Brown JA, Sykes PJ: Morbidity in the forearm flap donor arm. Br J Plast Surg 1987;40:207.
78. Ilankovan V, Avery BS, Putnam G: A technique to stabilize the radius after harvesting osteocutaneous flaps. Br J Oral Maxillofac Surg 1994;32:50.
79. Takato T, Harii K, Ebihara S, et al: Oral and pharyngeal reconstruction using the free forearm flap. Arch Otolaryngol Head Neck Surg 1987;113:873.
80. Jones BM, O'Brien C: Acute ischaemia of the hand resulting from elevation of a radial forearm flap. Br J Plast Surg 1985;38:396.
81. Hentz VR, Pearl RM, Grossman JAI, et al: The radial forearm flap: A versatile source of composite tissue. Ann Plast Surg 1987;19:485.
82. Hidalgo DA: Fibula free flap: A new method of mandible reconstruction. Plast Reconstr Surg 1989;84:71.
83. Reychler H, Ortabe JI: Mandibular reconstruction with the free fibula osteocutaneous flap. Int J Oral Maxillofac Surg 1994;23:209.
84. Weiland AJ: Clinical applications of vascularized bone grafts. *In* Friedlaender GE, Goldberg VM (eds): Bone and Cartilage Allografts. Park Ridge, IL, American Academy of Orthopaedic Surgeons, 1991, p 239.
85. Han CS, Wood MB, Bishop AT, et al: Vascularized bone transfer. J Bone Joint Surg Am 1992;74:1441–1449.
86. Anderson AF, Green NE: Residual functional deficit after partial fibulectomy for bone graft. Clin Orthop Relat Res 1991; 267:137.
87. Gilbert A: A free transfer of the fibula. Int J Microsurg 1979;5:100.
88. Minami A, Kaneda K, Itoga H, et al: Free vascularized fibular grafts. J Reconstr Microsurg 1989;5:37.
89. Bell FA: Patients' evaluation of mandibular skin graft vestibuloplasty. J Oral Surg 1976;34:707.
90. Rudolph R, Fisher JC, Ninnemann JC: Donor site healing. *In* Rudolph R, Fisher JC, Ninnemann JC (eds): Skin Grafting. Boston, Little, Brown, 1979, p 129.
91. Skouge JW: Techniques for split-thickness skin grafting. J Dermatol Surg Oncol 1987;13:841.
92. Dinner MI, Peters DR, Sherer J: Use of a semipermeable polyurethane membrane as a dressing for split-skin graft donor sites. Plast Reconstr Surg 1979;64:112.
93. Kravitz M, Green JA, Langston L, et al: Improperly sterilized fine-mesh gauze associated with donor site infections in skin-grafted burn patients. Am J Infect 1985;13:178.
94. Zingaro EA, Capozzi A, Pennisi VR: The scalp as a donor site in burns. Arch Surg 1988;123:652.
95. Hutchinson JJ, Lawrence JC: Wound infection under occlusive dressings. J Hosp Infec 1991;17:83.
96. Barnett AB, Oh R, Laub DR: Failure of healing of split-skin graft donor site in anhidrotic ectodermal dysplasia. Plast Reconstr Surg 1979;64:97.
97. Lesesne CB, Rosenthal R: A review of scalp split-thickness skin grafts and potential complications. Plast Reconstr Surg 1986;77:757.
98. Hjorting-Hansen E, Adawy AM, Hillerup S: Mandibular vestibulolingual sulcoplasty with free skin graft: A five year clinical follow-up study. J Oral Maxillofac Surg 1983;41:173.
99. Zoltie N: Forearm split-skin donor sites: Are they cosmetically acceptable? Ann Plast Surg 1988;21:11.
100. Stucker FJ, Shaw GY: An approach to management of keloids. Arch Otolaryngol Head Neck Surg 1992;118:63.
101. Lawrence WT: In search of the optimal treatment of keloids: Report of a series and a review of the literature. Ann Plast Surg 1991;27:164.
102. Datubo-Brown DD: Keloids: A review of the literature. Br J Plast Surg 1990;43:70.
103. Muir IF: On the nature of keloid and hypertrophic scars. Br J Plast Surg 1990;43:61.
104. Murray JC: Scars and keloids. Dermatol Clin 1993;11:697.
105. Murray JC: Keloids and hypertrophic scars. Clin Dermatol 1994;12:27.
106. Nemeth AJ: Keloids and hypertrophic scars. J Dermatol Surg Oncol 1993;19:738.
107. Zouboulis CC, Blume U, Buttner P, et al: Outcomes of cryosurgery in keloids and hypertrophic scars: A prospective consecutive trial of case series. Arch Dermatol 1993;129:1146.
108. Lo TC, Seckel BR, Salzman FA, et al: Single-dose electron beam irradiation in treatment and prevention of keloids and hypertrophic scars. Radiother Oncol 1990;19:267.
109. Larrabee W Jr, East CA, Jaffe HS, et al: Intralesional interferon gamma treatment for keloids and hypertrophic scars. Arch Otolaryngol Head Neck Surg 1990;116:1159.
110. Gold MH: Topical silicone gel sheeting in the treatment of hypertrophic scars and keloids: A dermatologic experience. J Dermatol Surg Oncol 1993;19:912.
111. Gold MH: A controlled clinical trial of topical silicone gel sheeting in the treatment of hypertrophic scars and keloids. J Am Acad Dermatol 1994;30:506.
112. Granstein RD, Rook A, Flotte TJ, et al: A controlled trial of intralesional recombinant interferon-gamma in the treatment of

keloidal scarring. Clinical and histologic findings. Arch Dermatol 1990;126:1295.
113. Chen HC, Ou SY, Lai YL: Combined surgery and irradiation for treatment of hypertrophic scars and keloids. Chin Med J (Engl) 1991;47:249.
114. Darzi MA, Chowdri NA, Kaul SK, et al: Evaluation of various methods of treating keloids and hypertrophic scars: A 10-year follow-up study. Br J Plast Surg 1992;45:174.
115. Doornbos JF, Stoffel TJ, Hass AC, et al: The role of kilovoltage irradiation in the treatment of keloids. Int J Radiat Oncol Biol Phys 1990;18:833.
116. Haq MA, Haq A: Pressure therapy in treatment of hypertrophic scar, burn contracture and keloid: The Kenyan experience. East Afr Med J 1990;67:785.
117. Supe SS, Supe SJ, Rao SM, et al: Treatment of keloids by 90Sr-90Y beta-rays. Strahlenther Onkol 1991;167:397.
118. Durosinmi-Etti FA, Olasinde TA, Solarin EO: A short course postoperative radiotherapy regime for keloid scars in Nigeria. West Afr J Med 1994;13:17.
119. Escarmant P, Zimmermann S, Amar A, et al: The treatment of 783 keloid scars by iridium 192 interstitial irradiation after surgical excision. Int J Radiat Oncol Biol Phys 1993;26:245.
120. Klumpar DI, Murray JC, Anscher M: Keloids treated with excision followed by radiation therapy. J Am Acad Dermatol 1994;31(pt 1):225.
121. Ship AG, Weiss PR, Mincer FR, et al: Sternal keloids: Successful treatment employing surgery and adjunctive radiation. Ann Plast Surg 1993;31:481.
122. Tang Y: Intra- and postoperative steroid injections for keloids and hypertrophic scars. Br J Plast Surg 1992;45:371.
123. Hall HD, O'Steen AN: Free grafts of palatal mucosa in mandibular vestibuloplasty. J Oral Surg 1970;28:565.
124. Hall HD: Mucosal grafts (palatal and buccal). J Oral Surg 1971;29:786.
125. Hillerup S: Preprosthetic mandibular vestibuloplasty with buccal mucosal graft. Int J Oral Surg 1982;11:81.
126. Maloney PL, Shepherd NS, Doku HC: Immediate vestibuloplasty with free mucosal grafts. J Oral Surg 1974;32:343.
127. Shepherd NS, Maloney PL, Doku HC: Fenestrated palatal mucosal grafts for vestibuloplasty. J Oral Surg 1975;33:34.
128. Hausamen JE, Samii M, Schmidsedr R: Repair of the mandibular nerve by means of autologous nerve after resection of the lower jaw. J Maxillofac Surg 1973;1:74.
129. Hill HL, Vasconez LO, Jurkewicz MJ: Method of obtaining a sural nerve graft. Plast Reconstr Surg 1978;61:177.
130. Noma H, Kakizawa T, Yamane G, et al: Repair of the mandibular nerve by autogenous grafting after partial resection of the mandible. J Oral Maxillofac Surg 1986;44:31.
131. Nunley JA, Ugino MR, Goldner RD, et al: Use of the anterior branch of the medial antebrachial cutaneous nerve as a graft for the repair of defects of the digital nerve. J Bone Joint Surg Am 1989;71:563.
132. Schultz JD, Dodson TB, Meyer RA: Donor site morbidity of greater auricular nerve graft harvesting. J Oral Maxillofac Surg 1992;50:803.
133. Fisher TR, Cox P: The sural nerve as autogenous nerve grafts. J Bone Joint Surg Br 1974;56:571.
134. Woods DD, LaBanc JP: Complications and morbidity associated with trigeminal nerve repairs. Oral Maxillofac Surg Clin North Am 1992;4:473.
135. McCormick SU, Buchbinder D, McCormick SA, et al: Microanatomic analysis of the medial antebrachial nerve as a potential donor nerve in maxillofacial grafting. J Oral Maxillofac Surg 1994;52:1022.

Chapter 9
COMPLICATIONS OF MANDIBULAR FRACTURES

by

Michael E. Koury

Introduction

Complications occur in 13% to 32% of mandibular fractures.[1–11] Complications associated with mandibular fracture include injuries that occur to distant structures as well as spinal injuries, intracranial trauma, and pulmonary emboli. More commonly, complications involve the mandible or adjoining structures. These problems may arise at the time of injury, during treatment, or throughout the healing process. Although a wide range of complications is discussed, this chapter focuses on those related to the mandible itself.

THE SUBJECTS DISCUSSED IN THIS CHAPTER ARE:

- Cervical spine and neurologic injuries
- Airway compromise
- Bleeding
- Lacerations
- Damage to teeth and alveolus
- Soft tissue infection
- Osteomyelitis
- Complications related to fracture union
  - Delayed union
  - Non-union
- Malocclusion and malunion
- Nerve damage
  - Causes
  - Treatment of nerve damage
- Parotid fistula and seroma
- Temporomandibular joint disorders
- Growth disturbances
  - Causes
  - Treatment of growth deformities

Cervical Spine and Neurologic Injuries

Because mandibular fractures are commonly caused by high-energy trauma, other injuries are often associated with them. Cervical spine injuries, intracranial bleeding, and internal carotid thrombosis are three of the more important.[12–14] Cervical spine injuries manifest as neck tenderness, decreased mobility, and neurosensory changes. Because 36% of patients with cervical spine injuries show no neurosensory symptoms, a cervical spine radiographic series is required for proper diagnosis. This series consists of anteroposterior and lateral as well as transoral views of the dens. All seven cervical vertebrae must be visualized to rule out injury to them. The patient wears a neck brace at all times until cervical vertebral injury is excluded.[12]

Intracranial bleeds and internal carotid thrombosis have similar presentations with a decreased level of consciousness, motor weakness, and sensory changes. CT scans and angiography differentiate the two conditions. Potentially severe consequences are associated with both conditions, and neurosurgical consultation is indicated.[13, 14]

Airway Compromise

Airway compromise with mandibular fractures may occur for several reasons. Instability of the chin segment with bilateral mandibular body fractures or destruction of the symphyseal region may allow the tongue to prolapse to the posterior pharynx.[15–18] Obstructive symptoms are prominent, with decreased breath sounds, stridor, paradoxic respiration, and cyanosis. Treatment includes positioning the patient on the side when conditions permit.[16] The tongue is controlled by means of anterior traction with a towel clamp or heavy suture.[15, 18] Oral or nasal airways are useful, and fracture fixation provides definitive control of fracture segment.[15] In some instances, endotracheal intubation may be necessary.

Aspiration of blood and particulate matter also may compromise the airway. Both teeth and partial dentures have been aspirated in some cases[19] (Fig. 9–1). The risk of aspiration is reduced by oral and pharyngeal suctioning and proper inspection and removal of all particulate matter from the oral cavity and airway.[15] Positioning the patient semiprone allows continued clearance of blood.[15, 18] Significant symptoms, such as with dyspnea, cyanosis, chest pain, spasmatic cough, and wheezing may be present. Once lodged, the foreign body may be relatively asymptomatic. Physical examination may show decreased vocal fremitus and breath sounds in affected lobes, stridor, and after-flow expiration. Teeth and bone are often superimposed on ribs and so are not evident on chest radiograph, but overinflation or, with time, atelectasis is seen. Without treatment, cough, hemoptysis, purulent sputum, fever, pneumonia, bronchiectasis, abscess, and empyema are possible. Treatment consists of bronchoscopic removal of the foreign body.[19, 20] Prophylactic antibiotics and steroids have not been shown to decrease morbidity or mortality.[20]

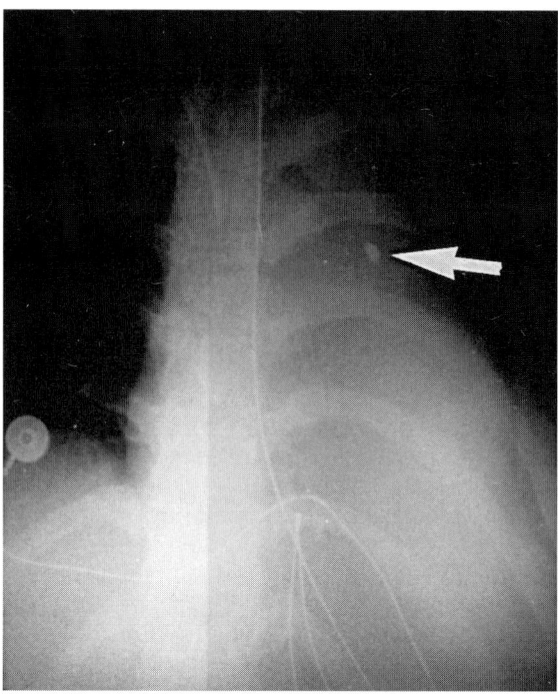

Figure 9–1. Radiograph showing tooth in left bronchus aspirated after mandibular fracture. Bronchoscopy was required for removal of the tooth.

Lingual swelling from either edema or hematoma formation may compromise the airway. Typically, swelling is self limiting, but with superimposed bleeding disorders, it may become significant. Treatment consists of placing pharyngeal airways when modest swelling occurs, and endotracheal intubation when airway compromise is possible.[18] Bleeding diathesis must be corrected. Usually, swelling subsides, allowing extubation within 4 or 5 days. With uncontrolled bleeding, tracheostomy may be needed to provide a patent airway for extended periods (Fig. 9–2).

Air emphysema is associated with tracheal, laryngeal, and bronchial injuries as well as mandibular fractures. Diagnosis rests on finding soft tissue swelling and crepitus on palpation of the neck, and on visualization, on lateral neck films, of air in the lateral pharyngeal and subcutaneous regions.[21, 22] Dysphagia, dysphonia, hyponasal speech, and airway compromise may occur.[21–23] With progression to a pneumomediastinum, air may be seen outlining the cardiac border and knob on an upright chest radiograph. Substernal pain, Hamman sign, and mediastinal crunching during systole may occur.[22] Air enters via mucosal tears overlying fractures of the body of the mandible and travels to the submandibular, lateral pharyngeal, lateral visceral, and pretracheal spaces. Inspiration, nose blowing, and sneezing are thought to cause its extension.[21, 22] Treatment consists of closure of intraoral wounds, reduction of the fractures, and prophylactic antibiotics.[21] The patient is observed closely for airway obstruction, be-

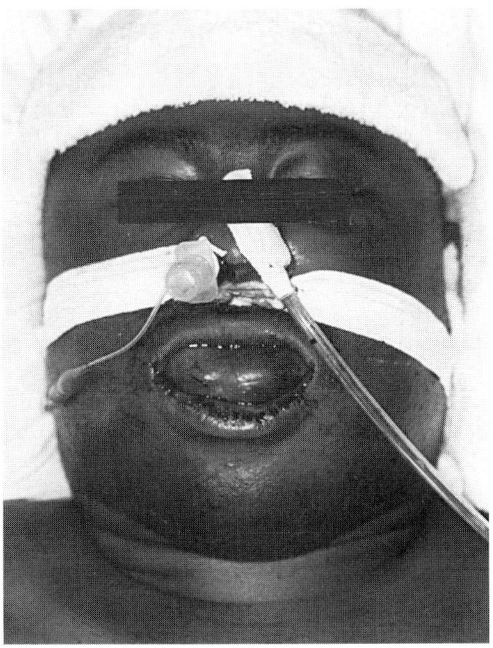

Figure 9–2. Significant tongue and neck swelling in patient with mandibular fracture and factor VIII deficiency requiring intubation.

cause intubation can be difficult and positive pressure is contraindicated.[24] Likewise, it is important to avoid coughing, sneezing, and nose blowing. Normally, resolution occurs in 72 hours.[21] Panendoscopy is utilized to rule out other injuries, including laryngeal fracture, tracheal and bronchial injury, and esophageal and pharyngeal perforation.[25]

Bleeding

Bleeding is common in mandibular fractures. Major facial lacerations occur in 7% of all fractures, and intraoral lacerations are common.[16] Soft tissue oozing is typical, but vessel bleeding may also occur. The inferior alveolar artery and the facial artery and vein are particularly susceptible. Severe, prolonged bleeding rarely occurs, and typically, control is obtained with pressure and laceration closure.[15] Occasionally, a vessel may need to be tied.[15, 17, 19] With brisk bleeding, endotracheal intubation may be needed to pack the airway without risk of airway compromise.[15] If bleeding obstructs visualization, and lacerations or fractures contraindicate blind nasal intubation, a surgical airway is needed. Generally, cricothyrotomy is preferred. Free air in the neck may indicate cricotracheal separation, however, in which case tracheostomy is indicated. Bleeding that does not respond to pressure or other local therapy is addressed with ligation of the external carotid artery or interarterial catheterization and embolization.[26]

Lacerations

Lacerations are associated with 7% to 30% of mandibular fractures.[16, 27] Internal structures are addressed prior to definitive closure of lacerations to improve access and avoid suture disruption. If treatment of the fracture is delayed, temporary single-layered skin and mucosal stitches are placed to close the wound.[16, 28] With soft tissue injury, tetanus immunization must be addressed, and antibiotics are started if the delay in closure is longer than 6 hours. The wound is meticulously débrided with pulsatile irrigation, and a multilayered closure is achieved after fracture treatment and conservative removal of tissue.[29]

Damage to Teeth and Alveolus

Trauma to teeth and alveolus frequently occur with mandibular fractures.[30] Lundin and associates[31] found that 23% of mandibular fractures were associated with tooth trauma. Avulsions, subluxations, and crown, root, and alveolar fractures occur, resulting in pulpal necrosis, root resorption, periodontal defects, infection, and alveolar bone loss[27, 30, 32] (Fig. 9–3). The rate of long-term loss of tooth vitality ranges from 25% to 41% in adults.[27, 33] In children, 35% of noncondylar fractures are associated with tooth avulsion, enamel hypoplasia, altered eruption, and cyst formation.[27, 34]

Tooth avulsion, fractures through the root apex, delayed treatment, closed apexes, and open reduction with internal fixation may compromise the vascular supply and cause pulpal necrosis.[26, 32, 34, 35] In one study, 38% of the teeth damaged in association with mandibular fractures required extraction. Fractures running through the root apex to the gingival margin carry the highest risk.[32] Fifty percent of teeth with fractures crossing the apex and 18% of those with fractures traversing other areas of the tooth become necrotic.[27] A delay in fixation longer than 48 hours is also correlated

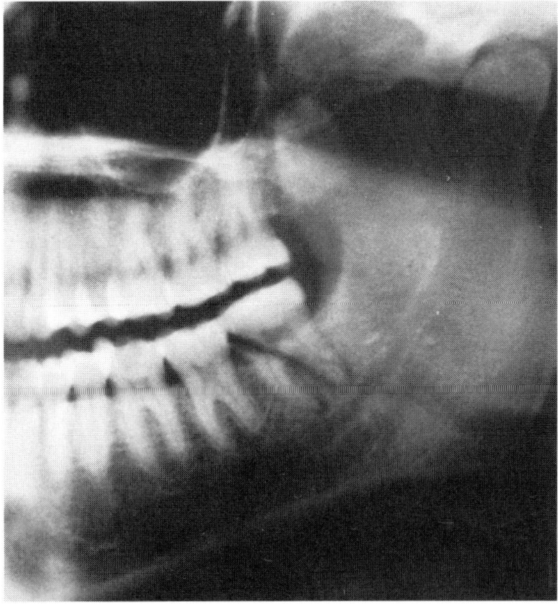

Figure 9–3. Radiograph showing a healed mandibular fracture at 6 weeks and root fracture resulting in infection. Patient was seen after primary trauma but was not treated. The root and mandibular fractures were missed on routine clinical and radiographic examinations.

with pulpal necrosis.[27, 36] On an average of 3 years after injury, 15% of the teeth in the line of a mandibular fracture treated within 48 hours demonstrated pulpal necrosis, as opposed to 37% thereafter.[27] Additionally, Kamboozia and Punnia-Moorthy[35] found a higher incidence of nonvital teeth, both in the line of and adjacent to the fracture, with open reduction and monocortical plate fixation than with maxillomandibular fixation. Greater manipulation, screw placement, and the open nature of the procedure were cited as probable causes of the loss of tooth vitality.

Progressive root resorption occurs in 0 to 11% of the teeth associated with fractures.[27, 32, 33] Internal root resorption is produced by pulpal necrosis. External resorption, which is more common, is classified as inflammatory or replacement.[32] Inflammatory resorption is caused by pulpal necrosis, and replacement resorption by damage to the periodontal ligament. Periodontal ligament damage occurs with avulsion, luxation, and fractures along the root surfaces.[37]

Periodontal bone loss occurs in 1% to 12% of mandibular fractures and is associated with poor fracture reduction and alveolar wall trauma.[27, 36] Vertical bone defects appear only when the fracture involves the periodontal membrane at the tooth cervix. Seventy-three percent of the vertical defects are related to poor reductions and not to initial traumatic displacement.[32] Nondislocated, well-reduced, and dislocated fractures showed 0, 11% and 26% rates of marginal bone loss, respectively.[36]

Fractures through developing tooth buds cause deformities of teeth, such as malformed crowns or roots and altered eruption, in 33% to 66% of children with mandibular fractures. Most malformations are not of functional or esthetic significance.[27]

Treatment of dental and alveolar sequelae depends on diagnosis. With pulpal necrosis, root canal therapy is indicated unless the tooth is compromised. In the latter case, extraction is the treatment of choice. Internal resorption requires root canal therapy. If perforation has resulted, calcium hydroxide fill, surgical retrofill, or extraction is needed.[38] Inflammatory resorption is treated with pulpectomy and calcium hydroxide fill. The filling is replaced every 3 months until the resorption stabilizes. Root canal therapy with gutta-percha can then proceed.[37] Replacement resorption of the root with bone is a slower process with a poorer prognosis. The tooth is extracted when resorption results in significant tooth mobility.[37] Periodontal defects are treated with a combination of scaling and root planing, periodontal surgery, and extraction, depending on the defect and tooth mobility. Lost teeth and alveolar bone are reconstructed simultaneously. Teeth may be replaced with implants, bridges, or removable prosthetics. If implants are selected, bone loss is addressed with grafting to improve contours, esthetics, hygiene, emergence profiles, and crown-to-root ratios. If substantial bone is present to anchor the implant, both bone and implants are placed simultaneously. For a patient without adequate host bone to anchor the implant, primary grafting is accomplished, with implant placement 3 to 4 months later.[39]

Soft Tissue Infection

Infection is the most common complication of mandibular fractures, occurring in 0.4% to 32% of cases.[1, 3, 4, 6, 9, 27, 40, 41] Cellulitis, abscess formation, osteomyelitis, and even necrotizing fasciitis and Ludwig angina occur.[42, 43] Infection has been associated with failure to use appropriate antibiotics, delayed treatment, angle fractures, noncompliance, teeth in the line of fracture, and mobility.[3, 6, 41, 44, 45]

Use of appropriate antibiotics in the treatment of mandibular fractures decreases the rate of infection. A high rate of infection (35%)[27] has been noted without their use, whereas two studies in particular have demonstrated their effectiveness.[44, 45] Twenty percent of patients who received one preoperative and one postoperative dose of cefazolin for the treatment of fractures of the mandibular parasymphysis, body, and angle developed infection, versus 60% of patients who received no antibiotics. Infection rates were reduced from 62% to 8% when antibiotics were used in open reductions.[45] Zallen and Curry,[44] in a randomized prospective study of antibiotic use in compound mandibular fractures, found infection rates of 50% in cases treated without antibiotics and 6% in cases treated with antibiotics. Higher infection rates occurred with both open and closed reductions when antibiotics were not administered.[46]

A delay in treatment is thought to increase the risk of infection.[3, 6, 47–49] A high preoperative infection rate is demonstrated when patients present for treatment 6 or more days after injury.[3, 45] These preoperative infections may persist postoperatively, but typically they resolve simply with primary immobilization and infection treatment.[3]

Several studies demonstrate that delayed treatment of fractures without clinical infection may risk postoperative infection.[40, 50, 51] Conversely, many studies have found no difference in infection rates when treatment was delayed.[3, 7, 45, 52, 53] A delay in treatment probably is associated with some risk of infection, for a number of reasons. Instability of the fracture segments leads to greater contamination of the wound and further damages soft tissue and bone.[54] Pulpal necrosis of teeth in the line of fracture increases with delays in treatment of over 48 hours and may contribute to infection.[27] A difference should be drawn, however, between delayed treatment and a delay in presentation. A patient who presents on the second day after injury is started on antibiotics, receives temporary immobilization with a bridal wire, and is taken to surgery late. This patient is not at the same risk as a patient who presents late with a mobile fracture and without having received antibiotics. A patient with subclinical infection may even benefit from preoperative antibiotics if fracture mobility is reduced.

Rates of infection have been found to differ by region of the fracture site. Infection of subcondylar fractures rarely occurs, and low incidence of infection is seen at the symphysis.[41, 45] Thick soft tissue at the condyle and ramus generally prevents open fractures, and muscle attachments at the symphysis, ramus, and condyle provide vascularity. Additionally at the symphysis, thick bone provides for advantageous fragment contact.

Conversely, the highest incidence of infection is at the angle.[3, 55, 56] With nonrigid fixation techniques, the infection rate is twice that of all fractures.[2] Angle fractures treated with rigid internal fixation (RIF) also are susceptible, particularly if treated intraorally and associated with teeth.[44] Maxillomandibular fixation (MMF) alone may poorly stabilize these fractures, because the proximal segment is not adequately immobilized. The mandible is thin, and resulting bone contact is limited.[56] Additionally, absolute rigidity with compression may be difficult to achieve, because of the biomechanical forces and thin bone in the region, particularly if third molars are removed.[51, 55, 57] Osteonecrosis is also thought to contribute to infection in this area.[8] Bone vascularity may be poor because limited marrow, often reduced by impacted teeth, is present.[55] Soft tissue trauma, swelling, surgical dissection, retraction injury, and surgical bone trauma with screw placement and compression may further disrupt the blood supply.[9]

Patient noncompliance with treatment may contribute to infection. Release of MMF and failure to follow diet restriction are the most commonly forms of noncompliance.[41, 57, 58]

Treatment of teeth in the line of the fracture has stirred much debate. Fractures associated with teeth incur a high infection rate compared with fractures at edentulous spaces.[3, 7, 37, 51] Contamination through a disrupted periodontal ligament or pulp chamber may occur. Melmed and Koonin[6] found that 83% of the infections with teeth at the fracture line resulted from carious teeth. Loss of vascular supply commonly occurs after tooth luxation, or when the root apex is involved in the fracture line, and may result in pulpal necrosis and infection.[37, 59] A low complication rate, however, has been associated with the retention of all teeth when antibiotics are administered. One study of 199 fractures, in which 85% were treated with closed techniques and retention of all teeth, found no complications were associated with impacted third molars or severely carious teeth. Thirty percent of the teeth with mobility, periapical radiolucency, pericoronal inflammation, or root fracture required extractions during treatment because of infection or odontalgia.[32] Additionally, no difference in infection rates is demonstrated when treatment involving teeth left without pathology is compared with treatment in which teeth were extracted when mobile, with root fractures, or with apical pathology.[3, 7]

Retention of teeth may actually improve results. Teeth may aid reduction of the fracture and prevent telescoping of the segments. Complete mesoangular and horizontal bony impactions, in particular, increase the abutment surface area and have a stabilizing effect on fractures.[60–62] Extraction of teeth in the line of fracture may also produce complications. Further bone fragmentation and soft tissue injury may result.[63] Removal of impacted molars especially require significant distraction of the fracture, cause mucosal tears, and convert a closed fracture into an open one.[64] Additionally, alveolar osteitis may occur.[63]

In most cases, teeth in the fracture line should be retained if no pathology is present.[27, 65, 66] Teeth with root fractures, apical pathology, cysts, significant mobility, or pericoronal inflammation, and those that inhibit fracture reduction should be removed.[67] Completely impacted third molars do not present an additional infection risk.[68] Additionally, the type of fixation may influence fracture treatment. Rubin and associates[69] found a higher infection rate for the retention of teeth in open reduction (44%) than for extraction of teeth in open reduction (19%) or closed reduction (20%). In light of these findings, greater consideration should be given to extraction of "borderline" teeth with open treatment.

Fixation failure in open fractures is a common cause of infection.[61] Closed treatment of closed fractures carries little risk of infection. Even closed mobile fractures do not become infected unless there is contamination from breaks in the soft tissue or hematogenous spread of bacteria.[70] Closed reduction of open fractures, however, incurs a significant risk. For treatment of angle fractures with closed reduction, an infection rate of 14% was observed.[7]

Some authors have reported a higher complication rate with open reduction of open fractures, whereas others have not.[3, 30, 33, 44] Larson and Nielsen,[27] in a study using primarily MMF, splints, and skeletal fixation, obtained a 0.4% infection rate; 20% of the fractures required wire fixation, which was placed from an extraoral approach. Fracture infections occurred only in case of osteosynthesis. Conversely, Bochlogyros[1] reported a 7% infection rate with no significant difference between rates in surgical and nonsurgical treatment.

Many advantages have been demonstrated for RIF, including a safer airway, better nutrition, ease of communication, less discomfort, easier physiotherapy, absence of claustrophobic episodes, improved hygiene, and less dependence on patient compliance.[41, 58, 71] The infection rate, however, has been questioned.[52] Comparative studies have shown high rates of infection with wire osteosynthesis and with RIF.[51, 56, 58, 72, 73] Luhr[73] found rates of 3.8% with closed reduction, 3.5% with compression plates, and 7.1% with wire osteosynthesis. In several studies, Ellis and colleagues[7–9, 57, 74] looked at a homogeneous population with angle fractures and evaluated different techniques, including MMF with closed reduction and with nonrigid fixation, two transoral minicompression plates, two transoral compression plates, transoral lag screws, and extraorally placed reconstruction plates. Infection rates ranged from 7.5% to 32%. Open reduction with wire and MMF incurred an intermediate (24%) infection rate compared with various RIF techniques. The lowest infection rate was obtained with the extraoral placement of reconstruction plates. Others have also found low complication rates with reconstruction plates, believing that such plates are more rigid and less technique sensitive.[56, 75]

In comparison with the low infection rates for extraorally placed reconstruction plates, good results have been obtained with tension band plates placed intraorally. Champy and associates[76] demonstrated a 3.8%

infection rate with this technique. Reasons for good results with this markedly different technique are unknown, but the limited dissection, simplicity, and favorable biomechanics of the technique may be responsible.

Fractures are treated similarly whether they become infected before or after fixation. Correction of underlying systemic factors, administration of antibiotics, and needed surgical therapy are undertaken. Patients are started on penicillin for empiric treatment.[52, 56] If Gram stain shows evidence of *Staphylococcus aureus*, a penicillinase-resistant penicillin is advised, and changes in antibiotic choice are guided by culture and sensitivity testing.[41, 60, 77] The fracture must then be immobilized. Traditionally, MMF or external fixation was recommended for the treatment of these fractures.[78] RIF is now an accepted and proven technique and is of benefit in patients who become infected because of a delay in seeking treatment.[70, 79] Fracture healing will occur predictably, although it may be delayed if infection persists.[79] Typically, infection resolves rapidly with stable RIF devices in place.[78–80]

Although compression and miniplate fixation have been used successfully with infected fractures, reconstruction plates with three screws in each segment are most reliable.[70, 76, 78] With reconstruction plates, screws can be placed farther from the involved bone, and osteolytic bone ends are not relied upon for rigidity.[1, 56] Additionally, mandibular shortening and deformity, which may occur when compression is used in the setting of interfragmentary bone loss, are avoided.[56, 78]

Timing and type of fixation are guided largely by the vascularity of the region. Infected fractures with mild to moderate cellulitis or spontaneously draining abscess can be drained and fixed primarily, whereas fractures with severe cellulitis or large abscess are best treated with incision and drainage, antibiotics, and immobilization with MMF for 3 to 4 days prior to RIF.[70]

With infection in previously fixed fractures, teeth, foreign bodies, and stability must be assessed.[70, 78, 81] Mobile teeth are extracted, and devitalized teeth are treated endodontically or extracted, depending on the condition of each tooth and the severity of the infection. Foreign bodies, including necrotic bone and loose hardware, are removed. RIF may become loose and fail because of use of insufficient hardware, loss of compression, improper biomechanics, or bone failure, necrosis, or trauma, and thus result in infection (Fig. 9–4).

With stable fixation, proper antibiotic coverage, and local wound care, the infection should resolve over the following 10 to 14 days. If significant infection still remains at this point despite appropriate antibiotic therapy, the patient is taken back to the operating room for exploration and treatment. Hardware is not removed if screws are tight and the plate is rigid. Typically, a loose screw or a piece of free, dead bone is found[70, 78, 82] (Fig. 9–5). Débridement of soft and hard tissue is achieved as necessary. If mobility is present, the fracture is stabilized either with a larger more rigid plate or with MMF if near union[54, 83] (Fig. 9–6). Rapid resolution of the infection typically occurs.[54, 56, 78, 82]

Alternatively, with minor persistent infection and stable fixation, the patient may be kept on antibiotic therapy for 8 to 10 weeks, until the fracture is healed and the hardware can be removed without further immobilization.[52, 62, 79, 80] Stable fixation with exposed hardware is treated similarly, with implant removal and wound closure after fracture healing. In cases with limited exposure, the wound may close through granulation.[70]

Infected fractures should be treated promptly, because osteomyelitis may result if treatment is delayed or inadequate.[84] Osteomyelitis occurs in 1% to 6% of mandibular fractures and is more common in patients with chronic disease.[1, 2, 60, 85, 86] Care should be taken to distinguish between infected fractures and true osteitis. Too often, cases of infection with sequestered bone are misdiagnosed as osteomyelitis. Bone may be devitalized by trauma or surgical therapy. Without marrow involvement, these cases are simply infected fractures, and they will respond quickly to fixation and conservative treatment.

Osteomyelitis

Osteomyelitis is an inflammatory reaction in bone and a disease of altered blood *supply*.[84, 87] Vessel inflammation and thromboses result in bone death and sequestrum formation. Highly vascular granulation tis-

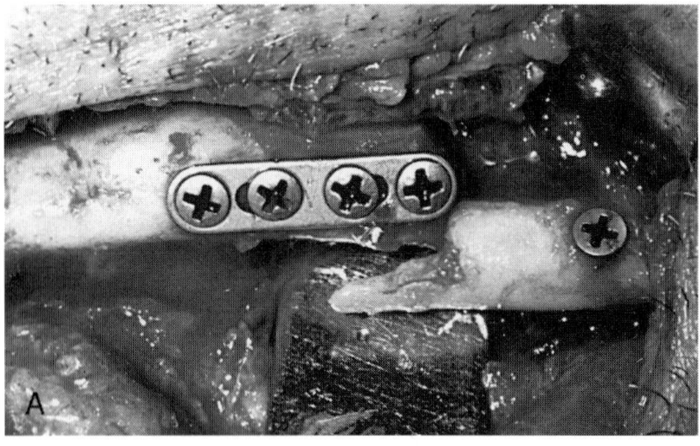

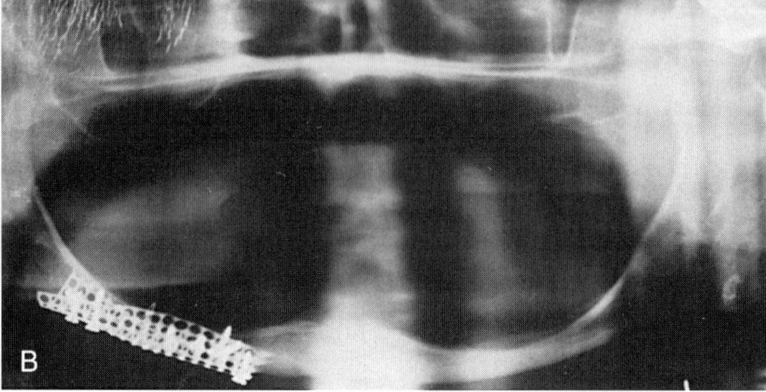

Figure 9–4. *A*, Early fixation failure resulting from screw placement too close to the fracture margin and in inadequate bone. *B*, The fracture is successfully refixed by using a titanium mesh tray and placing screws away from the fracture in sound bone.

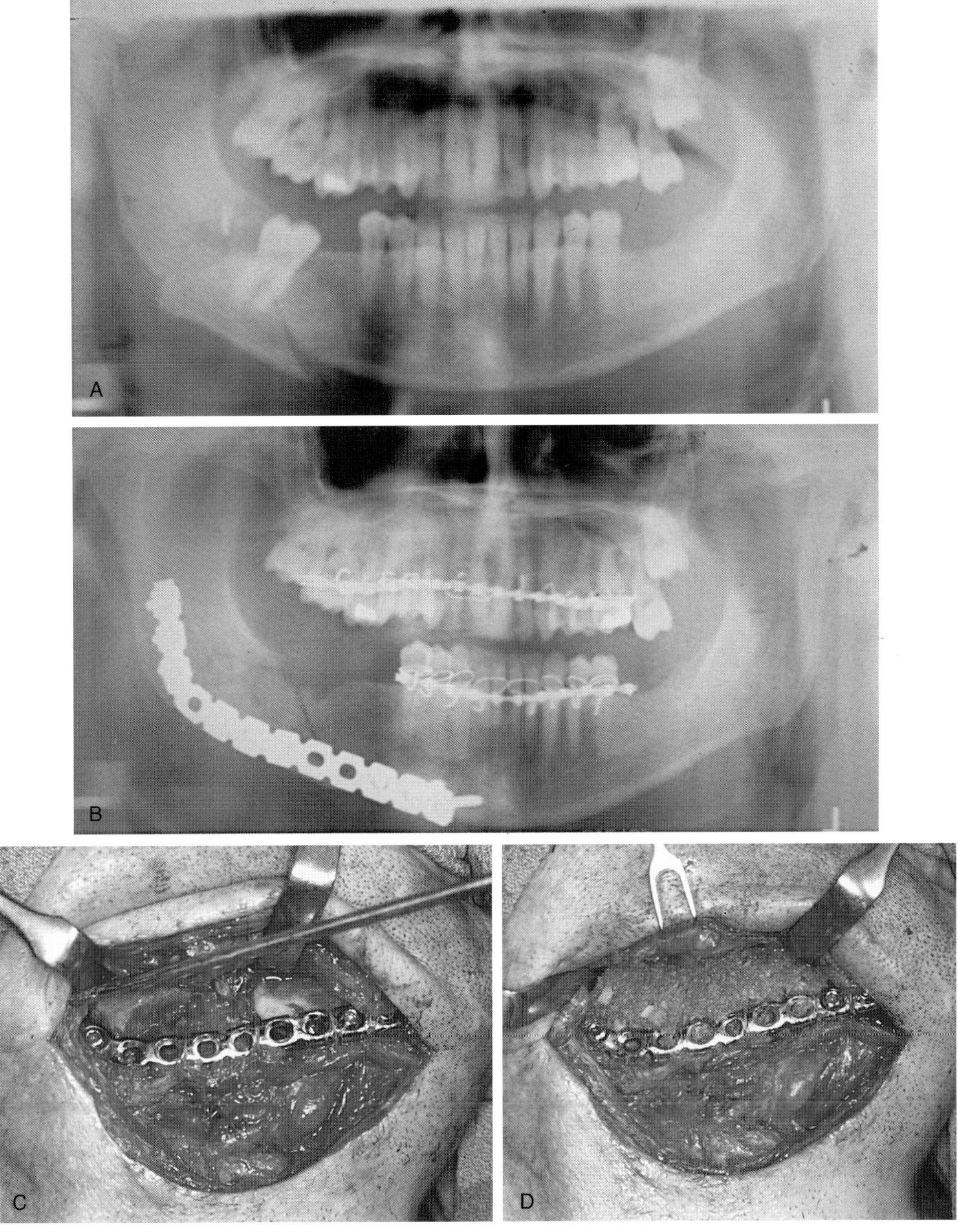

Figure 9–5. *A*, Right mandibular body fracture with single, large comminuted segment. *B*, Fixation of fracture with reconstruction plate. Note that the intervening segment is fixed to the plate with three screws. *C*, Fracture became infected and did not resolve with antibiotics, incision, and drainage. Patient was taken to surgery, and the plate was found to be stable but the comminuted segment to be mobile. Loose screws and segment were removed. This intraoperative photograph, taken 3 months later at the time of secondary bone grafting, demonstrates the defect. *D*, Particulate corticocancellous iliac crest bone graft condensed into bone defect.

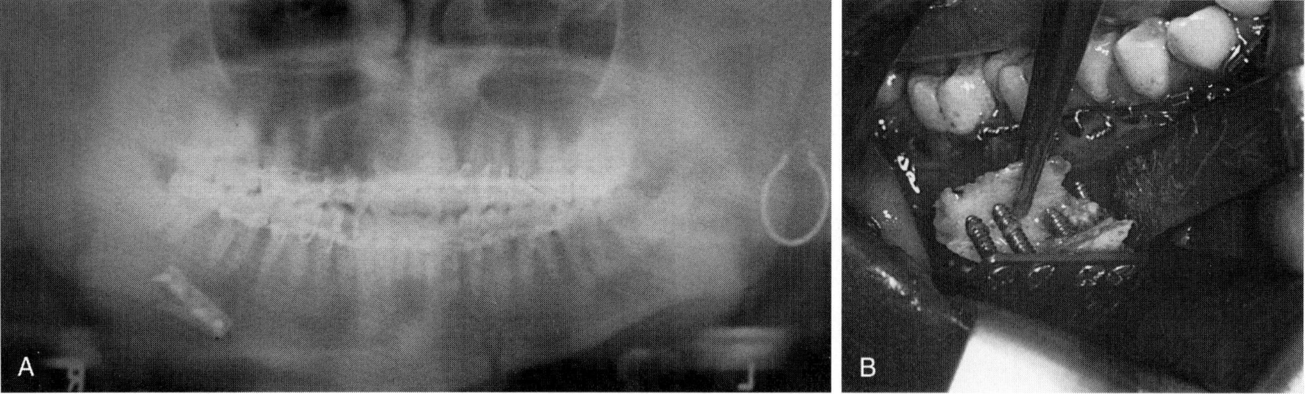

Figure 9–6. *A,* Infected right body fracture 6 weeks after treatment with maxillomandibular fixation (MMF) and positional bone plate. Osteolysis is noted around screws. *B,* All four screws were found to be loose. Necrotic bone fragment and hardware were removed. The fracture was somewhat mobile, and 2 to 3 additional weeks of MMF were required to achieve clinical union.

sue forms and becomes dense scar walling off dead bone and bacteria. Altered blood supply, scarring, and sclerotic bone formation inhibit antibiotic penetration and the immune response, making osteomyelitis more difficult to treat.[88, 89] Diagnosis can often be made at surgery, but bone biopsy with positive microbiologic and histologic findings is definitive.[88, 89] Biopsy shows inflammatory cells in the marrow space and necrotic bone.[84] Alternatively, technetium-99 diphosphate bone scans and radioactive indium–labeled white blood cell scans are very specific and sensitive for osteomyelitis when used together prior to surgical intervention.[90, 91] Radiographic evaluation shows mixed radiolucency and opacity after the process has been established for some time.[87]

Some authors believe that antibiotics alone will halt acute osteomyelitis without surgical intervention, even if fairly large sequestra are present, whereas others do not.[87, 92] Advocates of antibiotic therapy believe that the dead bone will gradually be resorbed and replaced by healthy bone.[6] Weeks of intravenous antibiotics are generally recommended.[92] This therapy typically is not indicated with fractures, however, in which both acute and chronic cases of osteomyelitis are addressed with surgery.

Surgical treatments include débridement, sequestrectomy, removal of scar tissue, and immobilization of the fragments.[55, 81, 84, 85, 92] For rapid resolution, all diseased bone, including both sclerotic and soft bone, must be removed.[84, 93] Accurate assessment of healthy bone can be determined only at surgery by visualizing normal bleeding. Conservative removal of diseased bone results in extended periods of fixation, antibiotics, and repeated surgical procedures.[94] Fixation of the fracture with intermaxillary, external, or rigid internal fixation may be utilized.[55] Rigid internal fixation with a reconstruction plate using four screws in each segment is beneficial because long periods of fixation are often needed for healing and reconstruction[55] (Fig. 9–7). The wound may be either packed open or closed primarily and treated with open or closed suction irrigation systems.[84] Giordano and associates[84] found that patients left the hospital sooner, had better cosmetic results, and needed fewer surgical interventions when treated with a closed irrigation system than when their wounds were packed open.

Antibiotic therapy is initiated after cultures are obtained. Intravenous antibiotics are given until all drainage has stopped, the white count has normalized, and fever, gross swelling, and erythema have resolved. Oral antibiotics are then given for 2 to 4 weeks longer.[89]

Antibiotic-impregnated polymethylmethacrylate beads have gained some support in the treatment of osteomyelitis of the maxillofacial region.[95–97] Local placement of such beads allows leaching of antibiotics into the affected area while minimizing systemic absorption.[96–98] Shortly after implantation, a 200:1 regional-to-blood concentration ratio has been demonstrated, and a 20 times higher local level may be obtained compared with therapeutic blood levels.[98, 99] Most of the antibiotic (70% to 90%) is released within 3 hours, and low levels are present at 4 days. Duration of effective antibiotic release has been variably reported, with local antibiotic levels present for 4 days to 3 weeks.[100–103] Gentamicin and tobramycin have primarily been used in the orthopedic arena, but other agents, including penicillin and clindamycin, may also be used.[96, 97, 100–102] Choice of antibiotics is made on the basis of expected sensitivity results, mode of action, and toxicity.[97, 101] The surgical procedure is unaltered by local antibiotic use, except that no drain is placed.[96, 97, 99] The beads are removed at 10 to 14 days unless secondary bone grafting is expected.[96, 97] In the latter case, the beads may be removed at the time of reconstruction, although considerable scar tissue will by then surround the beads.[97] Intravenous antibiotics are generally used to supplement the antibiotic beads for the first several days, particularly with extensive soft tissue involvement. Oral antibiotics are then continued for the balance of 6 weeks.[96, 97]

Although no comparative clinical studies are available showing better results with local bead therapy than with intravenous therapy in the maxillofacial region, antibiotic beads may be particularly useful in

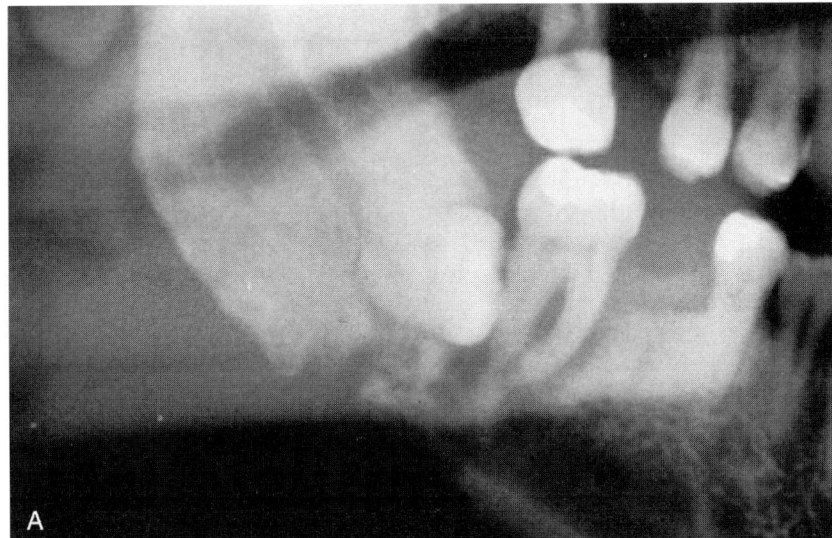

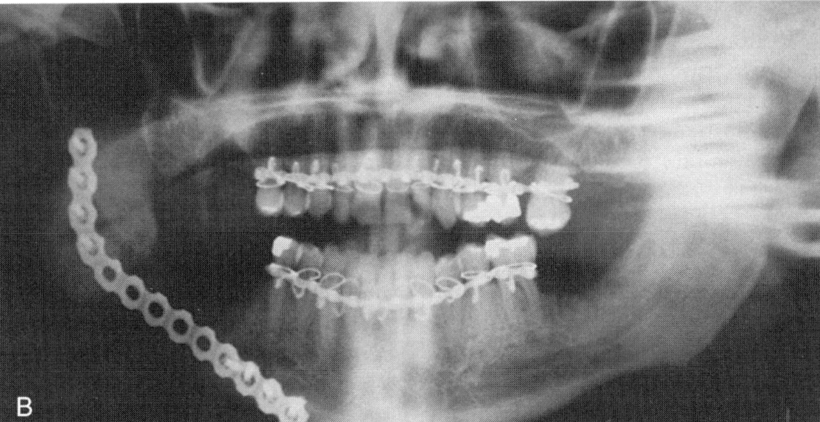

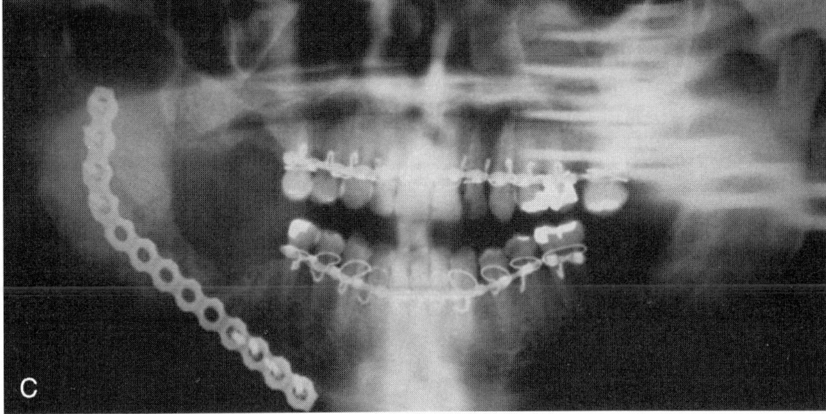

Figure 9–7. *A*, Fracture complicated by osteomyelitis in a patient who presented 4 weeks after initial trauma. *B*, Primary reconstruction via an intraoral approach with an internal fixation device placed at the time of initial débridement. *C*, Early healing of secondary corticocancellous bone graft placed 3 months after primary reconstruction.

poorly vascularized areas, where systemic antibiotics may penetrate poorly.[96, 97, 99] Infections complicated by significant scarring or sclerotic bone may be specific indications in the head and neck region.[96] Advantages of local antibiotics are decreased systemic toxicity, less dependence on patient compliance with outpatient therapy, and, possibly, fewer days of parenteral antibiotics with hospitalization.[97–99] Disadvantages include the need for a second procedure to remove the beads as well as the inability either to change antibiotics after receiving sensitivity results or to rapidly discontinue treatment at the onset of an allergic reaction.[100]

Non-unions, with or without residual infection, may result after the treatment of osteomyelitis. Reconstruction is discussed in the following section.

Complications Related to Fracture Union

Delayed Union

Delayed union, which occurs in 0 to 4.4% of mandibular fractures, is failure of the fracture to heal clinically by 2 months.[2, 3, 7, 41, 51, 104] By definition, delayed unions do go on to heal without additional surgical therapy. Infection, mobility, mandibular atrophy, increased age, and systemic illnesses are causes.[2, 81] A lower incidence of delayed union occurs with RIF (0 to 2.8%) than with nonrigid fixation (1% to 4.4%).[7, 41, 51] RIF actually masks delayed union with its inherent rigidity, and delayed union is not diagnosed until the hardware is removed. Failed RIF typically results in infected fractures or non-unions.

Non-union

A *non-union* is a fracture with arrested healing that requires further surgical therapy to achieve union. It is seen in 0 to 5% of mandibular fractures.[1, 3, 41, 63, 72, 86] Fracture mobility, repeated trauma, infection, wide fracture gap, soft tissue interposition, poor reduction, mandibular atrophy, decreased blood supply, and systemic disease can cause non-union.[86, 104, 105] Mobility is a common cause of non-union. Just as mobilization of the temporomandibular joint (TMJ) is important in preventing ankylosis, mobility of the fracture site favors production of fibrous tissue rather than bone.[86, 104, 105] In noncontaminated, closed fractures with excess mobility, a fibrous union or pseudoarthrosis results.[51] With open fractures, mobility typically results in infected non-unions. Repeat macrotrauma acts similarly to mobility and is involved in 20% of non-unions.[86]

More than 33% of the non-unions involve infection.[63, 86] As previously noted, mobility may lead to infection.[51] Conversely, with RIF or external fixation, infection may lead to mobility.[1, 50, 51, 86, 104, 105] Without union, fixation failure eventually occurs. Infection produces osteolysis around screws and resorption of the bone matrix at the fracture site.[86, 104, 105] The result is delayed healing and early failure of fixation. Thus, persistent infection increases the risk of non-union. With RIF, however, provided that fixation remains stable, union will occur.[41, 71] Clinically, the ability to resolve infections with stable hardware in place, and to achieve union when infection coexists with RIF explains why lower rates of non-union are found with RIF than with nonrigid techniques in comparative studies.[41, 72, 74]

Large fracture gaps may lead to non-union because of soft tissue collapse and insufficient bone formation.[86] Older individuals in particular may produce insufficient bone growth.[89] Large fracture gaps may be caused by infection, surgical intervention, high-energy wounds, cysts, unerupted teeth, or neoplasm.[86, 104, 105]

Other conditions may prevent adequate bone contact. Poor reduction or soft tissue trapping may separate the segments.[86, 104, 105] Edentulous fractures with significant loss of mandibular height produce a similar situation. A 10% non-union rate was reported in one series of edentulous fractures, in which 77% occurred in mandibles less than 10 mm in height.[106] With atrophic mandibles, little bone surface is available for apposition, and accurate reduction is difficult to achieve. Additionally, in older patients, poor healing occurs. Vascularity of the bone is reduced by early occlusion of the inferior alveolar artery.[106] Atrophic mandibles thus depend on the periosteal blood supply, which may be stripped by hematoma formation or surgical intervention.[107] Furthermore, atrophic mandibles are composed primarily of cortical bone, which is less cellular and heals slower than marrow.[105] Generally, 8 weeks of fixation is needed in patients older than 60 years.[86, 104, 105] Complicating this slow healing, immobilization is difficult because little ridge is exposed for splint abutment, poor buttressing of bone occurs, and there is little room for hardware placement[105] (Fig. 9–8). These factors contribute to a high rate of non-union.[8, 68, 104, 105]

The soft tissue bed must be adequate for healing. The blood supply carries the necessary oxygenation and nutrients to form callus and bone. Traumatic loss of soft tissue, scarring, stripping of periosteum, previous or repetitive trauma, or radiation may provide for a poor soft tissue bed and favor non-union.[82, 86, 104, 105]

Additionally, systemic abnormalities may interfere with the healing process. Anemia, diabetes mellitus, hyperparathyroidism, osteomalacia, Paget disease, chronic renal disease, hyperthyroidism, osteopetrosis, osteogenesis imperfecta, syphilis, vitamin B or C deficiency, Cushing syndrome, and chronic steroid use have been implicated.[86, 104, 105]

Delayed union manifests clinically as mobility and radiographically as irregular resorption and mottled segments.[105] Treatment involves additional immobilization of the fracture and control of infection and systemic disease.[104] Management of infection is achieved as previously discussed. With closed reduction, delayed union is realized with the release of fixation. Two scenarios are possible. In the first, the fracture is significantly mobile and requires additional immobilization. This presentation typically occurs in cases complicated by infection, a period of fixation loss, systemic disease, or old age. The second scenario involves a minor amount of mobility, and treatment consists of

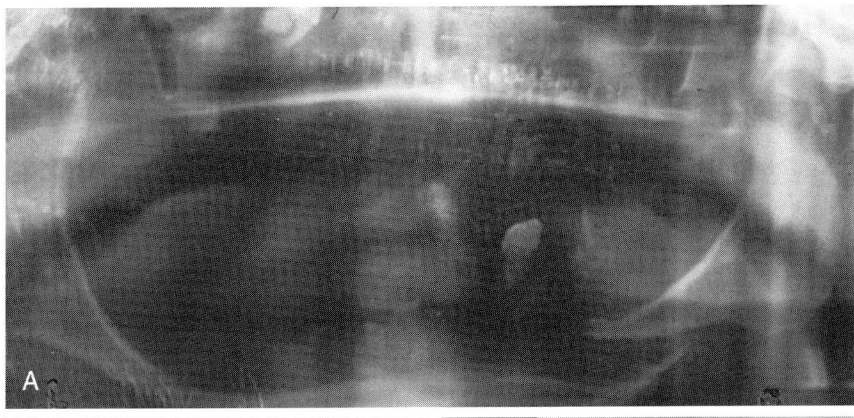

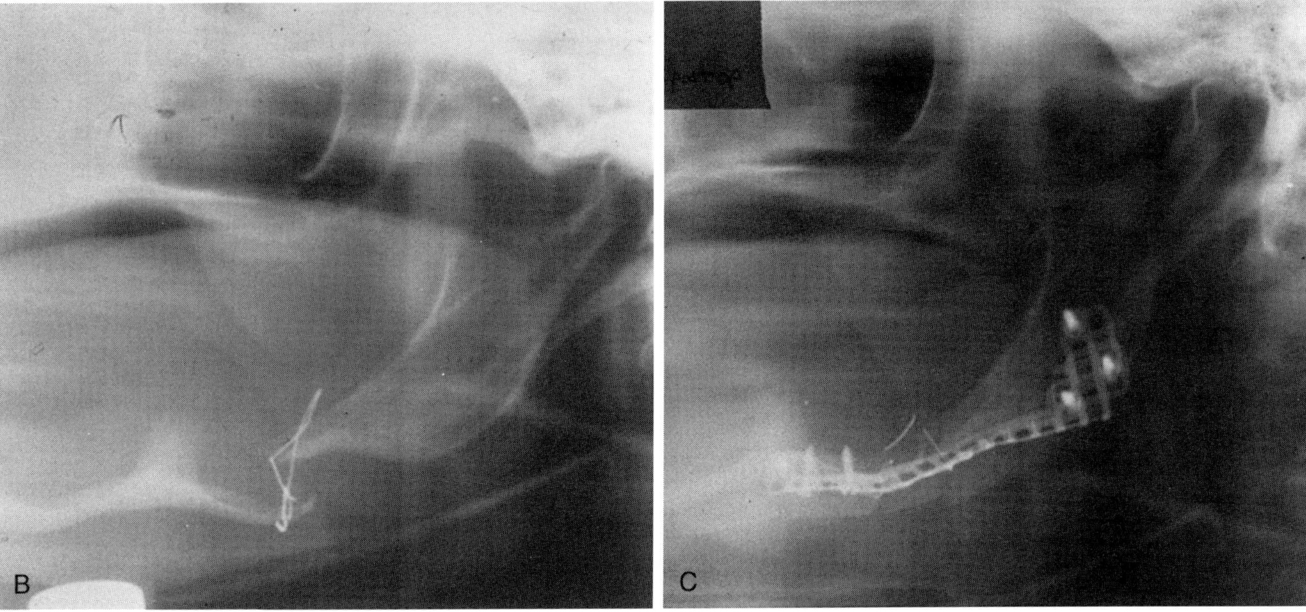

Figure 9–8. *A*, Displaced mandibular body fracture in severely atrophic mandible. *B*, The fracture was poorly stabilized by a figure-of-eight wire. *C*, The fracture was successfully refixed with wire mesh and primary bone grafting.

progressive stimulation of the bone. The patient is allowed to mobilize the mandible and wear night-time elastics to control the bite. Diet is slowly advanced to firmer foods as stabilization occurs over the following 2 to 3 weeks. Gradual loading stimulates the osteogenic matrix to ossify and achieve union.[104]

Treatment of non-union requires the evaluation of the patient's history and present condition. Compliance factors, the presence of infection and local pathology, and the quality and quantity of soft tissue are noted. Radiographically, the proximity, relationship, and cortication of the segments are examined.

A reactive, well-vascularized non-union does not require bone grafts if the gap is small.[54, 105] Treatment involves removing the intervening soft tissue, freshening and aligning segments, and restoring fixation.[105] A patient's ability to grow bone between fracture fragments is determined by patient age, vascularity of the fracture region, and height of the mandible. In younger patients with non-unions in well-vascularized areas, union generally occurs if the bone gap is 1 cm or less and extended periods of fixation are provided. Gaps larger than 1 to 1.5 cm may require bone grafting.[54, 108] Although MMF and external fixation are options, RIF prevents extended debilitation and is chosen if union may occur, a secondary procedure might be needed, or release of fixation or other forms of noncompliance contributed to the non-union.

Avascular non-unions have rounded, corticated margins and an avascular bed. Removal of the cortical margin, fixation, and placement of a particulate, cancellous bone graft is required.[3, 55, 109] MMF, external fixation, mesh trays, and RIF have all been utilized with success, but RIF provides the most versatility and stability, and the longest-lasting fixation.[55, 104, 109] Mesh trays give contour to the graft and often avoid immobilization but are more prone to hardware failure and provide less rigidity than RIF.[104] Interfragmentary mobility is a common cause of graft failure and may be a factor with mesh trays.[110] Both mesh trays and RIF may need to be removed for prosthetic reasons or to avoid stress shielding.[110]

Autogenous grafts are the best transplant material, and iliac crest is the most osteogenic.[104] With small defects, cancellous bone may be packed between the segments, but with larger defects, mesh trays or allogenic or autogenous rib, iliac crest, or mandible may be needed to confine the particles.[105, 110] Conversely, block grafts are easily immobilized by rigidly fixating them to plates or wiring them to the mandible. The disadvantage of solid grafts are that they are slow to remodel and to respond to the demands of function. Late resorption may lead to failure.[109] Additionally, transplanting a greater cellular density of osteocompetent cells has been shown to produce a greater bulk of new bone formation.[111] Because fewer osteocompetent cells are transferred with block grafts, a smaller-volume mandible often results.[109–111] With cancellous grafts, compression of particulate marrow increases the cellular density and produces substantial phase 1 graft bulk. Six to 10 mL of cancellous bone per centimeter of defect is needed.[111] Additionally, particulate cortical bone provides bone morphogenic protein for phase 2 bone healing and maintenance of graft volume.[111] The combination of autogenous cortical struts, compacted cancellous particles, and reconstruction plates has a high success rate.[110]

In most cases, preoperative model surgery and splint fabrication are needed to reposition segments and place the occlusion in the proper position. If the non-union is posterior to the dentition, a lateral cephalograph is utilized to trace the planned postoperative segment position. These two procedures allow the surgeon to estimate the intraoperative bone gap and the needed graft volume. Anterior iliac crest grafts provide a maximum of 50 mL of uncompressed bone to address defects up to 5 cm. Posterior iliac crest yields 2 to 2.5 times as much bone and is appropriate for defects larger than 5 cm.[111]

Infected non-unions are treated in much the same way as fractures complicated by osteomyelitis, that is, by removal of all infected tissue and fixation of the segments.[54, 94] Primary reconstruction with rigid plates with or without cancellous or block bone grafts has been used in this setting.[56, 81, 89, 93, 94] Primary reconstruction with bone offers several advantages. The infection leaves the soft tissue in a very vascular state compared with the scar tissue that develops with time. Additionally, the dissection is easier prior to scar formation, and a second insult may be avoided.[94] The disadvantage of primary bone grafting is the higher risk of graft loss secondary to persistent infection or dehiscence of friable infected tissue.[84, 93, 94] Morbidity is increased with a second graft harvest.

Obwegeser[93] and Obwegeser and Sailer[94] advocated bone grafting in the presence of osteomyelitis of the mandible if inflammation cannot be resolved without surgical intervention. In these studies, block grafts were used, and 12% were lost to infection.[102] Similarly, other local conditions that destroy bone and require surgical therapy, such as cysts and impacted teeth, may be treated at the time of bone grafting.[105] Successful primary grafting of infected defects requires the initiation of antibiotic therapy prior to surgery, the presence of tissue without significant distension, adequate quantity of nonfriable soft tissue for a tension-free closure, absolute immobilization of bone segments, and prevention of hematoma formation by placing a drain and filling all voids with cancellous bone.[93]

Alternatively, the infection may be treated prior to bone grafting. The advantages of this approach include a lower incidence of graft loss from infection and the possibility of avoiding grafting if bone regenerates.[84, 94] Disadvantages are the need for prolonged fixation and two surgical procedures. Surgical considerations are largely due to soft tissue scarring, which occurs as the infection resolves. Dissection is more difficult, increasing the hazard to the facial and inferior alveolar nerves, and compromised bed vascularity may inhibit graft take. Generally, 3 to 4 months elapse between resolution of the infection and bone grafting to allow time for scar maturation.[86, 89, 104] Overall, primary reconstruction with RIF and secondary bone grafting is the most predictable and most commonly used method (see Fig. 9–7).

Although the Obwegeser studies demonstrated successful bone grafting with the intraoral approach,[93, 94] extraoral grafting incurs a lower failure rate.[110] The latter approach is technically easier, particularly in the angle region, and with no mucosal perforation, percolation of saliva is avoided. With infected non-unions, oral contamination is less of a concern, and the extraoral approach may offer a smaller advantage.

With either approach, intervening fibrous tissue is removed from the graft bed and bone fragments to improve vascularity and mobilize the segments.[104, 105, 109] If not already present, or if hardware is loose and must be removed, a reconstruction plate is placed with at least four screws in each segment.[110, 112] A soft tissue pocket is created by suturing the periosteum or superficial layer of the deep cervical fascia to the reconstruction plate on the medial side. Allogeneic or autogenous rib or cortical iliac crest grafts may be utilized to provide superior and inferior walls to confine the graft in large defects. Cortical crib grafts are kept to a minimum, and holes are drilled in them to allow vascular ingrowth. Dead space is obliterated by densely packing cancellous bone.[93, 94] For grafting in the angle region, the periosteum and masseter are sutured over the graft and to the plate in order to avoid retraction and bunching of the soft tissue and to help confine the graft. An extraoral suction drain is then placed. A short period of MMF may help stabilize the vascular ingrowth and improve graft survival.[109] A second bone graft may be needed later to reconstruct the alveolus[83, 109] (Fig. 9–5).

Failure rates for conventional bone grafting range from 0 to 17%.[86, 109, 110] The most common complications are infection, non-union, dehiscence, and hardware failure.[104, 109, 110] Infection is minimized by ensuring that (1) the soft tissue is well vascularized, provides complete coverage, and is nonfriable; (2) fixation is stable; (3) intraoral wounds are well reepithelialized; and (4) all carious or periodontally involved teeth are treated or extracted prior to grafting. In significantly avascular regions, pedicled flaps or free grafting may be necessary to improve graft take.[109]

Vascularized bone grafts show good success with mandibular reconstruction and are best utilized in larger defects with concomitant soft tissue loss.[110, 111, 113] They are restricted by donor site bone volume and often produce poor form for prosthetic reconstruction. Additionally, significant morbidity is incurred, including permanent gait disturbances, prolonged rehabilitation, and loss of donor site contour.[109, 111]

Malocclusion and Malunion

Malunions occur when segments heal with improper alignment and result in malocclusions and facial deformities. The incidence of malunion ranges from 0 to 4.2%. This complication is associated with poor reduction, inadequate immobilization, delayed healing, poor patient compliance, and rigid fixation.* Poor reduction occurs particularly with inadequate anatomic references, such as missing and carious teeth, flat plane occlusion, segmental fractures of the maxilla, and multiple mandibular and dentoalveolar fractures. With inadequate dentition or segmental maxillary fractures, the maxilla is lost as a template for reduction, and arch form may be lost.[31] With posterior tooth loss and condyle, ramus, or angle fractures, vertical collapse with a loss in posterior facial height or freeway space occurs. Telescoping of midface fractures aggravates loss of posterior facial height.[115] Fractures proximal to the dentition may also have poor external reference and become unknowingly displaced without open reduction. With comminution, internal references are also lost[31, 114] (Fig. 9–9).

Improper fixation may lead to fracture displacement. Overtightening of buccal intermaxillary wires causes external rotation of segments with loss of lingual contacts and flaring of the inferior border of the mandible.[114, 115] Conversely, improper stabilization allows movement of the segments. Intermaxillary wires may be too loose, may loosen, or may fail, and periodontally involved teeth may drift or become luxated. A dentition with flat plane occlusion or many missing teeth may shift, and unfavorable segments posterior to the occlusion may undergo vertical rotation without fixation.[64] Poorly fixed atrophic mandibles in particular may heal improperly, and noncompliant patients may release fixation or fail to wear elastics for occlusal control of subcondylar fractures. Inadequate internal fixation may also allow movement of segments and result in malunion or may fail and lead to fracture infection or non-union.

Infection and mandibular atrophy are common causes of slow healing. Loss of stabilization and failure

*References 1, 2, 4, 6, 7, 31, 41, 60, 76, 114, 115.

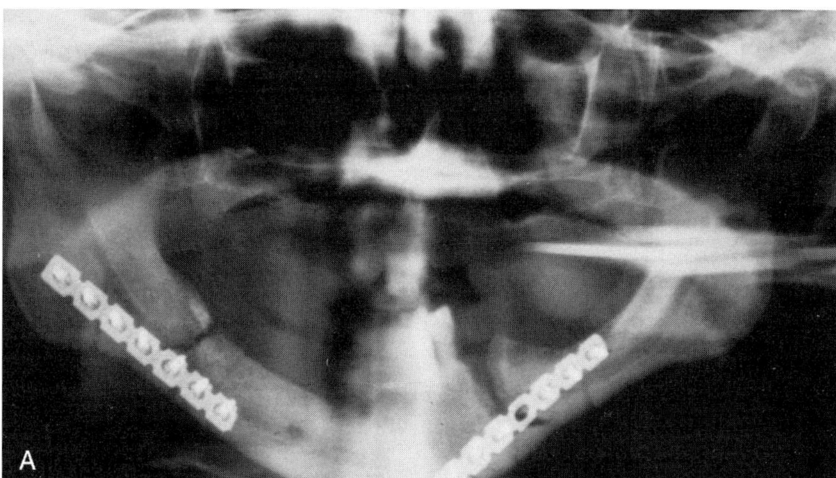

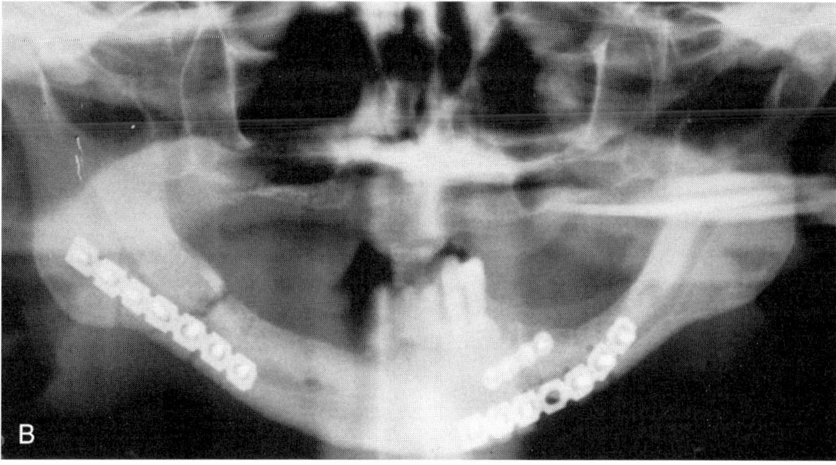

Figure 9–9. *A*, Radiograph demonstrates a poorly reduced left body fracture. No occlusal references, loss of a tooth at the fracture site, and comminution made reduction difficult. *B*, The patient was taken back to the operating room for proper reduction and refixation the following day.

to recognize the need for extended immobilization may lead to fracture displacement and malunion.[114]

Rigid internal fixation is more often associated with malunion than nonrigid techniques.[40, 45] MMF and tension band plating systems are semiflexible systems with low rates of malunion (0 to 0.5%), because the segments may be manipulated after fixation.[41, 60] In comparative studies, RIF has demonstrated higher malocclusion rates (4% to 5%).[41, 51] In particular, intraoral RIF of body and angle fractures is most problematic because of the technical difficulty involved with the approach.[52] The rigidity achieved prevents correction of technical errors without reoperation.[51, 72, 114, 115]

Treatment of malunions is best initiated early with refixation of fractures[115] (Fig. 9–9). All patients are evaluated after operation radiographically to assess results in three dimensions as well as clinically to detect occlusal and facial changes prior to discharge from the hospital. With swelling, facial contour evaluation is difficult. Posterior anterior facial radiographs may provide the only information about changes of facial width or asymmetry available at this time.[115]

Minor occlusal abnormalities may be treated nonsurgically, particularly if rigid fixation is not used. Elastic traction is used to stabilize the occlusion in subcondylar fractures as well as to improve minor interdigitation problems.[1, 26, 114] With rigid fixation, elastic traction produces only dental movement.[26] Occlusal equilibration may be utilized for fine tuning but, in general, is not undertaken unless models demonstrate that the grinding will produce the desired results without significant tooth destruction.[1, 41, 52] Additionally, fracture union must have occurred, and dental movements must have stabilized. Orthodontic treatment and prosthetic reconstruction are also options after clinical union.

Patients with severe malunions and gross malocclusions or facial deformities require surgical intervention. If possible, such patients are treated prior to the resolution of the initial swelling. Early intervention prevents two distinct episodes of swelling, scar tissue formation, and bone union and remodeling and allows treatment at the fracture sites without osteotomies.[52] Preoperative model evaluation and surgery are necessary for treatment planning and splint fabrication.[26] After bone union, reoperation may take place at the site of injury or at sites selected according to orthognathic principles. Typically, treatment consists of osteotomies at previous fracture sites if they are within the dental arch (Fig. 9–10). Fractures proximal to the dentition often are treated with ramus procedures. If significant movement of the uninvolved condyle is expected, contralateral ramus osteotomies may be needed to allow the temporomandibular joint to function in its newly adopted position.[115] Bone grafting may be necessary for significant collapse of segments, which may occur with infection or severe atrophy.[114]

A common deformity resulting from malunion after infection in the angle region consists of deviation of the chin to the affected side, crossbite, and loss of ipsilateral angle definition. This deformity results from loss of mandibular length secondary to infection. Treatment involves reestablishment of occlusion with a splint, osteotomy at the previous fracture site, proximal segment rotation, and bone grafting of the newly created defect. The proximal segment is handled variably. If the mandibular opening is inhibited by coronoid impingement secondary to segment rotation, the proximal segment is rotated clockwise to reestablish opening and angle definition. Rotation of the segment can be difficult because of muscle shortening and fibrosis.[105] If the mandibular opening is good, the proximal segment may be left in a less than completely rotated position, and the angle augmented with titanium mesh and bone at primary correction or with an allogeneic implant at a later date. Repositioning is the preferred method.

In some cases, facial deformity may be the only residual problem, because the occlusion was accepted or corrected by nonsurgical means or because the malunion occurred proximal to the dentition. Mandibular asymmetries, loss of posterior facial height, and facial width problems are most common. Although osteotomies at the malunion sites may be chosen, surgery can often be simplified, with equally good results, by the use of camouflage procedures. Horizontal osteotomy of the inferior border of the mandible, alloplastic angle augmentation, onlay bone grafting, or ostectomy may be useful.

Nerve Damage

Causes

Sensory nerve injury, particularly of the inferior alveolar and mental nerves, commonly occurs with mandibular fractures.[116] In 11% to 59% of displaced mandibular fractures, there is nerve injury at presentation.[102, 117, 118] Most injuries are neuropraxias and occur secondary to stretching or compression.[105, 116, 118, 119] Depending on the method and time of evaluation, the treatment used, and whether both high- and low-risk fractures were included in the series, dysfunction after treatment is reported in 1% to 47% of cases.[1, 27, 31, 118]

Sensory nerve damage occurs most frequently in the intrabony course of the inferior alveolar nerve. Injury is associated with displacement, extraction of third molars, open reduction, transcortical screw placement, osteomyelitis, and older patients.[1, 27, 118, 120, 121] Iizuka and Lindqvist[118] evaluated fractures through the mandible in the region of the inferior alveolar nerve. The overall rate of preoperative nerve dysfunction was 59%, with 26% noted in nondisplaced fractures. In displacement of less than 5 mm, the incidence of nerve dysfunction was 66%; in fractures displaced more than 5 mm, the incidence was 74%. Dislocation of the fracture site places traction on a small length of nerve because its ends are restricted in bone. Side-to-side movement of the segments at impact, prior to fixation, and during reduction may crush and further stretch the nerve.[1] Delay in seeking treatment increases the risk because of continued movement.[78]

Closed reduction generally yields low rates of nerve dysfunction, whereas surgical treatment may have a higher risk.[1, 27, 31, 118] For all treatments, Bochlogyros[1] found a 7.2% incidence of nerve dysfunction at 3

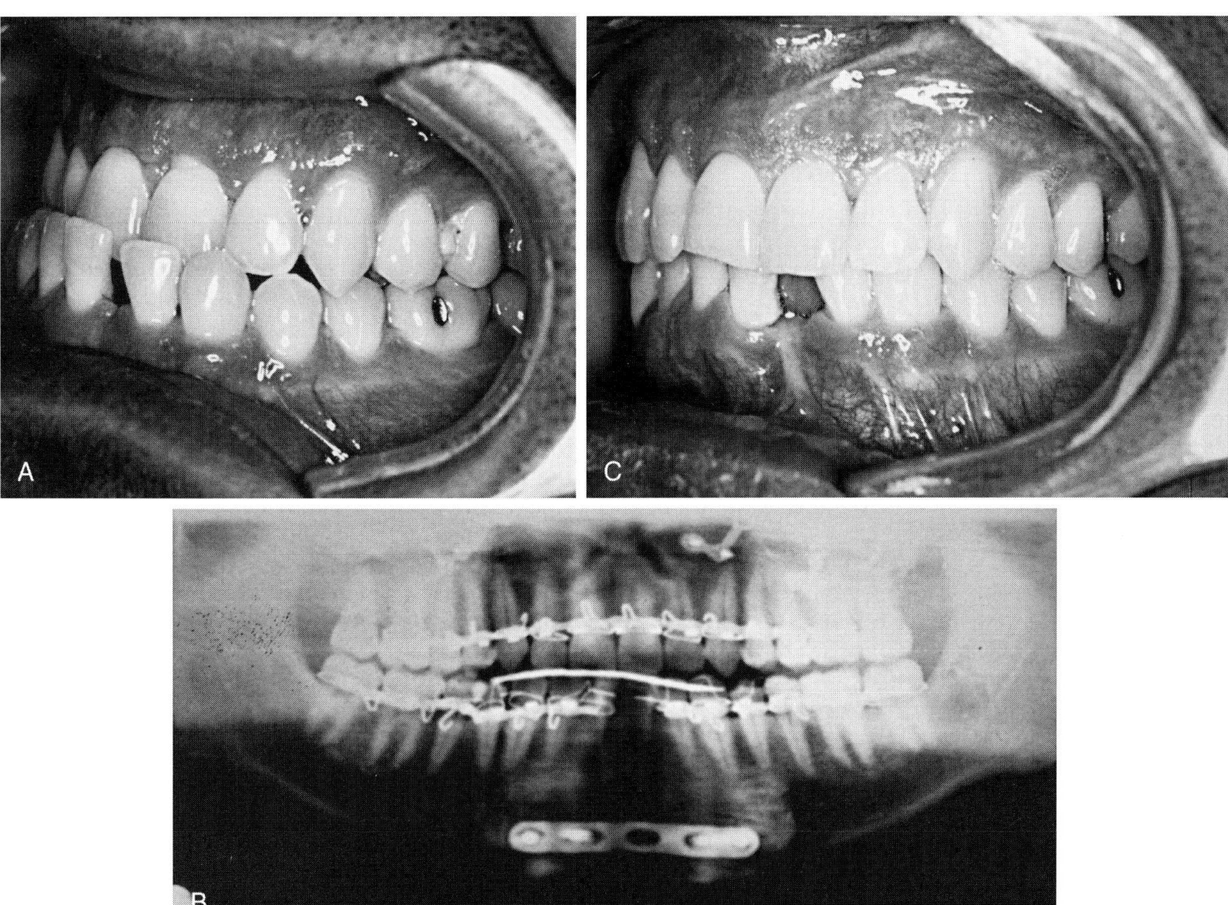

Figure 9–10. *A*, Three months after Le Fort III and mandibular fracture, this patient presented complaining of inability to open his mouth and an altered bite. Oral photograph shows class III occlusion, loss of lower central incisor, and constriction of the lower arch. *B*, Coronoid impingement, midface retrusion, and class III occlusion were treated with a modified Le Fort III osteotomy. The mandible was treated with a midline osteotomy and bone grafting at the edentulous space. The mandible is stabilized with a 2-mm plate and occlusal splint. *C*, Final occlusion after healing. Missing central incisor was later replaced with a bridge.

months—3.2% anesthesia, 2.6% hypesthesia, and 1.4% paraesthesia. Open reductions had a higher incidence of nerve dysfunction (10.8%) than closed reductions (5.1%). Surgery poses several risks. Dissection and retraction may injure the mental nerve, and the inferior alveolar nerve may be damaged with placement of fixation devices.[55] Extraction of third molars also risks injury to the inferior alveolar nerve if distraction of the segments or surgical instrumentation is necessary.[118]

Many authors have found high rates of sensory dysfunction with RIF (1% to 34%) compared with wire osteosynthesis.[1, 51, 118, 122–125] Bochlogyros[1] reported dysfunction rates of 10.8% for open reductions and 16.9% for RIF. Violation of the nerve may occur with instrumentation and screw placement. Because more exposure is needed with RIF, incisions are larger and retraction of the mental nerve is greater. Additionally, poorly adapted plates may cause distraction and overriding of the bony canals. Iizuka and Lindqvist[118] investigated the incidence of nerve dysfunction in the mandible using RIF placed primarily through an extraoral approach. They found that 91% of patients had immediate postoperative nerve dysfunction. At an average of 16 months postoperatively, 2% had hyperesthesia, 9% had marked hypesthesia, and 36% had clinically detectable dysfunction that was subjectively judged to be normal. Surgical manipulation was found to correlate with postoperative nerve dysfunction. Iizuka and Lindqvist[118] found the highest rates of dysfunction in atrophic mandibles treated with compression plates.[122] Atrophic mandibles leave little freedom for plate placement. Compression plates complicate the situation, because they bend little in the vertical plane and restrict screw positioning. Thus, such plates are more likely to overlie the nerve. In addition, older patients recover poorly and less completely after nerve injury.[120, 121, 126]

Although less commonly, other sensory nerves may be injured at the time of fracture, typically condyle fractures.[31] Chorda tympani, buccal, and auriculotemporal nerve injuries have been reported.[127]

Facial nerve dysfunction may also occur with mandibular fractures, but more commonly results iatrogenically from surgical access. Incidence of facial nerve palsy or paralysis, which is produced by traction, compression, or transection, ranges from 0 to 48% with the periauricular, retromandibular, and submandibular approaches.[2, 58, 60, 128–130]

Facial nerve dysfunction infrequently results from mandibular trauma but may occur in a variety of locations. Damage to the nerve in the fallopian canal can occur secondary to temporal bone fractures. Such fractures are associated with external auditory canal stenosis and sensorineural hearing loss. Delayed temporary facial nerve loss after condylar fractures may occur secondary to retrograde edema distal to the geniculate ganglion. Extracranial injury may also occur. Lateral dislocation of the condyle, with a proximal, contralateral fracture, may produce paresis secondary to damage distal to the stylomastoid foramen. Additionally, condylar neck fractures have caused complete transection in the retromandibular soft tissue.[131] More commonly, the facial nerve is involved in lacerations at a point along its soft tissue course.[27, 131]

Typically, facial nerve injuries result from overzealous retraction. Prevention of iatrogenic nerve injury involves using adequate incision length and approaches near the fracture site to minimize tension on soft tissues.[66, 130] Dissection injury is avoided with thorough knowledge of the regional anatomy and surgical approaches and utilization of good technique. Electrocautery, particularly monopolar, is avoided in the region of the nerve, and suture should be carefully placed with small bites in high-risk areas.

Treatment of Nerve Damage

Treatment of sensory nerve damage is covered in other sections of this chapter and so is not commented upon here.

Treatment of facial nerve damage depends on the cause, type, onset, and location of injury. Of nerve injuries caused by mandibular trauma, only delayed-onset injuries show complete, spontaneous recovery. Immediate facial paresis without a central cause is treated surgically. Loss of response with excitability testing indicates degeneration and the need for repair. Delayed onset with complete loss is handled variably. Excitability testing and electroneurography are utilized to evaluate progression of injury and degeneration.[131]

Localization of nerve injury is aided by the site of associated trauma and testing with audiogram, stapedial reflex, Schirmer test, nerve excitability, and electroneurography.[132] In a temporal bone fracture with no associated soft tissue lesions, a fallopian canal lesion is assumed, and decompression is undertaken.[131] Delayed onset with loss of stapedial reflex, changes in taste, and altered tearing supports a diagnosis of edema in the fallopian canal.[131] Steroids are given, and response is followed with excitability testing.[132] Associated injuries, lacerations, and condylar fractures and dislocations indicate the location of injury in soft tissue. If transection is suspected, early repair is initiated when the main trunk or cervicofacial or temporozygomatic branches are involved. Disruption of small branches of the zygomatic or buccal segments often produces little functional loss because of crossover connections. Branches distal to the lateral orbital rim and nasolabial groove do not require repair because of their small size.[132] Delayed reconstruction may need to be undertaken for poor soft tissue coverage or a contaminated wound. The distal stump is located with a nerve stimulator and tagged within 72 hours, before reactivity to nerve stimulation is lost.[132] When reconstruction is delayed, neurorrhaphy or grafting is best undertaken at 3 weeks.[131] Direct anastomosis is best, but if a large gap or undue tension exists, cable grafting of the cervical plexus, sural nerve, or lateral femoral cutaneous nerve is indicated.[133]

Most iatrogenic injuries of the facial nerve result in deficits of the marginal mandibular division, from the submandibular or retromandibular approach, or frontal branch, from the preauricular or coronal approach. Occasionally, other branches may be involved. Because damage typically results from stretching of small nerves, it is often not noticed at surgery. These injuries are managed expectantly and typically resolve in 3 to 6 months, although a small deficit may remain. In two studies, 11% and 29% of the deficits remained at 16 and 20 weeks, respectively.[128, 129] Known transections at the time of operation are repaired with 10-0 monofilament suture through the epineurium. Three to four sutures are placed in the nerve trunk, although one suture through the shaft of a fine peripheral nerve is sufficient.[133]

Results of primary or early secondary repair with end-to-end anastomosis or tension-free grafts result in good function in 80% of the cases, but synkinesis is common with main trunk injuries.[132, 134] Nonresolving injuries may be treated with a variety of procedures, including nerve crossover with hypoglossal or spinal accessory nerve, crossface sural nerve graft, regional muscle transfer, free muscle graft, muscle interdigitation, and facial stripping.[133] Of importance in the care of patients with facial paralysis is noting loss of orbicularis oculi function. Failure of the lids to close causes corneal drying and resulting ulceration. Eye drops must be used during the day, and the eye lubricated and taped closed at night to prevent injury.[132]

Parotid Fistula and Seroma

Parotid fistulas and seromas may occur any time a skin incision is made and dissection violates the gland or duct. They occur with lacerations, submandibular and retromandibular approaches to the mandible, and placement of external pin fixation devices.[71, 135] Interference with gland drainage and poor wound closure are causes of fistulas. Prevention involves atraumatic dissection through the parotid gland and meticulous closure of layers. The parotid duct should not be violated in the normal dissections to the mandible.

These entities must be differentiated from infection. Parotid fistulas produce clear, nonaromatic drainage without significant erythema, warmth, or other signs of infection (Fig. 9–11). Seromas often show prominent, localized swelling with minor erythema. Needle aspiration produces clear fluid.[135]

Treatment of seromas and fistulas involves aspiration of fluid and placement of a compressive dressing. Sero-

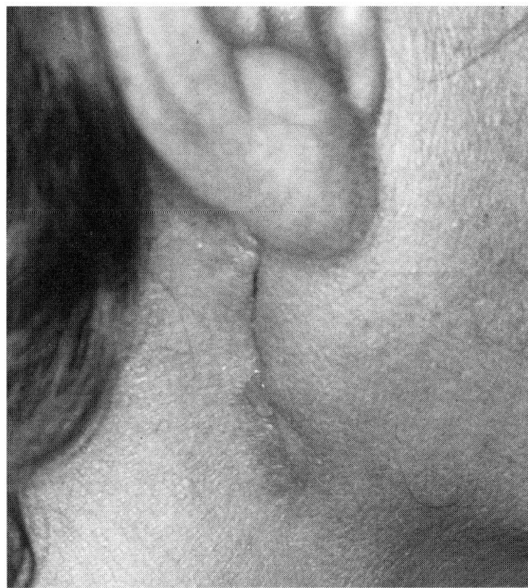

Figure 9–11. Parotid fistula after retromandibular approach to a subcondylar fracture. Resolution occurred over several days with the application of pressure dressings.

mas typically resolve in 2 to 3 days, whereas fistulas may take somewhat longer to stop draining. If a fistula is associated with an external fixation appliance, pins need not be removed until treatment is complete, although drainage may be somewhat bothersome. A bland diet and antisialagogues, such as propantheline, help minimize the output. After the removal of the pin fixation, spontaneous resolution typically occurs, but pressure dressings and antisialagogues may hasten closure.[135] In rare instances, reclosure of the wound, followed by application of pressure dressings, is necessary.

Temporomandibular Joint Disorders

Mandibular trauma may produce a variety of TMJ injuries, such as sprains, disk damage, and condyle fractures.[136–138] Sprains occur from damage to the ligaments and joint capsule and may result in disk displacement and dislocation. Joint effusions and hemarthrosis often are associated with soft tissue injury and typically resolve in 5 to 7 days.[136, 137] Disk damage may take the form of surface shredding, tearing, or complete destruction.[137] There may be fractures of the condylar surface, neck, subcondylar region, or glenoid fossa.[138]

These injuries alone or in combination produce disorders encompassing pain, dysfunction, degeneration, and limitation.[139] Pain may be associated with scarring and limitation of opening or impingement of soft tissue.[140, 141] Dysfunction involves alteration of condylar movement and is caused by irregular surfaces and changes in relationships between the disk and condyle, as well as adhesions.[136] Condyle fractures have been noted to cause popping and clicking in 4% to 32% of childhood condyle fractures at long-term follow-up.[34, 142–144] Condyle fracture produces shredding of the disk and joint surfaces 50% to 60% of the time, which are often greatest with dislocations and on the nonfractured side.[137] The disk tends to follow the proximal segment at the time of fracture displacement and repositioning, but with tearing of the ligaments and capsule, the disk and condyle may assume a new relationship and cause dysfunction.[138, 141, 143] Adhesions also are noted in fractured joints and may cause alteration in joint movement.[141]

Degeneration of the joint may occur with damage to the disk, altered loading, or devascularization of the proximal segment.[145] Damage and complete destruction of the disk may occur with condyle fractures, resulting in the loss of its stabilizing and protective properties.[137, 145] Increased loading of the condyle may occur with improper reduction and RIF of mandibular fractures. Incomplete reduction elongates the condyle and tips it onto the concave walls of the joint fossa, producing increased loading.[130, 146] Degenerative changes have been noted in condyles treated with RIF in the short term.[138, 146] Blood supply to the proximal segment in condyle fractures is chiefly via the lateral pterygoid. Complete detachment of the lateral pterygoid may also lead to resorption.[130, 138]

Limitation of mouth opening may be unilateral, resulting in deviation on opening and loss of ipsilateral lateral excursive movement, or bilateral, resulting in loss of interincisal opening and protrusion.[143] Deviation on opening occurs in 3% to 80% of condyle fractures.[144, 146–148] Causes include muscle fibrosis, scarring, adhesions, mechanical impingement, internal derangements, malposition of the condyle, lateral pterygoid dysfunction, and ankylosis. Immobilization of fractures, particularly condyle fractures, has been associated with a reduction in opening.[27, 31] Limitation of opening to less then 40 mm occurs 0.6% to 9% of the time.[1, 8, 27, 31, 138, 146] Immobilization may lead to muscle shortening and atrophy, fibrosis, loss of capsular plicae, and adhesions, all of which limit mouth opening.[140] Amaratunga[140] demonstrated a reduction of mouth opening with increased duration of MMF, compared with open reduction with wire osteosynthesis of noncondyle and coronoid fractures. At 6 months, groups with open reduction and immediate function and 3, 4, and 5 weeks of immobilization had mouth openings of 41, 38, 34, and 31 mm, respectively.

Good functional recovery of condyle fractures is typically seen with closed treatment.[147–149] Reported complications and rates are pain (1% to 2%), clicking (4%), limitation (0 to 7%), ankylosis (0 to 2%), and deviation on opening (2% to 20%).[147, 149–151] Closed rather than open treatment has been advocated.[147, 149] Takenoshita and associates[152] found that with closed treatment of condyle fractures, rehabilitation was faster and more complete than with open treatment. Severe displacement of mandibular fractures, however, may cause abnormal opening and dysfunction if not properly reduced. Excessive scarring, mechanical obstruction, internal derangements, or ankylosis may be responsible.[130, 138, 147]

Open reduction may offer some advantages to closed

treatment. In a randomized study, increased opening, less pain, and better function were found with wire osteosynthesis than with closed reduction.[153] Additionally, better condyle position has been demonstrated with open reduction and wire fixation.[149] With a more upright condyle position, compared with the typically anterior and medially tipped condyle that results with conservative treatment, the lateral pterygoid may better maintain its length and provide translation of the condyle. The result may be less deviation and asymmetry on opening. Open reduction without fixation, wire osteosynthesis, and RIF have all demonstrated better condyle translation than closed treatment.[130, 147, 153]

Condylar degeneration is avoided by reducing stresses placed on the condyle and preserving its blood supply. Rigid internal fixation of imperfectly fixed fractures may cause condylar loading, particularly if MMF is also used. Condylar degeneration has been noted when fractures are rigidly fixed.[138, 146] All 13 cases in one study demonstrated degeneration within 3 to 15 months of treatment; noise, but not pain or limitation, was correlated with the findings.[146] Simultaneous use of MMF may have contributed to the degeneration. Condylar fractures treated with wire fixation or no fixation do not commonly demonstrate degeneration unless blood supply to the proximal segment has been lost.[130, 146]

Loss of vascular supply to the proximal segment may cause osteolysis.[130, 138] Excess manipulation of the condylar segment, particularly with a preauricular approach, may detach soft tissue and the lateral pterygoid and is to be avoided.[130, 138] Meniscal disruption has also been suggested as a cause of degeneration.[138] Because the disk may not return to position with the condyle, some have suggested routine disk inspection and repositioning.[138, 143]

Ankylosis is estimated to occur in 0.2% to 0.4% of condyle fractures.[142, 154] True ankylosis involves a union between the condyle and the skull base; it is associated with immobilization, young age, high condyle fractures, infection, and loss of the disk.[155–160] Although prolonged immobilization in animals with surgical condylar fractures does not result in ankylosis, decreased function because of MMF or cerebral injury may do so in the clinical setting.[160–164]

Young age, particularly less than 10 years, is associated with ankylosis.[142, 154, 157, 158, 160] In the first 2 to 3 years of life, the condyle is very vascular, having a thin cortical shell, abundant marrow, and a short, thick neck. These factors predispose young children to comminution of condyle fractures. The marrow is a highly osteogenic material, and with the self-imposed immobilization that often occurs in the young, rapid fusion takes place.[154, 162, 163] Other factors, including high ongoing periosteal activity and metabolic rate, also contribute to ankylosis.[162, 163]

Hemarthrosis alone probably is not a significant risk for ankylosis. Although it is common after mandibular injury, blood does not cause articular cartilage changes or ankylosis even after repetitive exposure.[136, 140, 165]

The disk is believed to provide a key barrier to ankylosis.[159, 160] Although prolonged fixation, hemarthrosis, and condylar comminution alone do not normally result in ankylosis, animal studies have demonstrated that partial or complete removal of cartilage from the joint does.[159, 160, 166] Additionally, the disk is not often found during the surgical correction of ankylosis.[108, 156, 167] Thus, articular damage with disk loss may allow bone-to-bone contact and ankylosis.[168, 169] The disk may be lost through displacement, traumatic destruction, or infection. Infection destroys cartilage when granulation tissue forms and is a commonly cited cause of ankylosis.[137, 159, 160]

Posttraumatic TMJ disorders include pain, altered function, limitation, and degeneration. Physical examination is used to divide patients into three groups: those with ankylosis, those with hypermobility, and those with other disorders. Patients without ankylosis or hypermobility are treated with a trial of physiotherapy, antiinflammatory agents, splints, and other conservative measures to resolve pain and improve function, unless an obvious anatomic abnormality is noted on the screening panoramic radiograph or clinical examination. Patients for whom a reasonable course of conservative therapy fails may be surgical candidates if pain and dysfunction are significant. Arthroscopy is of value in treatment of adhesions and pain. Cases with significant fibrosis, degeneration, or disk damage or malposition require arthroplasty with or without soft tissue grafts. Patients who have functional problems with obvious anatomic causes may be treated primarily with condylar repositioning or arthroplasty[138] (Fig. 9–12).

Hypermobility disorders result from capsule and ligament damage. After failure of primary treatment of functional restriction and slow mobilization for soft tissue injury, MMF is accomplished for a period of 2 weeks with elastics or wire ligatures. The mandible is slowly returned to normal movement without use of passive exercises. If further dislocation occurs and is bothersome to the patient, surgical intervention may be undertaken. If a steep eminence is noted, eminectomy is an effective treatment that allows the condyle to return freely into the fossa. Repositioning or sclerosis of the joint ligaments and capsule may be appropriate in other cases.[139]

Patients with true ankylosis require surgical treatment. Preoperative coronal CT scanning with contrast demonstrates the presence and location of proliferative bone and large vessels. Assessment of CT scans allows evaluation of the risk of bleeding and dural injury and guides the level of osteotomy. Treatment options include gap arthroplasty, ascending ramus division, and costochondral grafting, all with or without interpositional grafts.[108] Arthroplasty successfully restores pain-free opening.[156, 168–170] A high osteotomy is desirable because improved function results, but a lower resection is often chosen to simplify the procedure and minimize bleeding and risk of dural injury.[130, 169] Proliferation of bone often obliterates normal anatomy. This bone is atypically hard and is located at the level of the condyle. The base of the neck often is less involved. In such cases, osteotomy is made at the deepest portion of the sigmoid notch and is extended to the

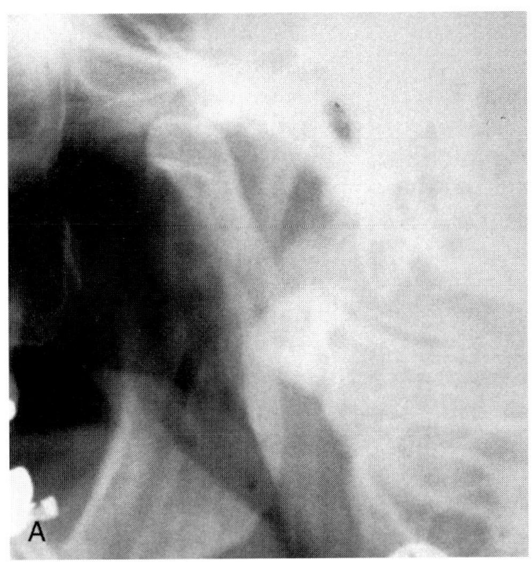

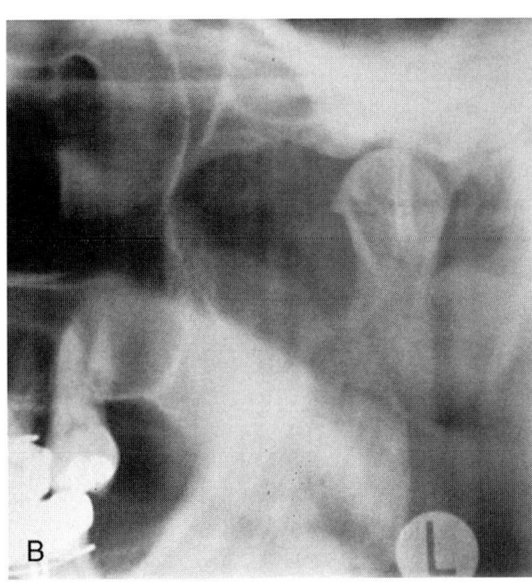

Figure 9–12. *A*, Patient presented 3 months after conservative treatment of a dislocated mandibular fracture. He complained of inability to open his mouth and preauricular pain. Panoramic radiograph shows the condyle out of the glenoid fossa. *B*, Patient was treated with open reduction without internal fixation and two weeks of maxillomandibular fixation. Panoramic radiograph demonstrates reduction of the condyle back into the glenoid fossa. The patient was rehabilitated to a pain-free opening of more than 40 mm over the next 6 weeks.

posterior border of the mandible.[170] Although with fibrous union, the condyle may be dissected out, no such attempt is made with a bony union. Bone removal at the height of the fossa risks perforation of the skull base and tympanic plate.[130, 170] If ankylosis involves the sigmoid fossa and coronoid process, the entire ramus is sectioned above the mandibular foramen.[156, 170] Patients undergoing unilateral gap arthroplasty are mobilized on the first postoperative day, and those undergoing bilateral procedures benefit from 5 days of immobilization.[170] Henderson[155] reported on 15 gap arthroplasties that resulted in postoperative openings between 20 and 35 mm.

The most common complication of gap arthroplasty is reankylosis.[155] Adequate resection (1 cm) and early mobilization are important preventive measures.[156, 168–170] Mobilization must be continued for extended periods, until stable opening and corticated bone margins are noted radiographically.[142, 171] Although reankylosis generally appears within 6 months, it may not be seen until 1.5 years after treatment.[171] Other complications of gap arthroplasty are posterior movement of the ramus, loss of posterior facial height, open bite, deviation on opening, and unstable occlusion.[108, 142, 171] Better movement and stability are obtained if the arthroplasty is performed close to the normal joint and if the occlusion is controlled at night with elastics and arch bars for 3 months after surgery.[171]

Some report limited success with gap arthroplasties, and the placement of interpositional material has been suggested to decrease reankylosis.[108, 138, 171, 172] In animals, soft tissue placed in static bone defects for 8 months without movement has prevented ossification.[171] Topazian[171] reported on 20 patients treated with gap arthroplasties, 5 of whom received interpositional grafts. Of the patients without interpositional grafts, 53% had reankylosis, compared with none of those who had the grafts. Temporalis muscle, cartilage, and dermis have been recommended as interpositional graft material, but there is no consensus.[108, 130, 173] Raveh and colleagues[130] advocate full removal of bone to the skull base and interposition of lyophilized costochondral cartilage. At an average of 3 years of follow-up, impressive results were obtained with no recurrences. The average preoperative and postoperative openings were less than 10 mm and greater than 40 mm, respectively.

Others advocate costochondral grafts, believing that a lower incidence of reankylosis results.[174–176] Grafts may also restore normal biomechanics by creating a definite posterior stop. This articulation provides a base for future osteotomies and allows partial correction of posterior facial height deficiencies and asymmetries.[177, 178] Additionally, growth potential in children and adaptability in adults is restored.[108, 178, 179]

Treatment with costochondral grafting involves aggressive removal of bone and scar tissue. Any remains of a displaced condyle are removed and, if present, the disk is repositioned. Typically, the disk is not present, and temporalis flaps may be utilized to act as an additional barrier.[172] Costochondral grafts are fixated with bone screws to the lateral aspect of the mandible after decortication of the graft and ramus on adjacent sides.[180] A contralateral ramus osteotomy may be needed if posterior facial height or anterior position of the mandible is altered significantly.[108] Depending on the stability of graft fixation, up to 2 weeks of MMF may be beneficial. A splint is used to stabilize and open the bite.[108, 167, 179, 180] The latter may be useful to offset the mild graft settling that may occur with loading.[167] Further bite opening may be useful to accomplish postoperative leveling of the occlusal plane by super-erupting the maxillary teeth.

Complications of costochondral grafting include ankylosis, lack of protrusive ability, non-union, fracture of the costochondral junction, exuberant overgrowth, infection, and donor site morbidity such as pneumothorax.[178, 180] As with gap arthroplasties, recurrence of ankylosis is the most common problem.[182, 183] Good opening tends to be maintained as long as mobilization exercises are utilized.[167, 183] Two studies demonstrated improved opening, from 9 mm (range 2 to 20 mm) to 27 mm (range 20 to 42 mm), and 16 mm (range 2 to 30 mm) to 31 mm (range 15 to 45 mm) with costochondral grafts.[167, 180] A 10-year follow-up of one study showed greater improvement with time.[184]

Most surgeons report deviation on opening and essentially no translation after costochondral grafts.[141, 167] Lindqvist and associates[180] noted deviation of 4.5 mm on opening and contralateral excursion of 3 mm (range 0 to 10 mm). But at the 10-year follow-up on 16 patients, however, 6 of whom had had ankylosis, improvements in lateral excursion and deviation on opening were demonstrated. The average translation on the operated side was 7 mm.[184]

Non-union, an uncommon complication of costochondral grafting, is avoided by decorticating the rib and mandible and using screw fixation.[180] Placement of a thin (<5 mm) cartilage cap, retention of a periosteal sleeve in children, and slowly progressive graft loading help prevent fracture of the costochondral junction.[167, 179]

With any technique, several principles must be followed to prevent reankylosis. At the time of surgery, adequate mobilization of the mandible must be accomplished by removal of all the bone and scar that are producing restriction. Considerable restriction is expected from soft tissue fibrosis and muscle contracture. Slow mechanical dilatation with a side-action mouth gag improves opening. Care is taken not to luxate teeth or fracture the jaw. Although an ultimate opening of greater than 30 mm in ankylosis cases has often been considered adequate, an opening of 40 mm must be achieved at operation.[142] Opening will not improve postoperatively, it will only be maintained or decrease.[169] If restriction persists after mechanical dilatation, an evaluation is made of the contralateral joint, coronoid processes, and soft tissue. Surgical treatment is undertaken until the desired opening is achieved.[169]

Coronoid hypertrophy often occurs in cases of ankylosis during growth and results in impingement of the zygomatic process.[155, 167, 172, 185] Coronoidectomy is the indicated treatment, but it is used cautiously. Considerable disability may result, because the temporalis muscle is important for controlling mandibular movements when normal lateral pterygoid function is lost.

After release of ankylosis, residual deformities may remain. Deformities are corrected with orthognathic procedures after stability of joint function has been demonstrated.[186] Cortication of the new condyle and a nonchanging opening are good indications of stability. Generally, 6 to 12 months is allowed for joint function to stabilize.

Approaches advocated for ankylosis release include the preauricular, Risdon, and coronal approaches.[156, 167, 169, 170, 186, 187] The preauricular approach allows direct access to the joint if a high osteotomy is undertaken.[130, 156] If coronoidectomy or a costochondral grafting is necessary, an additional approach must be used.[167] The Risdon approach decreases the risk to the facial nerve and is particularly useful for gap arthroplasties at the level of the sigmoid notch.[169, 170, 181] The coronal flap is useful in difficult cases needing extensive resection, particularly with the addition of coronoidectomy and costochondral grafting. A low incidence of facial nerve injury is noted because of the good access and little need for heavy retraction.[186]

Complications associated with correction of ankylosis include reankylosis, facial nerve damage, inferior alveolar nerve damage, bleeding, infection, and dural injury.[130, 155, 170, 176, 180] Tissue is often distorted in cases of ankylosis with scar tissue and proliferative bone formation. Adequate access, attention to existing anatomy, low osteotomies, and careful removal of scar and bone decrease the risk of complications.

Coronoid ankylosis or temporalis scarring may occur as an isolated finding and may be treated with coronoidectomy. Intraoral resection is generally preferred, followed by vigorous postoperative physiotherapy.[169]

Growth Disturbances

Causes

Growth disturbances occur primarily with condyle fractures and are related to ankylosis, young age, surgical scarring, and altered muscular activity.[27, 34, 157, 172, 188–191] Mandibular growth consists of both condylar elongation and appositional bone deposition at the posterior border of the ramus, coronoid tip, and alveolar process.[190, 191] In the past, the condyle was considered an active epiphyseal growth center, but now it is thought to behave in a more adaptive manner.[174, 185, 192–194] Transitional movement of the mandible is initiated by soft tissue, or the functional matrix, and the condyle grows to keep contact with the glenoid fossa.[167]

Disturbances of growth produce typical deformities. If one condyle is affected, a short, wide ramus, preangular notch, short body, ipsilateral fullness, and contralateral flatness result. Midline deviation, canting of the occlusal plane with vertical underdevelopment of the maxilla and alveolar process on the affected side, and dental compensations may be seen.[105, 185, 195] Bilateral condylar involvement results in a more or less symmetric retrognathic mandible, short posterior face height, and proclination of the mandibular incisors, or the bird-faced deformity.[108, 175]

Condylar trauma may cause 5% to 20% of all severe mandibular deficiencies or asymmetries.[34, 146] Growth changes occur in 3% to 52% of all pediatric condyle fractures.[188, 189] Both undergrowth and overgrowth are reported.[176, 189] Lund[189] identified 27 patients who had had unilateral condyle fractures as children; 30% demonstrated overgrowth of the fracture side, and 22% had undergrowth. Lindahl and Hollender[176] found deviation toward the fracture side only with dislocated fractures. Head and neck fractures tended to deviate toward, and subcondylar fractures away from, the fracture site. Overgrowth after condyle fracture is similar to that after pediatric long bone fractures.[176]

Age is correlated with growth disturbances, for several reasons. Ankylosis occurs more commonly, and more growth potential is present, at an early age. Deformities become progressively worse with growth.[191] Injuries occurring before the age of 3 years produce severe deformities, those after 6 years moderate deformities, and those after 12 years slight deformities.[162, 196]

Many theories have been postulated for growth restriction. Early ossification of epiphyseal cartilage, loss or destruction of the condylar cap, ankylosis, and loss of condylar translation have been suggested.[190, 197] A high correlation has been found between limited function and growth deficiency.[175, 190, 198] Because cartilage damage typically occurs with ankylosis, the question is whether the limited opening or damage to the cartilage produced the restricted growth. Sarnat[191] and Sarnat and Engel[185] produced growth deficiencies in animals by resecting the mandibular condyle. Mandibular opening was restored but growth was limited. Some growth still occurred under the influence of the tongue and pharynx. Other animal studies demonstrated the regeneration of the condyle to normal form but without cartilage, and restricted growth occurred.[199] In a similar study, Walker[200] found functional condyles with cartilage and normal growth after surgical condylar fracture and gross dislocation. Additionally, hemicondylectomies or autogenous transplants of condylectomized areas in animals show initial slowing of growth. Regeneration of the condylar cartilage then occurs, and normal growth resumes.[199] These findings have led some authors to conclude that the cartilaginous cap is necessary for growth, and that injuries to condyle cartilage or loss with dislocation reduces the capacity for complete remodeling and maintenance of normal skeletal joint relations.[105, 176]

Clinically, failure of the condyle to remodel to normal form has been associated with abnormal growth. Lindahl and Hollender[176] found that 80% of fracture cases in which normal skeletal relations of the joint were not attained via remodeling had growth deviations to the fracture side. Additionally, cases demonstrating no ankylosis but limited growth have been reported.[176]

Some authorities have questioned whether the condylar cartilage is necessary for normal growth.[201–203] Moss and Salentijn[203] believed that condylar cartilage responds in a compensatory fashion to stimulation from the functional matrix, and that the condyle serves only to maintain the temporomandibular articulation. Normal translation of the condyle may be the key factor.[188, 190, 204] Ankylosis may result in scarring and mechanical restrictions rather than damage to the growth center.[167, 188, 201] In cases with adequate opening but poor growth, translation may still be absent. Conversely, problems with restricted opening and intact translation, such as often occurs with false ankylosis, do not produce growth deformities.[156, 175]

Little or no lateral excursions are noted in patients with growth disturbances.[195] Engel and Brodie[190] presented 19 cases of growth arrest. Most were associated with loss of function, particularly translation of the affected condyle. Alteration in muscular activity may also prevent normal growth, because no mechanism for translation is present.[197] Functional appliances have been successful in restoring translation and growth in these cases.[188, 190, 197, 205]

Treatment of Growth Deformities

Treatment of growth defects depends on early recognition.[188] Clinical evaluation provides the best screening tool for growth disturbances, but photographs, radiographs, and models are needed to document their progression.[34, 175] Evaluation of interincisal opening, translation, asymmetry, mandibular retrognathia, and posterior facial height is required.[188, 190] Functional disturbances manifest before disturbances of facial growth. If altered function, asymmetry, mandibular retrusion, or short posterior facial height develops, baseline records are obtained, and the patient is followed with serial examinations including cephalometric radiographs, models, and photographs.[175] Presentation of ankylosis and growth deficiencies is usually delayed, so follow-up must be prolonged.[169]

Treatment options for growth deformities include ankylosis release with or without grafts, growth center transplants, functional appliances, serial lengthening procedures during growth, and osteotomies and camouflage after the cessation of growth.[180, 182, 188] Choice of treatment depends on patient age, joint function, and severity of the deformity. In general, early treatment of growth abnormalities is advocated to prevent further deformity.[141, 142, 156, 167, 183] If restricted opening without ankylosis is present, the patient is rehabilitated with active and passive physiotherapy and followed closely.[175] Mobilization may stimulate growth.[167] For restricted opening with ankylosis, early surgical treatment is indicated. Cooperation of very young patients can be a problem, but ankylosis release can generally be accomplished by age 5 or even younger.[142, 156, 206] Early release of ankylosis has the added benefit that less proliferative bone formation is present, making surgery easier.

Moss,[203] Sailer,[207] and others[142, 186, 188, 201] believe cartilage grafts are not required to restore normal growth. Still others believe that sufficient compensatory growth seldom occurs after osteoarthrotomy, and that growth arrest should be treated with a costochondral graft.[105, 181] If osteoarthrotomy is chosen, mobilization to normal opening is necessary.

If growth disturbances are noted and the joint is functional, an evaluation of translation is made. If active translation does not occur but passive translation does, a functional appliance may be tried. Favorable growth has been demonstrated with anterior positioning of the mandible with functional appliances.[188, 197, 205] Patients with growth arrest and adequate interincisal openings for whom functional appliance therapy fails or who do not demonstrate passive translation after physiotherapy are candidates for growth center transplants.

Costochondral grafts are currently the most supported treatment for growth restriction.[167, 179–184, 187] Such grafts grow and adapt commensurate with age by both intrinsic and extrinsic means.[167, 179, 181, 183, 187] Intrinsic growth may be responsible for the elongation that occurs without functional correction.[167, 181, 182] This same growth characteristic makes costochondral grafting unpredictable. Overgrowth may occur both during normal growth and during pregnancy.[167, 180, 181, 188] Undergrowth may also occur.

If normal opening is present in a young patient, serial lengthening procedures to minimize the deformity by preventing maxillary canting and alveolar growth restriction is a second option. Treatment involves overcorrection of the affected side with a splint placed at surgery to keep the posterior occlusion open. The splint is gradually thinned to allow tooth eruption and closure of the space.[162]

Conversely, in a patient with growth deformity seen at a late age, the deformity may be accepted and treated after the cessation of growth.[188] Cases of overgrowth caused by trauma typically are minor and may be treated in this fashion. If range of motion is good and stability is demonstrated, the joint is not violated. Rather, ramus procedures are utilized to lengthen the mandible. If significant joint pathology is present, ankylosis release or other treatment is undertaken as previously discussed. Costochondral grafts may provide a more stable stop for future orthognathic procedures, but simultaneous osteotomies are avoided. Osteotomies may interfere with joint rehabilitation and cause increased joint loading. Additionally, if graft resorption or joint changes take place, additional surgery is needed. Generally, 6 to 12 months is allowed to elapse before orthognathic and camouflage procedures are utilized.[162] The ideal age for secondary correction is 14 to 15 years.[188]

Conclusion

The oral and maxillofacial surgeon now has many options for treating mandibular fractures. Nevertheless, complication rates are significant. Although some techniques may be better than others, no one technique can be used in all situations. In most cases, more than one comparable option is available. The patient and fracture should be properly evaluated, and the best options selected. Risk and benefits of each are then presented to the patient. In most situations, both maxillomandibular fixation and rigid internal fixation are available to the patient. Successful implementation involves a thorough understanding of a technique and its limitations as well as the fixation requirements of the fracture. Only then can fractures be successfully treated and complications minimized.

References

1. Bochlogyros PN: A retrospective study of 1,521 mandibular fractures. J Oral Maxillofac Surg 1985;43:597.
2. Chuong R, Donoff RB, Guralnick WC: A retrospective analysis of 327 mandibular fractures. J Oral Maxillofac Surg 1983;41:305.
3. James RB, Kent JN: Prospective study of mandibular fractures. J Oral Surg 1981;39:275.
4. Busuito MJ, Smith DJ, Robson MC: Mandibular fractures in an urban trauma center. J Trauma 1986;26:826.
5. Olson BA, Fonseca RJ, Zeitler DL, et al: Fractures of the mandible: A review of 580 cases. J Oral Maxillofac Surg 1982;40:23.
6. Melmed EP, Koonin AJ: Fractures of the mandible: A review of 909 cases. Plast Reconstr Surg 1975;56:323.
7. Passeri LA, Ellis E, Sinn DP: Complication of nonrigid fixation of mandibular angle fractures. J Oral Maxillofac Surg 1993;51:382.
8. Ellis E, Karas N: Treatment of mandibular angle fractures using two mini dynamic compression plates. J Oral Maxillofac Surg 1992;50:958.
9. Ellis E, Sinn DP: Treatment of mandibular angle fractures using two 2.4mm dynamic compression plates. J Oral Maxillofac Surg 1993;51:969.
10. James RB, Fredrickson C, Kent JN: Prospective study of mandibular fractures. J Oral Surg 1981;39:275.
11. Wagner WF, Neal DC, Alpert T: Morbidity associated with extraoral open reduction of mandibular fractures. J Oral Surg 1979;36:859.
12. Hemmings KW: Fracture of the cervical spine complicating bilateral fractures of the mandible: A case report. Br J Oral Maxillofac Surg 1985;23:279.
13. Goldwasser MS, Lorson EL, Tucker DF, et al: Internal carotid artery thrombosis associated with a fracture. J Oral Surg 1978;36:543.
14. Mohamed B: Hemiplegia following mandibular fracture. Br J Oral Surg 1980;18:77.
15. Leigh F, Garfield F, Rowe NL, et al: Primary care. *In* Rowe NL, Williams JL (eds): Maxillofacial Injuries, vol I. New York, Churchill Livingstone, 1985, p 55.
16. Stanley RB: Pathogenesis and evaluation of mandibular fractures. *In* Mathog RH (ed): Maxillofacial Trauma. Baltimore, Williams & Wilkins, 1984, p 138.
17. Evans TW: General management of acutely injured patients. *In* Alling CC, Osbon DB (eds): Maxillofacial Trauma. Philadelphia, Lea & Febiger, 1988, p 17.
18. Kruger E, Schilli W: General principles of treatment in maxillofacial injuries. *In* Kruger E, Schilli W (eds): Oral and Maxillofacial Traumatology, vol I. Chicago, Quintessence, 1982, p 95.
19. McIntosh GC, Steadman RK, Gross BD: Aspiration of an unerupted permanent tooth during maxillofacial trauma. J Oral Maxillofac Surg 1982;40:448.
20. Bartlett JG, Gorbach SL: The triple threat of aspiration pneumonia. Chest 1975;68:560.
21. Oliver AJ, Diaz EM, Helfrick JG: Air emphysema secondary to mandibular fracture: Report of a case. J Oral Maxillofac Surg 1993;51:1143.
22. Henry CH, Hills EC: Traumatic emphysema of the head, neck and mediastinum associated with maxillofacial trauma: Case report and review. J Oral Maxillofac Surg 1989;47:876.
23. Peatfield RC, Edwards PR, Johnson NM: Two unexpected deaths from pneumothorax. Lancet 1979;1:356.
24. Gibney RTN, Finnegan B, Fitzgerald MX, et al: Upper airway obstruction caused by massive subcutaneous emphysema. Intensive Care Med 1984;10:43.
25. Haberkamp TJ, Levine HL, O'Brien G: Pneumomediastinum secondary to a mandible fracture. Otolaryngol Head Neck Surg 1989;101:104.
26. Kellman R, Williams E: Maxillofacial Trauma. *In* Krespi YP, Ossoff RH (eds): Complications in Head and Neck Surgery. Philadelphia, WB Saunders, 1993, p 322.
27. Larsen OD, Nielsen A: Mandibular fractures: A follow-up study of 229 patients. Scand J Plast Reconstr Surg 1976;10:219.
28. Alling CC: Soft-tissue injuries. *In* Alling CC, Osbon DB (eds): Maxillofacial Trauma. Philadelphia, Lea & Febiger, 1988, p 141.
29. Davies PKB, Shaheen O: Soft tissue injuries of the face and scalp: Fractures of the larynx. *In* Rowe NL, Williams JL (eds): Maxillofacial Injuries, vol I. New York, Churchill Livingstone, 1985, p 184.
30. Sowray FH: Localized injuries of the teeth and alveolar process. *In* Rowe NL, Williams JL (eds): Maxillofacial Injuries, vol I. New York, Churchill Livingstone, 1985, p 220.
31. Lundin K, Ridell A, Sandberg N, et al: Complications after jaw fractures. Acta Otolaryngol 1973;75:362.
32. Kahnber KE, Ridell A: Prognosis of teeth involved in the line of mandibular fractures. Int J Oral Surg 1979;8:163.
33. Andreasen JO: Fractures of the alveolar process of the jaw. Scand J Dent Res 1970;78:263.
34. McGuirt WF, Salisbury PL: Mandibular fractures—their effect on growth and dentition. Arch Otolaryngol Head Neck Surg 1987;113:257.
35. Kamboozia AH, Punnia-Moorthy A: The fate of teeth in mandibular fracture lines. Int J Oral Maxillofac Surg 1993;22:97.

36. Roed-Petersen B, Andreasen JO: Prognosis of permanent teeth involved in jaw fractures. Scand J Dent Res 1970;78:343.
37. Steiner JF, Grau WH: Management and complications of dentoalveolar trauma. Oral Maxillofac Surg Clin North Am 1990;2:515.
38. Hovland EJ, Dumsha TC: Problems in the management of tooth resorption. *In* Gutamen JL (ed): Problem Solving in Endodontics, ed 2. St. Louis, Mosby Year Book, 1992, p 190.
39. Collins TA: Onlay bone grafting in combination with Branemark implants. Oral Maxillofac Surg Clin North Am 1991;3:893.
40. Andersson L, Hultin M, Nordenram A, et al: Jaw fractures in the county of Stockholm (1978–1980). Int J Oral Surg 1984;13:194.
41. Theriot BA, Van Sickels JE, Triplett RG, Nishioka GJ: Intraosseous wire fixation versus rigid osseous fixation of mandibular fractures: A preliminary report. J Oral Maxillofac Surg 1987;45:577.
42. Falender LG, Barbieri D, Leban SG: Gas-producing necrotizing fasciitis following mandibular fracture. J Oral Maxillofac Surg 1989;47:856.
43. Hought RT, Fitzgerald BE, Latta JE, et al: Ludwig's angina: Report of two cases and review of the literature from 1945 to January 1979. J Oral Surg 1980;38:849.
44. Zallen RD, Curry JT: A study of antibiotic usage in compound mandibular fractures. J Oral Surg 1975;33:431.
45. Chole RA, James Y: Antibiotic prophylaxis for facial fractures. Arch Otolaryngol Head Neck Surg 1987;113:1055.
46. Rowe NL, Killey HG: Fractures of the Facial Skeleton. ed 2. Edinburgh, Churchill Livingstone, 1968, p 180.
47. Lewis GK, Perutsea SC: The complex mandibular fracture. Am J Surg 1959;97:283.
48. Maloney PL, Welch TB, Koku C: Early immobilization of mandibular fractures: A retrospective study. J Oral Maxillofac Surg 1991;49:698.
49. Eschelman LT: Prophylactic antibiotics in otolaryngologic surgery: A double blind study. Trans Am Acad Ophthalmol Otolaryngol 1971;75:387.
50. Philps R: Die geschlossene und offene Unterkieferfraktur. Eine retrospective studie zum Krankenfut von, 1976–1982 [Med Dissertation]. Universitat Basel, 1987.
51. Zachariades N, Papademetriou I, Rallis G: Complications associated with rigid internal fixation of facial bone fractures. J Oral Maxillofac Surg 1993;51:275.
52. Souyris F, Lamrache JP, Mirfakhrai AM: Treatment of mandibular fractures by intraoral placement of bone plates. J Oral Surg 1980;38:33.
53. Paterson JA, Cardo VA, Stratigos GT: An examination of antibiotic prophylaxis in oral and maxillofacial surgery. J Oral Maxillofac Surg 1970;28:753.
54. Prein J, Schmoker R: Treatment of infected fractures and pseudarthrosis of the mandible. *In* Spiessl B (ed): New Concepts in Maxillofacial Bone Surgery. New York, Springer-Verlag, 1976, p 169.
55. Levy RA, Smith RW, Odland RW, et al: Monocortical miniplate fixation of mandibular angle fractures. Arch Otolaryngol Head Neck Surg 1991;117:149.
56. Iizuka T, Lindqvist C, Hallikainen D, Paukku P: Infection after rigid internal fixation of mandibular fractures: A clinical and radiologic study. J Oral Maxillofac Surg 1991;49:585.
57. Ellis E: Treatment of mandibular angle fractures using the AO reconstruction plate. J Oral Maxillofac Surg 1993;51:250.
58. Dodson TB, Perrott DH, Kaban LB, et al: Fixation of mandibular fractures: A comparative analysis of rigid internal fixation and standard fixation techniques. J Oral Maxillofac Surg 1990;48:362.
59. Ridell A, Astrand P: Conservative treatment of teeth involved by mandibular fractures. Swed Dent J 1971;64:623.
60. Chan DM, Demuth RJ, Miller SH, Jastak JT: Management of mandibular fractures in unreliable patient populations. Ann Plast Surg 1984;13:298.
61. Schilli W: Compression osteosynthesis. J Oral Surg 1977;35:802.
62. Friedrich B, Klaue P: Mechanical stability and post-traumatic osteitis: An experimental evaluation of the relation between infection of bone and internal fixation. Injury 1977;9:23.
63. Shetty V, Freymiller E: Teeth in the line of fracture: A review. J Oral Maxillofac Surg 1989;47:1303.
64. Spiessl B: Osteosynthese des unterkiefers. Manual der AO-Prinzipien. New York, Springer-Verlag, 1988, p 199.
65. Schneider SS, Stern M: Teeth in the line of mandibular fractures. J Oral Surg 1971;29:107.
66. Neal DC, Wagner WF, Alpert B: Morbidity associated with teeth in line of mandibular fractures. J Oral Surg 1978;36:859.
67. Marker P, Eckerdal A, Smith-Sivertsen C: Incompletely erupted third molars in the line of mandibular fractures. Oral Surg Oral Med Oral Pathol 1994;78:425.
68. Rink B, Stoehr K: Weisheitszahne im Brucspalt. Stomatol DDR 1978;28:307.
69. Rubin MM, Koll TJ, Sadoff RS: Morbidity associated with incompletely erupted third molars in the line of mandibular fractures. J Oral Maxillofac Surg 1990;48:1045.
70. Koury M, Ellis E: Rigid internal fixation for the treatment of infected mandibular fractures. J Oral Maxillofac Surg 1992; 50:434.
71. Kellman RM: Repair of mandibular fractures via compression plating and more traditional techniques: A comparison of results. Laryngoscope 1984;94:1560.
72. Hoffman WY, Barton RM, Price M, Mathes SJ: Rigid internal fixation versus traditional techniques for the treatment of mandible fractures. J Trauma 1990;30:1032.
73. Luhr HG: Compression plate osteosynthesis through the Luhr system. *In* Kruger E, Schilli W (eds): Oral and Maxillofacial Traumatology. Chicago, Quintessence, 1982, p 319.
74. Ellis E, Ghali G: Lag screw fixation of mandibular angle fractures. J Oral Maxillofac Surg 1991;49:234.
75. Schwimmer A: Discussion: Treatment of mandibular angle fractures using the AO reconstruction plate. J Oral Maxillofac Surg 1993;49:255.
76. Champy M, Lodde JP, Schmitt R, et al: Mandibular osteosynthesis by miniature screwed plates via a buccal approach. J Maxillofac Surg 1978;6:14.
77. Topazian RG: Osteomyelitis of the jaws. *In* Topazian RG, Golberg MH (eds): Oral and Maxillofacial Infections, ed 2. Philadelphia, WB Saunders, 1987, p 211.
78. Johansson B, Krekmanov L, Thomsson M: Miniplate osteosynthesis of infected mandibular fractures. J Craniomaxillofac Surg 1988;16:22.
79. Beckers HL: Treatment of initially infected mandibular fractures with bone plates. J Oral Surg 1979;37:310.
80. Rittmann WW, Perren SM: Cortical Bone Healing after Internal Fixation and Infection. New York, Springer-Verlag, 1974.
81. Fischer-Brandies E, Dielert E: The infected mandibular fracture. Arch Orthop Trauma Surg 1984;103:337.
82. Buchbinder D, Weber W: Discussion: Rigid internal fixation for the treatment of infected mandibular fractures. J Oral Maxillofac Surg 1992;50:443.
83. Spiessl B: Internal Fixation of the Mandible: A Manual of AO:ASIF Principles. New York, Springer-Verlag, 1989, p 245.
84. Giordano AM, Foster CA, Boies LR, Maisel RH: Chronic osteomyelitis following mandibular fractures and its treatment. Arch Otolaryngol 1982;108:30.
85. Shakenovsky BN, Ripamonti U, Lownie JF: Chronic osteomyelitis of the jaws. Int J Oral Maxillofac Surg 1986;15:352.
86. Mathog RH, Boises LR: Nonunion of the mandible. Laryngoscope 1976;86:908.
87. Daramola JO, Ajagbe HA: Chronic osteomyelitis of the mandible in adults: A clinical study of 34 cases. Br J Oral Surg 1982;20:58.
88. Wannfors K, Hammarstrom L: Infectious foci in chronic osteomyelitis of the jaws. Int J Oral Surg 1985;14:493.
89. Koury ME, Perrott DH, Kaban LB: The use of rigid internal fixation in mandibular fractures complicated by osteomyelitis. J Oral Maxillofac Surg 1994;52:1114.
90. Al-Sheikh W, Sfakianakis GN, Mnaymneh W, et al: Subacute and chronic bone infections: Diagnosis using In^{111}, Ga^{67} and TC^{99m} MDP bone scintigraphy and radiography. Radiology 1985;155:501.
91. Schauwecker DS: Osteomyelitis: Diagnosis with In^{111} labeled leukocytes. Radiology 1989;171:141.
92. Khosla VM: Current concepts in the treatment of acute and chronic osteomyelitis: Review and report of four cases. J Oral Surg 1970;28:210.
93. Obwegeser HL: Simultaneous resection and reconstruction of parts of the mandible via the intraoral route in patients with and without gross infection. Oral Surg 1966;21:693.

94. Obwegeser HL, Sailer HF: Experiences with intra-oral partial resection and simultaneous reconstruction in cases of mandibular osteomyelitis. J Oral Maxillofac Surg 1978;6:34.
95. Ludwig Von H, Haneke A: Ein neues Verfahren in der Behandlung der Osteomyelitis. Dtsch Z Mund Kiefer-Gesichts-Chir 1978;2:190,192.
96. Grime PD, Bowerman JE, Weller PJ: Gentamicin impregnated polymethylmethacrylate beads in the treatment of primary chronic osteomyelitis of the mandible. Br J Oral Maxillofac Surg 1990;28:367.
97. Chisholm BB, Lew D, Sadasivan K: The use of tobramycin impregnated polymethylmethacrylate beads in the treatment of osteomyelitis of the mandible. J Oral Maxillofac Surg 1993;51:444.
98. Alpert B, Colosi T, Von Fraunhofer JA, Seligson D: The in vivo behavior of gentamicin-PMMA beads in the maxillofacial region. J Oral Maxillofac Surg 1989;47:46.
99. Alpert B, Seligson D: Discussion: The use of tobramycin impregnated polymethylmethacrylate beads in the treatment of osteomyelitis of the mandible. J Oral Maxillofac Surg 1993;51:449.
100. Levin P: The effectiveness of various antibiotics in methylmethacrylate. J Bone Joint Surg Br 1975;57:234.
101. Picknell B, Mizen L, Sutherland R: Antibacterial activity of antibiotics in acrylic bone cement. J Bone Joint Surg Br 1977; 59:302.
102. Hoff S, Fitzgerald R, Kelly P: The depot administration of penicillin G and gentamicin in acrylic bone cement. J Bone Joint Surg Am 1981;63:798.
103. Hill J, Klenerman L, Trustey S, et al: Diffusion of antibiotics from acrylic bone-cement in vitro. J Bone Joint Surg Br 1977;59:197.
104. Mathog RH: Nonunion of the mandible. Otolaryngol Clin North Am 1983;16:533.
105. Leopard P: Complications. *In* Rowe NL, Williams JL (eds): Maxillofacial Injuries, vol II. New York, Churchill Livingstone, 1985, p 730.
106. Bruce RA, Strachan DS: Fractures of the edentulous mandible: The Chalmers J. Lyons Academy study. J Oral Surg 1976;34:973.
107. Bradley JC: A radiological investigation into the age changes of the inferior dental artery. Br J Oral Surg 1975;13:82.
108. Evans AJ, Burwell RG, Merville L, et al: Residual deformities. *In* Rowe NL, Williams JL (eds): Maxillofacial Injuries, vol II. New York, Churchill Livingstone, 1985, p 843.
109. Boyne PJ, Zarem H: Osseous reconstruction of the resected mandible. Am J Surg 1976;132:49.
110. Assael LA: Mandibular reconstruction using cortical bone grafts packed with cancellous marrow and a reconstruction plate. Oral Maxillofacial Surg Clin North Am 1991;3:223.
111. Marx RE: Philosophy and particulars of autogenous bone grafting. Oral Maxillofac Surg Clin North Am 1993;5:599.
112. Schwimmer A: Discussion: Treatment of mandibular angle fractures using the AO reconstruction plate. J Oral Maxillofac Surg 1991;51:255.
113. Reuther JF, Meier JL: Microvascular surgical tissue transfer for reconstruction in the head and neck area. Oral Maxillofac Clin North Am 1993;5:687.
114. Macintosh RB: Malunion and malocclusion in mandibular fractures. *In* Mathog RH (ed): Maxillofacial Trauma. Baltimore, Williams & Wilkins, 1984, p 186.
115. Ellis E, Tharanon W: Facial width problems associated with rigid fixation of mandibular fractures: Case reports. J Oral Maxillofac Surg 1992;50:87.
116. Merrill RG: Decompression for inferior alveolar nerve injury. J Oral Surg 1964;22:291.
117. Kruger E: Conservative therapy. *In* Kruger E, Schilli W (eds): Oral and Maxillofacial Traumatology. vol I. Chicago, Quintessence, 1982, p 273.
118. Iizuka T, Lindqvist C: Sensory disturbances associated with rigid internal fixation of mandibular fractures. J Oral Maxillofac Surg 1991;49:1264.
119. Seddon HJ: Nerve lesions complicating certain closed bone injuries. JAMA 1947;135:691.
120. Campbell RL, Shamaskin RG, Harkins SW: Assessment of recovery from injury to inferior alveolar and mental nerves. Oral Surg 1987;64:519.
121. Zaytown HS, Philips C, Terry BC: Long term neurosensory deficits following transoral vertical ramus and sagittal split osteotomies for mandibular prognathism. J Oral Maxillofac Surg 1986;44:193.
122. Tu HK, Tenhulzen D: Compression osteosynthesis of mandibular fractures. J Oral Maxillofacial Surg 1985;43:585.
123. Lindqvist C, Kontio R, Pihakari A, et al: Rigid internal fixation of mandibular fractures. Int J Oral Maxillofac Surg 1986;15:657.
124. Ardary WC: Prospective clinical evaluation of the use of compression plates and screws in the management of mandible fractures. J Oral Maxillofac Surg 1989;47:1150.
125. Raveh J, Vuillemin T, Ladradch K, et al: Plate osteosynthesis of 367 mandibular fractures: The unrestricted indications for the intraoral approach. J Craniomaxillofac Surg 1987;15:244.
126. Meyer RA: Applications of microneurosurgery to the repair of trigeminal nerve injuries. Oral Maxillofac Surg Clin North Am 1992;4:405.
127. Allen FG, Young AH: Lateral displacement of the intact mandibular condyle. Br J Oral Surg 1969;7:24.
128. Weinberg S, Kryshtalskyj B: Facial nerve function following temporomandibular joint surgery using the preauricular approach. J Oral Maxillofac Surg 1992;50:1048.
129. Ellis E, Dean J: Rigid fixation of mandibular condyle fractures. Oral Surg 1993;76:6.
130. Raveh J, Ladrach K, Vuillemin T, et al: Indications for open reduction of dislocated, fractured condylar process: Evaluation and management of conservatively treated cases. *In* Worthington P, Evans JR (eds): Controversies in Oral and Maxillofacial Surgery. Philadelphia, WB Saunders, 1994, p 173.
131. Goin KW: Facial nerve paralysis secondary to mandibular fracture. Laryngoscope 1980;90:1777.
132. Adkins WY, Osguthorpe JD: Management of trauma of the facial nerve. Otolaryngol Clin North Am 1991;24:587.
133. Gullane PJ, Cheng K: Extratemporal facial reanimation. *In* Paparella MM, Shumrick DA, Gluckman JL, et al (eds): Otolaryngology, ed 3, vol IV. Philadelphia, WB Saunders, 1991, p 2849.
134. Hausamen JE, Neukam FW: Autogenous microneurosurgery in the oral and maxillofacial region. Oral Maxillofac Surg Clin North Am 1993;5:613.
135. Laskin JL: Parotid fistula after the use of external pin fixation: Report of case. J Oral Surg 1978;36:621.
136. Schule H: Injuries of the temporomandibular joint. *In* Kruger E, Schilli W (eds): Oral and Maxillofacial Traumatology, vol II. Chicago, Quintessence, 1986, p 48.
137. Goss AN, Bosanquet AG: The arthroscopic appearance of acute temporomandibular joint trauma. J Oral Maxillofac Surg 1990;48:780.
138. Kent JN, Neary JP, Silvia C, et al: Open reduction of fractured mandibular condyles. Oral Maxillofac Surg Clin North Am 1990;2:69.
139. Alling CC: Mandibular fractures. *In* Alling CC, Osbon DB: Maxillofacial Trauma. Philadelphia, Lea & Febiger, 1988, p 283.
140. Amaratunga NA: Mouth opening after release of maxillomandibular fixation in fracture patients. J Oral Maxillofac Surg 1987;45:383.
141. Walker RV: Discussion: Open reduction of condylar fractures of the mandible in conjunction with repair of discal injury. J Oral Maxillofac Surg 1988;46:262.
142. Nwoku AL: Rehabilitating children with temporomandibular joint ankylosis. Int J Oral Surg 1979;8:271.
143. Choung R, Piper MA: Open reduction of condylar fractures of the mandible in conjunction with repair of discal injury. J Oral Maxillofac Surg 1988;46:257.
144. Thomson HG, Garmer AW, Lindsay WK: Condylar neck fractures of the mandible in children. Plast Reconstr Surg 1964;34:452.
145. Bradley P: Injuries of the condylar and coronoid process. *In* Rowe NL, Williams JL (eds): Maxillofacial Injuries, vol II. New York, Churchill Livingstone, 1985, p 338.
146. Iizuka T, Lindqvist C, Hallikainen D, et al: Severe bone resorption and osteoarthrosis after miniplate fixation of high condylar fractures. Oral Surg 1991;72:400.
147. Blevins C, Gores RJ: Fractures of the mandibular condyloid process: Results of conservative treatment in 140 patients. J Oral Surg 1961;19:392.

148. Levant BA: Mental anesthesia and its prognosis. Br J Oral Surg 1967;4:206.
149. MacLennan WD: Consideration of 180 cases of typical fractures of the mandibular condylar process. Br J Plast Surg 1952;5:122.
150. Members of the Chalmers J Lyons Club: Fractures involving the mandibular condyle: A post treatment survey of 120 cases. J Oral Surg 1947;5:45.
151. Kromer H: Closed and open reduction of condylar fractures. Dent Record 1953;73:569.
152. Takenoshita Y, Ishibaski H, Oka M: Comparison of functional recovery after nonsurgical and surgical treatment of condylar fractures. J Oral Maxillofac Surg 1990;48:1191.
153. Worsaae N, Thorn JJ: Surgical versus nonsurgical treatment of unilateral dislocated low subcondylar fractures: A clinical study of 52 cases. J Oral Maxillofac Surg 1994;52:353.
154. Allison N, Brooks B: Ankylosis: An experimental study. Surg Gynecol Obstet 1914;19:568.
155. Henderson MS: Ankylosis of the jaw. Surg Gynecol Obstet 1918;27:451.
156. Kazanjian VH: Ankylosis of the temporomandibular joint. Surg Gynecol Obstet 1938;67:333.
157. Amaratunga NA: Mandibular fractures in children—a study of clinical aspects, treatment needs, and complications. J Oral Maxillofac Surg 1988;46:637.
158. Posnick JC, Wells M, Pron GE: Pediatric facial fractures: Evolving patterns of treatment. J Oral Maxillofac Surg 1993;51:836.
159. Laskin DM: Role of the meniscus in the etiology of post-traumatic temporomandibular joint ankylosis. Int J Oral Surg 1978;7:340.
160. Topazian RG: Etiology of ankylosis of temporomandibular joint: Analysis of 44 cases. J Oral Surg 1964;22:227.
161. Pepper L, Zide MF: Mandibular condyle fracture and dislocation into the middle cranial fossa. Int J Oral Surg 1985;14:278.
162. Rowe NL: Fractures of the jaws in children. J Oral Surg 1969;27:497.
163. Waite DE: Pediatric fractures of jaw and facial bones. Pediatrics 1973;51:551.
164. Adekeye EO: Pediatric fractures of the facial skeleton. J Oral Surg 1980;38:355.
165. Hoaglund FT: Experimental hemarthrosis. J Bone Joint Surg Am 1967;49: 285.
166. Wheat PM, Evaskus DS, Laskin DM: Effects of temporomandibular joint meniscectomy in adult and juvenile primates. J Dent Res 1977;58:39.
167. Politis C, Fossion E, Bossuyt M: The use of costochondral grafts in arthroplasty of the temporomandibular joint. J Craniomaxillofac Surg 1987;15:345.
168. Gray RL: Coronocondylar ankylosis in childhood due to infection. Br J Oral Surg 1969;7:40.
169. Straith CL, Lewis JR: Ankylosis of the temporo-mandibular joint. Plast Reconstr Surg 1948;3:464.
170. Walker RV: Arthroplasty of the ankylosed temporomandibular joint. Trans Cong Int Assoc Oral Surg 1973;4:279.
171. Topazian RG: Comparison of gap and interposition arthroplasty in the treatment of temporomandibular joint ankylosis. J Oral Surg 1966;24:405.
172. Bowerman J: Reconstruction of the temporomandibular joint for acquired deformity and congenital malformation. Br J Oral Maxillofac Surg 1987;25:149.
173. Dingman RO, Grabb WC: Reconstruction of both mandibular condyles with metatarsal bone grafts. Plast Reconstr Surg 1964;34:441.
174. Lindahl L: Condylar fractures of the mandible. Int J Oral Surg 1977;6:166.
175. MacIntosh RB, Henny FA: A spectrum of application of autogenous costochondral grafts. J Maxillofac Surg 1977;5:257.
176. Lindahl L, Hollender L: Condylar fractures of the mandible. Int J Oral Surg 1977;6:153.
177. Rowe NL: Ankylosis of the temporomandibular joint. J Coll Surg Edinb 1982;27:209.
178. MacIntosh RB: Current spectrum of costochondral and dermal grafting. *In* Bell WH (ed): Modern Practice in Orthognathic and Reconstructive Surgery, vol II. Philadelphia, WB Saunders, 1992, p 894.
179. Poswillo DE: Biological reconstruction of the mandibular condyle. Br J Oral Maxillofac Surg 1987;25:100.
180. Lindqvist C, Pihakari A, Tasanen A, Goran H: Autogenous costochondral grafts in temporomandibular joint arthroplasty. J Maxillofac Surg 1986;14:143.
181. Ware WH, Brown SL: Growth center transplantation to replace mandibular condyles. J Maxillofac Surg 1981;9:50.
182. Ware WH, Taylor RC: Growth center transplantation to replace damaged mandibular condyles. J Am Dent Assoc 1966;73:128.
183. Kennett S: Temporomandibular joint ankylosis: The rationale for grafting in the young patient. J Oral Surg 1973;31:744.
184. Lindqvist C, Jokinen J, Paukku P, Tasanen A: Adaptation of autogenous costochondral grafts used for temporomandibular joint reconstruction. J Oral Maxillofac Surg 1988;46:465.
185. Sarnat RG, Engel MB: A serial study of mandibular growth after removal of the condyle in the macaca rhesus monkey. Plast Reconstr Surg 1951;7:364.
186. Dingman RO: Ankylosis of the temporomandibular joint. *In* Mathog RH (ed): Maxillofacial Trauma. Baltimore, Williams & Wilkins, 1984, p 212.
187. Figueroa AA, Gans BJ, Pruzansky S: Long term follow up of a mandibular costochondral graft. Oral Surg 1984;58:257.
188. Proffit WR, Vig KWL, Turvey TA: Early fracture of the mandibular condyles: Frequently an unsuspected cause of growth disturbances. Am J Orthod 1980;78:1.
189. Lund K: Mandibular growth and remodeling processes after condylar fracture. Acta Odontol Scand 1974;32:suppl 64.
190. Engel MB, Brodie AG: Condylar growth and mandibular deformities. Surgery 1947;22:976.
191. Sarnat BG: Facial and neurocranial growth after removal of the mandibular condyle in the macaca rhesus monkey. Am J Surg 1957;94:19.
192. Beekler DM, Walker RV: Condyle fractures. J Oral Surg 1969;27:563.
193. Meikle MC: In vivo transplantation of the mandibular joint of the rat: An autoradiographic investigation into cellular changes at the condyle. Arch Oral Biol 1973;18:1011.
194. Poswillo D: Experimental reconstruction of the mandibular joint. Int J Oral Surg 1974;3:400.
195. Anderson, MF, Alling CC: Subcondylar fractures in young dogs. Oral Surg 1965;19:263.
196. Ramba J: Fractures of facial bones in children. Int J Oral Surg 1985;14:472.
197. Coccaro PJ: Restitution of mandibular form after condylar injury in infancy. Am J Orthod 1969;55:33.
198. Walker DG: Mandibular condyle: 50 cases demonstrating arrest in development. Dent Pract 1957;7:160.
199. Peskin S, Laskin DM: Contribution of autogenous condylar grafts to mandibular growth. Oral Surg 1965;20:517.
200. Walker RV: Traumatic mandibular condylar fracture dislocations. Am J Surg 1960;100:850.
201. Poswillo DE: The late effects of mandibular condylectomy. Oral Surg 1972;33:500.
202. Collins DA, Becks H, Simpson ME: Growth and transformation of the mandibular joint in the rat. Am J Orthodontics 1946;32:443.
203. Moss ML, Salentijn L: The compensatory role of the condylar cartilage in mandibular growth: Theoretical and clinical implications. Dtsch. Zahn Mund Kieferheilkd Zentralbl 1971;56:5.
204. Broadbent HB: A new x-ray technique and its application to orthodontics. Angle Orthodontist 1931;1:45.
205. Hotz RP: Functional jaw orthopedics in the treatment of condylar fractures. Am J Orthod 1978;73:365.
206. Burket LW: Congenital bony temporomandibular ankylosis and facial hemiatrophy. JAMA 1936;106:1719.
207. Sailer HF: Experiences with intra-oral partial resection and simultaneous reconstruction of the mandible in pre-operatively noninfected cases. J Maxillofac Surg 1974;2:173.

Chapter 10
COMPLICATIONS IN THE TREATMENT OF MIDFACE FRACTURES

by

Richard H. Haug
Jon P. Bradrick
Jackson P. Morgan III

Introduction

Complications have been recognized as realistic sequelae of midface trauma surgery.[1, 2] Although their occurrence is disappointing to both patient and surgeon, the recognition, evaluation, and open discussion of these problems are the only means by which clinicians can hope to prevent or to avoid them. The purpose of this chapter is to describe the most common and morbid complications associated with the treatment of midface fractures and the ways to avoid them intraoperatively. Comorbid injury and lifesaving measures associated with midface trauma are the subjects of other texts.[3, 4]

THE SUBJECTS DISCUSSED IN THIS CHAPTER ARE:

- Evaluation
- Nasal fractures
  - Septal deviation, synechiae, and hematoma
- Naso-orbital-ethmoidal injuries
  - Telecanthus
  - Saddle defects
  - Enophthalmos and proptosis
  - Dacryocystitis and epiphora
- Ocular injuries
  - Blindness
  - Corneal abrasion
  - Ruptured globe
  - Retinal detachment
  - Lens dislocation
- Maxillary fractures
  - Malocclusion
  - Maxillary sinusitis
- Zygomatic fractures
- Frontal sinus and frontal bone fractures
  - Frontal sinusitis
- Panfacial fractures
  - Anesthesia and paresthesia
  - Contour deformity
  - Nonunion
  - Unsightly scars
  - Wound infection and foreign body reaction
- Concomitant injuries in midface fractures
  - Cerebrospinal fluid leak
  - Intracranial injury
  - Anosmia
  - Psychiatric effect of trauma
- Chronic pain
- Avulsed tissues
  - Teeth
  - Bone
  - Soft tissues

Evaluation

Although some postoperative problems may not be prevented, such as blindness caused by co-injury or tissue loss due to avulsion, the vast majority can be avoided or minimized by performing a good history and clinical examination, conducting a thorough imaging evaluation (Fig. 10–1), and providing an all-inclusive treatment plan.

Assessing the nature of the injury can yield important clinical information. High-energy impacts tend to cause more comminution, whereas low-energy impacts tend to yield simple single fractures, thus requiring different treatment modalities. A thorough "hands-on" clinical examination supported by a complete imaging survey provides the precise diagnosis required to formulate an appropriate treatment plan. The treatment plan should include techniques designed to minimize and address problems if they occur.

Tables 10–1 to 10–5 list the most common complications of midface fractures. Most of these complications, including their prevention and treatment, are discussed in this chapter, but several complications listed in the tables are discussed elsewhere in this book. A discussion of the management of late postoperative sequelae of facial injuries appears in Chapter 20.

Nasal Fractures

Because of its prominence on the face and its central location, the nose is one of the most commonly fractured bones of the body, but reports of the complications of nasal fracture treatment appear infrequently in the surgical literature. The most often reported problems are imperfect postoperative contours, ranging in incidence from 20% to 80% of all open or closed treatments (Table 10–1).[5–8] These are usually associated with insufficient reduction of the nasal septum and resultant septal deviation.[5–8] Respiratory obstruction, when a complaint, is also related to septal deviation or the development of synechiae between the septum and concha.

Table 10–1. Complications Associated with Nasal Fractures

Contour irregularities
Septal deviation
Difficulty breathing
Septal hematoma
Synechiae

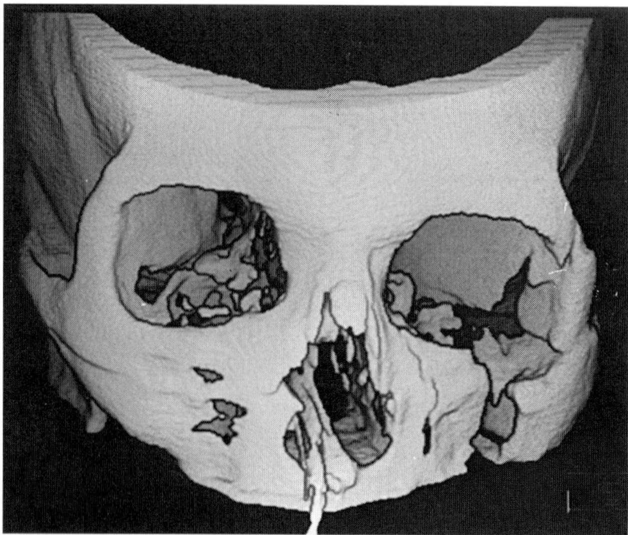

Figure 10–1. Three-dimensional reconstructions of computed tomographic scans aid in the diagnosis and total appreciation of fracture geometry.

Septal Deviation, Synechiae, and Hematoma

The vast majority of postoperative problems associated with the treatment of nasal fractures involve the septum.[5–9] These are usually due to a failure to diagnose the problem on clinical examination. Good lighting and a long speculum help to ensure the identification of septal deviation (Fig. 10–2) and hematoma.

Hematomas should be incised and drained; otherwise, they may become infected and cause a perforation of the septum. Treatment is accomplished with the local or topical administration of an anesthetic agent followed by incision of the hematoma parallel to the floor of the nose. The hematoma is then evacuated, and anterior nasal packing is utilized to decompress the space and achieve hemostasis. The use of appropriate prophylactic antibiotics is encouraged.

When a deviated septum is visualized preoperatively, adequate reduction and stabilization will ensure good contour. Asch forceps should be utilized to lift the fractured nasal bones up and out. A Goldman elevator or Walsham forceps may then be used to refine the contours of the nasal bones. The Asch forceps is then used to straighten or morselize the nasal septum

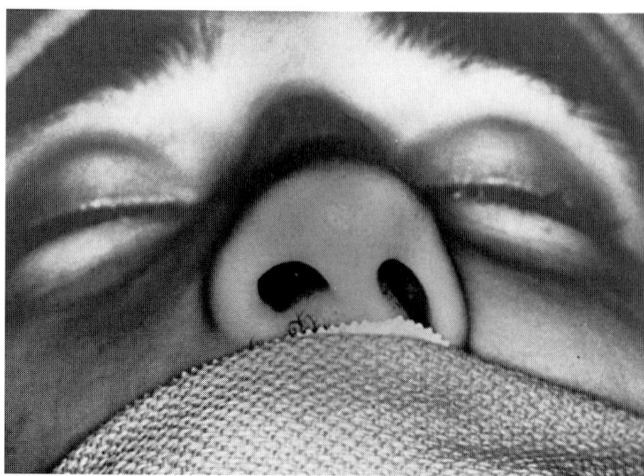

Figure 10–2. Septal deviation from an inadequately diagnosed and treated fracture.

from posterior to anterior, and from superior to inferior. The nose should be packed in layers from posterior to anterior and superior to inferior with bacitracin-impregnated gauze. The packing should remain in place for 2 to 5 days.

Synechiae are unions or adhesions of the mucosa of the septum to the nasal concha caused by improper reduction of the nasal septum. They may be treated by a simple release with scissors under local anesthesia followed by nasal packing. If this measure fails, an intranasal incision and submucosal resection of the septum are required.

Naso-orbital-ethmoidal Injuries

Lying immediately posterior to the nasal bones are the naso-orbital-ethmoidal structures. With high-energy impacts to the nose, these structures are invariably injured. The thin and complicated osseous anatomy make this region difficult to repair. Telecanthus and saddle defects of the nasal bridge are the most commonly reported sequelae of naso-orbital-ethmoidal injury (Table 10–2).[10–12] Included with contour irregularities are septal deviations. Unsightly scars may occur as comorbid events. Failure to properly treat the medial orbital wall and floor will result in enophthalmos and diplopia.[10] Despite the complexity of the nasolacrimal apparatus, it becomes obstructed in less than 18% of naso-orbital-ethmoidal injuries.[10, 13] Because of the thin nature of the skin overlying these structures, visible or palpable hardware is occasionally a problem. Less common postoperative complications are frontal sinusitis and cerebrospinal fluid leaks. Uncommon ocular injuries, which may occur during periorbital surgery, include blindness, corneal abrasions, ruptured globes, retinal detachment, and lens dislocations.[14]

The presence of retinal detachment or globe injury is a contraindication to the manipulation of the midfacial bones, in the opinion of some ophthalmologists.[15] In such cases, immediate intervention by closed technique is preferred, with consideration of secondary reconstruction of the facial bones. Blindness is not a contraindication for midfacial repair. It is extremely important to reconstruct the orbital osseous structures in anticipation of a prosthetic reconstruction.

Table 10–2. Complications Associated with Naso-orbital-ethmoidal Fractures

Saddle defect
Telecanthus
Septal deviation
Unsightly scars
Enophthalmos
Diplopia
Nasolacrimal obstruction
Visible or palpable hardware
Cerebrospinal fluid leak
Sinusitis
Ocular injury

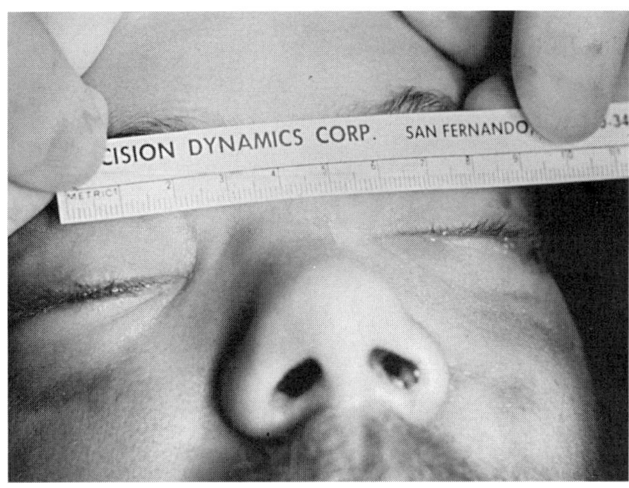

Figure 10–3. Traumatic telecanthus.

Telecanthus

The intercanthal distance in males is 31.7 (±2.8) mm and in females 30.8 (±2.2).[16] When a naso-orbital-ethmoidal fracture occurs, the canthal ligaments and osseous structures frequently become displaced, resulting in traumatic telecanthus or widening beyond the acceptable values (Fig. 10–3). Although minimally invasive, closed reduction of these injuries cannot adequately address this problem. Open reduction with internal fixation is the only method to ensure proper treatment. Gull-wing and bitemporal incisions are the best incisions to gain access to these structures. After appropriate exposure, the type of naso-orbital-ethmoidal injury should be assessed.[10] The osseous structures should be initially reapproximated. A wire placed posterior to the canthal ligaments may be necessary to ensure proper alignment.[10] The fracture can then be stabilized with an assortment of titanium microplates (Fig. 10–4*A*). The postoperative inner intercanthal distance should be verified by measurement prior to closure of the incisions.[16]

Saddle Defects

Gross fragmentation and displacement of the naso-orbital-ethmoid region commonly results in osseous structures that are irretrievable, unidentifiable, or too small to reconstruct. Failure to provide anatomic form to this area invariably results in a saddle defect of the nose, because of absence of contour of the dorsal region. Under these circumstances, augmentation grafting with a cantilevered cranial bone graft and lag screw fixation provide reasonable postoperative aesthetic results.[17]

Through a bitemporal flap, the void in the dorsum of the naso-orbital-ethmoid region may be visualized. An outer table calvarial bone graft should be harvested according to the technique described by Markowitz and Allan.[18] The graft should then be contoured to fit intimately with the stable osseous structures of the

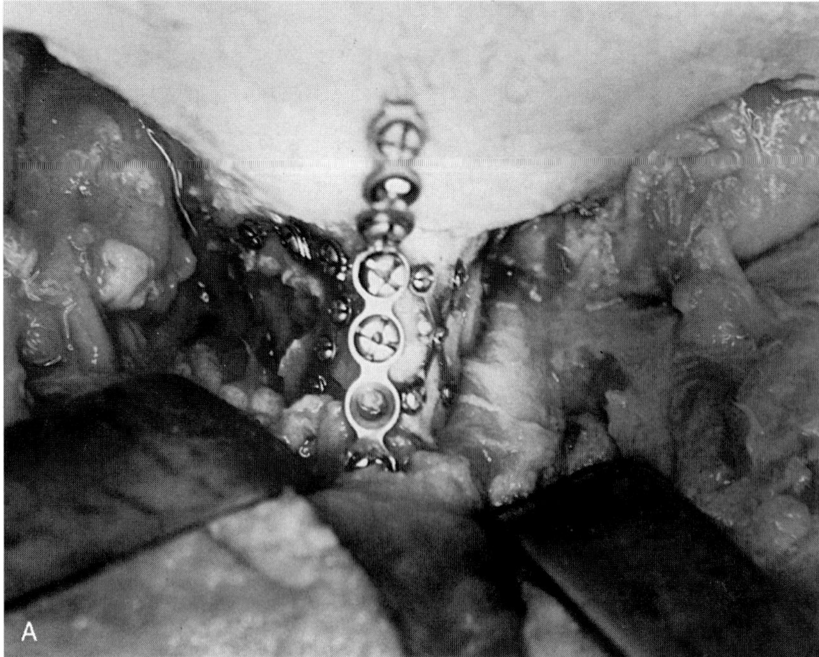

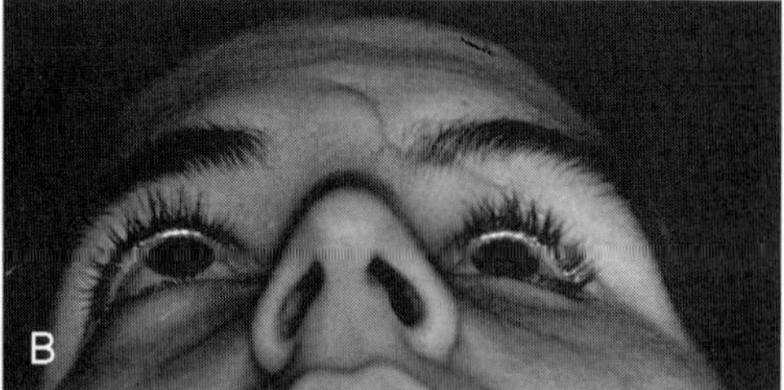

Figure 10–4. *A*, Successful repair of the nasal-orbital-ethmoidal region with titanium microplates. *B*, Postoperative enophthalmos in a patient whose orbital floor fracture was inadequately treated.

frontal bone and then continued to the lateral crura to ensure coverage of the nasal septum. The graft should then be fixated with 1.3-mm lag screws.[19] Symmetry, projection, and contour should be reassessed prior to closure.

Enophthalmos and Proptosis

Postoperative enophthalmos and proptosis (occasionally with associated diplopia) are known complications associated with orbital, zygomatic, and naso-orbital-ethmoid fractures (Fig. 10–4*B*). Computed tomographic scanning with coronal or sagittal sections is invaluable in assessing the status of both the hard and soft tissues of the orbit (Fig. 10–5). This assessment should complement the performance of a good clinical examination. If an orbital wall or floor defect is suspected, it should be explored and examined via an open approach. If a defect is noted, it must be repaired. Cranial bone, Medpore (Porex Medical, Fairburn, GA), Supramid (S. Jackson Inc, Alexandria, VA), and titanium mesh are satisfactory materials for use in the reconstruction of these defects. They can be easily affixed via the use of microscrews. After reconstruction of the defect, a forced duction test should be performed to assure that the inferior rectus, inferior oblique, and medial rectus muscles are not entrapped. After this test, and before swelling and edema ensue, the proper anterior-posterior position of the globe should be assessed (Fig. 10–6).

Immediate postoperative proptosis may be the result of a retrobulbar hematoma, diminished orbital volume due to an inadequately reduced fracture, or reconstruction of the orbital floor with too thick an implant. A clinical assessment reveals flattening on the affected side or asymmetry if the fracture was improperly reduced. If a retrobulbar hematoma is present, tense proptosis, pupillary dilatation, swelling, ophthalmoplegia, and pain are noted. An unattended, retrobulbar hematoma can lead to retinal artery obstruction or optic nerve compression and blindness.[20–22] A lateral canthotomy is a simple procedure to relieve the intraorbital pressure. It is performed by placing one blade of a sharp scissors into the conjunctiva lateral to the globe at the junction of the upper and lower lid and the other blade through the skin medial to the orbital rim. The blades are then closed, the tissues incised, and the blades then advanced, opened, and removed. The or-

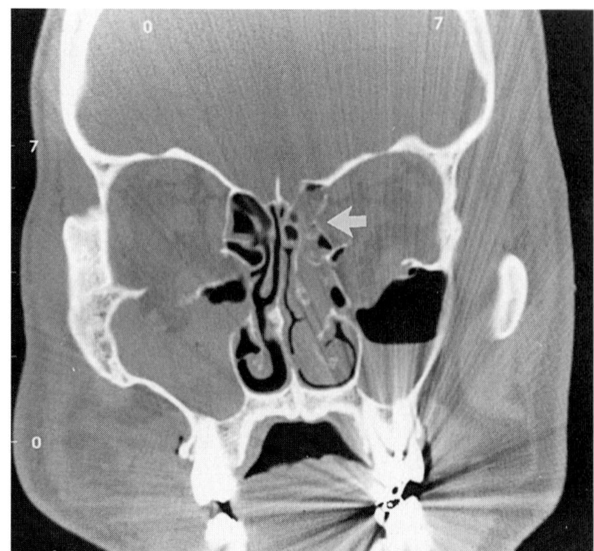

Figure 10–5. Coronal section of a computed tomographic image revealing bilateral orbital floor fractures with orbital contents herniated into the antra. Note the displaced left medial wall fracture *(arrow)*.

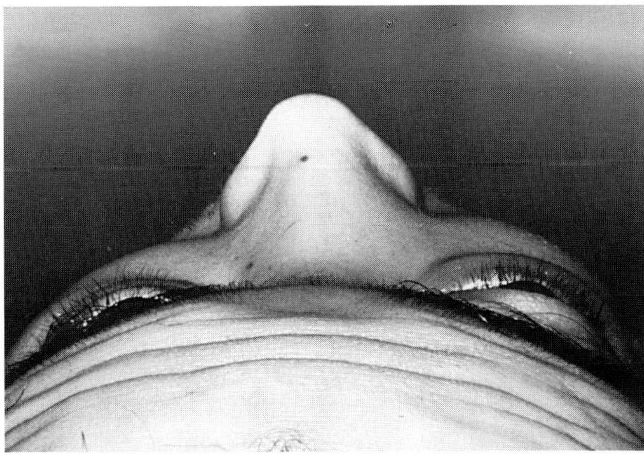

Figure 10–6. The proper antero-posterior position of the globe is best assessed with the lids retracted and the lenses visualized from above. The malar prominences may also be assessed in this manner.

bital septum must be perforated in order to gain access to the hematoma, which can then be evacuated.

Dacryocystitis and Epiphora

Injuries to the nasolacrimal system may occur in naso-orbital-ethmoidal injuries. When present, nasolacrimal injuries are most commonly accompanied by traumatic telecanthus.[23] The best method of preventing this type of complication is the open reduction, exploration, and careful fixation of the naso-orbital-ethmoidal fracture at the time of the primary repair. Assessment of the nasolacrimal system at the time of repair is difficult and should be avoided unless obvious laceration or injury is identified. The surgeon should resist the temptation to intubate the nasolacrimal duct with canalicular intubation tubes, because their subsequent fixation may render the tubes irretrievable.

If epiphora does occur, and it appears to be associated with scar contracture or lid laxity, improvement can usually be gained with lower lid massage. If the condition does not improve, a dacryocystorhinostomy should be performed after documentation of the obstruction by dacryocystography. If dacryocystitis is present along with the obstruction, it should first be treated with a 7 day course of antibiotics and a 4 week delay of surgical intervention.[23]

The dacryocystorhinostomy is performed by creating a subciliary skin incision adjacent to the puncta. Incising the orbicularis muscle should be avoided. Entry through the lacrimal fossae into the nose should be accomplished with rotary instrumentation in order to trephine through the bone, thereby preserving the nasal mucosa. The mucosa can then be incised and sutured to the remnants of the lacrimal sac. Canalicular intubation tubes should be placed for a period of 6 to 12 weeks in order to ensure patency (Fig. 10–7). The tubes should be sutured to the nasal mucosa to achieve proper position during healing.

Ocular Injuries

Uncommon ocular injuries that occur during periorbital surgery are blindness, corneal abrasions, ruptured globes, retinal detachment, and lens dislocations.[14]

Blindness

Blindness, an unusual complication of the repair of zygomatic and orbital fractures, occurs with a frequency of less than 3 in 1,000.[22, 24] The cause is either impingement of the optic nerve by bone fragments or, more frequently, obstruction of the retinal artery by retrobulbar hematoma or arteriospasm.[20, 22, 24] During the first half-hour postoperatively, the patient should be observed for the presence of vision. If vision is absent, the patient should be carefully examined for proptosis and, via a funduscope, for constricted arteries and dilated veins. If proptosis is noted, the retrobulbar hematoma should be evacuated as described previously for proptosis.

If proptosis is not present, the retinal artery should be treated for arteriospasm or obstruction. Rowe[20] recommends that the supraorbital artery be identified, dissected free, and cannulated with a 22-gauge angiocatheter. Papaverine should be injected until the vessels dilate (40 to 80 mg). The canula should remain in place, and a saline drip of 1 liter containing 80 mg of papaverine and 10,000 units of heparin should be given at a rate of up to 10 drops per minute for 24 hours.[20] The patient should receive 200 mL of a 20% solution of mannitol in order to reduce the volume of the aqueous and vitreous humors, and then 500 mg of acetazolamide to reduce further humor production.[20] Anderson and colleagues[25] also suggest a course of steroid therapy. They recommend the administration of 3.0

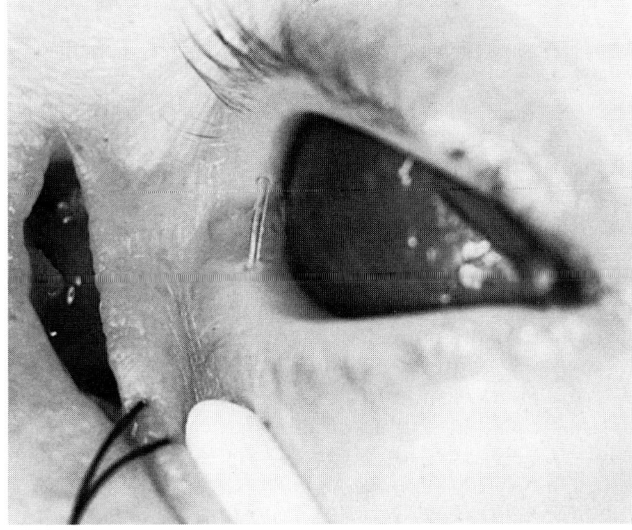

Figure 10–7. Insertion of a canalicular silicone tube during the performance of a dacryocystorhinostomy. Note that the tube bridges the gap between the superior and inferior lacrimal puncta; the other ends of the tubes are exiting the nose through the newly created nasal lacrimal orifice.

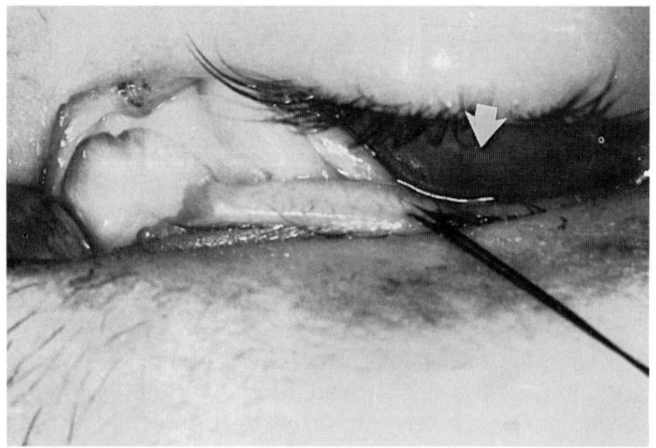

Figure 10–8. The use of proper ocular lubricants and corneal protectors (*arrow*) minimizes iatrogenic injury during periorbital surgery.

to 4.0 mg/kg of dexamethasone phosphate initially, followed by 1.0 to 3.0 mg/kg every 6 hours.[25] If this type of medical therapy is not effective within the first half-hour, as indicated by vessel dilatation and confirmed funduscopically, then impingement of the optic nerve by osseous fragments should be suspected. A computed tomographic scan in coronal sections confirms the diagnosis.

Although it would seem that further manipulation of the zygoma and orbital fracture would correct optic nerve impingement, access to the optic canal cannot be achieved with this approach. Either intracranial exploration of the optic canal, through the jugum of the lesser wing of the sphenoid and orbital plate of the frontal bone, or transnasal exploration through the ethmoid sinuses provides the desired access for visualization and treatment. This procedure is best performed by an experienced neurosurgeon or ophthalmologic surgeon.

Corneal Abrasion

Whenever surgery is performed periorbitally, abrasions or ulcerations of the cornea can occur. They result in pain, blurred vision, and even the need for a corneal transplant. Corneal injury is best prevented by protecting the cornea with well-lubricated corneal protectors (Fig. 10–8). Lacri-Lube (Allergan, Inc, Irvine, CA) is an effective lubricant. Use of corneal protectors prevents damage from excessive manipulation of the eyelids or from uncontrolled instrumentation. Temporary tarsorrhaphy sutures are also helpful.

Corneal ulcerations can be caused by an array of antimicrobial skin preparations, especially those that contain detergents or alcohols. These ulcerations can cause isolated defects but more commonly result in damage to the entire cornea, requiring transplantation. Organic mercurials, chlorhexidine, hexachlorophene, alcohols, tinctures, and scrubs should be avoided for periorbital antimicrobial skin preparation at all costs.[26] Povidone-iodine (10%) solution, although not ideal, is currently the safest and best suited for this anatomic region.[26] If a corneal abrasion occurs, an ophthalmologist should be consulted.

Ruptured Globe

Rupture of the globe is a very rare but devastating complication in trauma. Its intraoperative occurrence is invariably the result of the manipulation of a globe that was injured preoperatively. Because most globe ruptures are hidden, however, by hemorrhagic and edematous conjunctiva or Tenon fascia, they are extremely difficult to diagnose before surgery. Nevertheless, a good clinical examination of the globe should be performed in all patients with periorbital fractures. Hyphema, pupillary irregularities, white pupils, and lacerations are signs of globe damage and require the attention of an ophthalmologist.[14, 27] If a globe is inadvertently ruptured during a periorbital surgical procedure, all manipulation must be discontinued. The eye should be protected without pressure. Intravenous antibiotics should be administered to prevent endophthalmitis; gentamicin and the cephalosporins are good choices.[15] Immediate repair by an ophthalmologic surgeon is preferred.

Retinal Detachment

Intraoperative retinal detachment is another injury that results from a preexisting condition.[15] Symptoms of retinal detachment are defects in the peripheral visual field, flashes of light, and showers of black specks. If these symptoms occur postoperatively, a funduscopic examination, with confirmation of the diagnosis by ultrasonography or computed tomography, is in order. Early treatment by an ophthalmologic surgeon via photocoagulation or cryosurgery is preferred.

Lens Dislocation

Dislocation of the lens into the vitreous cavity or anterior chamber during midface fracture surgery occurs from a pre-existing injury.[15] If a lens dislocation occurs intraoperatively, the procedure should be terminated. Immediate examination and repair by an ophthalmologic surgeon is in order.

Maxillary Fractures

The maxillae, along with the palatine bones, form the foundation of the midface, about which mastication, phonation, deglutition, breathing, and moisturizing and warming of the air all occur. Failure to restore complete anatomic contour results in septal deviation and overcontoured or undercontoured zygomatic arches (12% to 33%).[27–32] The improper verification of the occlusion, especially in the use of rigid internal fixation, invariably results in a malocclusion (13% to 38% incidence of complication in the treatment of maxillary fracture).[27, 28] A variety of general complications can occur with maxillary fractures (Table 10–3), many of which are discussed elsewhere in this chapter.

Table 10–3. Complications Associated with Maxillary Fractures

Infraorbital nerve paresthesia
Enophthalmos
Infected hardware or wires
Exposed hardware or wires
Deviated septum
Altered vision
Overcontoured zygomatic arch
Malocclusion
Epiphora
Foreign body reactions
Scars at incision or fixation sites
Sinusitis
Anosmia
Non-union
Cerebrospinal fluid leak

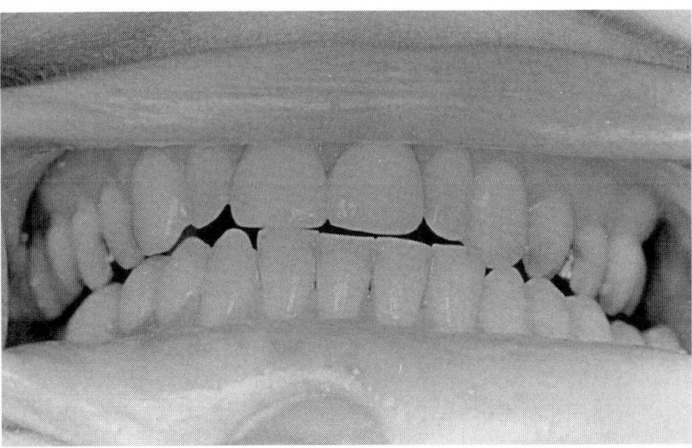

Figure 10–10. Postoperative malocclusion secondary to condylar distraction. The occlusion should be verified for maximum intercuspation with the condyles seated in the fossae, much the same as an anatomic articulator.

Malocclusion

When the technique of closed reduction with maxillomandibular fixation is used to treat a maxillary fracture, the incidence of malocclusion is minimal.[27] When it does occur, the usual cause is patient noncompliance with the fixation. Admonition and education are the only solutions. When open reduction and rigid internal fixation are used to treat a maxillary fracture, however, the incidence of postoperative malocclusion is higher (Fig. 10–9).[28] Postoperative occlusal equilibration and orthodontic movement can be employed to correct minor malocclusions, but reoperation may be required.

In order to avoid this complication, prevention is best. This requires the placement of stable maxillomandibular fixation with arch bars, not merely Ivy loops or Stout wires, prior to the open reduction and fixation of the fracture. After anatomic reduction and manipulation of the maxillomandibular complex such that the condyles are passively seated, fixation with miniplates and screws should be attempted. The zygomaticomaxillary buttresses should first be affixed bilaterally, and then the nasomaxillary buttresses bilaterally. Completion of unilateral fixation rather than bilateral fixation from posterior to anterior may unseat the condyles and result in occlusal prematurities. After fixation has been applied to the buttresses, the maxillomandibular fixation should be released and the occlusion verified with the condyles seated in the fossae, much as occlusion is verified on an anatomic articulator. If a malocclusion exists (Fig. 10–10), the fixation should be completely removed and then reapplied in a slightly different location.

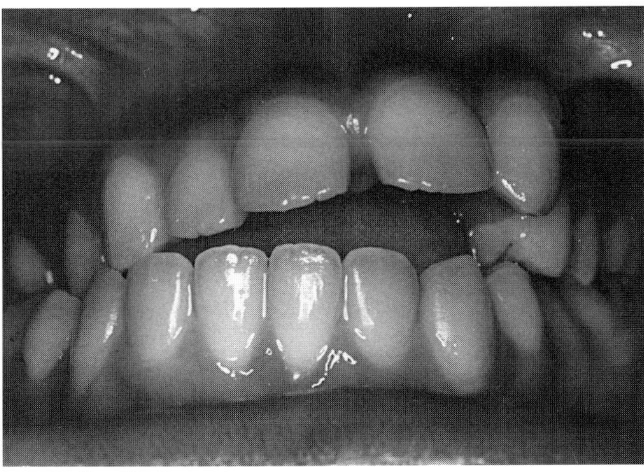

Figure 10–9. A malocclusion noted postoperatively in a patient with a multiple-piece midface fracture.

Maxillary Sinusitis

Maxillary sinusitis is a relatively infrequent complication of maxillary fractures (Fig. 10–11).[27–32] It is routinely treated with enteral antibiotics and decongestants. A 7-day course of amoxicillin and clavulanate

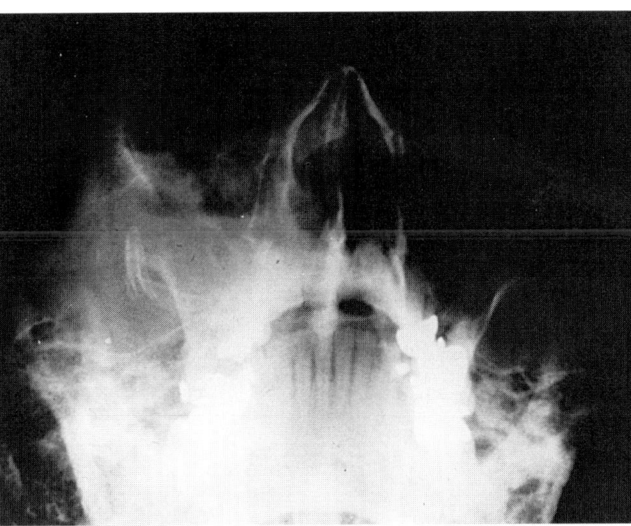

Figure 10–11. This Water's view radiograph reveals a unilateral maxillary sinusitis subsequent to the plate fixation of a midface fracture.

500 mg PO TID; 0.4% oxymetazoline nose drops, one spray each nostril q8h; and pseudoephedrine 30 mg q12h, is generally successful. If the sinusitis is persistent or recurs, the osteum is invariably obstructed, and a nasal antrostomy is in order.

The nasal antrostomy can be performed using either topical or local anesthetics placed under the inferior concha. A hemostat or antral rasp is placed into the nasal aperture against the lateral wall of the nose, inferior to the inferior concha, and then is directed superiorly and laterally. It is pushed into the antrum and manipulated. Suction should be at hand to aspirate hemorrhage or purulent material. Antral mucoceles and pyoceles are rare sequelae to midfacial trauma and may be removed via a Caldwell-Luc procedure or functional endoscopic sinus (FES) surgery.

Zygomatic Fractures

Lying superior to the maxillae and palatine bones, and lateral to the naso-orbital-ethmoid region, are the zygomas, which provide form and permit function. The most common finding in zygoma fractures (18% to 56% incidence) is infraorbital nerve paresthesia, which may not resolve postoperatively (Table 10–4).[14, 20, 31–35] Second in frequency is flattened facial contour from inadequately reduced zygomatic arches or inadequate malar projection (3.6% to 26%).[20, 31–35] Failure to adequately evaluate and explore the floor of the orbit may result in both enophthalmos and diplopia (5% to 26%).[14, 31–35] Infected antral hematomas associated with the fracture may result in sinusitis. Infected, palpable, or visible hardware and wires are uncommon complications of the placement of such devices. The presence of unsightly scars and ectropion may result from the incisions required to gain access for reduction and stabilization of zygoma fractures or from lacerations overlying the fractured bone (37% to 42%).[21, 36] When present, abducens nerve palsy causes inadequate abduction of the eye; this is considered an infrequent comorbid event.[37] Blindness, reported to occur in 3 per 1,000 cases of zygoma fracture, results from either orbital apex syndrome or obstruction of the retinal artery.[20, 22, 24] Most of these complications are discussed in this chapter. Prevention and treatment of ectropion are discussed in Chapter 20.

Table 10–4. Complications Associated with Zygomatic Fractures

Infraorbital nerve paresthesia
Flattened zygomatic arch
Enophthalmos
Diplopia
Sinusitis
Visible or palpable hardware or wires
Infected hardware or wires
Ectropion
Unsightly scars
Abducens nerve palsy
Ocular injury

Table 10–5. Complications Associated with Frontal Sinus Fractures

Contour irregularities
Chronic pain
Supraorbital nerve paresthesia
Sinusitis
Mucocele
Pyocele
Meningitis
Cerebrospinal fluid leak
Visible or palpable hardware

Frontal Sinus and Frontal Bone Fractures

The frontal bone houses the frontal sinus and forms the supraorbital rim and orbital roof. The most common complaints of patients who have undergone surgical treatment of fractures of this bone are of contour irregularities, voids, or depressions (Table 10–5 and Fig. 10–12).[38–43] Next in frequency is the complaint of chronic pain. Occasionally, because of concurrent injury or the surgical approach, supraorbital nerve paresthesia persists postoperatively.[43] Long-term problems (6 months to 15 years after the injury) include the development of mucoceles and pyoceles.[38, 43] Sinusitis may develop from improperly managed nasofrontal ducts. If persistent, this sinusitis may erode the posterior table and cause meningitis.[38–43] Rarely does a cerebrospinal fluid leak persist postoperatively.

Frontal Sinusitis

Mucoceles or pyoceles of the frontal sinus are potentially devastating long-term postoperative complications. They can erode the anterior as well as the posterior table and thus cause neurologic problems.

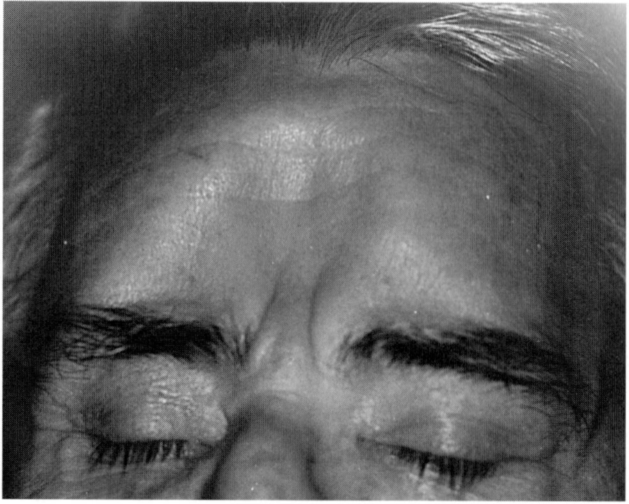

Figure 10–12. A forehead defect secondary to an unrepaired fracture of the anterior table of the frontal sinus and supraorbital rims.

Mucoceles or pyoceles invariably occur by the proliferation of sinus mucosa trapped in the fracture when it was reduced. The key to the prevention of such problems is the meticulous removal of all sinus mucosa from the fractured segments during reduction and stabilization.

Frontal sinusitis in the postoperative setting is usually the result of malfunctioning nasofrontal ducts. To prevent it, the patency of the nasofrontal ducts must be verified intraoperatively.[43] After access to the sinus has been obtained, the duct should be visualized and a 1.5-inch, 18-gauge polytetrafluoroethylene angiocatheter inserted, followed by injection of methylene blue or indigo carmine dye. Patency of the duct is verified by exudation of dye from the patient's nasal aperture (Fig. 10–13) or collection of dye in the patient's hypopharynx. If the duct is not patent, a new duct must be created or the sinus obliterated.[43]

Panfacial Fractures

Panfacial fractures are common occurrences in the polytraumatized patient and may involve any two or more of the facial structures previously mentioned. These types of injuries are therefore prone to any of the complications listed in Tables 10–1 to 10–5. Each anatomic unit must be evaluated and treated individually, with the approach that the sum of the units results in the patient's facial form and abilities to function.

Anesthesia and Paresthesia

Supraorbital Nerve

Persistent postoperative anesthesia or paresthesia of the supraorbital nerve is an uncommon complication of the management of naso-orbital-ethmoid fractures, supraorbital rim fractures, and frontal sinus fractures. It is best avoided by the use of a bitemporal or coronal incision.[44] When the bitemporal incision is performed properly, the supraorbital nerve as well as the facial nerve branches are protected and preserved. If further retraction is required, the supraorbital nerve may be removed from its foramen by creation of an osteotomy inferior to the foramen with small chisels or a rongeur (Fig. 10–14). Even further release can be provided by preauricular extensions and division of the scalp periosteum in the midline of the flap.

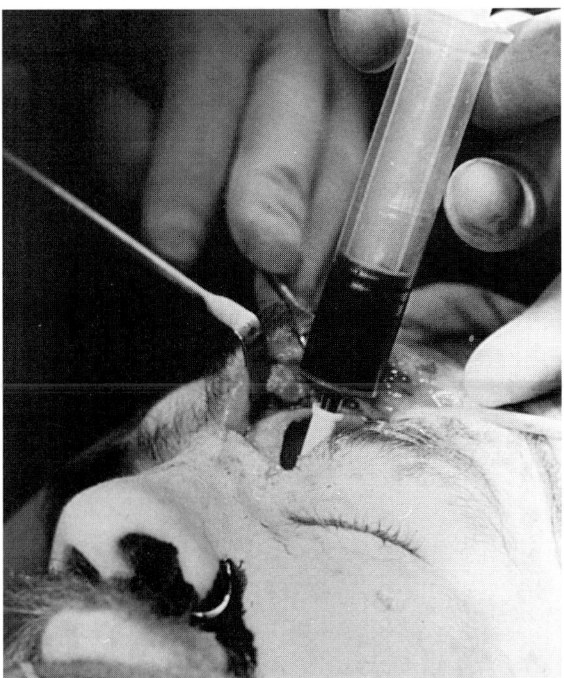

Figure 10–13. Evaluation of the patency of the nasofrontal duct by the introduction of a Teflon catheter. Verification of duct patency is by exudation of methylene blue dye from the nasal aperture.

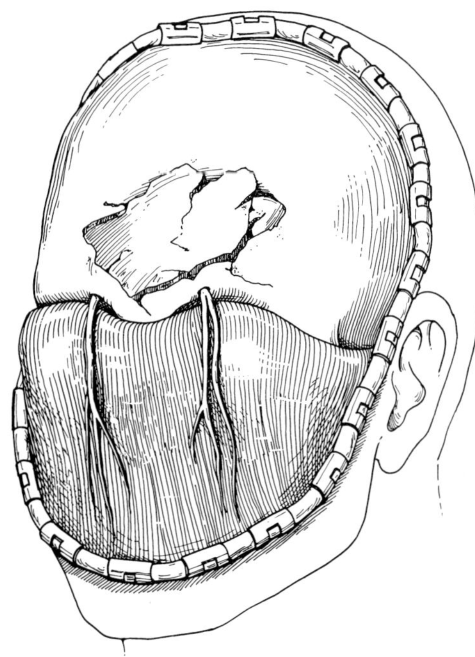

Figure 10–14. The proper reflection of a bitemporal flap preserves the supraorbital nerve and creates excellent access for visualization and treatment of upper midface fractures. (*From* Haug RH: Midface fractures I. Atlas of the Oral and Maxillofacial Surgery Clinics of North America 1993;1:2.)

If a bilateral suprabrow incision is chosen for access (Fig. 10–15), care must be taken to locate and preserve the nerves.[44] After the incision is made through the cutaneous tissues and fibers of the orbicularis oculi muscle, blunt and sharp dissection is performed until the supraorbital nerve and foramen are located. The nerve is then retracted while a periosteal incision is made and a subperiosteal flap reflected. Release of the periosteum and connective tissue helps to preserve the nerve by eliminating tension during retraction.

Infraorbital Nerve

Anesthesia or paresthesia of the infraorbital nerve is most likely a comorbid event.[27–28] Infraorbital anesthesia is the most common finding associated with maxillary fractures (14% to 24% incidence) (see Table 10–1).[27–29] Yet certain precautions can be taken to prevent iatrogenic anesthesia. In treating a zygoma fracture with infraorbital paresthesia, anatomic osseous reduc-

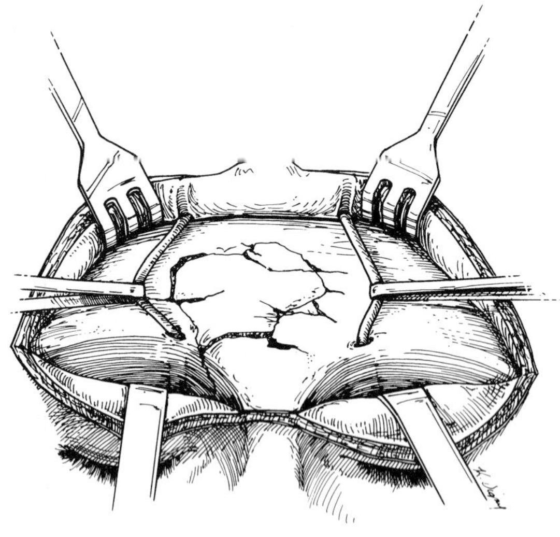

Figure 10–15. The proper reflection of a suprabrow flap ensures preservation of the supraorbital nerve by careful exploration and release from the flap. (From Haug RH: Midface fractures I. Atlas of the Oral and Maxillofacial Surgery Clinics of North America 1993;1:8.)

tion to minimize impingement of the nerve is critical. For treating maxillary or central midface fractures, circumvestibular incisions or maxillary degloving incisions are frequently employed. Care must be taken in these approaches to identify, preserve, and protect the nerve.[44]

The circumvestibular incision is created through mucosa and periosteum from molar to molar, approximately 1.0 cm superior to the attached gingiva, followed by a subperiosteal dissection until the fracture site is visualized or the infraorbital nerve is encountered. Often, the fracture can be visualized and treated without locating the nerve. If greater surgical access is required, however, the infraorbital foramen and nerve should be isolated, released from the flap, and protected (Fig. 10–16).

If even further access is required, a maxillary degloving incision may be performed.[45] This procedure incorporates an intranasal connection of bilateral intercartilaginous incisions, bilateral pyriform rim incisions, and a complete transfixion incision. The incisions are then connected via soft tissue dissection to an intraoral maxillary circumvestibular incision. The nasal skin, tip, alar cartilages, and anterior membranous septum from the nasal bones and lateral cartilages are then mobilized (Fig. 10–17). This exposure provides direct access to and exceptional visualization of midface structures up to the nasofrontal suture without cutaneous incisions (Fig. 10–18). Exploration of the orbital floor is possible, as is repair of inferior rim fractures with alternate side-to-side retraction of the infraorbital nerve. The maxillary degloving incision, when coupled with a bitemporal incision, provides access to virtually every midfacial fracture while protecting the sensory nerve supply. Because of the greater tissue reflection created by the maxillary degloving incision, retraction damage to the infraorbital nerve is a real risk. The surgeon should resist the temptation to release the infraorbital nerves from the inferior orbital rims in a manner similar to supraorbital nerve release from the supraorbital rim for bitemporal exposure. The thickness of the bone of the inferior orbital rim and the distance of the inferior orbital foramen from the rim preclude simple release without excessive bone removal. Release of the periosteal sheath from the underlying nerve provides the additional retraction required, but the greater risk to the nerve must be appreciated.

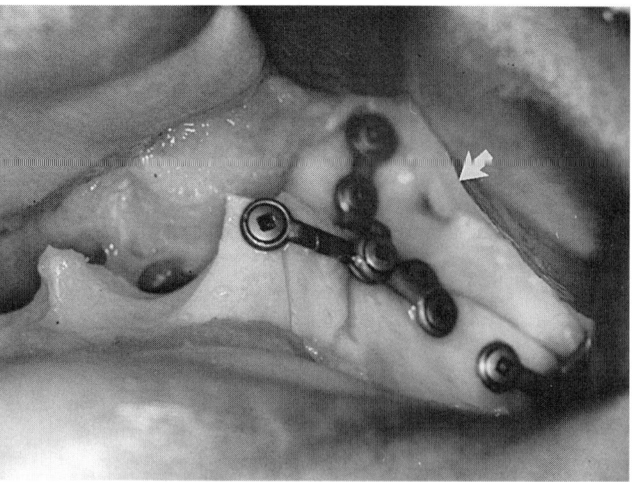

Figure 10–16. The circumvestibular incision provides access to lower-level midface fractures. Note the infraorbital nerve retraction on the patient's left *(arrow)*.

Contour Deformity

Overcontoured and undercontoured facial bones are uncommon complications of the treatment of midfacial fractures (Fig. 10–19). They can result from imperfect reduction or unstable fixation. Isolated fractures with minimal fragmentation or displacement can be rou-

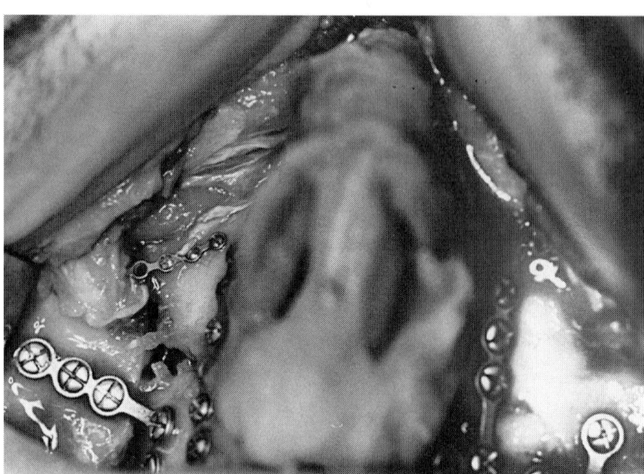

Figure 10–17. The maxillary degloving incision connects intranasal incisions and intraoral incisions. It provides universal access to midface fractures with preservation of the infraorbital nerves.

tinely treated with closed reduction or wire osteosynthesis. When multiple fractured bones and gross comminution exist, however, open assessment and rigid internal fixation are recommended. No replacement exists for a careful hands-on clinical examination, but computed tomography has evolved into an integral component of the diagnosis of midfacial fractures. The modality is unparalleled in assessing both soft and hard tissue injury and developing a treatment plan.

In order to assess the extent of the fractures as well as their anatomic reduction, open access is preferred. Numerous incisions for access to facial fractures exist, but the midface degloving incision (described in the section on anesthesia and paresthesia) coupled with a bitemporal incision provides universal access to the entire midface. This approach ensures complete visualization for fracture assessment as well as access for fixation.

Wire osteosynthesis may be useful for isolated injuries, but the small plate-and-screw systems offer much greater postoperative stability, preventing overcontouring and undercontouring by postoperative displacement. However, these devices are unforgiving after placement. The clinician must assess the fracture for proper anatomic reduction and contour, and then reassess before wound closure.

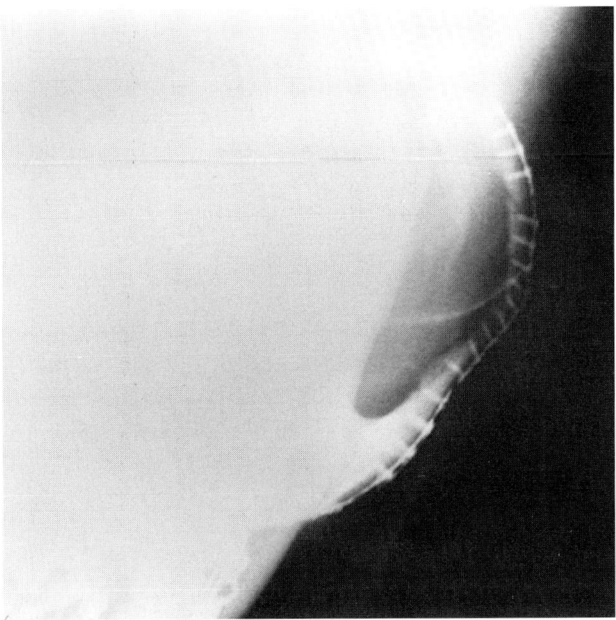

Figure 10–19. A submental vertex radiographic view of an overcontoured zygoma.

Nonunion

Nonunion is a very uncommon complication in the treatment of midface fractures. Nonunions of the non–stress-bearing bones of the zygoma, nose, and frontal bone have little consequence unless coupled with infection or chronic pain. If infection or pain exists, the fibrous and necrotic tissues should be débrided and the unstable bones rigidly stabilized. If voids exist that compromise form or function, bone grafting with cranial bone is preferred.

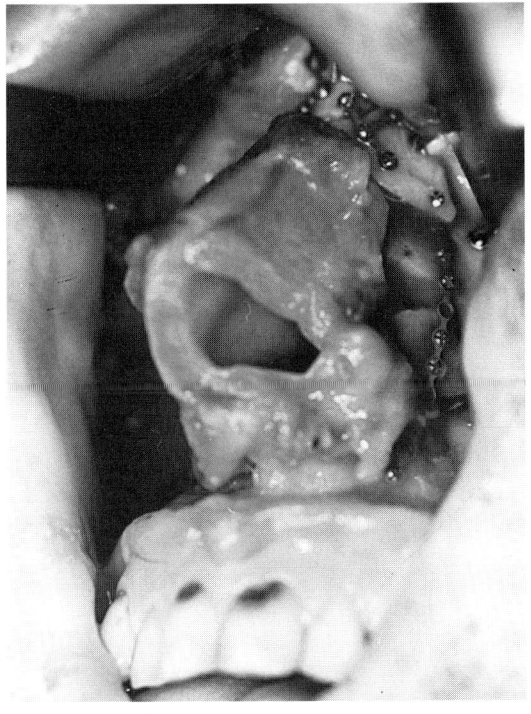

Figure 10–18. Midfacial degloving incision. Note the bone plate placement along the nasal bones and frontal process of the maxilla.

The maxilla possesses a difficult problem in that it is a bone constantly placed into function. The etiology for maxillary nonunion is the perpetual movement that is produced by mastication, phonation, or deglutition with nonrigid stabilization. The causes include patient noncompliance with treatment through release of maxillomandibular fixation, bruxism during maxillomandibular fixation, and function against inadequate rigid fixation. The principles of buttress reconstruction discussed previously should be adhered to, and 1.5- or 2.0-mm plates and screws should be used. If a nonunion does occur, removal of the fixation and placement of bone grafts with a rigid fixation system are required. Aggressive movement of the jaw by the patient should be discouraged during healing.

Unsightly Scars

A complete discussion of soft tissue wound healing appears in Chapter 4. The management of mature, unsightly scars is discussed in Chapter 20. The focus of this section is intraoperative considerations to limit adverse sequelae.

The Bitemporal (Coronal) Incision

When the incision is designed for a bitemporal (coronal) flap, the development of male-pattern baldness should be anticipated. Two philosophies regarding incision design exist. One incorporates a curvilinear inci-

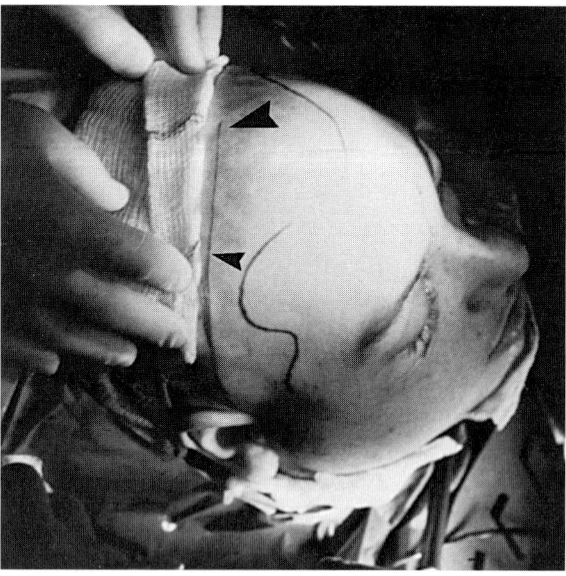

Figure 10–20. The proper placement of the bitemporal incision *(arrows)* from preauricular region to preauricular region over the vertex of the cranium.

sion 2.0 to 3.0 cm posterior to the hairline from the crest of the cranium to either preauricular region. The advocates of this incision claim a better cosmetic result in anticipation of progressive male-pattern baldness.

The other philosophy involves a vertical incision over the vertex from preauricular region to preauricular region. The advocates of this design claim that even if a poor scar results, it cannot be visualized when placed in this fashion (Fig. 10–20). In addition, a straight vertical incision extending over the vertex of the scalp may result in less paresthesia of the periincisional skin, because an incision placed here lies in a "watershed" between the anterior and posterior sensory innervations of the scalp. Only smaller terminal sensory nerve fibers are violated, thereby resulting in an improved prognosis for return of normal sensation along the incision line. The incision should be created parallel to the hair follicles so as not to damage them. In addition, the excessive use of electrocautery along the incision line may damage hair follicles, creating a noticeable margin of alopecia. Consideration should be given to alternative approaches in patients who have alopecia or who are already bald.[44, 46]

Periorbital Incisions

Unsightly scars associated with periorbital incisions are bothersome to the patient and quite difficult for the surgeon to repair secondarily. Lateral brow incisions are falling out of vogue because they cannot be hidden cosmetically and because damaged hair follicles are unsightly and impossible to correct (Fig. 10–21). The placement of incisions within skin creases and parallel rather than perpendicular to Langer lines offers the best results.[44, 46] Upper blepharoplasty and transconjunctival approaches provide the most aesthetic access,

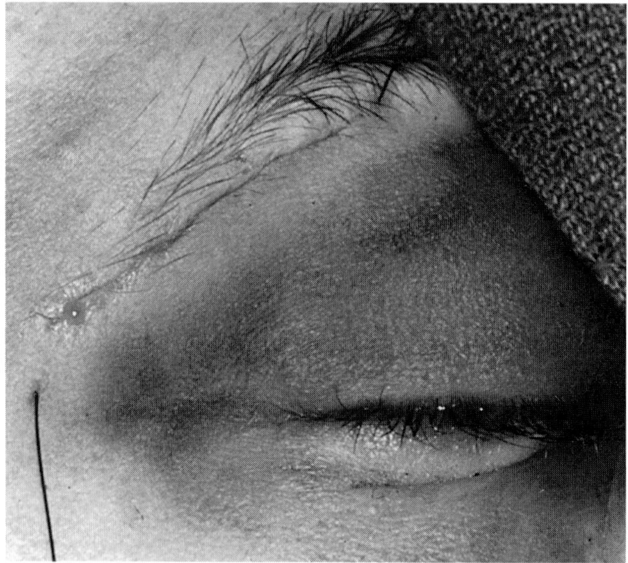

Figure 10–21. The unaesthetic appearance of the traditional lateral brow incision.

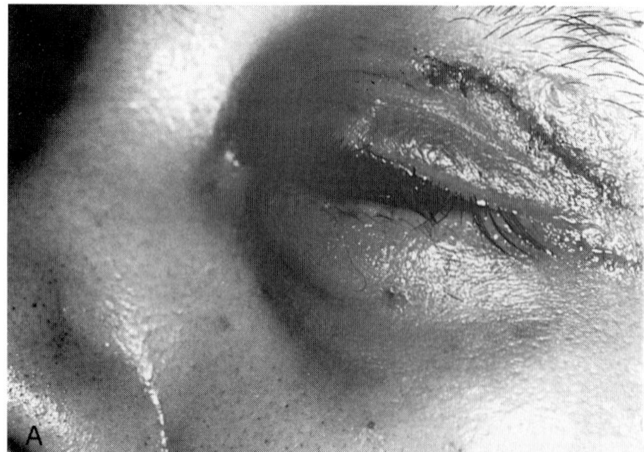

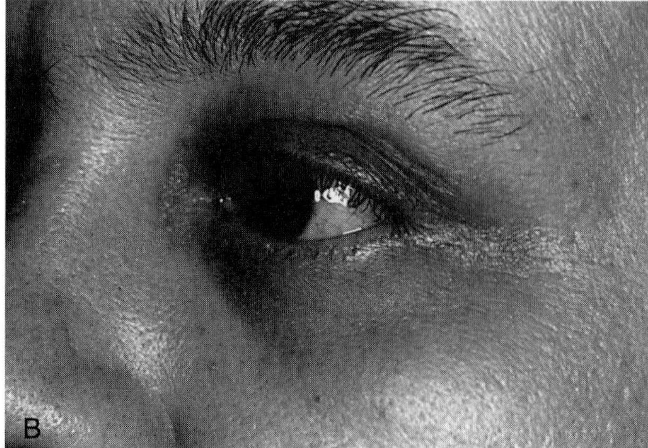

Figure 10–22. *A,* The appearance of an upper lid blepharoplasty incision and lower lid transconjunctival incision with lateral canthotomy extension 1 week postoperatively. *B,* The 6-week postoperative appearance of the same patient. Note the enhanced aesthetics of these approaches.

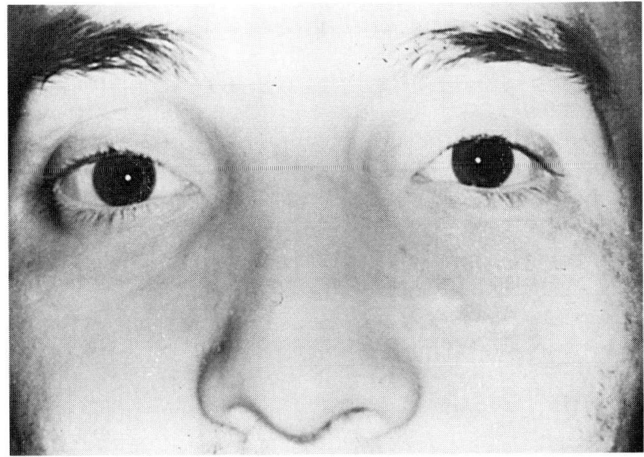

Figure 10–23. The poor scar that invariably occurs with medial orbital rim incisions.

and the subciliary approach with a lateral canthal extension offers a reasonable alternative (Fig. 10–22).[44, 46]

Because of the thin nature of the skin in the medial orbital and lateral nasal regions, the Lynch incision and "open sky" approach are best avoided (Fig. 10–23). The bitemporal incision is the best alternative for naso-orbital-ethmoidal injuries.[44, 46]

Scars from Suspension Devices

There are practitioners who find that closed reduction with maxillomandibular fixation supported by skeletal suspension is a minimally invasive alternative to open reduction.[47] Some surgeons even continue to use lead plates and buttons for the reduction of edema and stabilization of the soft tissues in naso-orbital-ethmoidal injuries. Unfortunately, these devices tend to produce unfavorable scars (Fig. 10–24). Scars may be avoided or at least minimized by placing Xeroform gauze padding (Sherwood Medical, St. Louis, MO) between the skin and the plate or button as a cushion (Fig. 10–25). Gauze dressings should be changed every 3 to 7 days for the duration of the suspension. If a scar does occur, it may be modified by simple dermabrasion techniques.

Wound Infection and Foreign Body Reaction

Wound infections have been reported as uncommon complications (less than 10% of cases) in the repair of midface fractures.[27–30, 32] Foreign body reactions have been attributed to the use of implantable devices (wires, screws and plates, implants).[27]

Wound Infections

Surgical wound infections are to be expected with any type of surgery. Cellulitis is best treated with antibiotic therapy alone, whereas an abscess requires antibiotic therapy along with incision, drainage, and culture and sensitivity testing. Antibiotic regimens, as discussed in the next section, should be adhered to.

Wires

Suspension devices and osteosynthesis wires provide nonrigid supplementation of maxillomandibular fixation and are usually placed at multiple sites. Thus, the sacrifice of an individual wire does not routinely affect the overall stability of the system. If cellulitis develops about a wire (Fig. 10–26), it should be treated first with 5 to 7 days of enteral antibiotics. Cephalosporins remain good choices for cutaneous wounds, and penicillin is best for intraoral wounds. If the cellulitis resolves, the wire may remain for the course of healing. If not, the wire should be removed, and antibiotic therapy continued for an additional 5 days. If an abscess develops, the patient should be placed on antibiotics, the wire removed using local anesthesia (and/or intravenous sedation), and an incision with drainage performed along with sampling for culture and sensi-

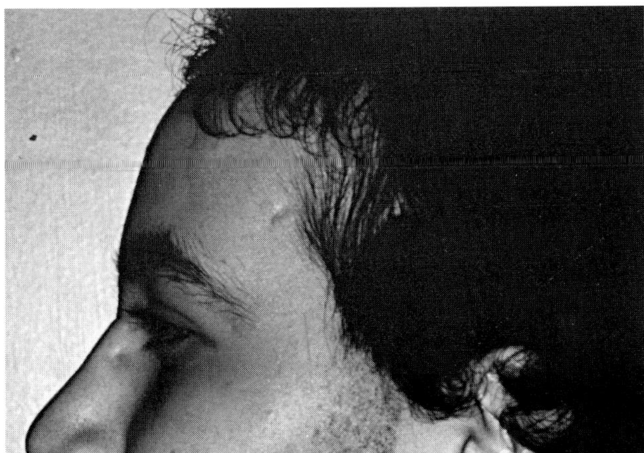

Figure 10–24. Pullout wires with lead bolsters or buttons commonly leave unaesthetic scars. Note depressions in the temporal and nasal areas.

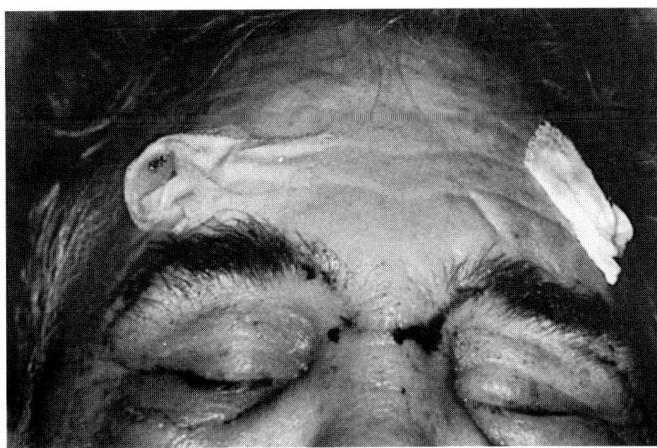

Figure 10–25. Xeroform padding placed under cutaneous buttons that are secured to skeletal fixation wires.

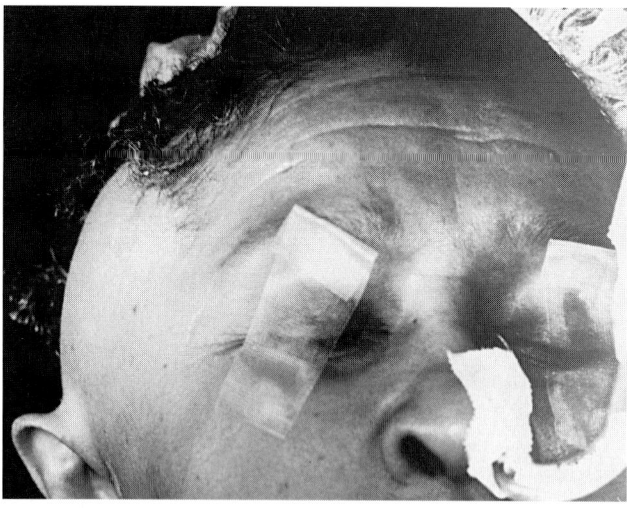

Figure 10–26. A temporal abscess associated with a circumzygomatic skeletal pullout wire.

tivity testing of the offending bacteria. A drain may be placed until the abscess becomes nonproductive.

Plates and Screws

Rigid internal fixation devices provide stability to a bone while in function, and their survival during the entire course of healing is important. Complications associated with the use of rigid internal fixation are discussed in Chapter 14.

Orbital Floor Implants

Infected orbital floor implants are potentially morbid occurrences and provide the practitioner with complex decisions. Implants may become infected within days after surgery or many years postoperatively; thus, continued patient contact is important (Fig. 10–27). A patient who develops an infection about the orbital floor implant should be admitted to the hospital for intravenous antibiotic therapy.[48] Using general anesthesia, the implant should be removed through the incision with which it was inserted. Silastic (Dow Corning, Midland, MI) implants are easily removed. Medpore (Porex, Fairburn, GA) are more difficult to remove, and wire mesh are the most difficult. The patient should remain on antibiotic therapy for 7 to 10 days. Repair of the orbital floor should be delayed until after the infection has resolved. After resolution of the infection with its associated edema, the need for secondary reconstruction can be assessed.

Concomitant Injuries in Midface Fractures

Cerebrospinal fluid leaks and anosmia have been associated with midface injury as comorbid events.[29, 31] Although rare, these complications must be addressed properly for good long-term results.

Cerebrospinal Fluid Leak

The presence of a cerebrospinal fluid leak along with a frontal sinus, naso-orbital-ethmoid, or LeFort-level fracture should not prohibit its repair. In fact, the early reduction and fixation of the associated facial fractures routinely stops the leak. Under no circumstances should nasal packing be performed to control a CSF leak. If it is persistent, a craniotomy with direct repair of the dura is indicated.

Intracranial Injury

The presence of intracranial injury does not prevent the repair of midfacial fractures but may require modification in management.[49] The anesthetic technique should not include medications that increase intracranial pressure or aggravate pneumoencephaly. Procedures that will cause bucking or Valsalva maneuvers should be eliminated. Rigid fixation techniques should be employed to protect the airway in the neurologically impaired patient, eliminating the potential for airway compromise found with maxillomandibular fixation.

Anosmia

Anosmia is considered a comorbid event for which minimal improvement occurs. Reapproximation of the naso-ethmoid region is the only hope for any improvement.

Psychiatric Effects of Trauma

The structures of the midface are involved in sight, smell, deglutition, respiration, and phonation. Perhaps even more important, the midface is the focal point of

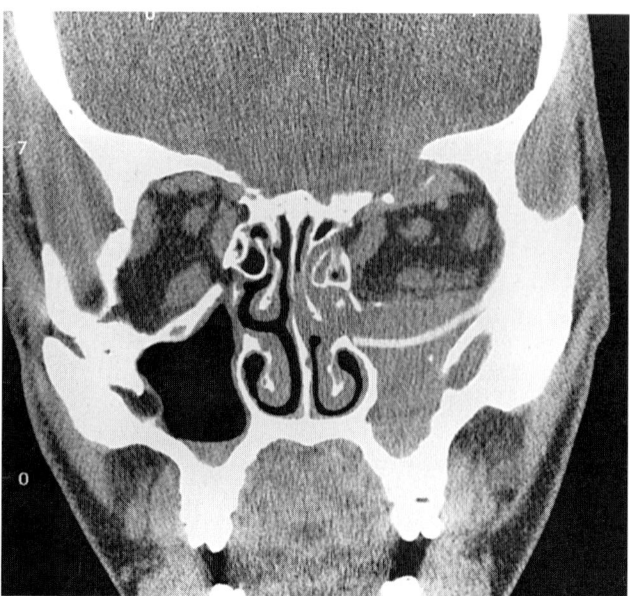

Figure 10–27. CT scan of an infected Silastic orbital floor implant 3 years after its insertion.

the facial aesthetic form and thus provides the foundation of self-image. Other body parts can be masked after injury; the midface cannot. Thus, disfiguring injury to this anatomic region can have profound psychiatric manifestations. Even beyond the anguish associated with congenital anomalies, whose victims have known no other quality of life, is that suffered by the individual whose entire life was previously normal and who overnight becomes grossly disfigured or functionless. This acute change can bring about severe depression, denial, and psychiatric disorders. The maxillofacial surgeon must be understanding, sensitive, and empathetic. Showing respect, honesty, and support perioperatively is helpful. If psychiatric problems are suspected, appropriate consultation with a psychologist or psychiatrist is recommended.[50]

Chronic Pain

Chronic pain associated with the treatment of midfacial fractures is a frustrating problem for both the patient and the surgeon. Fortunately, the incidence of this complication is low, and although the pain may affect any of the facial bones, the pneumatized structures of the frontal sinus and maxilla seem to be affected more often. Narcotic analgesics are effective in the short-term postoperative phase (from hospital discharge to 8 weeks), but nonsteroidal anti-inflammatory analgesics are preferred for the long-term postoperative phase (up to 6 months after discharge). Patients with persistent pain must be evaluated for infection or necrosis of the repaired structures as well as the possibility of neuroma or foreign body granuloma formation. These disorders should be treated on an individual basis. Chronic pain with no identifiable etiology may be due to deafferentation or have psychogenic causes. Affected patients may be best treated by referral to the appropriate chronic pain specialist. Biofeedback, stellate ganglion blocks, physical therapy, and pharmacologic modification may be helpful. In our group's experience, when all other modalities fail, removal of hardware has been noted to improve the patient's perception of pain.

Avulsed Tissues

Teeth

With the advent of osseointegration and improvements in dental materials, the loss of teeth in trauma has become a minor concern. Attention should be paid, however, to the maintenance (if possible) of the remaining bone and soft tissues. A temporary prosthesis may be placed even before the soft tissue wounds have healed. Implants should be placed 3 months or more after the fracture has consolidated, in order to provide a satisfactory osseous base. Dentoalveolar trauma and complications are discussed in Chapter 11.

Bone

When bone is avulsed in midface fractures, consideration should be given to location, volume, and function of the missing tissue. Secondary reconstruction is a satisfactory alternative, but immediate microvascular reconstruction with a radial forearm flap is also an effective and useful modality.[51] The advantages of this latter approach are immediate repair, minimal cosmetic defect, and improved patient self-image. Its disadvantages are that a microvascular team must be called upon at a moment's notice, the reconstructive procedure along with the trauma repair takes many hours, and contamination and edema may prohibit or compromise graft placement. Massive injuries, such as those encountered in high-energy gunshot wounds, should be repaired in a secondary procedure.

Soft Tissues

Repair of avulsed soft tissues has a number of alternatives, depending upon volume lost, function of the structure, and quality of the underlying tissues. Simple local flap advancement meets the needs of small defects. Skin grafting is an acceptable alternative for large wounds with good underlying tissues (Fig. 10–28). Wound pexy can minimize the volume to be repaired in large defects (Fig. 10–29).[52] When the underlying osseous tissues have been avulsed, microvascular cable grafts or composite grafts are effective.[53]

Summary

Avoiding complications in midface fractures requires that a thorough clinical examination be performed, a complete and accurate diagnosis be made, and the simplest treatment plan that will address the problems be executed. The patient must be assessed and reassessed preoperatively, intraoperatively, and postoperatively.

Although simple isolated fractures may best be treated by closed or minimally invasive approaches, panfacial fractures and fractures with comminution are better treated by wide-open surgical access and then

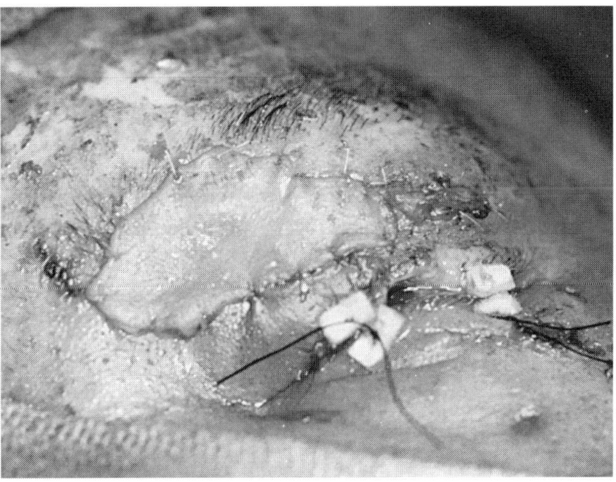

Figure 10–28. A split-thickness skin graft harvested from the postauricular area to reconstruct a traumatic defect of the upper left eyelid. The eyelids have temporary tarsorrhaphy sutures.

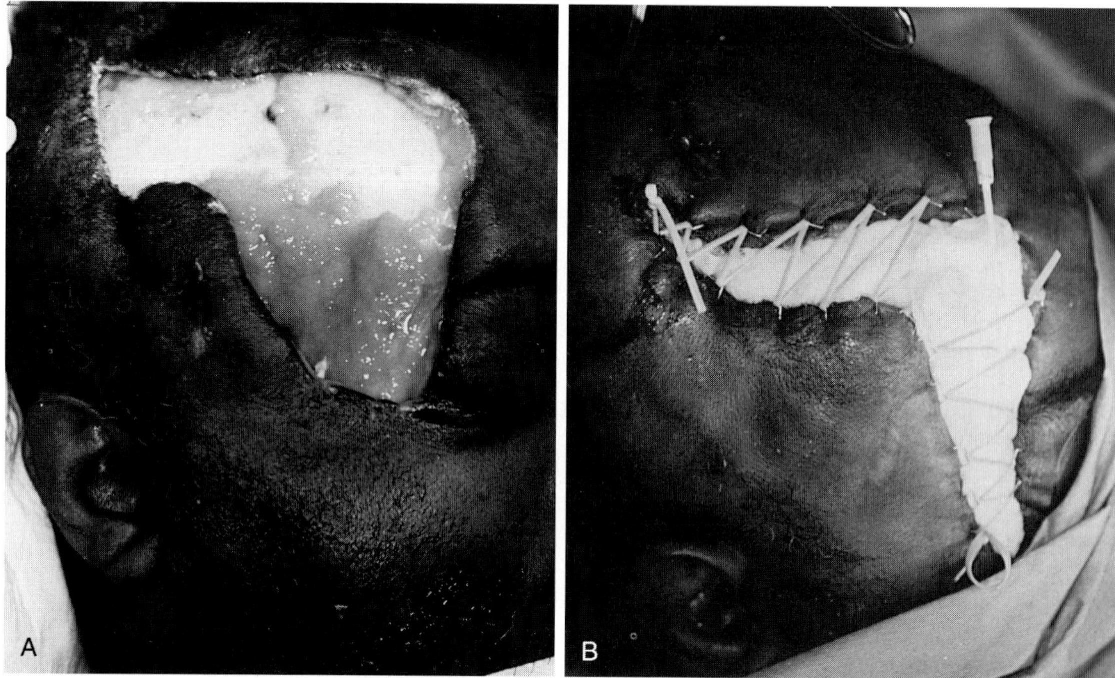

Figure 10–29. *A*, An infected scalp laceration with retraction of the flap precluding primary tissue reapproximation. *B*, Galeapexy and superficial elastic traction sutures with appropriate dressing changes eventually allowed this wound to be closed primarily.

stabilized by rigid techniques. The osseous structures provide the foundation for soft tissue drape, but intimate attention must be paid to the quality of the repair of soft tissues. Adherence to the principles described in this chapter assists the surgeon in obtaining the desired result with few complications.

References

1. Kaban LB: Complications, poor results and treatment failures: Diagnosis, prevention and management. Oral Maxillofac Surg Clin North Am 1990;2:416.
2. Helfrick JF, Kelly JF: Parameters of care for oral and maxillofacial surgery. J Oral Maxillofac Surg 1992;50(supp2):1.
3. Moore EE: Early Care of the Injured Patient. Philadelphia, BC Decker, 1990.
4. Alexander RH, Proctor HJ: Advanced Trauma Life Support. Chicago, American College of Surgeons, 1993.
5. Haug RH, Prather JL: The closed reduction of nasal fractures: An evaluation of two techniques. J Oral Maxillofac Surg 1991;49:1288.
6. Harrison DH: Nasal injuries: Their pathogenesis and treatment. Br J Plast Surg 1979;32:57.
7. Crowther JA, O'Donoghue GM: The broken nose: Does familiarity breed contempt? Ann R Coll Surg Edin 1987;69:259.
8. Illum P, Kristensen C, Jorgensen K, et al: Role of fixation in the treatment of nasal fractures. Clin Otol 1983;8:191.
9. Altreuter RW: Nasal trauma. Emergency Med Clin North Am 1987;5:300.
10. Markowitz BL, Manson PN, Sargent L, et al: Management of the medial canthal tendon in nasoethmoid orbital fractures: The importance of the central fragment in classification and treatment. Plast Reconstr Surg 1991;87:843.
11. Ellis E: Sequencing treatment for naso-orbital-ethmoidal fractures. J Oral Maxillofac Surg 1993;51:543.
12. Hardesty RH, Coffey AJ: Secondary craniomaxillofacial deformities: Current principles and management. Clin Plast Surg 1992;19:275.
13. Gruss JS: Naso-ethmoid-orbital fractures: Classification and role of primary bone grafting. Plast Reconstr Surg 1991;87:843.
14. Perrott DH, Kaban LB: Management of zygomatic complex fractures. *In* Peterson LJ, Indresano AT, Marciani RD, et al (eds): Principles of Oral and Maxillofacial Surgery. Philadelphia, WB Saunders, 1992, p 484.
15. Deutsch TA, Feller DB: Paton and Goldberg's Management of Ocular Injuries, Philadelphia, WB Saunders, 1985.
16. Freihofer HP: Inner intercanthal and interorbital distances. J Maxillofac Surg 1980;8:324.
17. Sargent LA: Naso-ethmoid-orbital fractures. Problems in Plastic and Reconstructive Surgery 1991;1:426.
18. Markowitz NR, Allan PG: Cranial bone harvesting: A modified technique. J Oral Maxillofac Surg 1989;47:1113.
19. Graft P, Sargent LA: Membranous bone healing and techniques in cranial bone grafting. Clin Plast Surg 1989;16:11.
20. Rowe NL: Fractures of the zygomatic complex and orbit. *In* Rowe N, Williams JL: Maxillofacial Injuries, vol I. New York, Churchill Livingstone, 1985, p 538.
21. Ellis E: Fractures of the zygomatic complex and arch. *In* Fonseca RJ, Walker RV (eds): Oral and Maxillofacial Trauma. Philadelphia, WB Saunders, 1991, p 435.
22. Wood GD: Blindness following fracture of the zygomatic bone. Br J Oral Maxillofac Surg 1986;24:12.
23. Gruss JS, Hurwitz JJ, Nik NA, et al: The pattern and incidence of nasolacrimal injury in naso-orbital-ethmoid fractures: The role of delayed assessment and dacryocystorhinostomy. Br J Plast Surg 1985;38:116.
24. Ord RA: Postoperative retrobulbar hemorrhage and blindness complicating trauma surgery. Br J Oral Surg 1981;19:202.
25. Anderson RC, Panje WR, Cross CE: Optic nerve blindness following blunt forehead trauma. Ophthalmology 1982;89:445.
26. Morgan JP, Haug RH, Kosman JW: A review of antimicrobial skin preparations for the maxillofacial region. J Oral Maxillofac Surg 1996;54:89
27. Haug RH, Prather J, Bradrick JP, et al: The morbidity associated with 50 maxillary fractures treated by closed reduction. Oral Surg Oral Med Oral Pathol 1992;73:659.
28. Haug RH, Adams JA, Jordan RB: Comparison of the morbidity associated with maxillary fractures treated by maxillomandibular

and rigid internal fixation. Oral Surg Oral Med Oral Pathol Oral Rad Endol 1995;80:629.
29. Sofferman RA, Danielson PA, Quatela V, et al: Retrospective analysis of surgically treated LeFort fractures: Is suspension necessary? Arch Otolaryngol 1983;109:446.
30. Steidler NE, Cook RM, Reade PC: Incidence and management of major middle third facial fractures at the Royal Melbourne Hospital. Int J Oral Surg 1980;9:92.
31. Morgan BDG, Madan DK, Bergerot JPC: Fractures of the middle third of the face—a review of 300 cases. Br J Plast Surg 1972;25:147.
32. Heimgartner-Candinas B, Heimgartner M, Jonutis A: Results of treatment of midfacial fractures. J Maxillofac Surg 1978;6:293.
33. Helfrick JF: Complications of midface injury. Oral Maxillofac Surg Clin North Am 1990;2:551.
34. Ellis E, El-Attar A, Moos KF: An analysis of 2,067 cases of zygomatico-orbital fractures. J Oral Maxillofac Surg 1985;43:167.
35. Martin BC, Trabue JC, Leech TR: An analysis of the etiology, treatment and complications of fractures of the malar compound and zygomatic arch. Am J Surg 1956;92:920.
36. Converse JM: Discussion of a randomized comparison of four incisions for orbital floor fractures. Plast Reconstr Surg 1981;67:736.
37. Porto DP, Duvall AJ: Long term results with nasofrontal duct reconstruction. Laryngoscope 1986;96:856.
38. Rucker CW: Paralysis of the third, fourth and sixth cranial nerves. Am J Ophthalmol 1958;46:787.
39. Helmy ES, Koh RL, Bays RA: Management of frontal sinus fractures. Oral Surg Oral Med Oral Pathol 1990;69:137.
40. Duvall AJ, Porto DP, Lyons D, et al: Frontal sinus fractures. Arch Otolaryngol Head Neck Surg 1987;113:933.
41. Larson CH, Adkins WY, Oscuthorpe JD: Post-traumatic frontal and frontoethmoid mucoceles causing reversible visual loss. Otolaryngol Head Neck Surg 1983;91:691.
42. Larabee WF, Travis LW, Tobb HG: Frontal sinus fractures: Their suppurative complications and surgical management. Laryngoscope 1980;90:1810.
43. Haug RH: Management of frontal sinus and frontal bone fractures. *In* Peterson LJ, Indresano AT, Marciani RD, et al (eds): Principles of Oral and Maxillofacial Surgery, vol I. Philadelphia, JB Lippincott, 1992, p 575.
44. Haug RH, Buchbinder D: Incisions for access to craniomaxillofacial fractures. Atlas of the Oral and Maxillofacial Surgery Clinics of North America 1993;1:1.
45. Epply BL, Custer PL, Sadove AM: Cutaneous approaches to the orbital skeleton and periorbital structures. J Oral Maxillofac Surg 1990;48:842.
46. Casson PR, Bonanno PC, Converse JM: The midface degloving procedure. Plast Reconstr Surg 1977;53:102.
47. Powers M, Betts N: Devices which support dental fixation. Atlas of the Oral and Maxillofacial Surg Clinics of North America 1994;1:57.
48. Browning CW: Alloplastic materials in orbital repair. Am J Ophthalmol 1967;63:955.
49. Conforti PJ, Haug RH, Likavec M: The management of the maxillofacial trauma patient with closed head injury. J Oral Maxillofac Surg 1993;51:298.
50. Nordlichit S: Facial disfigurements and psychiatric sequelae. NY State J Med 1979;79:1282.
51. Coleman JJ: Osseous reconstruction of the midface and orbits. Clin Plast Surg 1994;21:113.
52. Zide MF: Pexing and presuturing for closure of traumatic soft tissue injuries. J Oral Maxillofac Surg 1994;52:698.
53. Shestak KC: Soft tissue reconstruction of craniofacial defects. Clin Plast Surg 1994;21:107.

Chapter 11
DENTOALVEOLAR TRAUMA

by

Michael Miloro
Peter E. Larsen

Introduction

Dentoalveolar injuries are encountered frequently by the oral and maxillofacial surgeon; yet in general, the possible complications resulting from either the injury or its treatment are commonly overlooked. Complications related to dentoalveolar trauma can be divided into late and early phases. Early complications are usually the result of undiagnosed injuries or improper treatment. In addition to these etiologic factors, late complications can also be the result of pathologic processes unique to the dentoalveolar unit.

THE SUBJECTS DISCUSSED IN THIS CHAPTER ARE:

- History, physical examination, and diagnosis
- Classification of dentoalveolar injuries
- General management guidelines and early complications
- Specific treatment protocols and early complications
  - Aspiration or ingestion of teeth
  - Injuries to the hard dental tissues and the pulp
  - Injuries to the periodontal tissues
  - Injuries to supporting bone
- Stabilization and fixation techniques and complications
  - Semirigid splinting
  - Rigid splinting
- Long-term complications and treatment
  - Pulpal necrosis
  - Pulp canal obliteration
  - Infection
  - Root resorption
  - Loss of marginal bone support
  - Damage to the underlying permanent teeth
  - Crown discoloration

Perhaps one of the more common injuries encountered by the oral and maxillofacial surgeon involves damage to the teeth and their supporting alveolar structures. Although these injuries usually occur alone, they may be associated with a variety of other facial fractures[1] in the multiple-trauma patient.[2] Many possible etiologic factors may be responsible for dentoalveolar trauma, including motor vehicle accidents, interpersonal violence, falls, sports-related injuries,[3] self-inflicted injury in the semicomatose patient,[4] iatrogenic injury during dentoalveolar surgery, and direct laryngoscopy during general anesthetic intubations.[5–7]

The dentition may be injured by *direct trauma* to the teeth themselves, or by *indirect trauma* secondary to blunt trauma to the face (e.g., chin) resulting in sudden and forceful contact of the mandibular teeth with the maxillary dentition. In general, direct trauma usually results in damage to the anterior teeth, and indirect trauma leads to damage to the posterior dentition. Commonly, dental trauma affects one tooth,[8] but multiple teeth are often involved. Trauma to the primary dentition predominantly involves the supporting structures, and injuries to the permanent teeth result in crown fractures.[9] It has been well documented that trauma to the maxillary central incisors, both primary and permanent, results from the relative prominence of their position within the oral cavity.[10, 11] A variety of factors are associated with a higher incidence of trauma to these teeth, including increased protrusion and overjet and insufficient lip closure over the incisors.[12, 13] Many studies have shown that dentoalveolar trauma is twice as common in patients with protrusive maxillary incisors.[9, 12]

The incidence of dentoalveolar trauma varies according the age of the patient, the etiologic event, and the presence or absence of other injuries, but various reports cite figures from 4% to 30% among pediatric populations.[14–16] Males are twice as likely as females to sustain injury to the permanent teeth (owing to more involvement in contact sports and aggressive behavior),[15, 17, 18] but the difference is less marked in the incidence of trauma to primary dentition.[19] In the pediatric population, the frequency of dental injuries increases as a child begins to walk.[20] The clinician must be alert to the possibility of child abuse in patients who have multiple injuries to various parts of the body in characteristic patterns and for whom discrepancies are apparent between the history and the physical findings.[21–23]

HISTORY, PHYSICAL EXAMINATION, AND DIAGNOSIS

The primary survey of the multiple-trauma patient with facial injuries includes the maxillofacial region, specifically with regard to airway management. As a result, dentoalveolar trauma may be regarded as a medical emergency, in so far as it affects the airway of the patient.[24] Once the airway has been secured, the patient is assessed for evidence of other life-threatening injuries and managed appropriately. Subsequently, in the secondary survey of specific areas of the body, the maxillofacial region is carefully examined for evidence of other injuries.

A comprehensive history should be obtained about the specifics of the mechanism of injury as well as the events surrounding it. Important information should be obtained regarding the preinjury status of the dentition, including dentoskeletal deformities, malocclusions, crossbites, and missing teeth. The mechanism of action might give clues about the injury, such as trauma to the chin that results in an associated mandibular subcondylar fracture and malocclusion. One critical aspect of the history of dentoalveolar trauma involves the time between injury and clinical presentation. In general, the earlier these injuries are treated, the better the eventual prognosis.[17]

A complete physical examination of the maxillofacial region should be performed, assessing both extraorally and intraorally. A meticulous examination of the dentition should involve assessment of the occlusion and determination of the presence of fractured teeth, missing teeth, or displaced teeth with documentation of the direction of displacement. The presence of a malocclusion may indicate dental trauma or skeletal fractures. All teeth, or portions of teeth, must be accounted for either at the scene of the injury or at the time of presentation. Teeth or tooth fragments may be located within the soft tissues of the lips, cheeks, floor of mouth, palate, or neck or within confined cavities such as the maxillary sinus, nasal cavity, and orbit. Teeth or fragments may also have been swallowed or aspirated into the esophagus, epiglottis, trachea, carina, or mainstem bronchi. A complete radiographic examination of the head, neck, chest, abdomen, and pelvis must be obtained to document the presence or absence of teeth or tooth fragments.[25, 26]

A variety of other diagnostic modalities may be used in the assessment of dentoalveolar trauma. Tooth mobility should be documented, as well as sensitivity or dullness to percussion, which may indicate a partially avulsed tooth or an alveolar fracture. Vitality testing may be performed in a number of ways. Thermal sensitivity to an ice chip, ethyl chloride, or warmed gutta-percha can be used,[27] but electric pulp testing may be easier to perform in the emergent setting, and perhaps easier to interpret. It should be recognized that any test of pulpal vitality shortly after dental trauma may be difficult to interpret, because acute neural disruption may cause decreased responses over the short term. The value of pulp testing lies in serial examinations after injury, which may indicate prognosis for long-term recovery and potential long-term complications.

Radiographic examination of dentoalveolar injuries can begin with routine head and neck plain films, including cervical spine radiographs, that may have been obtained for the assessment of other injuries. The common dentofacial radiographs, however, are panoramic, occlusal, and periapical views of involved areas. A panoramic radiograph can yield information regarding the status of the entire dentition, fractures of the mandible and maxilla, air-fluid levels in the maxillary sinus, the presence of foreign bodies, and a gross assessment of dentoalveolar injury, although a clear depiction of details is not possible, especially in the anterior jaws. The periapical radiographs are perhaps the most valuable in demonstrating the details of dental injuries, such as minimally displaced root fractures, associated alveolar fractures, and widening or absence of periodontal ligament spaces. An occlusal radiograph provides a greater area of view, is easy to perform, and yields detail similar to those of periapical films in depicting root fractures, alveolar fractures, and the presence of foreign bodies in the soft tissues.[28]

Classification of Dentoalveolar Injuries

A variety of classification systems have been developed to categorize injuries to the teeth and their supporting structures.[14, 17, 29–31] The two most commonly used classification systems are shown in Tables 11–1 and 11–2. This chapter presents management considerations according to the classification scheme proposed by Andreasen and Andreasen[17] (Table 11–2). The classification of dentoalveolar injuries becomes clinically useful for many reasons. The particular classification of injury aids in determining prognosis as well as the most appropriate treatment options. Additionally, a universal agreement upon classification enables clear communication among dentists, dental specialists, and physicians. The relative incidences of these injuries are shown in Table 11–3.

General Management Guidelines and Early Complications

As a result of the history, clinical examination, and radiographic evaluation, a preliminary diagnosis can be established and a treatment plan proposed. This plan should take a variety of factors into account, such as systemic as well as regional, head and neck injuries, the specific dentoalveolar injury, patient age, previous medical history, damage to the primary or permanent dentition, anticipated patient compliance with therapy, oral hygiene and periodontal status of the remaining dentition, tooth vitality, residual alveolar bony support, and soft tissue injuries, all of which serve as modifying variables.

As a general rule, the management of dentoalveolar injuries should begin promptly following diagnosis, because unnecessary delay could adversely affect the prognosis. After the assessment of other injuries, including tooth and jaw fractures (which potentially could be approached through existing lacerations), soft tissue wounds are addressed. Wound edges are reapproximated primarily if possible. The sequence of closure begins intraorally and proceeds extraorally, with copious irrigation.

In addition to the preceding treatment recommendations, consideration should be given to tetanus prophylaxis if clinically indicated, along with antibiotic coverage and chlorhexidine rinses. The patient should be advised about a soft diet. Close follow-up, both clinical and radiographic, is mandatory, because infections can be an early complication of dentoalveolar trauma.

Table 11–1. Ellis Classification of Dentoalveolar Injuries (1970)

Class I	Simple crown fracture with little or no dentin affected
Class II	Extensive crown fracture with considerable loss of dentin, but with the pulp not involved
Class III	Extensive crown fracture with considerable loss of dentin and pulp exposure
Class IV	A tooth devitalized by trauma with or without loss of tooth structure
Class V	Teeth lost as a result of trauma
Class VI	Root fracture with or without the loss of crown structure
Class VII	Displacement of the tooth with neither root nor crown fracture
Class VIII	Complete crown fracture and its replacement
Class IX	Traumatic injuries of primary teeth

Data from Ellis RG, Daury KW: The Classification and Treatment of Injuries to the Teeth of Children, ed 5. Chicago, Year Book Medical, 1970.

Specific Treatment Protocols and Early Complications

Aspiration or Ingestion of Teeth

A tooth, teeth, or dentoalveolar segment may be aspirated or ingested during an acute traumatic episode. These objects tend to lodge in the oropharynx or epiglottal region and are preferentially swallowed as opposed to aspirated. Because an aspirated foreign body may become a medical emergency, however, diligent examination is necessary to account for all missing teeth and to rule out their aspiration into the tracheobronchial tree. This is best done by a complete physical examination, with questions regarding the presence of teeth or tooth fragments at the scene of the trauma, head and neck radiographs, chest film (Fig. 11–1), abdominal films, and endoscopy (laryngoscopy, esophagoscopy, and/or bronchoscopy), with a pulmonary consultation and the use of antibiotic therapy if indicated. Teeth commonly lodge in the right main-stem bronchus, but they may be elsewhere, including the gastointestinal tract. Ingested teeth usually cause no untoward sequelae, and they can be observed radiographically until they have passed through the gastrointestinal tract.

Injuries to the Hard Dental Tissues and the Pulp

Crown Infraction

Crown infractions, which are merely "cracks" or incomplete fractures in the enamel surface without loss of tooth substance, are often difficult to diagnose, and

Table 11–2. Andreasen Classification of Dentoalveolar Injuries (1981)—Modification of the WHO System (1978)[31]

I. Injuries to the Hard Dental Tissues and the Pulp	
Crown infraction	An incomplete fracture (crack) of the enamel without loss of tooth substance
Uncomplicated crown fracture	A fracture confined to the enamel or involving enamel and dentin, but not exposing the pulp
Complicated crown fracture	A fracture involving enamel and dentin, and exposing the pulp
Uncomplicated crown-root fracture	A fracture involving enamel, dentin, and cementum, but not exposing the pulp
Complicated crown-root fracture	A fracture involving enamel, dentin, and cementum, and exposing the pulp
Root fracture	A fracture involving dentin, cementum, and the pulp
II. Injuries to the Periodontal Tissues	
Concussion	An injury to the tooth-supporting structures *without* abnormal loosening or displacement of the tooth but with marked reaction to percussion
Subluxation (loosening)	An injury to the tooth-supporting structures *with* abnormal loosening but without displacement of the tooth
Intrusive luxation (central dislocation)	Displacement of the tooth into the bone This injury is accompanied by comminution or fracture of the alveolar socket
Extrusive luxation (peripheral dislocation, partial avulsion)	Partial displacement of the tooth out of its socket
Lateral luxation	Displacement of the tooth in a direction other than axially This is accompanied by comminution or fracture of the alveolar socket
Exarticulation (complete avulsion)	Complete displacement of the tooth out of its socket
III. Injuries to the Supporting Bone	
Comminution of alveolar socket	Crushing and compression of the alveolar socket This condition is found together with intrusive and lateral luxation
Fracture of alveolar socket wall	A fracture confined to the facial or lingual socket wall
Fracture of alveolar process	A fracture of the alveolar process that may or may not involve the alveolar socket
Fracture of mandible or maxilla	A fracture involving the base of the mandible or maxilla and often the alveolar process (jaw fracture) The fracture may or may not involve the alveolar socket
IV. Injuries to the Gingiva or Oral Mucosa	
Laceration of gingiva or oral mucosa	A shallow or deep wound in the mucosa resulting from a tear, and usually produced by a sharp object
Contusion of gingiva or oral mucosa	A bruise usually produced by impact from a blunt object and not accompanied by a break in the mucosa, usually causing submucosal hemorrhage
Abrasion of gingiva or oral mucosa	A superficial wound produced by rubbing or scraping of the mucosa, leaving a raw, bleeding surface

Adapted from Andreasen JO, Andreasen FM: Textbook and Color Atlas of Traumatic Injuries to the Teeth, ed 3. St Louis, CV Mosby, 1994.

they rarely require specific immediate treatment. It should be recognized that these cracks may indicate damage to the underlying supporting structures, and associated dentoalveolar injuries must be ruled out. As a rule, enamel infractions in the permanent dentition do not require treatment. A late complication of a crown infraction, however, is pulpal necrosis. Therefore, periodic vitality testing should be performed to monitor for signs of pulpal changes. Patients may desire cosmetic restoration in cases of anterior crown infractions.

Table 11–3. Incidence of Dentoalveolar Injuries

Type of Injury	Incidence in Primary Dentition (%)	Incidence in Permanent Dentition (%)
Crown fractures	4–38	26–76
Crown-root fractures	2	5
Root fractures	2–4	0.5–7
Luxation injuries	62–69	15–40
Avulsion injuries	7–13	0.5–16
Alveolar fractures	7	16

Crown Fractures

Crown fractures that involve enamel only may require recontouring sharp edges or cosmetic restoration. Periodic vitality testing is indicated. Crown fractures account for one fourth to three fourths of dental injuries in the permanent dentition and for up to 40% in the primary dentition.

With dentin exposure, a prompt (within 24 hours) attempt should be made to cover the exposed dentin with a calcium hydroxide–based material and provide an acid-etched composite restoration. This technique

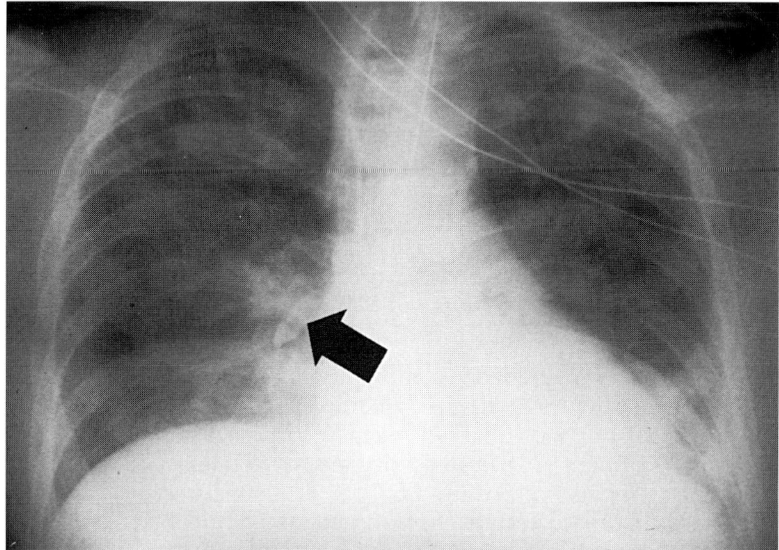

Figure 11–1. Chest radiograph showing a tooth lodged in the right mainstem bronchus (*arrow*).

allows for the deposition of secondary dentin. This urgency in treatment is necessary to prevent posttraumatic pulpal necrosis.

There are several options in the management of crown fractures with pulpal exposure. For such a fracture in the permanent dentition, maintenance of the tooth is paramount, and extraction is reserved as a last resort. Pulp capping may be performed within 24 hours after injury, and only with small pulpal exposures.[32] A cervical pulpotomy, which removes only 2 to 4 mm of pulpal tissue in the region of the exposure, can be used between 24 and 96 hours after injury for recently erupted teeth with incompletely closed apices, because there is sufficient pulpal tissue to allow for secondary dentin formation as well as root development and apex closure, with the use of calcium hydroxide paste.[32–38] A conventional pulpotomy, in contrast, removes pulpal tissue to the level of the cemento-enamel junction. Either pulpotomy procedure should be considered temporary, and endodontic therapy is subsequently indicated, because calcium hydroxide pulpotomies can result in pulp canal obliteration with resultant inability to perform endodontic therapy if the tooth becomes symptomatic. In mature teeth with fully formed apices, significant pulpal exposure, and delayed presentation (more than 96 hours), pulpectomy is indicated, with total pulpal extirpation and endodontic filling with gutta-percha.

With regard to the primary dentition, pulpal exposure usually warrants extraction, because of the relatively small tooth size and large pulp chambers, as well as a lack of patient cooperation, although pulp capping, pulpotomy, or pulpectomy procedures may be performed.

Serial follow-up examinations are indicated in all cases of dental trauma. It should be recognized that normal pulpal sensibility may be transiently decreased for 6 to 8 weeks following trauma; therefore, pulp vitality testing during this period is unreliable. Radiographs should be obtained in approximately 6 weeks and then as guided by clinical examination.

Crown-Root Fractures

Crown-root fractures account for 5% of injuries to the permanent dentition and 2% to the primary dentition. The majority of primary teeth with crown-root fractures should be extracted.[39] The management of these injuries in the permanent dentition depends on the level of fracture—specifically, whether it occurs in the coronal, middle, or apical third of the tooth. Coronal fractures usually necessitate removal of the fractured segment, possible crown lengthening procedures, pulpectomy, and prosthetic restoration. Pulpal necrosis has a lower incidence with fractures of the middle and apical thirds; therefore, attempts should be made to reduce and stabilize the fractured segments. This fixation is maintained for 8 to 16 weeks. If the segments have not healed by this time, extraction is indicated. Additionally, the option of hemisection should be considered in selected cases.[40] Failure to recognize or properly treat crown-root fractures can lead to infection and surrounding bone loss.

Root Fractures

With regard to root fractures in the primary dentition, it may be appropriate to remove the mobile crown segment and leave the root segment in place to be resorbed by eruption of the permanent dentition, in order to prevent injury to the underlying, developing succedaneous tooth.

As with crown-root fractures, treatment of root fractures in the permanent dentition[41] is guided by the level of the fracture. Fractures in the apical third of the root require minimal treatment if nonmobile. For fractures in the coronal portion of the root, (1) the coronal segment is stabilized rigidly, (2) both segments are removed, or (3) the apical segment is maintained with endodontic therapy and prosthetic restoration. The prognosis for middle-third root fractures depends on the extent of displacement and the mobility of the segments.[42] The fractured segments must be realigned and rigidly fixed for 2 to 4 months. Any vertical root fracture is usually managed with surgical extraction. Serial clinical and radiographic evaluations are indicated for all root fractures, and if the segments do not heal after an appropriate fixation period, extraction is indicated. Infection and bone loss are potential complications.

Injuries to the Periodontal Tissues

Concussion

A *concussion* is defined as an injury to the tooth-supporting structures without abnormal loosening or displacement but with marked reaction to percussion. Minimal treatment is indicated for concussive injuries, although selective opposing occlusal adjustment to eliminate continued trauma from occlusion should be considered, as well as periodic vitality testing. Long-term complications of pulpal necrosis warrant endodontic therapy.

Subluxation (Loosening)

A *subluxation* is an injury with abnormal mobility but without clinical or radiographic evidence of tooth displacement. Usually, conservative treatment with soft diet and occlusal adjustments is all that is necessary for subluxation injuries. For a tooth with significant mobility, splinting to adjacent teeth for 10 to 14 days may be required. Failure to properly treat subluxation may lead to tooth loss.

Intrusive Luxation (Central Dislocation)

Intrusive injury ranges from minimal tooth displacement to complete tooth impaction within the alveolus. Treatment of intrusive injuries is controversial,[43] but suggested therapeutic modalities include (1) no treatment, allowing the tooth to erupt spontaneously, (2) gentle orthodontic repositioning over 3 to 4 weeks,[44] and (3) immediate surgical repositioning and splinting to adjacent teeth. Endodontic therapy may also be necessary.

Management of the intruded deciduous tooth is also controversial. Some surgeons advocate the spontaneous eruption of the tooth or orthodontic guidance, because removal might jeopardize the permanent tooth.[45] Others, however, prefer prompt extraction, because the retained deciduous tooth is likely to damage the underlying succedaneous tooth.[46]

Extrusive Luxation (Peripheral Dislocation, Partial Avulsion)

The treatment for the traumatically extruded or displaced permanent tooth is prompt digital repositioning and nonrigid splint stabilization for 10 to 14 days, in order to allow some physiologic movement within the alveolus and to prevent ankylosis. Routine follow-up examinations are necessary, because a high percentage of these injuries require endodontic therapy.[47] Associated gingival lacerations should be sutured.

The management of an extruded primary tooth is controversial, with some authorities advocating observation, and others recommending immediate extraction to prevent injury to the underlying permanent tooth.[17] Perhaps the most appropriate approach should be to extract the tooth, because children can be uncooperative, and it is difficult to stabilize a tooth and expect the child to comply with a liquid or soft diet.

Lateral Luxation

Lateral luxation commonly involves the maxillary central incisor, such that the crown is displaced lingually and the root is displaced labially through the apical alveolar plate. Usually, the tooth can be digitally repositioned and stabilized for 2 to 8 weeks, depending on the degree of displacement as well as on the extent of the associated alveolar fracture. As with intrusive injuries, there is a 10% incidence of marginal bone loss. Periodic evaluation is necessary to assess the need for endodontic therapy stemming from necrosis.

Exarticulation (Complete Avulsion)

The most important prognostic indicator for the avulsed tooth is the time the tooth has been out of the alveolus.[48–51] The major complication of exarticulation is root resorption. It has been shown that 90% of teeth reimplanted within 30 minutes from injury had no evidence of root resorption, but that more than 95% of teeth reimplanted after 2 hours showed root resorption.[49] Additionally, the care and method of storage for the avulsed tooth are critical factors in the success of reimplantation. If possible, temporary reimplantation by the patient is advisable; however, if this is not possible, the patient should be instructed to store the tooth in saliva or in a container with milk or a special solution. Milk serves to preserve the viable periodontal fibroblasts and cementoblasts and therefore to prolong the time the tooth can remain outside the alveolus.[52–54] The tooth should be manipulated by the crown only, with every attempt made to avoid direct contact with the root surface. The root can be gently irrigated to remove blood and debris.

To reduce complications such as root resorption, infection, and instability, the following factors should be considered prior to reimplanting an avulsed tooth:[17]

1. The avulsed tooth should be without advanced periodontal disease.
2. The alveolar socket should be reasonably intact in order to provide a seat for the avulsed tooth.
3. There should be no orthodontic considerations, such as significant crowding of the teeth.
4. The extraalveolar period should be considered; i.e., periods exceeding 2 hours are usually associated with marked root resorption.
5. The stage of root development should be evaluated. Survival of the pulp is possible in teeth with incomplete root formation if replantation is accomplished within 2 hours after injury.

The tooth should be replanted and stabilized with a nonrigid splint for 10 to 14 days.[55] In the event of a concomitant alveolar fracture, a rigid splint should be used for 3 to 4 weeks.[17] A postimplantation radiograph should be obtained to verify the position of the tooth within the alveolus. The tooth should be relieved from the occlusion, and the patient instructed about a soft diet.

Standard management considerations for avulsed teeth have changed significantly, in terms of methods of tooth storage, treatment of the root surface, treatment of the pulp, and length of splinting time. Krasner[56] has proposed a specific treatment regimen for the avulsed tooth, based upon whether the tooth is primary or permanent, whether the apex is open or closed, and the amount of time passed since the avulsion occurred (extraoral time); this regimen is shown in Table 11–4.

Injuries to Supporting Bone

Comminution of the Alveolar Socket or Fracture of the Alveolar Socket Wall

Both alveolar socket comminution and alveolar socket wall fracture are common in lateral luxation injuries and usually occur in the anterior of the jaw. These fractures are difficult to diagnose radiographically but may be palpated manually during mobility assessment of the involved tooth. Treatment consists of digital repositioning, with pressure placed over the involved alveolar fracture site, followed by splint placement and immobilization for 3 to 4 weeks, with the patient instructed about a soft diet.

Fracture of the Alveolar Process

Alveolar process fracture may present a diagnostic dilemma, because radiographic examination may be

Table 11–4. Specific Treatment Regimen for Avulsed Teeth

Apex	Extraoral Time (min)	Treatment
		Permanent and Primary Teeth
Closed	<15	1. Rinse or soak tooth with physiologic saline or Hank's Balanced Solution* to remove debris. 2. Flush socket with sterile saline to remove debris. 3. Reimplant tooth and functionally splint for a maximum of 2 weeks. 4. Remove pulp within 1 week.
	15–120	1. Soak tooth in Hank's Balanced Solution* for 30 minutes. 2. Flush socket with sterile saline to remove debris and blood clot. 3. Reimplant tooth and functionally splint for a maximum of 2 weeks. 4. Remove pulp within 1 week.
	>120	1. Perform root canal treatment extraorally. 2. Soak tooth in a saturated citric acid solution for 5 minutes. 3. Rinse off citric acid with physiologic saline, and soak tooth in a 1% stannous fluoride solution for 5 minutes. 4. Reimplant tooth and functionally splint for 2 weeks.
		Permanent Teeth
Open	<15	1. Rinse or soak tooth with physiologic saline or Hank's Balanced Solution* to remove debris. 2. Soak tooth in a 5% doxycycline solution for 5 minutes. 3. Flush socket with sterile saline to remove debris and blood clot. 4. Reimplant tooth and functionally splint for a maximum of 2 weeks. 5. Test for return of normal vitality response every month.
	15–120	1. Soak tooth in Hank's Balanced Solution* for 30 minutes. 2. Soak tooth in a 5% doxycycline solution for 5 minutes. 3. Flush socket with sterile saline to remove debris and blood clot. 4. Reimplant tooth and functionally splint for a maximum of 2 weeks. 5. Test for return of normal vitality response every month.
	>120	1. Remove pulp extraorally. 2. Soak tooth in a saturated citric acid solution for 5 minutes. 3. Rinse off citric acid with physiologic saline, and soak tooth in a 1% stannous fluoride solution for 5 minutes. 4. Soak tooth in a 5% doxycycline solution for 5 minutes. 5. Dry canal with paper points and place calcium hydroxide in root canal. 6. Flush socket with sterile saline to remove debris and clot. 7. Functionally splint for a maximum of 2 weeks. 8. Check for radiographic evidence of apexification.

*In Save·A·Tooth, The Emergency Tooth Preserving System (Biological Rescue Products, Inc., Philadelphia, PA).[69, 70]
Adapted from Krasner P: Modern treatment of avulsed teeth by emergency physicians. Am J Emerg Med 1994;12:241.

inconclusive. The clinical examination for such injuries involves assessment of the common sites: the labial surface of the anterior maxillary alveolus and either the labial or lingual apical regions of the mandibular arch. Alveolar process fractures may involve one or more teeth, and the diagnosis becomes more apparent when a segment containing two or more teeth is jointly mobile. The primary treatment goal involves maintenance of the blood supply to the fractured osseous segment to prevent necrosis. The area should be irrigated gently to remove small fragments of bone or other foreign body debris. Usually, a closed reduction of the alveolar fracture along with repositioning of the involved teeth is the appropriate treatment. Occasionally, interferences in the apical region may prevent manipulation of the osseous segment into proper orientation, and an open reduction may be indicated with or without the use of internal fixation. Soft tissue injuries should be carefully repaired. Stabilization with rigid splinting for 4 weeks is required. Additionally, any occlusal interferences should be relieved completely. There is an urgency to the treatment of these injuries, because the incidence of pulpal necrosis and periapical inflammation is reduced significantly if the teeth and alveolar segments are splinted within 1 hour after injury.[17]

Early complications of alveolar process fracture include infection and hard and soft tissue necrosis. The severity of the injury most often dictates the complications. Other complications, such as tooth mobility and malocclusion, can be avoided by following the recommended protocol.

Stabilization and Fixation Techniques and Complications

The main objective of splinting for luxation or avulsion injuries is to stabilize the dental segment in order to allow pulpal and periodontal healing *(soft tissue healing).* The luxated or avulsed tooth should be stabilized for 2 weeks or less,[57, 58] with a splint that allows physiologic movement.[59] Stabilization of an associated bony fracture must be rigid (no physiologic movement) and should be maintained for a longer time (approximately 4 weeks) to allow for *bone tissue healing.* Failure to achieve adequate stabilization can lead to nonunion malocclusion. The requirements for an acceptable splint have been established.[17] An ideal splint for an avulsed or luxated tooth

- Allows direct application in the mouth without delay for laboratory procedures
- Does not traumatize the tooth during application
- Immobilizes the injured tooth in a normal position
- Provides adequate fixation throughout the entire period of immobilization
- Neither damages the gingiva nor predisposes to caries
- Does not interfere with occlusion or articulation
- Does not interfere with endodontic therapy if needed
- Preferably fulfills aesthetic demands

A variety of options exist for the management of dentoalveolar injuries with different indications and applications as well as the preference of the surgeon employing them.

Semirigid Splinting

One popular technique is the application of an acid-etched composite resin splint with or without an accessory wire (or fish line) bridge (Fig. 11–2). Such a splint may be used for the single or multiple luxation injury as well as an associated alveolar fracture. The acrylic serves as a semirigid splint, which allows physiologic movement of the teeth within the alveolus, thereby preventing the development of bony ankylosis. As commonly employed for avulsed primary teeth, a silk suture may be placed over the crown of a tooth in a figure-of-eight fashion, engaging the buccal and lingual gingivae. The major complication of this technique is instability due to poor acid-etch technique or not using an accessory wire. Also, one must evaluate the occlusion following placement of the composite on mandibular anterior teeth, to prevent trauma from the opposing arch.

Rigid Splinting

The use of Erich arch bars with wire ligature fixation is a common technique for an avulsed or luxated tooth with associated alveolar fractures, which require rigid stabilization. The major complication of this technique is tooth extrusion. Therefore, the circumdental wires should be placed incisally to the cingulum of the teeth to prevent extrusive forces as they are tightened. Many other interdental wiring techniques have been used.[60] The Essig wire is indicated for multiple luxations with or without an associated alveolar fracture. Other wiring techniques are loop wiring, figure-of-eight wiring, and Risdon wires, primarily for the patient with mixed dentition.

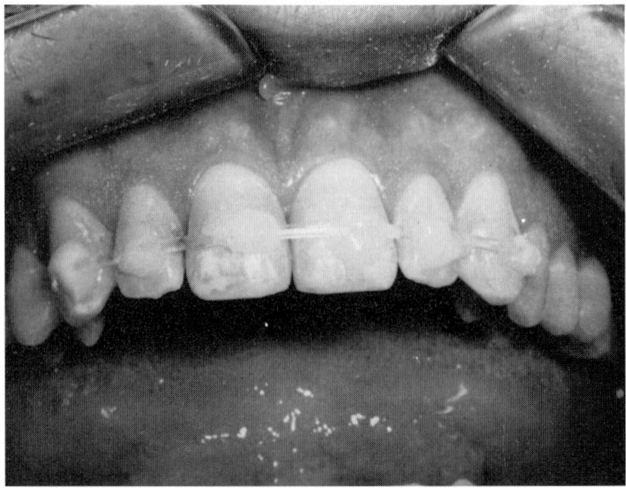

Figure 11–2. Semirigid splint fabricated with 50-lb test monofilament fishing line stabilized with acrylic resin.

Table 11–5. Classification of Pulpal Response After Tooth Reimplantation

I	Regular tubular reparative dentin
II	Irregular reparative dentin with diminished tubular structures
III	Irregular reparative dentin with encapsulated cells (osteodentin)
IV	Irregular immature bone
V	Regular lamellated bone or cementum
VI	Internal resorption
VII	Aplasia (pulp degeneration and necrosis)

Long-Term Complications and Treatment

A wide range of dentinal and pulpal responses may occur following replantation of avulsed teeth.[61, 62] Their classification is shown in Table 11–5.

In considering the periodontal reactions to exarticulation and reimplantation, Andreasen and colleagues[17, 63, 64] have shown the following possible histologic outcomes:

Healing with a Normal Periodontal Ligament. This response represents the normal spontaneous recovery of the periodontal supporting attachments to the tooth.

Healing with Ankylosis (Replacement Resorption). The development of ankylosis of permanent teeth usually does not present a major problem and needs to be addressed only if resorption has led to mobility and requires extraction of the involved tooth.

Inflammatory Resorption. One of the major complications associated with exarticulation injuries is root resorption. Histologically, there is resorption of cementum and dentin with associated inflammation of the periodontal ligament. Radiographic signs of resorption may be evident as early as 2 weeks after injury, usually in the apical third of the root.[49] Inflammatory root resorption usually becomes evident within the first year, but a more rapid course may result in loss of the tooth as early as 3 months after reimplantation. It must be remembered that rigid splinting may increase the amount of root resorption.[64] Reimplanted teeth with complete root formation should undergo endodontic therapy, which may arrest the process of root resorption.[65] Andreasen and Andreasen[17] recommend root canal therapy within 2 weeks of reimplantation, except in teeth with wide-open apices, to allow the undisturbed reattachment of periodontal ligament fibers.

Pulpal Necrosis

In general, any type of dentoalveolar injury, including crown and root fractures, luxations, and avulsions may result in a variety of possible adverse outcomes. Pulpal necrosis may occur after 15% to 95% of luxation injuries of the permanent dentition[66, 67] (Table 11–6). The incidence in the primary dentition is similar to that in the permanent dentition. Pulpal necrosis is usually asymptomatic but may be associated with pain upon mastication. Also, there may be mobility, tooth discoloration (especially in primary teeth), or fistula formation.

The interpretation of vitality testing in the acutely traumatized tooth may be difficult, but an obvious change from a positive to a negative response is likely to signify pulpal necrosis. The most common radiographic finding is periapical rarefaction, which usually develops within 2 months of injury.

The type of injury is the most important factor in the development of pulpal necrosis. Avulsion of a tooth results in a 100% incidence of pulpal necrosis if the tooth is out of the alveolus for more than 2 hours.[17] Of the luxation injuries, intrusive injury results in the highest frequency of pulp necrosis, followed by extrusive luxations and subluxations.[68, 69] Overall, the incidence of pulpal necrosis following luxation injuries in teeth with open apices is 8%, and with closed apices is 38%.[70]

Pulpal necrosis may also result from fractures of the teeth. The incidence of pulpal necrosis following enamel fractures is less than 5%, dentin exposure re-

Table 11–6. Incidence of Complications (%) After Dentoalveolar Trauma

Type of Injury	Pulp Necrosis	Pulp Canal Obliteration	Root Resorption	Loss of Supporting Bone
Crown infraction	0–3.5	0	0	—
Enamel fracture	0.2–1.0	0.5	0.2	—
Enamel-dentin fracture	1–6	0	0	—
Root fracture	20–44	69	60	—
Luxation	15–95	6–35	1–18	10
Concussion	3	—	—	—
Subluxation	6	—	—	—
Extrusive luxation	26	—	—	—
Lateral luxation	58	—	—	—
Intrusive luxation	85	—	—	—
Exarticulation	—	—	75–95	—
Alveolar fracture	5–38	2–24	0–4	11–18

Adapted from Andreasen JO, Andreasen FM: Textbook and Color Atlas of Traumatic Injuries to the Teeth, ed 3. St Louis, CV Mosby, 1994.

sults in a 7% incidence, and pulp exposures and root fractures result in a 20% to 30% incidence.[17] The incidence of pulpal necrosis increases significantly if treatment is delayed for more than 24 hours.[71, 72] Overall, these injuries are associated with an incidence of pulpal necrosis between 5% and 10%,[66, 73] depending on the amount of dentin exposed as well as on the associated dentoalveolar injury. For example, the incidence of pulpal necrosis and pulp canal obliteration increases with crown fractures in the permanent dentition with open or closed apices from concussion, subluxation, extrusion, lateral luxation, and intrusion injuries. Crown fractures with pulpal exposure result in pulpal necrosis in approximately 25% to 30% of cases.[74] With crown-root fractures in the coronal third, the incidence of pulpal necrosis approaches 50%, whereas with those in the middle or apical third, it is 15% to 20%. The incidence of pulpal necrosis with root fractures is usually between 20% and 25%, but partial or complete pulpal canal obliteration may be much more common.[75] The diagnosis of pulpal necrosis warrants either endodontic therapy or tooth extraction.

Pulp Canal Obliteration

Pulp canal obliteration results from accelerated secondary dentin deposition (Fig. 11–3) and commonly (6% to 35%) follows avulsive or luxation injuries to the permanent dentition.[73, 76] The obliteration can be *partial*,[77] in which the apical portion of the canal remains visible, or *total*, in which the entire pulp chamber and canal are absent.[78] Clinically, the tooth has a yellow crown discoloration, and vitality is decreased or absent.

Radiographically, the obliteration begins in the coronal portion of the tooth and progresses apically, although there is a persistent narrow pulp chamber, even when total obliteration is apparent radiographically.

Pulpal necrosis may occur secondary to pulp canal obliteration but is uncommon (approximately 1% incidence).[79] There is controversy regarding the management of pulp canal obliteration, with some authorities advocating prompt endodontic therapy for prophylactic reasons and others utilizing frequent careful clinical and radiographic assessments to identify the first signs and symptoms of pulpal necrosis and then performing root canal therapy if indicated. Obviously, performing endodontic therapy on a tooth with pulp canal obliteration is technically difficult and may require several appointments; however, the success of endodontic therapy is approximately 80%.[80] Primary teeth with pulp canal obliteration should be extracted.[81]

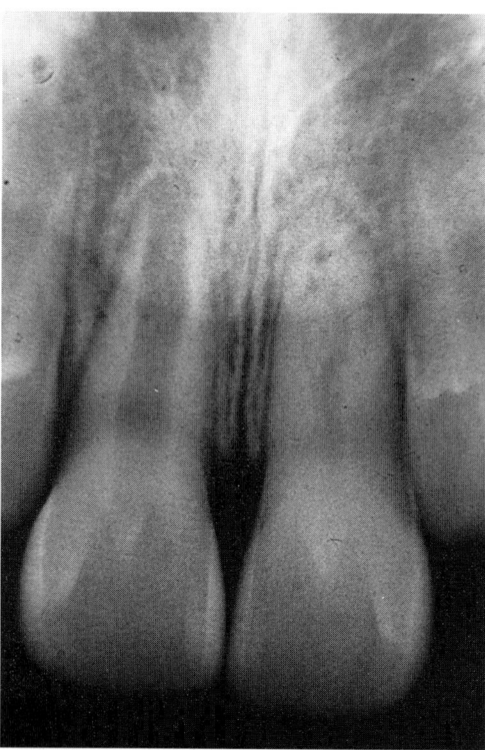

Figure 11–3. A permanent central incisor demonstrating pulp canal obliteration.

Infection

Although infection may follow any facial injury, its occurrence with an isolated dentoalveolar injury is usually low. There is the potential that foreign bodies or bony spicules that were inadequately débrided may result in a localized cellulitis or abscess. Additionally, the oral hygiene of the patient significantly influences the incidence of infection. Inability to stabilize and fix a loose tooth or dentoalveolar segment likely results in fibrous tissue formation, with a malunion or nonunion, and possible infection secondary to mobility problems. This may ultimately result in the loss of the tooth/or dentoalveolar segment.

Root Resorption

External Root Resorption

The development of external root resorption (Fig. 11–4) is a potential complication of any type of dentoalveolar trauma but is most commonly associated with luxation injuries. Presumably, the resorptive process results from damage to the periodontal tissues, root surface, and pulp, leading to an inflammatory response and subsequent resorption of the root via the exposed dentinal tubules. Radiographically, the resorptive process is characterized by a progressively increased radiolucency of the root surface as well as the surrounding alveolar bone. Generally, these radiographic changes occur between 2 and 12 weeks after injury. The incidence of resorption has been shown to vary between 75% and 95% following exarticulation injuries.[17] Although a variety of factors may contribute to the development of root resorption, the length of time the tooth is out of the alveolus is the most critical. The use of various treatment solutions for avulsed teeth prior to reimplantation has been shown to decrease the incidence of resorption.[82] In general, the treatment and prognosis depend on the type of resorption. Andreasen and Andreasen[17] have classified external root resorption into three distinct types, surface, replacement, and inflammatory.

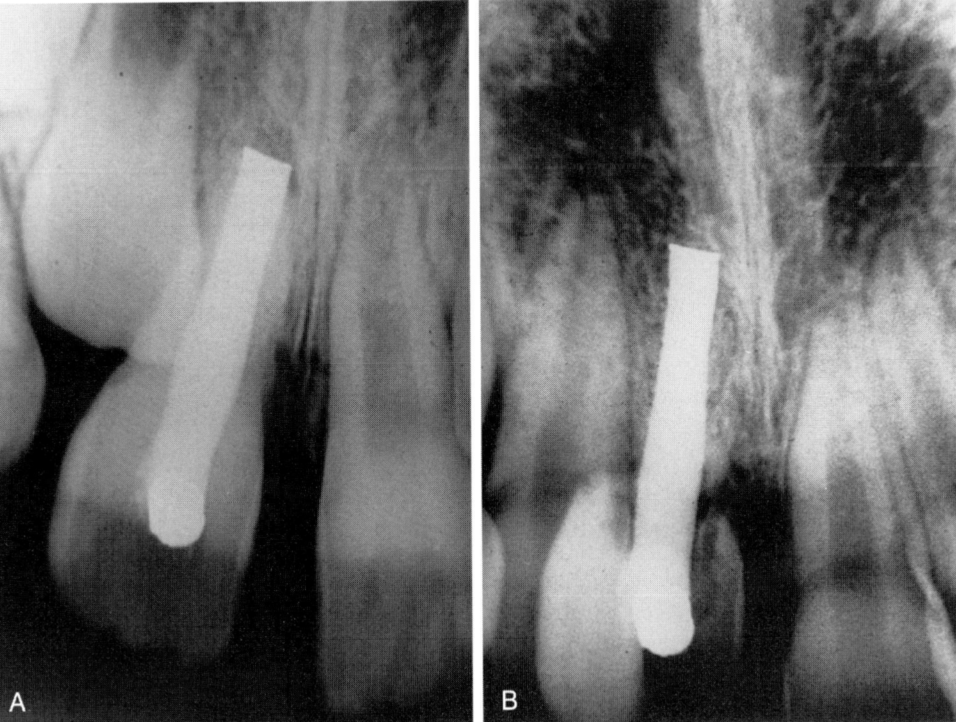

Figure 11–4. *A,* A permanent central incisor that was avulsed and reimplanted after placement of gutta percha. *B,* At 3-year follow-up, external replacement resorption has destroyed the entire root.

Surface Resorption. Root fractures lead commonly to external or surface resorption but uncommonly to external and internal replacement and inflammatory resorption. Surface resorption is characterized by superficial resorption of cementum and the development of lacunae, with subsequent replacement by newly formed cementum. Surface resorption is usually self-limited and undergoes spontaneous resolution. This injury is difficult to visualize radiographically and usually does not affect prognosis.

Replacement Resorption. Replacement resorption, or ankylosis, occurs when there is a direct union between bone and root surface cementum, and it commonly follows luxation injuries. Radiographically, there is loss of the periodontal ligament space and continued root resorption. This process likely inhibits physiologic movement of the tooth and prevents continued eruption. In cases with progressive infraocclusion of the ankylosed tooth, orthodontic or prosthetic reconstruction may be considered, but surgical extraction is usually indicated.

Inflammatory Resorption. The inflammatory resorptive pattern results in external resorption of both cementum and dentin with inflammatory changes in the periodontal tissues (Fig. 11–5). In general, this type of resorption is more common in primary teeth, because of the presence of thin dentinal walls and wide-open dentinal tubules.[68] Primary teeth with inflammatory root resorption should be extracted.[17] The treatment of choice for permanent teeth is endodontic therapy to remove the necrotic pulp and bacteria. The use of calcium hydroxide has been shown to be beneficial in the healing and arrest of inflammatory resorption,[83] and should be used prior to filling the canal with gutta-percha.

Internal Root Resorption

Internal root resorption (Fig. 11–6) is less common than external root resorption. This type of resorption occurs commonly after root fractures, but extremely uncommonly following luxation injuries.[84, 85] Radio-

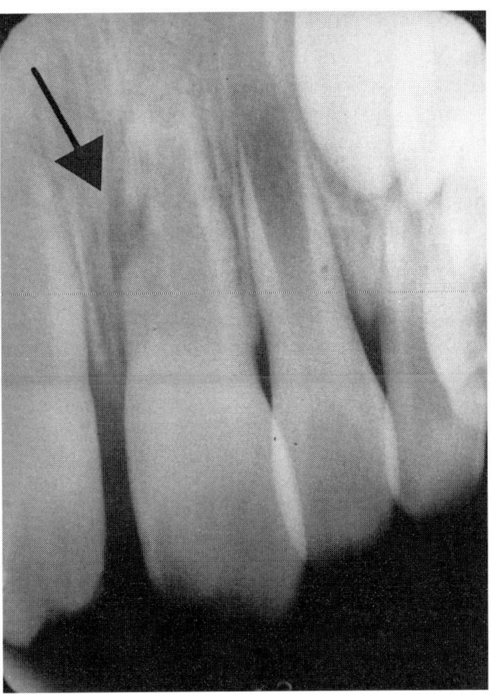

Figure 11–5. An example of external inflammatory resorption on the mesial root surface of the central incisor (*arrow*).

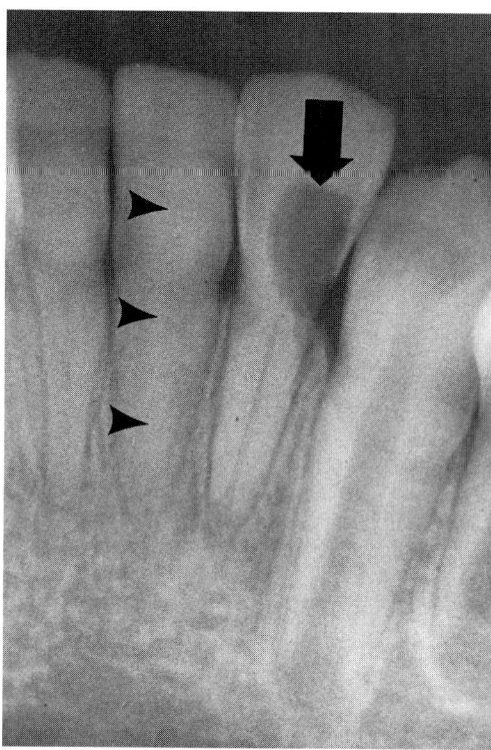

Figure 11–6. Radiograph demonstrating internal root resorption of the mandibular lateral incisor (*arrow*) and pulp canal obliteration of the central incisor (*arrowheads*).

graphically, a diagnostic dilemma exists, because a suggestion of internal resorption might prove to be superimposed external resorption if the radiograph was taken from another direction. Internal resorption is classified into two types, replacement and inflammatory.

Replacement Resorption. A replacement resorptive pattern is characterized by an irregular enlargement of the pulp chamber with replacement by bone and resultant canal obliteration. There is continued bony remodeling, which results in dentinal resorption. Most cases of internal resorption should be treated with routine endodontic therapy. The prognosis for these injuries is not known.

Inflammatory Resorption. Radiographically, this type of resorption is characterized by dentin resorption in an oval pattern with an associated inflammatory response of the pulpal tissues. This pattern continues until the pulp is extirpated endodontically.

Endodontic therapy should be instituted as soon as the diagnosis of internal resorption has been made, in order to arrest the progressive nature of this process. Primary teeth with internal resorption should be extracted to avoid a potential pathologic root fracture and subsequent difficult extraction. Prognosis for inflammatory resorption is not known.

Loss of Marginal Bone Support

Dentoalveolar injuries result in damage to the periodontal tissues, including the marginal supporting periodontium. The resulting inflammatory response causes resorption of the traumatized marginal crestal bone and interim replacement by granulation tissue. Over the next 2 months, the periodontium is repaired, with the development of new bone, as well as the reattachment of periodontal ligament fibers. The development of localized infection, as a result of poor oral hygiene or for other reasons, may alter this sequence, and permanent loss of marginal bone support may occur. Marginal bone loss occurs approximately 10% of the time with luxation injuries.

Damage to the Underlying Permanent Teeth

Trauma to the primary dentition may result in a variety of changes within the primary tooth, including pulpal necrosis, crown discoloration, pulp canal obliteration, and ankylosis. Such changes may lead to secondary damage to the underlying permanent tooth, possibly causing permanent crown discoloration, crown malformations with enamel hypoplasia[86] (Fig. 11–7), root developmental delay, dilaceration of the roots,[87] or delayed or prevented eruption of the permanent tooth. Inflammatory changes with necrosis of the pulp of the primary tooth may occur because of hypomineralization or dilaceration upon the tooth's exposure to the oral cavity.[88] Areas of hypomineralization should be treated with a composite restoration soon after eruption. Premature loss of a primary tooth presents potential problems related to space maintenance for eruption of the permanent tooth. If necessary, the space can be maintained through appliances, orthodontics, or prosthetic methods.

Crown Discoloration

Color changes to the crown of a tooth occur commonly following trauma, because of the accumulation

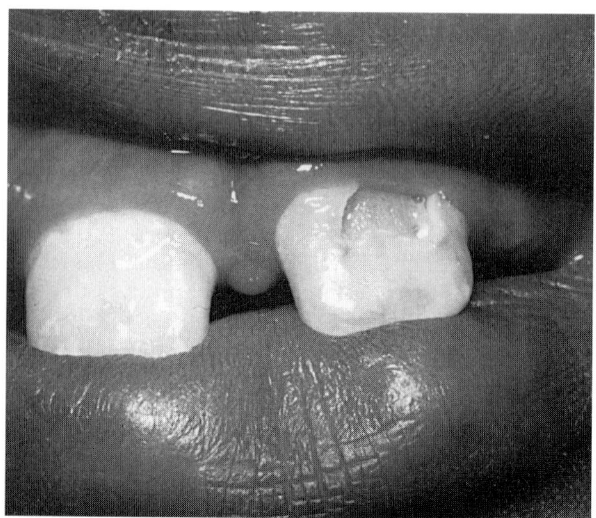

Figure 11–7. Enamel hypoplasia of a permanent central incisor secondary to an intrusion of a primary incisor.

of erythrocytes in the pulp chamber. Although there are no specific color patterns for individual injuries, and variations occur between primary and permanent teeth, most changes begin with a pink appearance due to hemoglobin. As the hemoglobin is metabolized, a variety of other changes may occur. Early color changes may be reversible,[89] but later discolorations are usually irreversible. These later color changes include a yellow discoloration, which may indicate pulp canal obliteration, and a gray color, which might suggest pulpal necrosis. Transillumination may reveal decreased lucency of a tooth owing to pigment accumulation. Crown discoloration can occur in the absence of radiographic changes but may be an indication for endodontic therapy in order to perform nonvital bleaching with sodium perborate for aesthetic reasons.[90, 91] Results have been acceptable or good in approximately 80% of treated teeth; in approximately 30% of cases, discoloration recurs within 5 years.[92]

References

1. Silvennoinen U, Lindqvist C, Oikarinen K: Dental injuries in association with mandibular condyle fractures. Endodont Dental Traumatol 1993;9:254.
2. Dierks EJ: Management of associated dental injuries in maxillofacial trauma. Otolaryngol Clin North Am 1991;24:165.
3. Ellis E, Moos Kf, El-Attar A: Ten years after mandibular fractures: An analysis of 2137 cases. Oral Surg Oral Med Oral Pathol 1985;59:120.
4. Piercell MP, White DE, Nelson R: Prevention of self-inflicted trauma in semicomatose patients. J Oral Surg 1974;32:903.
5. Lockhart PB, Feldbau EV, Gabel RA, et al: Dental complications during and after tracheal intubation. J Am Dent Assoc 1986;112:480.
6. Wareing MJ, Fisher EW, Manning RH, et al: The extraction and re-implantation of teeth for difficult laryngoscopy. J Laryngol Otol 1994;108:44.
7. Watanabe S, Suga A, Asakura N, et al: Determination of the distance between the laryngoscope blade and the upper incisors during direct laryngoscopy: Comparisons of a curved, angulated straight, and two straight blades. Anesth Analg 1994;79:638.
8. Grundy JR: The incidence of fractured incisors. Br Dent J 1959;106:312.
9. Andreason JO: Etiology and pathogenesis of traumatic dental injuries: A clinical study of 1,298 cases. Scand J Dent Res 1970;78:329.
10. Berkowitz R, Ludwig S, Johnson R: Dental trauma in children and adolescents. Clin Pediatr 1980;19:166.
11. Lewis TE: Incidence of fractured anterior teeth as related to their protrusion. Angle Orthod 1959;29:128.
12. McEwen JD, McHugh WD, Hitchin AD: Fractured maxillary central incisors and incisal relationships. J Dent Res 1967;46:1290.
13. Forsberg CM, Tedestam G: Etiological and predisposing factors related to traumatic injuries to permanent teeth. Swed Dent J 1993;17:183.
14. Ellis RG, Daury KW: The Classification and Treatment of Injuries to the Teeth of Children, ed 5. Chicago, Year Book Medical, 1970.
15. Andreason JO, Ravn JJ: Epidemiology of traumatic dental injuries to primary and permanent teeth in a Danish population sample. Int J Oral Surg 1972;1:235.
16. O'Mullane DM: Some factors predisposing to injuries of permanent incisors in school children. Br Dent J 1973;134:328.
17. Andreasen JO, Andreasen FM: Textbook and Color Atlas of Traumatic Injuries to the Teeth, ed 3. St Louis, CV Mosby, 1994.
18. Camp JH: Diagnosis and management of sports-related injuries to the teeth. Dent Clin North Am 1991;35:733.
19. Schreiber CK: The effect of trauma on the anterior deciduous teeth. Br Dent J 1959;106:340.
20. Levine N, Paedo D: Injury to the primary dentition. Dent Clin North Am 1982;26:461.
21. Laskin DM: The battered-child syndrome. J Oral Surg 1973; 31:903.
22. Laskin DM: The recognition of child abuse. J Oral Surg 1978;36:349.
23. Schwartz S, Woolridge E, Stege D: Oral manifestations and legal aspects of child abuse. J Am Dent Assoc 1977;95:586.
24. American College of Surgeons: Advanced Trauma Life Support Course for Physicians. Chicago, American College of Surgeons, 1992.
25. Assael LA, Ellis EE: Soft tissue and dentoalveolar injuries. In Peterson LJ, Ellis EE, Hupp J, Tucker M (eds): Contemporary Oral and Maxillofacial Surgery. St Louis, CV Mosby, 1988.
26. Woodcock JA: The diagnosis and management of the fractured tooth. Part 1: Diagnosis. Dental Update 1991;18:283.
27. Mumford JM: Evaluation of gutta-percha and ethyl chloride in pulp-testing. Br Dent J 1964;116:338.
28. Margarone JE, Hall R: Management of alveolar and dental fractures. In Peterson LJ, Ellis EE, Hupp J, Tucker M (eds): Principles of Oral and Maxillofacial Surgery. Philadelphia, JB Lippincott, 1992.
29. Sweet CA: A classification and treatment for traumatized anterior teeth. J Dent Child 1955;22:144.
30. Basrani E: Fractures of the Teeth. Philadelphia, Lea & Febiger, 1985.
31. Application of the International Classification of Diseases and Stomatology, IDC-DA, ed 2. Geneva, World Health Organization, 1978.
32. Powers MP: Diagnosis and management of dentoalveolar injuries. *In* Fonseca RJ, Walker RV: Oral and Maxillofacial Trauma. Philadelphia, WB Saunders, 1991.
33. Martin DM, Crabb HSM: Calcium hydroxide in root canal therapy: A review. Br Dent J 1977;142:277.
34. Aponte AJ, Hartsook JT, Crowley MC: Indirect pulp capping success verified. J Dent Child 1966;33:164.
35. Attalla MN, Noujaim AA: Role of calcium hydroxide in the formation of reparative dentin. Can Dent Assoc J 1969;35:267.
36. Steiner JC, Van Hassel HJ: Experimental root apexification in primates. Oral Surg Oral Med Oral Pathol 1971;31:409.
37. Cukjati JF: Intracanal calcium hydroxide therapy—the Webber technique. J Vet Dent 1992;9:26.
38. Fuks AB, Gavra S, Chosack A: Long-term followup of traumatized incisors treated by partial pulpotomy. Pediatr Dent 1993;15:334.
39. Josell SD, Abrams RG: Traumatic injuries to the dentition and its supporting structure. Pediatr Clin North Am 1982;29:717.
40. Burke FJ: Hemisection: A treatment option for the vertically split tooth. Dental Update 1992;19:8.
41. Yates JA: Root fractures in permanent teeth: A clinical review. Int Endodont J 1992;25:150.
42. Hovland EJ: Horizontal root fractures: Treatment and repair. Dent Clin North Am 1992;36:509.
43. Mamber EK: Treatment of intruded permanent incisors: A multidisciplinary approach. Endodont Dental Traumatol 1994;10:98.
44. Steiner JF, Grau WH: Management and complications of dentoalveolar trauma. Oral Maxillofac Surg Clin North Am 1990;2:515.
45. Jacobsen I: Clinical follow-up study of permanent incisors with intrusive luxation after acute trauma. J Dent Res 1983;62:486.
46. Sowray JH: Localized injuries of the teeth and alveolar process. *In* Rowe NL, Williams JL (eds): Maxillofacial Injuries. Edinburgh, Churchill Livingstone, 1985, p 214.
47. Antrim DD, Bakland LK, Parker MW: Treatment of endodontic urgent care cases. Dent Clin North Am 1986;30:559.
48. Andreasen JO: Periodontal healing after replantation of traumatically avulsed human teeth: Assessment by mobility testing and radiography. Acta Odontol Scand 1975;33:325.
49. Andreasen JO, Hjorting-Hansen E: Replantation of teeth I: Radiographic and clinical study of 110 human teeth replanted after accidental loss. Acta Odontol Scand 1966;24:263.
50. Camp JH: Replantation of teeth following trauma. *In* McDonald RE, Hurt WC, Gilmore HW, et al (eds): Current Therapy in Dentistry, vol VII. St Louis, CV Mosby, 1980.
51. Grossman LI, Ship II: Survival rate of reimplanted teeth. Oral Surg 1970;29:899.
52. Courts FJ, Mueller WA, Tabeling HJ: Milk as an interim storage medium for avulsed teeth. Pediatr Dent 1983;5:183.

53. Patel S, Dumsha TC, Sydiskis RJ: Determining periodontal ligament (PDL) cell vitality from exarticulated teeth stored in saline or milk using fluorescein diacetate. Int Endodont J 1994;27:1.
54. Blomlof L, Lindskog S, Andersson L, et al: Storage of experimentally avulsed teeth in milk prior to replantation. J Dent Res 1983;62:912.
55. Camp JH: Treatment of the avulsed tooth. J Am Dent Assoc 1980;107:706.
56. Krasner P: Modern treatment of avulsed teeth by emergency physicians. Am J Emerg Med 1994;12:241.
57. Kehoe J: Splinting and replantation after traumatic avulsion. J Am Dent Assoc 1986;112:224.
58. Hammarstrom L, Pierce A, Blomlof L, et al: Tooth avulsion and replantation: A review. Endodont Dental Traumatol 1986;2:1.
59. Tronstad L: Root resorption: Etiology, terminology, and clinical manifestations. Endodont Dental Traumatol 1988;4:241.
60. Dawoodbhoy I, Valiathan A, Lalani ZS, et al: Splinting of avulsed central incisors with orthodontic wires: A case report. Endodont Dental Traumatol 1994;10:149.
61. Anderson AW, Sharav Y, Massler M: Periodontal reattachment after tooth replantation. Periodontics 1968;6:161.
62. Anderson AW, Sharav Y, Massler M: Reparative dentine formation and pulp morphology. Oral Surg 1968;26:837.
63. Andreasen JO, Hjorting-Hansen E: Replantation of teeth II: Histologic study of 22 replanted anterior teeth in humans. Acta Odont Scand 1966;24:287.
64. Andreasen JO: The effect of splinting upon periodontal healing after replantation of permanent incisors in monkeys. Acta Odont Scand 1975;33:313.
65. Barbakow FH, Austin JC, Cleaton-Jones PE: Experimental reimplantation of root-canal filled and untreated teeth in the vervet monkey. J Endodont 1977;3:89.
66. Stalkane I, Hedegard B: Traumatized permanent teeth in children aged 7–15 years. Part II. Swed Dent J 1975;68:157.
67. Andreasen JO: Luxation of permanent teeth due to trauma: A clinical and radiographic follow-up study of 189 injured teeth. Scand J Dent Res 1970;78:273.
68. Skieller V: The prognosis for young teeth loosened after mechanical injuries. Acta Odont Scand 1960;18:171.
69. Eklund G, Stalhane I, Hedegard B: A study of traumatized permanent teeth in children aged 7–15 years. Part III: A multivariate analysis of post-traumatic complications of subluxated and luxated teeth. Swed Dent J 1976;69:179.
70. Andreasen FM, Vestergaard Pedersen B: Prognosis of luxated permanent teeth—the development of pulp necrosis. Endodont Dental Traumatol 1985;1:207.
71. Cvek M: A clinical report on partial pulpotomy and capping with calcium hydroxide in permanent incisors with complicated crown fracture. J Endodont 1978;5:232.
72. Klein H, Fuks A, Eidelman E, et al: Partial pulpotomy following complicated crown fracture in permanent incisors: A clinical and radiographic study. J Pedodont 1985;9:142.
73. Zadik D, Chosack A, Eidelman E: The prognosis of traumatized permanent anterior teeth with fracture of the enamel and dentin. Oral Surg 1979;47:173.
74. Cvek M: Endodontic treatment of traumatized teeth. *In* Andreasen, JO (eds): Traumatic Injuries of the Teeth, ed 2. Copenhagen, Munksgaard, 1981.
75. Zachrisson BU, Jacobsen I: Long-term prognosis of 66 permanent anterior teeth with root fracture. Scand J Dent Res 1975;83:345.
76. Ravn JJ: Follow-up study of permanent incisors with enamel fractures as a result of an acute trauma. Scand J Dent Res 1981;89:213.
77. Shuler SE, Howell BT, Green DB: Unusual pattern of pulp canal obliteration following luxation injury. J Endodont 1994;20:460.
78. Jacobsen I, Kerekes K: Long-term prognosis of traumatized permanent anterior teeth showing calcifying processes within the pulp cavity. Scand J Dent Res 1977;85:588.
79. Andreasen FM, Yu Z, Thomsen BL, Anderson PK: Occurrence of pulp canal obliteration after luxation injuries in the permanent dentition. Endod Dental Traumatol 1987;3:103.
80. Cvek M, Granath LE, Lundberg M: Failures and healing in endodontically treated non-vital anterior teeth with post-traumatically reduced pulpal lumen. Acta Odont Scand 1982;40:223.
81. Jacobsen I, Sangnes G: Traumatized primary anterior teeth: Prognosis related to calcific reactions in the pulp cavity. Acta Odont Scand 1978;36:199.
82. Nasjleti CE, Caffesse RG, Castelli WA, et al: Effect of fibronectin on healing of replanted teeth in monkeys: A histologic and autoradiographic study. Oral Surg Oral Med Oral Pathol 1987;63:291.
83. Cvek M: Prognosis of luxated non-vital maxillary incisors treated with calcium hydroxide and filled with gutta percha. Endodont Dental Traumatol 1992;8:45.
84. Andreasen FM, Andreasen JO: Resorption and mineralization processes following root fracture of permanent incisors. Endodont Dental Traumatol 1988;4:202.
85. Andreasen FM: Pulpal healing after luxation injuries and root fracture in the permanent dentition. Endodont Dent Traumatol 1989;5:11.
86. Andreasen JO, Ravn JJ: Enamel changes to permanent teeth after trauma to their primary predecessors. Scand J Dent Res 1973;81:203.
87. VanGool AV: Injury to the permanent tooth germ after trauma to their deciduous predecessor. Oral Surg Oral Med Oral Pathol 1973;35:2.
88. VanGool AV: Injury to the permanent tooth germ after trauma to the deciduous predecessor. Oral Surg Oral Med Oral Pathol 1973;35:2.
89. Andreasen FM: Transient apical breakdown and its relation to color and sensitivity changes after luxation injuries to the teeth. Endodont Dental Traumatol 1986;2:9.
90. Frank AL: Bleaching of vital and non-vital teeth. *In* Cohen S, Burns RC (eds): Pathways of the Pulp, ed 2. St Louis, CV Mosby, 1980.
91. Rotstein I, Zalkind M, Mor C, et al: In vitro efficacy of sodium perborate preparations used for intracoronal bleaching of discoloured non-vital teeth. Endodont Dental Traumatol 1991;7:177.
92. Holmstrup G, Palm AM, Lambjerg-Hansen H: Bleaching of discoloured root-filled teeth. Endodont Dental Traumatol 1988;4:197.

Chapter 12

COMPLICATIONS ASSOCIATED WITH TREATMENT OF HEAD AND NECK CANCER

by

Meredith August

Introduction

Patients with oral and oropharyngeal cancer often contend with severe functional, anatomic, and aesthetic deficits after treatment. These problems may be related to surgical treatment of the primary tumor or neck, radiation treatment of the primary tumor or neck, or chemotherapy. The size and location of the primary tumor and the presence or absence of disease in the neck also have a major impact on morbidity. This chapter discusses the diagnosis, management, and strategies for prevention of complications associated with treatment of head and neck cancer.

THE SUBJECTS DISCUSSED IN THIS CHAPTER ARE:

- Complications associated with surgical treatment of the primary tumor
  - Speech deficits
  - Swallowing dysfunction and aspiration
  - Neurologic dysfunction
  - Wound breakdown and fistula formation
  - Complications of reconstruction plates
- Complications associated with surgical treatment of the neck
  - Shoulder dysfunction and pain
  - Edema
  - Phrenic nerve injury
  - Thoracic duct injury
  - Cranial nerve injury
  - Carotid artery rupture
- Complications associated with radiation treatment for head and neck cancer
  - Osteoradionecrosis
  - Endocrine abnormalities
  - Atherosclerosis
  - Neck and shoulder function
  - Trismus
  - Oral side effects and complications
  - Visual impairment
  - Radiation neuritis
- Complications associated with chemotherapy for head and neck cancer

Complications Associated with Surgical Treatment of the Primary Tumor

Patients with oral and oropharyngeal cancer often manifest severe functional problems after treatment. Because the size and location of the tumor dictate the extent of the resection, the sacrifice of important contiguous structures is often mandated by the disease and the principles of oncologic safety. Loss of tongue and floor of mouth musculature, removal of bone and associated muscle attachments, and the sacrifice of both sensory and motor cranial nerves greatly affect aesthetics, speech, swallowing, and nutritional status as well as psychosocial function. The use of bulky and adynamic distal flaps for immediate reconstruction can further compound functional problems, especially articulation and the oral phase of swallowing. Wound dehiscence, often associated with radiation therapy, and contamination of wounds with oral contents can lead to persistent fistulization and more devastating complications. Scar contracture, of both the skin and the muscles of mastication, creates additional problems with mobility and resultant trismus.

Speech Deficits

Various measures of speech intelligibility have been utilized in postoperative oral cancer patients to better appreciate the deficits associated with tongue and floor of mouth resections. Pauloski and colleagues[1] assessed the speech of patients who received anterior tongue and floor of mouth resections with distal flap closure. All patients had mandibular preservation. This group found a 50% drop in intelligibility after surgery that did not appear to improve over time. In more heterogeneous groups of patients, the speech deficit was found to correlate with the amount of tongue resected as well as removal of tongue substance from the posterior third (tongue base). Longitudinal follow-up revealed that the level of speech patients demonstrated 3 months after healing was characteristic of their status at 1 year. Of note is that in the majority of cases, the only speech therapy the patients received was given within 1 month of surgery.

The major functional consideration with tongue resection is the resultant decrease in mobility. Glossectomies may be closed primarily, left to granulate secondarily, skin grafted, or closed with local flaps, regional pedicled flaps, or free flaps. These decisions are based on the size of the ablative defect and the need for additional soft tissue. In cases of partial glossectomy involving the anterior two thirds of the tongue, primary closure often results in the least functional impairment. With greater than half of the anterior two thirds of the tongue removed, a skin graft or flap may be indicated, especially when the anterior floor of the mouth is also resected (Fig. 12–1). The residual portion of the tongue should not be used as a flap or sutured to the floor of the mouth or anterior mandible, because doing so results in significant mobility problems and dramatic changes in articulation (Fig. 12–2). Tongue base resections that interfere with the tongue-palatal contact may lead to nasopharyngeal incompetence, hypernasality, and air escape with speaking. Primary closure in the region of the tongue base may result in tethering of the tongue to the cheek with resultant mobility problems as well.

In a recent review of the functional consequences of partial glossectomy, Dios and associates[2] reviewed deglutition, oral suction, and speech in 11 patients an average of 18 months after partial glossectomy for treatment of squamous cell carcinoma. They were compared with healthy volunteer controls. Significant deficits were noted in the duration of bolus deglutition and suction in the patient population. The ingestion rate was found to correlate with the area of the tongue removed. In general, these investigators found that the intelligibility of speech in glossectomized patients was fairly good. Deficits in this area similarly correlated with the quantity of tissue extirpated. In patients who underwent secondary operations to mobilize the remaining tongue, speech returned to near-normal levels. It has been reported that even in cases of more radical glossectomies, some speech rehabilitation is possible if

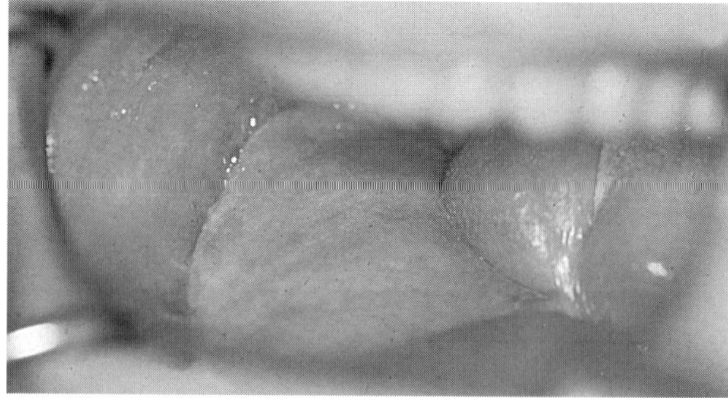

Figure 12–1. Free flap insertion after partial glossectomy and resection of the floor of the mouth.

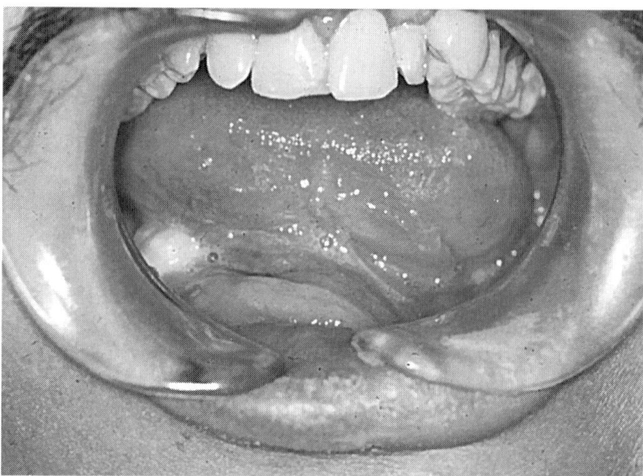

Figure 12–2. Ventral aspect of tongue sutured to residual alveolus, resulting in significant tethering and limitation of tongue mobility.

the larynx is preserved. Problems with chronic low-grade aspiration, however, can compromise the patient's pulmonary status.

Swallowing Dysfunction and Aspiration

Deficits in the swallowing mechanism following resection of tumors in the oral cavity and oropharynx have been extensively studied. Swallowing is a mixed voluntary and involuntary activity in which a synchronized system of muscle contractions and relaxations allows for the propulsion of a bolus from the oral cavity into the stomach. The oral phase is largely voluntary and depends on saliva to prepare the bolus after adequate chewing and on the tongue to compress the bolus against the hard palate, shaping it, further lubricating it, and squeezing it into the oropharynx. The pharyngeal phase of swallowing, largely involuntary, results in elevation of the larynx and inhibition of respiration as the swallow is completed.

Immediately postoperatively, patients undergoing resection of head and neck tumors experience some swallowing dysfunction or aspiration secondary to swelling, muscle dysfunction, and altered anatomy. Because of this problem, the tracheostomy is often utilized at the time of operation to separate the airway from the pharynx temporarily and allow for adequate tracheal suctioning and assisted ventilation, if needed. Aspiration can result in life-threatening pulmonary problems. Symptoms such as cough, fever, recurrent tracheobronchitis, atelectasis, pneumonia, and empyema have all been described. Patients may demonstrate weight loss, cachexia, and dehydration. The frequency and severity of aspiration increase with mechanical impairment of the larynx and pharynx following ablative surgery and are worsened by neurologic deficits and decreasing levels of consciousness.

With persistent swallowing dysfunction and aspiration, various diagnostic methods are used to better understand the nature of the problem and determine which phases of the swallowing cycle are involved. Direct fiberoptic laryngoscopy can identify defects in laryngeal motion, pooling in the hypopharynx, poor contractility of the pharyngeal musculature, or obstruction from a large flap or mass lesion. Electromyography can determine mechanical and neural dysfunction. Most commonly, the modified barium swallow study can identify subtle changes within the swallowing cycle (Fig. 12–3). The swallowing effort can be analyzed, and adynamic areas and areas of obstruction and dyssynchrony as well as the frequency and severity of aspiration can be identified. The optimal head position for swallowing and the most efficacious consistency of bolus are also noted and can guide rehabilitation. Swallowing therapy can be beneficial in many instances. The method of food introduction, quantity and consistency of food, and other parameters can be altered and the study repeated. In patients who fail to obtain improvement with these efforts, nasogastric tubes or gastrostomies may be required for the long term.

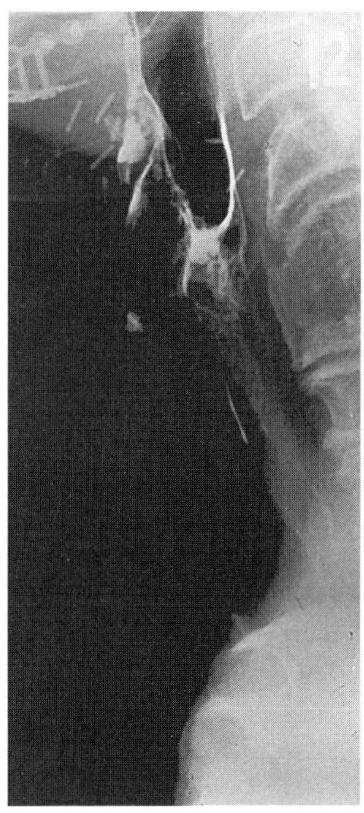

Figure 12–3. Modified barium swallow demonstrating aspiration in head and neck cancer patient after resection.

Neurologic Dysfunction

Neurologic dysfunction following treatment of squamous cell carcinoma of the oral cavity commonly involves sacrifice of the lower division of the trigeminal nerve as well as facial nerve weakness. Impairment of cranial nerves IX, X, XI, and XII is discussed further in the section on complications of neck treatment.

The loss of cranial nerve V produces a sensory deficit that may further compound speech and swallowing problems. The already reduced tongue volume may now be both tethered and insensate. Limited ability to create an adequate oral seal is seen with denervation of the muscles of mastication. With loss of the lower branches of the facial nerve, orbicularis and buccinator function is impaired (Fig. 12–4). Cranial nerve IX provides sensation to the tonsillar region, palate, posterior third of the tongue, and the pharynx as well as motor function to part of the soft palate and pharyngeal constrictor muscles. With loss of this nerve's function, the gag reflex is impaired, and the uvula is found to deviate. Dysfunction of the vagus nerve results in the most severe swallowing disabilities and predisposes to aspiration. The motor function to the larynx is provided peripherally by the recurrent and superior laryngeal nerves. The superior laryngeal nerve also provides sensory innervation to the supraglottic portion of the larynx. Thus, both motor and sensory impairments may result from its damage and make aspiration more likely. Cranial nerve XII gives motor innervation to the tongue. Loss of its function worsens articulation and the swallowing problems seen with glossectomy and floor of mouth resection.

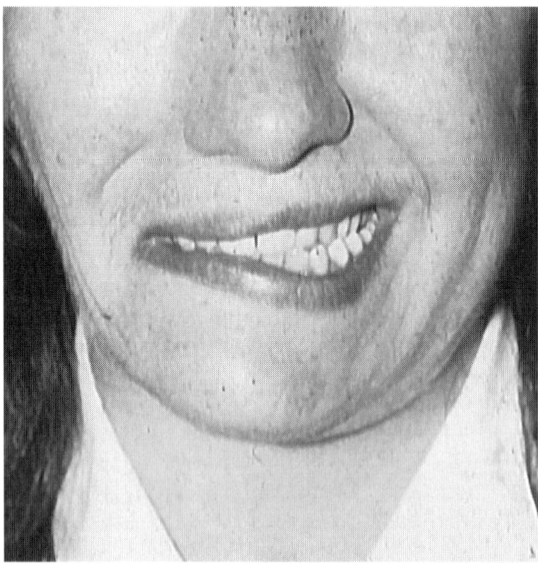

Figure 12–4. Marginal mandibular injury and resultant deficit.

Wound Breakdown and Fistula Formation

Intraoral wound breakdown is often associated with radiation therapy and can result in contamination of deep spaces within the neck by saliva and other oral contents (see section on complications of surgical treatment of the neck). The use of regional musculocutaneous and axial flaps that have cutaneous portions with inconsistent vascularity similarly predisposes to intraoral wound breakdown if the blood supply is compromised by torsion of the pedicle. Marginal necrosis of the distal portion of the flap may progress to frank wound breakdown. Free transfer of well-vascularized tissue provides more consistent soft tissue coverage, especially in the patient undergoing radiation therapy, and similarly provides thinner and more pliable oral lining following large resections and has the added advantage of providing sensate tissue upon which dental prostheses can function. Despite the associated donor site morbidity, free tissue transfer is rapidly becoming the technique of choice for the closure of large ablative defects.

Complications of Reconstruction Plates

The use of rigid plating systems to restore mandibular continuity following resection of tumors that involve bone and contiguous structures has found wide acceptance (Fig. 12–5). Spiessl and coworkers[3] first reported the use of a three-dimensional, bendable plate for bridging mandibular defects. Since 1979, many reports have described similar techniques and refinements. Complications associated with both stainless steel and titanium reconstruction plates have been reported. Lavertu and associates[4] considered both early and late complications associated with reconstruction plates and dealt with functional and cosmetic aspects of their use as well. They found a 44% rate of early complications, which included wound dehiscence and plate exposure. Of note is that 10 of 12 patients who developed early complications had received previous radiation therapy. Late complications were pain, plate exposure, infection, loose screws, and plate fracture; 63% of patients had at least one late complication. Plate exposure occurred in 5 of 17 patients, loose screws were found in 2 of 17 patients, and one plate fractured 27 months after reconstruction. The cosmetic results in this group were described as "excellent" or "good" in 96% of patients, and 89% of patients had postoperative speech deemed "sufficient for communication." Unfortunately, no patients were fitted for dental prostheses and none was allowed to resume a solid diet.

Boyd and colleagues,[5] reviewing the use of metallic reconstruction plates in conjunction with radial forearm fasiocutaneous flaps, reported an overall failure rate of 33.3%. Failures were intraoral and extraoral exposure of the plate in 4 of 15 patients and one plate fracture. Three of the failures occurred in anterior mandibular reconstructions. The researchers concluded that these symphyseal reconstructions are particularly vulnerable to breakdown. Often, the remaining mandibular segments are displaced superiorly by the unsupported action of the temporalis muscles. The plate is superiorly displaced, often above the patulous and incompetent lower lip, and can thus erode through the flap. The failures in this group occurred an average of 14.3 months postoperatively. Lindqvist and coworkers[6] reviewed 34 primary alloplastic mandibular reconstructions as part of the treatment of oral malignancies. They reported that 35% of reconstruction plates were removed because of complications, such as chronic infection, plate exposure, plate fracture, screw loosening, and fistula formation. Complications were observed from between 3 and 24 months postoperatively, and all patients received radiation therapy.

Complications Associated with Surgical Treatment of the Neck

The radical neck dissection as first described by Crile[7] in 1906 was long considered the only oncologi-

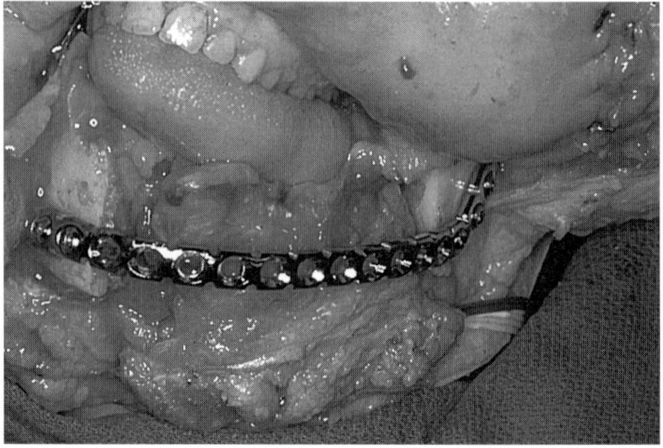

Figure 12–5. Mandibular reconstruction after ablative surgery using reconstruction bone plate.

cally safe operation for the treatment of lymph node metastasis to the neck from various head and neck primary malignancies. The concept of en bloc removal of major cervical lymph node groups along with contiguous anatomic structures was both conceptually and anatomically logical. In addition, the radical neck dissection, with its sacrifice of the spinal accessory nerve, sternocleidomastoid muscle, and internal jugular vein, is still considered a technically simpler operation than the modified and functional procedures that are more common today.

Shoulder Dysfunction and Pain

Shoulder dysfunction and pain were long associated with the radical neck dissection. In 1961, Nahum and colleagues[8] more formally described what has come to be known as the *shoulder syndrome,* which consists of pain in the shoulder; limited abduction of the shoulder; anatomic deformities such as scapular flaring, shoulder droop and protraction; and abnormal electromyograms of the trapezius muscle. With sacrifice of the spinal accessory nerve and denervation of the trapezius muscle, the scapula can no longer be stabilized. It tends to flare out at the vertebral border, slip forward and downward, and thereby limit the ability of the shoulder to move in full active range of motion. With longitudinal follow-up, Sobol and coworkers[9] found little improvement in the functional disability associated with the radical dissection and persistence of pain. Objective parameters they used to study shoulder function were physical measurements of range of motion (abduction and flexion) as well as measurements of strength and posture, electromyography of the trapezius muscle compared with the unoperated side, and the subjective perception of pain and dysfunction as elicited by questionnaire. Despite active physical therapy, little improvement was documented longitudinally in this group of patients.

Debate still rages regarding the merits and oncologic safety of preserving the spinal accessory nerve. Both Lingeman and associates[10] and Skolnik and colleagues[11] have shown good evidence for the safety of its preservation in appropriately selected cases, most often in patients with clinically negative necks. Recalling the anatomy of the nerve and its relationship to the major lymph node groups in the neck can aid in proper case selection for nerve sparing (Fig. 12–6). The accessory nerve emerges from the base of the skull lateral and superficial to the internal jugular vein. It passes through the sternocleidomastoid muscle and into the posterior triangle of the neck. If there is obvious lymph node involvement in either the jugulodigastric area or the posterior triangle, the nerve must be sacrificed.

The reduced functional disability associated with nerve preservation has been extensively studied. Leipzig and associates[12] followed 109 patients prospectively and found a significantly higher incidence of shoulder dysfunction in patients whose nerve had been more completely dissected or severed. Sobol and coworkers,[9] in addition to studying patients who had undergone classical radical neck dissections, reviewed those who had modified radical dissections with preservation of the 11th cranial nerve as well as those who had supraomohyoid dissections with preservation of the 11th cranial nerve, sternocleidomastoid muscle, and internal jugular vein. In this prospective study, 35 patients undergoing 44 neck procedures were evaluated preoperatively and postoperatively using the aforementioned objective and subjective criteria. Baseline range of motion, strength, posture, and electromyography (EMG) measurements were obtained and were repeated at 16 weeks and again at 1 year postoperatively. The EMG scores were designated as normal, slightly impaired, moderately impaired, or severely impaired. The latency and amplitude of the muscle were compared with those in healthy age-matched controls. Of note is that no patients in the supraomohyoid dissection group demonstrated severe or moderate EMG abnormalities 1 year after surgery. Even at 16 weeks, 56% of this group had normal EMG scores compared with none in the radical dissection group and 30% in the modified dissection group. In addition, the supraomohyoid dissection group showed a statistically significant improvement in shoulder abduction and flexion with and without 1.5-lb weights when measured at 16 weeks. Protraction and shoulder droop were significantly less. The modified radical dissection group showed gradual improvement over the year that patients were followed. Seven of eight patients in the modified radical dissection group showed improvement in all parameters, whereas the radical neck dissection group continued to show progressive deterioration.[9]

Shoulder function following neck dissection is thus seen to be a complex and multifactorial problem. Although the spinal accessory nerve is usually regarded as the sole innervation of the trapezius muscle, anatomists have described varying motor and sensory connections that form a plexus with the 11th cranial nerve and account for the variability in motor innervation and function of the muscle. Contributions to innervation include fibers from the great auricular nerve, phrenic nerve, and brachial plexus branches as well as branches from the second, third, and fourth cervical nerves. With preservation of the 11th cranial nerve, even in cases of extensive dissection, time appears to be the most important factor in improvement of shoulder disability.

Edema

Ligation of the internal jugular vein is part of the classic neck dissection for the treatment of malignant disease. This maneuver, combined with the removal of the lymphatic channels that drain the head, can result in both facial and intracerebral edema. Simultaneous bilateral neck dissections, in which both veins are sacrificed, are often staged. This issue remains controversial. Prolonged papilledema and several reported cases of blindness have appeared in the literature.[13] Three studies, however, have demonstrated only transient increases in cerebrospinal fluid (CSF) pressure following bilateral vein ligation.[14–16] Abundant collateral venous drainage of the head occurs through vertebral, paraver-

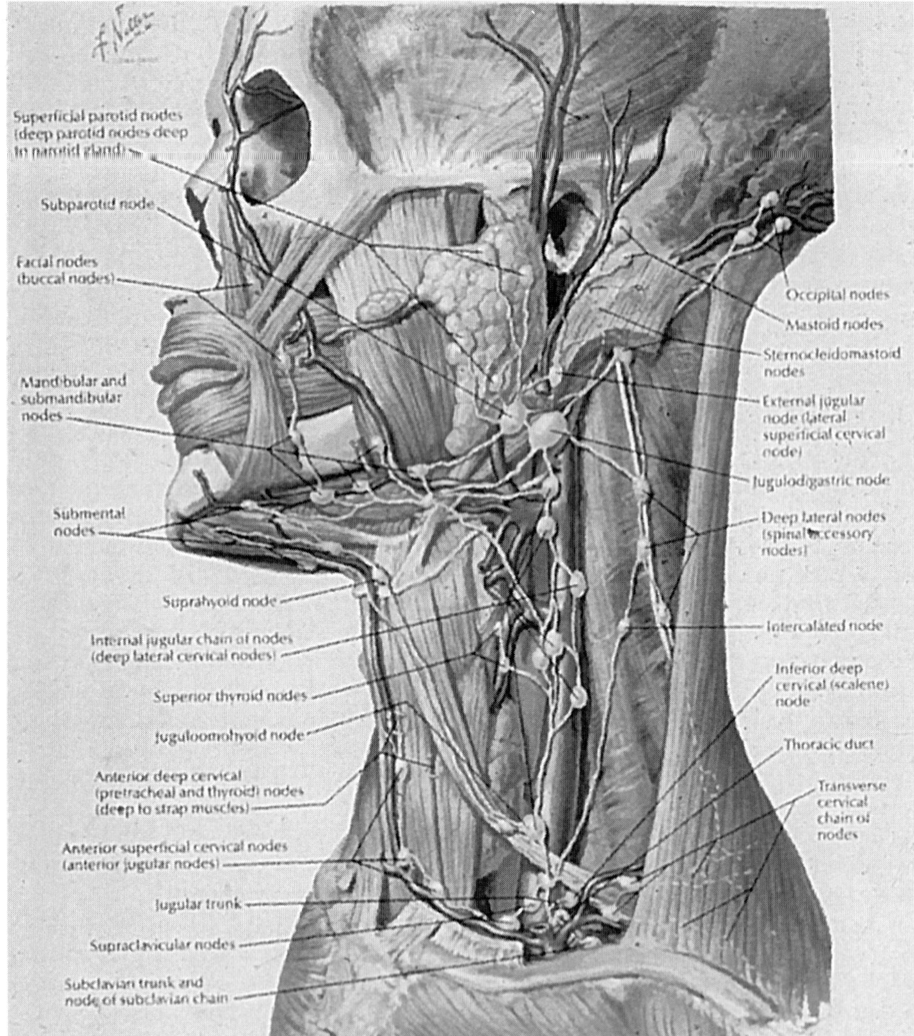

Figure 12–6. Relation of spinal accessory nerve to the major lymph node groups in the neck. (From Netter, Frank H: *In* Colacino, Sharon (ed): Atlas of Human Anatomy. West Caldwell, NJ, Ciba-Geigy.)

tebral, emissary, and ophthalmic veins. Although the associated morbidity of bilateral radical neck dissections may be acceptable, most surgeons advocate staging the second dissection to allow for collateral venous and lymphatic drainage. In a nonirradiated patient, 3 weeks is thought to be the minimal waiting period. In irradiated patients, severe facial edema can be seen even following unilateral radical neck dissection. Radiation certainly increases the incidence and severity of lymphatic obstruction. Engorgement of the parapharyngeal venous plexus can lead to severe supraglottic edema and airway compromise postoperatively. In the irradiated population, careful preoperative assessment of the pharyngeal mucosa is imperative, and tracheostomy is often indicated.

Modification of the radical neck dissection often involves sparing of the internal jugular vein. Sparing the vein minimizes edematous involvement of the face and, in conjunction with preservation of the sternocleidomastoid muscle, provides good soft tissue coverage of the carotid artery, thus obviating local muscle flap coverage or dermal grafting for carotid protection. In cases of wound dehiscence, however, the retained jugular vein becomes vulnerable to erosion. Reported cases of jugular vein rupture have followed the development of initially undetected wound breakdown with contamination of the neck by saliva and oral contents.[17] These seem to be similar factors predisposing to carotid artery rupture, although in cases of venous erosion, previous radiation therapy seems to play a smaller role, with half the reported cases occurring in nonirradiated patients. Cases of venous rupture were characterized by the presence of repeated small bleeds from the site of breakdown rather than the single sentinel bleed described for carotid artery rupture. Methods of preventing this vascular complication involve good soft tissue coverage of the retained vein (and underlying artery) and early recognition of wound breakdown and pharyngocutaneous fistula formation.

Phrenic Nerve Injury

Phrenic nerve injury during neck dissection usually represents surgical misadventure rather than direct tumor extension into the vicinity of the nerve. Sensory branches of C2–C3 and C3–C4 of the cervical plexus pierce the deep layer of the superficial fascia of the neck en route to the skin. They are routinely transected during neck dissection. These nerves must be well visualized before transection and ligated away from their exit from the intermuscular septum and deep fascia. Ligation avoids pulling the phrenic nerve, the longest branch of the cervical plexus, up into the specimen. The phrenic nerve is also vulnerable low in the neck. Here, it lies on the scalenus anticus muscle and must be identified before the jugular vein, omohyoid muscle, and the contents of the posterior triangle are divided.

There is an overall 8% reported incidence of phrenic nerve injury and resultant diaphragmatic paralysis following neck dissection. The diagnosis is usually made after a postoperative chest radiograph is obtained (Fig. 12–7). Ipsilateral elevation of the diaphragm at least one intercostal space above the unaffected side is the radiologic indicator. The diagnosis is then often confirmed with fluoroscopy. The signs of phrenic nerve injury are (1) diminished, absent, or paradoxic movement of the diaphragm on inspiration, (2) mediastinal shifting toward the contralateral side with inspiration, and (3) paradoxic movement of the diaphragm under conditions of augmented load (e.g., coughing). The symptoms associated with diaphragmatic paralysis may well be subtle. Respiratory, cardiac, and gastrointestinal symptoms have been reported in the literature, though they are usually not severe. De Jong and Manni[18] reviewed 176 patients undergoing neck dissections—136 radical and 40 conservative. Sixty of the patients in this group had received preoperative radiation therapy. Eleven patients were found to have permanent paralysis of the diaphragm postoperatively, and three demonstrated paralysis that resolved within 3 weeks of surgery. Careful evaluation of the operative reports demonstrated higher incidence of complicating factors in cases of phrenic nerve injury. Soft tissue fibrosis, edema, tumor infiltration near the nerve, diffuse bleeding with ligation, and electrocoagulation in the vicinity of the nerve were mentioned in the operative notes. Respiratory symptoms in these patients included cough, dyspnea, chest pain, and cyanosis thought to be secondary to a reduction in lung volume (measured as a 7% decrement). The cardiac symptoms—palpitations, tachycardia, and extrasystoles—were thought to be secondary to the displacement of the mediastinum. The gastrointestinal complaints included pain in the abdomen, nausea, and vomiting and similarly were thought to be due to the superior displacement of abdominal contents. Overall, pulmonary function tests demonstrated a 25% decrease in vital capacity, a 20% decrease in ventilation-perfusion ratios and, as mentioned, a 7% decrease in lung volume.

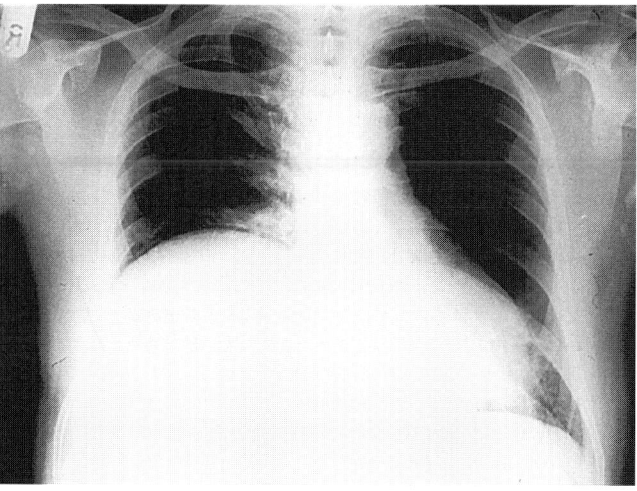

Figure 12–7. Elevation of the right hemidiaphragm secondary to phrenic nerve injury on the ipsilateral side.

These data agree closely with those reported by Simpson and colleagues[19] and Swift,[20] who documented 11% and 10% incidences, respectively, of phrenic nerve injury secondary to radical neck dissection with a similar spectrum of symptoms.

Thoracic Duct Injury

Injury to the thoracic duct during neck dissection with the associated development of chylous fistulas has a reported incidence of 1% to 2% and is thought to occur primarily in the left neck. Involvement of the accessory duct in the right neck, although less common, has also been described. An unrecognized and uncontrolled chyle leak may result in massive plasma loss and hypoalbuminemia as well as loss of fatty acids and triglycerides.

Early recognition and treatment with adequate drainage and pressure dressings are usually sufficient to control the leak. Persistent drainage of more than 500 mL per day warrants reexploration of the neck. Nutritional support with medium-chain triglycerides compensates for losses as the drainage continues. Most surgeons emphasize the importance of preventing this complication.[21] After the internal jugular vein is ligated, attention should be given to the presence of any lymphatic leak. Before wound closure, the patient can be placed in the Trendelenburg position; with the administration of increased intrathoracic positive pressure by the anesthesiologist, a lymphatic leak should be apparent. Reported cases of massive chylothoraces have associated mortality rates as high as 7.5%, owing to the intense inflammatory reaction of the lung parenchyma.[22] Delayed lymphocele formation, with evidence of an expansile mass and overlying skin erythema, has also been reported.[23] This complication needs to be differentiated from hematoma and seroma formation.

Cranial Nerve Injury

Potential injury to the hypoglossal nerve during neck dissection that involves the submandibular triangle causes functional impairment of the intrinsic tongue musculature as well as the hyoglossus, styloglossus, and genioglossus muscles. In standard neck dissections, every effort is made to identify and preserve this nerve unless it is directly involved with tumor. The hypoglossal nerve, with contributions from the cervical plexus in the ansa hypoglossi, also innervates the thyrohyoid, sternohyoid, sternothyroid, and omohyoid muscles. Palsy of cranial nerve XII thus results in paralysis of the ipsilateral tongue as well as interference with elevation and depression of the larynx, which are so important to the swallowing mechanism. The nerve is particularly vulnerable to injury as it crosses the occipital artery, superficial to the external carotid and lingual arteries.[22] Extreme care must be exercised in dissecting the carotid sheath in this region. Ligation or cautery of the ranine veins may also result in injury.

The marginal mandibular branch of the facial nerve and its vulnerability in the submandibular triangle are well known. It lies deep to both the platysma muscle and the superficial layer of the deep cervical fascia. Medial to the facial artery, the ramus mandibularis usually lies above the lower border of the mandible and is less susceptible to injury. Preservation of this nerve and its innervation of the musculature of the lower lip spares patients significant facial deformities postoperatively (see Fig. 12–4).

Carotid Artery Rupture

Perhaps the most dreaded of surgical complications is rupture of the carotid artery. Fortunately unusual, this vascular complication carries a high mortality rate, reportedly between 18% and 50%.[24] Various large studies have shown carotid artery rupture to occur in approximately 3% of patients undergoing neck dissection.[25] Previous radiation therapy to the neck is most common in these cases. A large review by Heller and Strong[26] found that 56 of 63 (88%) patients with carotid artery hemorrhage had previously received radiation therapy. Marchetta and associates[27] documented a 7% rate of carotid rupture in 36 patients previously treated with irradiation, as opposed to none in 18 nonirradiated patients. Radiation therapy has been demonstrated to cause thrombosis of the vasa vasorum, premature atherosclerotic changes in large arteries, and progressive weakening of the vessel walls and thinning of the vessel media and fibrosis of the adventitia.

Swain and colleagues[24] developed an experimental model for carotid artery rupture to better elucidate those factors thought to be etiologic. They studied four clinical conditions in a dog model: blood supply, infection, desiccation of the vessel, and salivary contamination. Their results demonstrated that blood supply and infection were the most strongly implicated factors in carotid artery rupture. If the blood supply to the vessel was intact (nonirradiated animals), neither salivary contamination nor desiccation caused rupture. Similarly, in a nonirradiated vessel with an intact blood supply, clinical infection did not cause rupture.

Major postoperative complications commonly precede carotid artery rupture. Heller and Strong[26] found that 39 of 63 patients demonstrated substantial necrosis of cervical skin flaps. Unplanned fistulas developed in 40 of their patients. Only five patients in their group demonstrated neither complication but were found, at the time of surgical exploration, to have undetected wound sepsis or mucosal breakdown with salivary contamination of the neck. Coupled with a history of radiation therapy, these clinical results agree with those obtained in the animal model by Swain and colleagues.[24]

Exsanguinating hemorrhage of the artery is usually preceded by less dramatic sentinel bleeding. Identifying patients at risk and acting rapidly before hypovolemic shock supervenes can well be life-saving and can reduce the significant neurologic morbidity associated with rupture. The area of greatest risk of rupture is the common carotid artery in the midportion of the neck and the carotid bulb. If the artery becomes exposed in an irradiated patient, immediate coverage is mandatory. Although treatment is controversial, elective ligation does not significantly improve survival or decrease neurologic consequences. Coleman[28] advocates débridement of the neck to remove necrotic and infected material. A muscle or musculocutaneous flap is then utilized to cover the vessel. If adequate neck débridement requires removal of a portion of the vessel, the excised segments must similarly be covered by muscle to avoid further bleeding from avascular and necrotic vessel segments.

Once frank vessel rupture has occurred, repair is not possible, and the vessel should be regarded as an infected foreign body. Control of hemorrhage and fluid resuscitation are first undertaken, followed by proximal and distal artery resection and ligation. Coleman[28] advocates resolution of orocutaneous or pharyngocutaneous fistulas, if possible, at the same time. As mentioned previously, the vessel stumps should be well covered with extracervical muscle. Heller and Strong[26] reported that 16 of 50 patients (32%) with carotid artery hemorrhage died without ever leaving the hospital. The mortality rate was comparable, however, for those undergoing elective ligation in anticipation of hemorrhage, with 5 of 13 patients (38%) not leaving the hospital alive. These latter patients succumbed to either irreversible shock or massive neurologic injury. This study found no significant difference in the incidence of stroke in patients who hemorrhaged and those who underwent elective ligation. Permanent neurologic sequelae most commonly were hemiparesis and aphasia. This has been reported to occur with an incidence of between 12% and 50% in association with carotid artery rupture.

With the advent of newer and more sophisticated techniques to assess the adequacy of collateral cerebral blood flow, advocates of elective ligation and elective balloon embolization of the carotid artery have reported better survival and morbidity data. An indirect measure of cerebral blood flow can be obtained through ophthalmoplethysmography. This procedure measures the filling pressure of the retinal arteries, a reflection of the blood pressure in the internal carotid system. Diagnostic angiography combined with carotid cross-compression or balloon occlusion, which can be performed with a patient awake, gives significant information about neurologic status during trial occlusion. In addition, measurement of carotid backflow pressure can be obtained by using a double-lumen catheter. Zimmerman and associates[29] reported six cases of elective occlusion in patients at risk for carotid artery rupture. All patients had demonstrated prodromal arterial bleeding. Balloon embolization was successful in all patients in stopping bleeding, and there were no cases of rebleeding. No patients died as a result of the occlusion. Three patients experienced transient neurologic impairment, and one patient remained permanently hemiparetic. This was a small series, but as the technique continues to improve, this method of treatment may better the prognosis of this subset of patients.[30]

Complications Associated with Radiation Treatment for Head and Neck Cancer

Ionizing radiation has been used successfully for the treatment of head and neck tumors for more than 60 years. Although associated complications and the effects on normal tissue (bone, skin, salivary glands) are often described, well-documented incidence rates are difficult to ascertain. Most discussions of radiation-associated complications describe both acute problems, often noted within weeks of completion of therapy, and later effects, which involve damage to more slow-growing tissue and are noted 6 to 12 months after treatment. The so-called stochastic effects of radiation, such as the induction of secondary neoplasia, have also been described.[31]

Some researchers make a distinction between the side effects of radiation on normal tissue and actual complications. These problems, however, represent a continuum. The commonly described problems of xerostomia, loss of taste, epilation of the skin, and mucositis are unavoidable and, with proper patient education, are managed with supportive measures. Some of the more serious complications, such as soft tissue ulceration, the development of orocutaneous fistulas, and osteoradionecrosis, may be the result of overly aggressive treatment or faulty technique. For major complications, one must look critically at the treatment modality employed, the time-dose fraction program utilized, the size of the radiation portals, the extent and location of disease, as well as the patient's age and nutritional status to best understand the factors involved. In addition, combined surgical and radiation treatment may have an additive effect, in that tissue with already compromised vascularity is being irradiated.

Osteoradionecrosis

Bony necrosis can be a devastating consequence of radiation treatment (Fig. 12–8). The incidence of osteoradionecrosis was higher in the era preceding the use of megavoltage radiation produced by telecobalt machines and linear accelerators. The pathophysiology of osteoradionecrosis has been well worked out.[32] Radiation causes destruction of both osteocytes and osteoblasts and thereby limits the formation of new osteoid tissue. In addition, significant changes occur in the irradiated blood vessels. Small vessels are thickened by myointimal fibrosis thought to be secondary to endothelial cell damage. Histologic studies have also shown a disruption of the internal elastica with overlying thrombus formation. Both factors result in vessel narrowing or occlusion and diminution of blood supply.

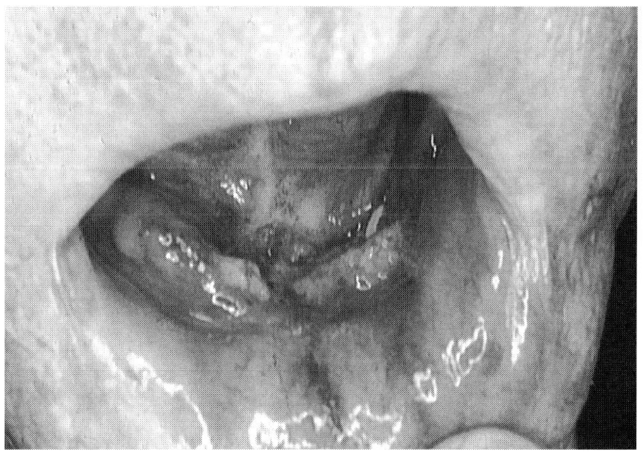

Figure 12–8. Osteoradionecrosis and resultant fracture of the exposed portion of the mandible.

Damaged bone is highly susceptible to secondary infection and demonstrates a limited capacity to heal, even from minor trauma such as movement of overlying denture prostheses.

The incidence of osteoradionecrosis is variably reported as between 0 and 37% in the literature.[33] Most workers agree that etiologic factors are: (1) the anatomic site of the tumor, (2) tumor dose, (3) radiation technique, and (4) pretreatment dental status of the patient. Each of these is discussed individually. Secondary causes are a history of trauma and prosthesis movement. The incidence of osteoradionecrosis is far greater in the mandible than in the maxilla, because of the mandible's greater bone density, greater absorption of radiation, and, especially, restricted localized blood supply, which is often completely within the field of treatment.

The greatest risk for developing osteoradionecrosis is reported to be associated with treatment of tumors of the tongue, floor of the mouth, and alveolar ridge. These anatomic sites often require total bone exposure to be greater than 60 Gy, a dose associated with higher incidence of necrosis.[34] Radiation techniques that limit bony exposure are associated with lower reported rates of osteoradionecrosis. The use of the intraoral cone for treatment of these anatomic sites within the oral cavity has been advocated extensively by Foyos and Lampe[35] and Wang and associates.[36] With the use of cones of variable sizes and shapes, the electron beam is delivered to the primary lesion, which receives a total dose of approximately 75 Gy, but associated bony involvement is limited (Fig. 12–9). The mandibular dose remains less than 60 Gy. A review by Wang and Biggs[37] demonstrated no occurrence of persistent ulceration or osteoradionecrosis in 196 patients so treated from 1975 to 1993.

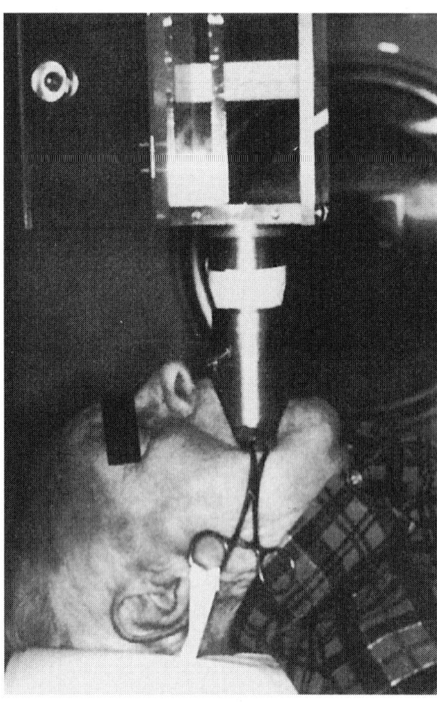

Figure 12–9. Intraoral electron cone boost technique. (From Wang CC, Kelly J, August M, et al: Early carcinoma of the oral cavity: A conservative approach with radiation therapy. J Oral Maxillofac Surg. 1995; 53:687–690.)

Relationship between the pretreatment dental status of irradiated patients and the subsequent development of osteonecrosis has been extensively studied, although controversy still exists regarding optimal management. Murray and coworkers[38] reported a twofold increase in the development of osteonecrosis in dentate patients, whereas Beumer and associates[39] described a fourfold increase. The periodontal ligament, gingiva, and pulpal tissues all represent potential sites for the passage of microorganisms from the oral cavity into the bone. If significant dental disease exists before treatment, it should be eradicated. If extractions are required, most workers recommend waiting at least 10 days before commencing radiation treatment, to allow for surface coverage of exposed bone at the time of extraction. Alveolectomy and primary closure should be attempted at the time of extraction.[40] Makkonen and coworkers[41] reviewed 92 cases of patients who were treated with multiple dental extractions prior to starting radiation therapy. Radiation was delayed until the extraction sites were completely healed. No cases of osteoradionecrosis developed in these patients. Most researchers agree that elective post-treatment extractions are best avoided and that endodontic treatment and subsequent restoration of teeth are preferable. Maintenance of optimal hygiene and the liberal use of topical fluoride are now routine parts of dental care in irradiated patients.

Endocrine Abnormalities

The development of endocrine abnormalities as a consequence of radiation treatment has been most extensively reviewed in the neurosurgical literature in cases of hypothalamic and pituitary exposure. Samaan and colleagues[42] reviewed 166 patients treated with primary radiation therapy for carcinoma of the nasopharynx and paranasal sinuses, 110 of whom received neck irradiation with a median dose to the thyroid of 5000 rads. Patients were followed for up to 5 years. Forty-eight of the 110 patients demonstrated evidence of primary hypothyroidism on biochemical testing that consisted of serum thyroid-stimulating hormone, total serum T_4, serum T_3, and resin uptake measurements. Although the majority of patients were not clinically symptomatic, Samaan and colleagues[42] advocate long-term follow-up to determine whether thyroid function continues to deteriorate. Just how sensitive the thyroid gland is to radiation damage and what dose is required to induce hypofunction are not known. In addition, the latency period and time course have not been well worked out.

Favus and coworkers[43] reported on the incidence of thyroid carcinoma as a late consequence of head and neck radiation. They reviewed 1,056 patients who had been treated in the 1940s and 1950s. All patients had been treated for infectious or inflammatory disease of the upper respiratory tract and had received an average of 200 KV exposure of the anterior skin of the neck. The mean latency period between treatment and examination in this group was 27 years. Palpable nodular thyroid disease was found in 16.5% of patients. Technetium-99m imaging demonstrated that an additional 10.7% had thyroid lesions; surgery performed in 71% of this subgroup revealed carcinoma in 33%. Tumors were of the papillary, follicular, or mixed histologic type. Of note in this group is that 174 patients had taken thyroid replacement hormone in the past. Favus and coworkers[43] concluded that a significant prevalence of nodular thyroid disease, both benign and malignant, persists for more than 30 years after radiation treatment. These lesions may be undetected by physical examination alone.

Parathyroid abnormalities have similarly been reported in patients receiving radiation to the neck.[44] Dosage and latency data are unfortunately scant in this group as well. Case reports of the development of parathyroid adenomas and hyperparathyroidism appear in the literature. Holten and Petersen[45] studied patients treated with neck irradiation for malignant disease to determine parathyroid function in the early years following treatment. Fifty patients with head and neck cancer were identified. Levels of iPTH, calcium, phosphate, T_3, T_4, and TSH were checked before treatment and then every 3 to 4 months for 36 months. All patients in this study received treatment with telecobalt to parallel, opposite fields. The dose to the parathyroid glands differed according to the tumor location and extension, with the majority receiving between 63 and 66 Gy of exposure. No cases of hyperparathyroidism developed in any of these patients during the observational period. A slight, though not clinically significant, trend toward increased iPTH was noted in this group. No alteration in serum calcium was found, however.

This area needs further investigation with longer periods of observation.

Atherosclerosis

Much has been written about radiation changes induced in small blood vessels. Large-vessel disease and the premature development of atherosclerotic carotid disease have also been described and studied.[46] Call and associates[47] demonstrated atherosclerosis with associated round cell infiltration in irradiated carotid arteries. These lesions could be induced with doses in excess of 50 Gy and were associated with long latency periods. In most reported cases, the interval from radiation exposure to the development of neurologic symptoms was greater than 15 years. Several case reports have described progressive carotid artery narrowing within 3 years of therapeutic radiation to the neck and without angiographic evidence of atherosclerosis.[48] These cases contrast strikingly with those of progressive atherosclerosis, which commonly demonstrate diffuse involvement of the arteries in the radiation port. The pathophysiology in these rapidly progressive cases is thought to be thrombotic in nature and secondary to myointimal fibrosis and disruption of the endothelial lining of the vessel with resultant thrombus formation in the absence of severe stenosis. Conomy and Kellermeyer[49] studied cases at autopsy and noted the presence of carotid bifurcation thrombosis in the absence of stenosis in patients who had been irradiated. The prognosis for patients who develop cerebral ischemic symptoms within only a few years of radiation is variable and somewhat hard to predict. The development of devastating infarctions as well as of transient monocular blindness has been reported.[50] Patients with hypercoagulable states and hypercholesterolemia appear to be at higher risk. It is now commonly recommended that this patient population be followed with noninvasive carotid studies beginning 5 years after radiation exposure.

Neck and Shoulder Function

The changes in neck and shoulder motion in patients treated with neck dissection has been discussed in some detail earlier in this chapter. Progressive muscle fibrosis following radiation treatment further limits normal motion, most notably flexion, extension, and lateral bending of the neck (Fig. 12-10). Nowak and coworkers[51] studied 126 patients in prospective fashion to better understand the effect of surgery, radiation, and combined treatment on neck and shoulder mobility. The movement of the head was expressed in degrees of motion, and active flexion, extension, lateral rotation, and lateral bending were assessed. Shoulder motion was evaluated by measuring passive and active flexion, extension, abduction, adduction, external rotation, internal rotation, and scapular elevation. All patients were evaluated both before and after treatment. The greatest limitation was demonstrated in patients who had undergone radical neck dissection followed by pedicle flap reconstruction and postoperative radiation. In patients treated with radiation therapy alone, a significant decrease in head mobility was observed, with good preservation of shoulder function. Short and colleagues[52] similarly demonstrated minimal functional disability with both shoulder elevation and abduction in eight patients treated with radiation therapy alone.

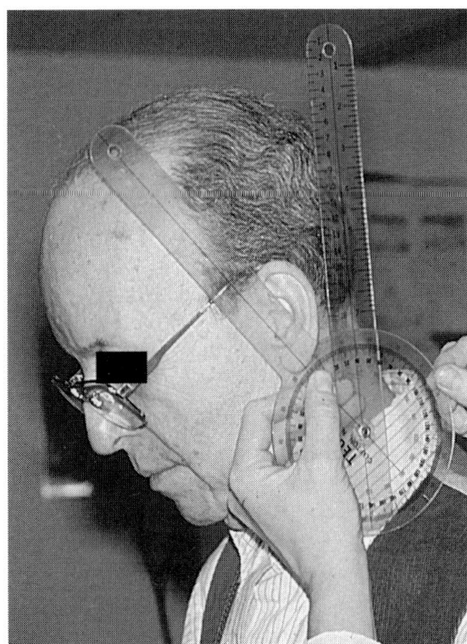

Figure 12–10. Limitation of flexion as measured with a goniometer in patient who received neck radiotherapy as part of head and neck cancer therapy.

Trismus

Trismus is yet another manifestation of progressive muscle fibrosis secondary to radiation therapy of the facial region. It is most commonly a late complication of therapy, often observed a year or more after completion of treatment. Trismus can be a progressive problem further compounding the maintenance of oral health and dental rehabilitation. Because all the muscles of mastication are commonly involved, management by simple coronoidectomy is usually disappointing. Opening exercises and vigorous physical therapy instituted early appear to be helpful in the motivated patient.

Oral Side Effects and Complications

The oral side effects of head and neck irradiation can greatly affect quality of life. Severe xerostomia, altered taste, dysphagia, increased problems with oral infection, and mucosal changes are common sequelae of treatment.

Kuter and associates[53] studied the oral side effects of radiation in four specific groups of patients. In group I patients, the radiation fields included all of the major salivary glands. In group II patients, radiation fields included more than 50% of the parotid glands. Less than 50% of the parotid glands was treated in group III patients. In group IV patients, treatment of the larynx included no major salivary glands within the radiation field. All patients in the study received radiation using either cobalt 60 or 8-MV photon beams via parallel opposing portals. The secretion rate, sodium concentration, pH, and concentration of *Candida* in saliva were studied. In addition, clinical manifestations such as dryness, taste impairment, dysphagia, salivary secretion, and composition were evaluated. Kuter and associates[53] concluded that salivary function is extremely sensitive to radiation, with most of the loss of function occurring after 10 to 20 Gy of exposure. An associated rise in salivary sodium level on the order of 50% was found in groups I to III. This finding was thought to be secondary to damage to the acinar and ductal systems as well as to leakage through damaged mucosa. Of note is that objective decreases in measured salivary flow rates correlated well with subjective complaints of xerostomia in these patients. Associated loss of taste was a more gradual problem, with 50% of patients reporting this after 20 to 30 Gy of exposure. These data agree with results of previous studies, which similarly showed that salivary gland tissue is more sensitive to radiation damage than gustatory tissues.[54] Symptoms of dysphagia were reported in all the treatment groups and occurred after 30 Gy in groups III and IV and after 50 Gy in groups I and II. This finding would indicate that dysphagia is found secondary to not xerostomia alone, but rather to a combination of dryness, mucosal inflammation, and edema as well as secondary infection (e.g., candidiasis). In cases of severe dysphagia, esophageal stenosis may be the etiology. This is often associated with retrosternal burning, vomiting, and weight loss and may require the interruption of treatment. As the dose of radiation gradually increases, there is a concurrent increase in oral yeast flora and a decrease in salivary pH, further compounding problems with swallowing.

Stucchi and colleagues[55] have proposed a grading system for radiation effects on normal tissue. They consider changes that appear within 1 month of treatment to be *acute.* Acute skin reactions are described as mild (erythema, dry desquamation, brown pigmentation, hair loss), moderate (blistering, moist desquamation, crust formation), or severe (deep blisters, areas of necrosis) (Fig. 12–11). Similarly, acute mucosal changes range from erythema and edema to frank necrosis and breakdown. In their study, late changes are defined as changes that manifest at least 12 months after treatment is begun. Late skin changes are dryness, hair loss, thinning, pachydermia, and development of telangiectasia. Late mucosal changes are dryness, atrophy, telangiectasia, sclerosis, and chronic edema.

The late effects on connective tissue consist of nonelasticity, edema, and severe fibrosis as well as the development of ulcers and fistula formation. Late salivary gland changes range from hyposalivation to asialorrhea. Late effects on the head and neck musculature range from retraction with functional loss to frank trismus. Regarding the radiation effects on normal tissue in this manner greatly aids in following patients longitudinally and in appropriately evaluating and counseling them both before and after treatment.

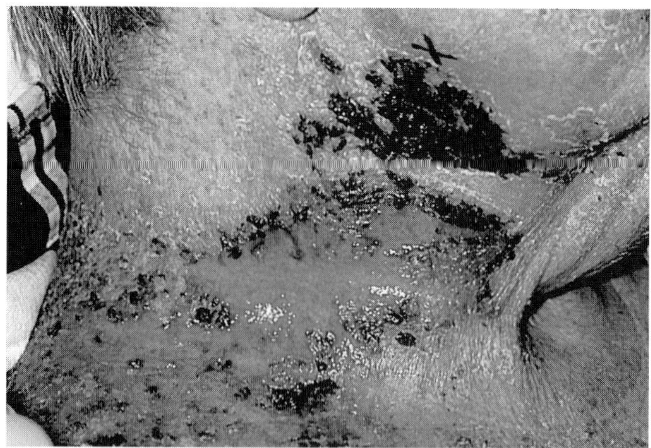

Figure 12–11. Severe desquamation of neck skin secondary to radiotherapy.

Visual Impairment

Radiation to the visual apparatus may accompany the treatment of tumors of the maxilla, maxillary sinus, orbit, and ethmoid and sphenoid sinuses.[56] Reported complications include the development of radiation keratitis, cataract formation, and optic neuritis with progressive visual loss. The incidence of radiation damage to the optic nerve and chiasm is related to both the total dose and the fraction size. Because fraction sizes of 250 rad per fraction may lead to blindness, whenever possible fraction size should be kept below this level.

Radiation Neuritis

Radiation neuritis of other cranial nerves is a reported complication of treatment of head and neck tumors.[57] The occurrence is uncommon, and the incidence can be markedly reduced if the total dose to neural structures is kept below 7000 rad in 7 weeks. Similarly, radiation-induced transverse myelitis is now a rare sequela of radiation treatment if total dosage to the spinal cord is kept below 5000 rad in 5 weeks.

Complications Associated with Chemotherapy for Head and Neck Cancer

Chemotherapy remains an important part of adjuvant therapy for advanced cancers of the head and neck as well as of the treatment of recurrent tumors. For patients who present with late-stage disease, the prognosis is guarded, with most series demonstrating a less than 25% 5-year survival rate. The value of treating head and neck cancer patients with chemotherapy before surgery or radiation therapy remains controversial. The National Cancer Institute contracts program showed no benefit from the addition of chemotherapy (56% and 59% of patients alive at 2 years despite treatment),[58] whereas several more aggressive pilot studies have demonstrated a better 2-year survival.[59]

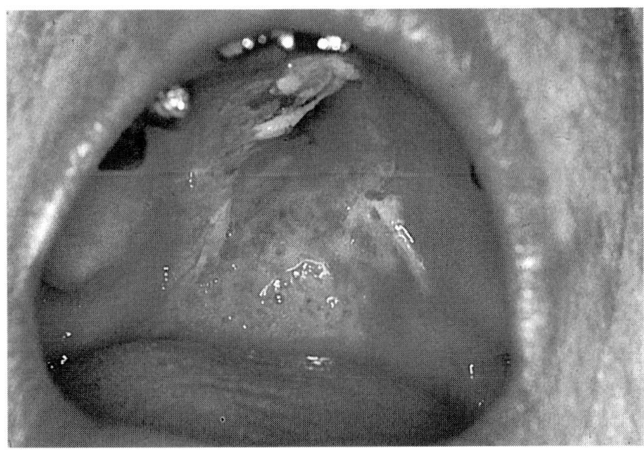

Figure 12–12. Chemotherapy-induced mucositis in patient being treated for recurrent squamous cell carcinoma of the oral cavity.

The chemotherapeutic agents most commonly employed for the treatment of head and neck epidermoid carcinoma are cisplatin, bleomycin, 5-fluorouracil (5-FU), methotrexate, and vincristine. In the treatment of recurrent disease, median survival of 4 to 6 months has been reported with the use of weekly methotrexate.[60] No survival advantage was demonstrated for the use of higher methotrexate doses with leucovorin rescue. A later report has demonstrated a 70% response rate in recurrent or metastatic disease using a combination of cisplatin and 5-FU[55]; however, median survival was only 7 months in this group. Addition of bleomycin to the regimen did not appreciably alter survival time.

The toxicity associated with each of the preceding agents is well documented. Nausea, vomiting, diarrhea, stomatitis (Fig. 12–12), and shortness of breath are commonly reported. If associated gastrointestinal symptoms are severe, intravenous nutritional support may be required. Renal toxicity is usually characterized by a transient elevation in blood urea nitrogen and creatinine, which almost always reverses itself and rarely results in the need for electrolyte repletion. Hematologic toxicity is generally reported as mild for most regimens reviewed. Leukopenia is more severe in multiagent protocols. Thrombocytopenia is very mild throughout treatment.

Stomatitis of a serious nature (grade 3 or 4) is reported in 25% of patients and needs to be managed with appropriate supportive care. Ototoxicity is usually minimal. High-frequency hearing loss is most commonly reported but is usually less than 10 dB. Hypertension during infusion has been noted with the use of cisplatin. Systolic blood pressures of greater than 200 mm Hg may require treatment. Persistent dyspnea without obvious cause has been reported. More catastrophic problems, such as myocardial infarction and septic shock, are fortunately rare.

References

1. Pauloski BR, Rademaker AW, McConnell FM, et al. Speech and swallowing function after anterior tongue and floor of mouth resection with distal flap reconstruction. J Speech Hear Res 1993;36:267–276.
2. Dios PD, Feijoo JF, Ferreiro MC, et al. Functional consequences of partial glossectomy. J Oral Maxillofac Surg 1994;52:12–14.
3. Spiessl B, Prein J, Schmoker R. Anatomic reconstruction and functional rehabilitation of mandibular defects after ablative surgery. *In* Spiessl B (ed): New Concepts in Maxillofacial Bone Surgery. Berlin, Springer-Verlag, 1976, pp 160–166.
4. Lavertu P, Wanamaker JR, Bold EL, et al. The AO system for primary mandibular reconstruction. Am J Surg 1994;168:503–507.
5. Boyd JB, Morris S, Rosen IB, et al. The through-and-through oromandibular defect: Rationale for aggressive reconstruction. Plast Reconstr Surg 1994;93:44–53.
6. Lindqvist C, Soderholm AL, Laine P, et al. Rigid reconstruction plates for immediate reconstruction following mandibular resection for malignant tumors. J Oral Maxillofac Surg 1992;50:1158–1163.
7. Crile GW. Excision of cancer of the head and neck. JAMA 1906;47:1780–1786.
8. Nahum AM, Mullally W, Marmor L. A syndrome resulting from radical neck dissection. Arch Otolaryngol 1961;74:424–428.
9. Sobol S, Jensen C, Sawyer W, et al: Objective comparison of physical dysfunction after neck dissection. Head Neck 1990; 12:342–345.
10. Lingeman R, Helmus C, Stephens R, et al. Neck dissection: Radical or conservative? Ann Otol Rhinol Laryngol 1977;86:737–744.
11. Skolnik E, Yee K, Friedman M, et al. The posterior triangle in radical neck dissection. Arch Otolaryngol 1976;102:1–4.
12. Leipzig B, Suen J, English J, et al: Functional evaluation of the spinal accessory nerve after neck dissection. Am J Surg 1983;146:526–530.
13. Marks S, Jaques D, Hirata R, et al: Blindness following bilateral radical neck dissection. Head Neck 1990;12:342–345.
14. Sugarbaker E, Wiley H: Intracranial pressure studies incident to resection of the internal jugular veins. Cancer 1951;12:342–345.
15. Royster HP: The relation between internal jugular vein pressure and cerebrospinal fluid pressure in the operation of radical neck dissection. Ann Surg 1953;137:826–832.
16. Jones RK: Increased intracranial pressure following radical neck surgery. Arch Surg 1951;63:599–603.
17. Wurster C, Krespi Y, Sisson G, et al: A new complication of modified neck dissection: Internal jugular vein blowout. Otolaryngol Head Neck Surg 1985;93:812–814.
18. de Jong AA, Manni JJ: Phrenic nerve paralysis following neck dissection. Eur Arch Otorhinolaryngol 1991;248:132–134.
19. Simpson SA, Gordon SS, Jorgens J, et al: Roentgen changes following radical neck dissection. Radiology 1956;67:704–713.
20. Swift TR: Involvement of peripheral nerves in radical neck dissection. Arch Otolaryngol 1970;119:694–698.
21. Fitz-Hugh GS, Cowgill R: Chylous fistula, complication of neck dissection. Arch Otolaryngol 1970;91:543.
22. Coleman JJ: Complications in head and neck surgery. Surg Clin North Am 1986;66:149–167.
23. Chantarasak DN, Green MF: Delayed lymphocele following neck dissection. Br J Plast Surg 1989;42:339–340.
24. Swain RE, Biller HF, Ogura JH: An experimental analysis of causative factors and protective methods in carotid artery rupture. Arch Otolaryngol 1974;99:235–241.
25. Ketchum AS, Hays JC: Spontaneous carotid artery hemorrhage after head and neck surgery. Am J Surg 1965;110:649–655.
26. Heller KS, Strong EW: Carotid arterial hemorrhage after radical head and neck surgery. Am J Surg 1979;138:607–610.
27. Marchetta FC, Sako K, Maxwell W: Complications after radical head and neck surgery performed through previously irradiated tissues. Am J Surg 1967;114:835.
28. Coleman JJ: Treatment of the ruptured of exposed carotid artery: A rational approach. S Med J 1985;73:262–267.
29. Zimmerman MC, Mickel RA, Kessler DJ, et al: Treatment of impending carotid rupture with detachable balloon embolization. Arch Otolaryngol Head Neck Surg 1987;113:1169–1175.
30. Gonzalez CF, Moret J: Balloon occlusion of the carotid artery prior to surgery for neck tumors. Am J Neuroradiol 1990;11:649–652.

31. Bertoni SF, Bignardi M, Clottoli GB, et al: Proposed evaluation scale for damage to healthy tissues as a result of radiotherapy of chest, head and neck cancers. Int J Tiss React 1987;9:509–513.
32. Marx RE: Osteoradionecrosis of the jaws: Review and update. HBO Rev 1984;5:78–126.
33. Bedwinek JM, Chavoski LJ, Fletcher GH, et al: Osteonecrosis in patients treated with definitive radiotherapy for squamous cell carcinomas of the oral cavity and naso- and oropharynx. Radiology 1976;119:665–667.
34. Morrish RB, Chan E, Silverman S, et al: Osteoradionecrosis in patients irradiated for head and neck cancer. Cancer 1981; 47:1980–1983.
35. Foyos JV, Lampe I: Peroral irradiation of carcinoma of the oral tongue. Radiology 1969;93:387.
36. Wang CC, Kelly JP, August M, et al: Early carcinoma of the oral cavity: A conservative approach with radiation therapy. J Oral Maxillofac Surg 1995;53:687–690.
37. Wang CC, Biggs PJ: Technical and radiotherapeutic considerations of intra-oral cone electron beam radiation therapy for head and neck cancers. Semin Radiat Oncol 1992;2:171–179.
38. Murray CG, Herson J, Daly TE, et al: Radiation necrosis of the mandible: A 10 year study. Dental factors, onset, duration and management of necrosis. Int J Radiat Oncol Biol Phys 1980;6:549–553.
39. Beumer J, Harrison R, Sanders B, et al: Preradiation dental extractions and the incidence of bone necrosis. Head Neck Surg 1983;5:514–521.
40. Greenspan D: The side effects of radiation therapy and chemotherapy on the oral structures. Oral Maxillofac Surg Clin North Am 1993;5:347–353.
41. Makkonen TA, Kiminki A, Makkonen TK, et al: Dental extractions in relation to radiation therapy of 224 patients. Int J Oral Maxillofac Surg 1987;16:56–64.
42. Samaan NA, Schultz PN, Yang KP, et al: Endocrine complications after radiotherapy for tumors of the head and neck. J Lab Clin Med 1987;364–372.
43. Favus MJ, Schneider AB, Stachura ME, et al: Thyroid cancer occurring as a late consequence of head and neck irradiation. N Engl J Med 1976;294:1019–1025.
44. Tamura K, Shimaoka K, Spaulding S, et al: Association between primary hyperparathyroidism and previous irradiation. J Surg Oncol 1982;19:193–196.
45. Holten I, Petersen LJ: Early changes in parathyroid function after high-dose irradiation of the neck. Cancer 1988;62:1476–1478.
46. Silverberg GD, Britt RH, Goffinet DR: Radiation-induced carotid artery disease. Cancer 1978;41:130–137.
47. Call GK, Bray PF, Smoker WR, et al: Carotid thrombosis following neck irradiation. Int J Radiat Oncol Biol Phys 1989;635–640.
48. Hayward RH: Arteriosclerosis induced by radiation. Surg Clin North Am 1972;52:359–366.
49. Conomy JP, Kellermeyer RW: Delayed cerebrovascular consequences of therapeutic radiation. Cancer 1975;36:1702–1708.
50. Nardelli E, Fiaschi F, Ferrari G: Delayed cerebrovascular consequences of radiation to the neck. Arch Neurol 1978;35:538–540.
51. Nowak P, Parzuchowski J, Jacobs J: Effects of combined modality therapy of head and neck carcinoma on shoulder and head mobility. J Surg Oncol 1989;41:143–147.
52. Short SO, Kaplan JN, Laramore G: Shoulder pain and function after neck dissection with or without preservation of the spinal accessory nerve. Am J Surg 1984;148:478–502.
53. Kuter A, Ben-Aryeh H, Berdicevsky I, et al: Oral side effects of head and neck irradiation: Correlation between clinical manifestations and laboratory data. Int J Oncol Biol Phys 1986;12:401–405.
54. Mossman KL: Quantitative radiation dose-response relationships for normal tissues in man: Response of the salivary glands during radiotherapy. Radiat Res 1983;95:392–398.
55. Stucchi F, Bertoni F, Bignardi M, et al: Proposed evaluation scale for damage to healthy tissues as a result of radiotherapy of chest, head and neck cancers. Int J Tissue React 1987;9:509–513.
56. Shukovsky LJ, Fletcher GH: Retinal and optic nerve complications in a high dose irradiation technique of ethmoid sinus and nasal cavity. Radiology 1972;104:629–634.
57. Cheng VST, Schultz MD: Unilateral hypoglossal nerve atrophy as a late complication of radiation therapy of head and neck carcinoma: A report of four cases and review of the literature on peripheral and cranial nerve damages after radiation therapy. Cancer 1975;35:1537–1544.
58. Rowland KM, Taylor SG, Spiers ASD, et al: Cisplatin and 5-FU infusion in advanced recurrent cancer of the head and neck. Eastern Cooperative Oncology Group Pilot Study. Cancer Treat Rep 1986;70:461–464.
59. Amrein PG, Fabian RL: Treatment of recurrent head and neck cancer with cisplatin and 5-FU vs. the same plus bleomycin and methotrexate. Laryngoscope 1992;102:901–906.
60. Woods RL, Fox RM, Tattersall MHN: Methotrexate treatment of squamous cell head and neck cancers: Dose-response evaluation. Br Med J 1981;286:600–602.

Chapter 13
COMPLICATIONS OF ORTHOGNATHIC SURGERY

by

Robert A. Bays

Introduction

Few surgical procedures are as satisfying for the surgeon and patient as a well-done orthognathic correction. On the other hand, few procedures are as difficult to do well. Generally, if the result of an orthognathic operation is less than perfect, one or more of the problems described herein have occurred. In this chapter, I discuss these complications with an attempt to assist in prevention whenever possible. Nowhere is the adage "An ounce of prevention is worth a pound of cure" more applicable.

This chapter is organized according to procedures, although I recognize that many complications are common to several operations. The assumption is that the reader is interested in the potential pitfalls of a specific operation when consulting this reference, rather than all of the causes of a particular complication—such as nerve injury. This discussion is of interest to all surgeons, but particularly, the neophyte orthognathic surgeon should learn that despite the best intentions, complications occur and thinking about prevention is important.

Although certain aspects of orthognathic complications have been widely discussed in the literature (e.g., relapse), others have often been relegated to discussions in the surgeons' lounge. Literature sources are cited when there are quality data to support a particular concept or statement; however, much of this presentation about the prevention and treatment of orthognathic mishaps is derived from my own experience as well as that of my colleagues and residents over the last 20 years.

THE SUBJECTS DISCUSSED IN THIS CHAPTER ARE:

Mandibular Procedures

Preoperative Factors That May Adversely Affect Outcomes

Orthodontic preparation, evaluation of maxillary and chin midlines, recognition of *significant* temporomandibular joint abnormalities, surgical splint construction, and patient expectations may all adversely affect the outcome of a mandibular orthognathic procedure.

Orthodontic preparation may be inappropriate or inadequate because of lack of communication (between surgeon and orthodontist) before orthodontic treatment or because of an inability to achieve preoperative goals and a failure to recognize that they have not been met. In mandibular surgery, considerations of extraction should be decided before orthodontics is initiated.[1] If maxillary extractions are considered, will they compromise upper lip support and facial aesthetics? Also, the amount of mandibular advancement may be diminished by four bicuspid extractions. Mandibular extractions without maxillary extractions performed to maximize advancement may leave maxillary second molars unopposed after surgery.

Inability to level the curve of Spee is a relative problem. So long as an adequate tripod of occlusal stability (six anterior teeth and posterior molars) can be achieved at the time of surgery, much leveling can be done postoperatively.

In prognathic cases, dental compensations may be inappropriately increased orthodontically rather than reduced.[2] This may occur if orthodontic treatment is initiated in the growing child with class III deformity in the hope that surgery will not be necessary. Ultimately, it may become obvious that the mandible is growing beyond the maxilla, and the surgeon is consulted. Delay is wise in this situation. Discontinuance of orthodontic treatment and observation of growth for one to several years is the course of choice. Only in the severest of class III deformities, in which psychological problems exist, is it recommended that surgical treatment precede cessation of growth. In these cases, it is even more important that dental compensations are eliminated, not exaggerated.

Arch width incompatibilities must be assessed by the orthodontist and surgeon preoperatively. If orthodontic-orthopedic expansion is attempted and results in excessive tipping of the teeth rather than true skeletal enlargement, transverse relapse and open bite may develop after completion of orthognathic treatment. This will also result in autorotation of the mandible down and back (clockwise), simulating anteroposterior (AP) relapse. In the long term, it may be difficult to determine whether the open bite and anteroposterior changes are orthodontic or surgical.

If the pretreatment decision is made to attempt nonsurgical expansion, and if it subsequently fails to achieve the desired result, the expansion must be reversed prior to surgery, and a surgical plan for expansion must be developed. The options for surgical expansion are surgical rapid palatal expansion (SRPE) and multipiece maxillary osteotomy. A complete discussion of the indications for each is not possible here, but because SRPE is usually performed before orthodontic therapy, pretreatment planning is essential to avoid this late-appearing dilemma.

Any interdental osteotomy requires sufficient space between the roots to accomplish the cut without damaging the roots or the periodontium. Ideally, the orthodontist should know from the surgeon at the beginning of treatment where these osteotomies will be performed so that proper root divergence can be achieved. Occasionally, the site of interdental osteotomy may change as orthodontic treatment progresses from between canine and first premolar tooth to between canine and lateral incisor. Therefore, the best plan is to achieve ideal root parallelism to permit flexibility in the final planning stages.

Certain orthodontic tooth movements are known to be unstable, such as extrusion of maxillary anterior teeth. They should be avoided in the preoperative phase.

Finally, there should be no active archwires at the time of surgery. Specifically, there must not be any changes in tooth position between the time that the surgical models are taken for splint construction and the actual surgical procedure.

In mandibular surgery, the *maxillary midline* will not change, but the *chin midline* may change when mandibular movements are asymmetric. If the chin midline is coincident with the facial midline preoperatively, but the planned movement is asymmetric, the movement will leave the chin deviated from the preoperative position. In some cases, the maxillary midline may be slightly deviated to one side, or the maxillary occlusal plane may be canted. If the combination of asymmetric mandibular movement, slight maxillary midline deviation, and cant leads to a chin movement in the same direction, the result may be aesthetically unacceptable. Of course, if the cumulative effects of these movements offset one another, the chin will be positioned appropriately. Preoperative evaluation of all of these factors avoids unexpected outcomes.

It is beyond the scope of this chapter to discuss a comprehensive approach to the patient who is undergoing *orthognathic* surgery with temporomandibular joint problems. Suffice it to say that minor temporomandibular disorder (TMD) complaints should be documented, slightly significant complaints should be discussed with the patient and orthodontist to form a plan if they are exacerbated, and significant TMD problems should be addressed before orthognathic treatment. Wisdom lies in recognizing the difference.

Surgical splints, or wafers, that are made on a semiadjustable articulator from facebow-mounted models should allow the mandible to be rotated in and out of occlusion without interferences. If the intention is to wire the splint in place and let the patient function into it for a period of time postoperatively, it is essential that the depressions for the lower teeth are not so deep that they interfere with the path of closure. This may also be important at the end of surgery after rigid fixation has been applied to test the accuracy of the mandibular position. Intraoperatively, if an occlusal prematurity exists upon closure into the splint, it may not be certain whether this problem is due to poor splint construction, to warping of the splint as it is ligated to the arch wire, or to inaccurate mandibular positioning. In such cases, the splint should be removed, at least temporarily, and the occlusion checked without it. It is almost always a bad idea to grind on the splint to allow the mandible to better occlude into it. Doing so usually represents burying one's head in the sand. If the jaw is not positioned properly, this reality will emerge when the splint is removed.

It is also beyond the scope of this discussion to address the subject of preoperative psychological evaluation. Are preoperative computer-generated video imaging predictions helpful or deceiving? Are psychological or personality inventories useful in assessing *patient expectations*? The answers to these questions are not well known. The best guiding principle is to make an effort to get to know each patient. Talk to the patient and the family. They will talk to the clinician who listens.

Intraoperative and Postoperative Complications and Their Prevention

Preventive, intraoperative, and **postoperative** concerns in mandibular operations are combined and categorized according to specific procedures.

Bilateral Sagittal Split Osteotomy (BSSO)

The most commonly reported complications for the BSSO are as follows:

- Bad splits[3–6]
- Nerve injury[3, 5–17]
- Bleeding[3, 5, 6]
- Proximal segment malpositioning[3, 5, 12, 18–20]
- Condylar resorption[21–25]
- Interfragmentary incompatibilities[5, 26, 27]
- Distal segment interferences with large setbacks (rare)[2]

The subject of postoperative open bites is discussed with vertical ramus osteotomy. Relapse, for the purpose of this discussion, is not considered a complication, but rather an inevitability. Especially with BSSO, relapse to some degree occurs in every case. In this section, I consider bad splits, proximal segment malpositioning, and condylar resorption.

Bad Splits

Prevention. Proper corticotomy technique is the first line of prevention. The bur or saw blade must be angled parallel to the mandibular occlusal plane for the medial ramus cut. Removal of the internal oblique ridge with a large bur facilitates tremendously visualization of the medial cut[28] (Fig. 13–1*A* and *B*). Visualization of the lateral ramal cortex as the medial corticotomy is made prevents placing the medial cut too superiorly and risking a horizontal ramus fracture. The vertical lateral corticotomy of the mandibular body should penetrate only the cortex and exactly half of the inferior border. The corticotomy that connects the medial ramus and the lateral body corticotomies should be as lateral as possible while still remaining inside the lateral cortex, and it should be angled laterally to facilitate a lateral direction to the chisel (Fig. 13–1*C*).

An access bevel is placed on the anterior lip of the vertical corticotomy to allow the chisel to slide just under the lateral cortex as it is driven from top to bottom of the vertical cut and through the inferior border[28] (Fig. 13–1*D*). The access bevel and a strong lateral direction to the sharp chisel permit excellent visualization of the inferior border cut.

Next, the medial cut should be enhanced with the sharp chisel under direct vision so that any subsequent stress placed upon it will result in a split along the desired lines. Finally, a sharp cement spatula chisel can be driven up and down the connecting cut with strong lateral pressure to "skin under" the lateral cortex, thus avoiding the neurovascular bundle while gently separating the proximal fragment from the distal fragment.

As the split begins to open up, the lines of separation can be inspected. If they are not as planned, the surgeon may be able to "regroup" before the bad split has occurred. Also, the neurovascular bundle can be visualized, and if it tends to remain in the proximal fragment, it can be teased out before the split has been completed, thereby reducing the stretch placed upon it. After the position of the neurovascular bundle has been secured, the inferior border is cut directly from above through the splitting osteotomy. With this controlled technique, no heavy prying forces are placed on the segments.

Mandibular third molars, especially impacted ones, probably increase the risk of a bad split[4] and inferior alveolar nerve injury.[6] Therefore, it is strongly recommended that they be removed at least 9 months before sagittal split of the mandible. If third molars are in the mandible at the time of osteotomy, they should not be removed by conventional techniques. In fact, it is recommended that the osteotomy be conducted just as described and, if the third molar is in the path of the connecting cut, that it simply be drilled through without allowing it to alter the direction or extent of the cuts. The only variation that is necessary is that if the third molar is in the line of the connecting cut, the bur cut that goes through the molar should completely penetrate it, so that the chisel will easily divide it into a large medial portion and a thin lateral portion. The parts of the third molar can be removed after the split has been completed. The larger medial part of the molar may need to be divided between the crown and the root to avoid stressing the posterior aspect of the distal fragment, because a fracture just posterior to the second molar in the distal fragment is at risk.

Intraoperative Considerations. The incidence of unfavorable splits with the BSSO has been reported to be 3% to 20%.[26] This wide range is probably due to different definitions of a bad split, variations in tech-

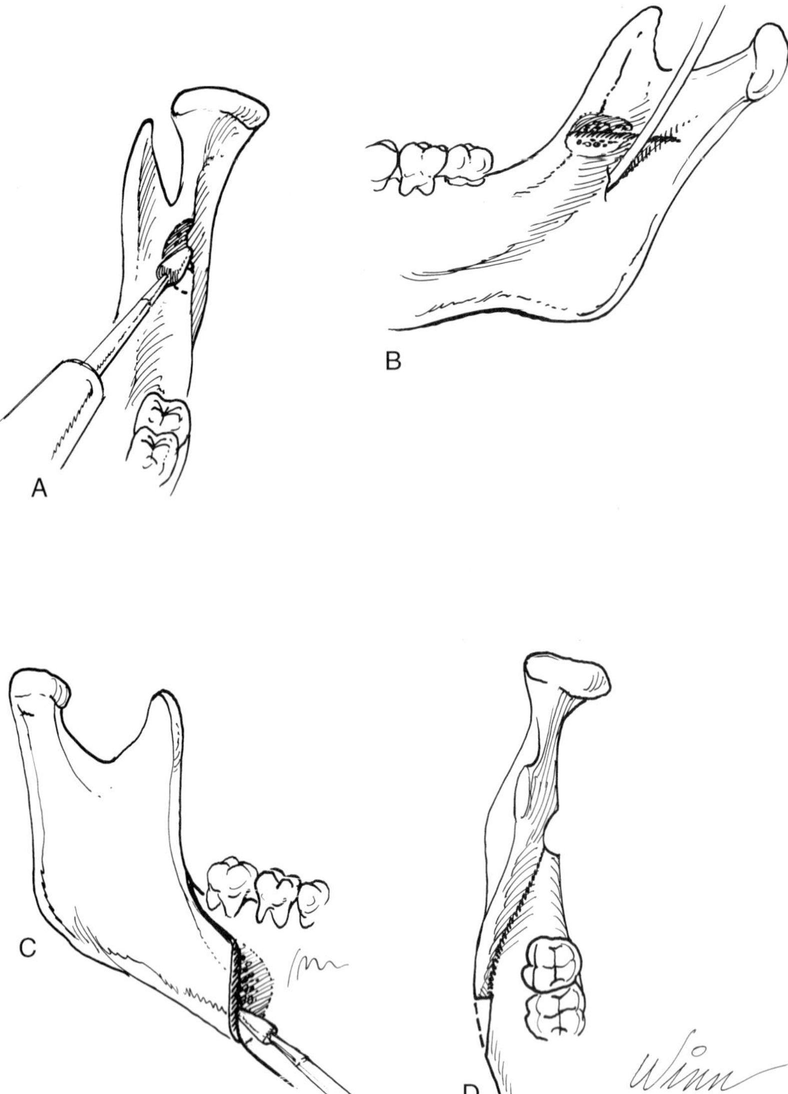

Figure 13–1. Bilateral sagittal split osteotomy (BSSO). *A*, Access bevel through internal oblique ridge to improve visualization of the medial cortex. *B*, Medial view of the access bevel and improved visualization of the mandibular fossa. *C*, Lateral placement of the connecting osteotomy to enhance ability to successfully split the mandible. Also, note the access bevel anterior to the vertical corticotomy. *D*, Additional view of the access bevel at the vertical corticotomy, which improves the opportunity to drive a chisel just under the lateral cortex through the inferior border, thereby ensuring a proper split at the anteroinferior aspect of the BSSO.

nique, and the experience of the operator. Intuitively, one would expect factors such as the presence of third molars, incomplete or poorly placed corticotomies, and excessive prying to contribute to this problem.

Although it may be attractive to regard the management of a bad split during BSSO as similar to that of a comminuted mandibular fracture, there is an important difference. In orthognathic surgery, the distal segment is to be relocated to a new position. Therefore, conservative measures appropriate to deal with a comminuted traumatic ramus fracture may be inadequate, especially when the distal segment is not returned to the original position.

If a bad split occurs, the first decision to be made is whether to proceed with the operation by relocating the distal segment to the planned postoperative occlusion or to abort the procedure and return the segments to their preoperative positions. Although it may be easier to make this decision if the complication occurs on the first side, even if the bad split occurs on the second side, returning the mandible to the original preoperative position, fixing the segments, and allowing them to heal carries less risk of developing a weak bony union than proceeding with the advancement. Nevertheless, with modern rigid fixation systems, many experienced operators would complete the operation and employ a more stable fixation system than usual. In large advancements, this decision may be risky without benefit of bone grafting. The presence of third molars in the mandible increases the probability of a bad split and reduces both the bone-to-bone contact between the segments and the bony area available for rigid fixation.

Several bad splits and techniques for stabilizing them are illustrated in Figures 13–2 to 13–8. Although there are a myriad of techniques for management of bad splits, a basic tenet is that the most proximal, stable segment containing the condyle should be rigidly fixed to the intact distal segment. Piecing multiple sections together in chain-link fashion is less than acceptable. The reason is that each bridging fixation device (wires or plates) that crosses a fractured segment represents a

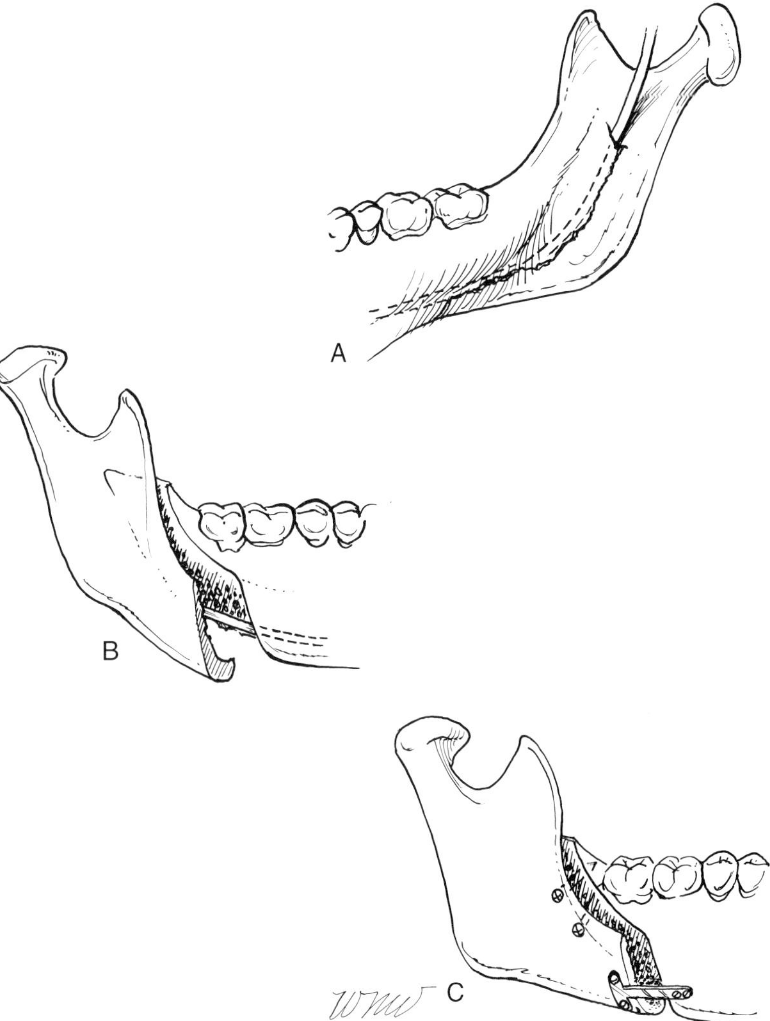

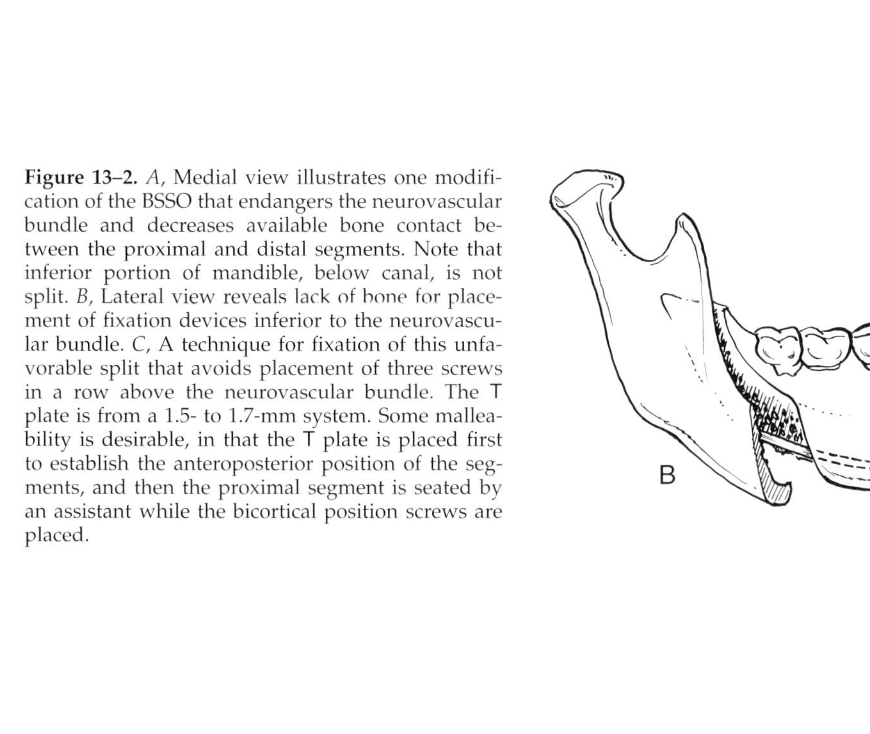

Figure 13–2. *A*, Medial view illustrates one modification of the BSSO that endangers the neurovascular bundle and decreases available bone contact between the proximal and distal segments. Note that inferior portion of mandible, below canal, is not split. *B*, Lateral view reveals lack of bone for placement of fixation devices inferior to the neurovascular bundle. *C*, A technique for fixation of this unfavorable split that avoids placement of three screws in a row above the neurovascular bundle. The T plate is from a 1.5- to 1.7-mm system. Some malleability is desirable, in that the T plate is placed first to establish the anteroposterior position of the segments, and then the proximal segment is seated by an assistant while the bicortical position screws are placed.

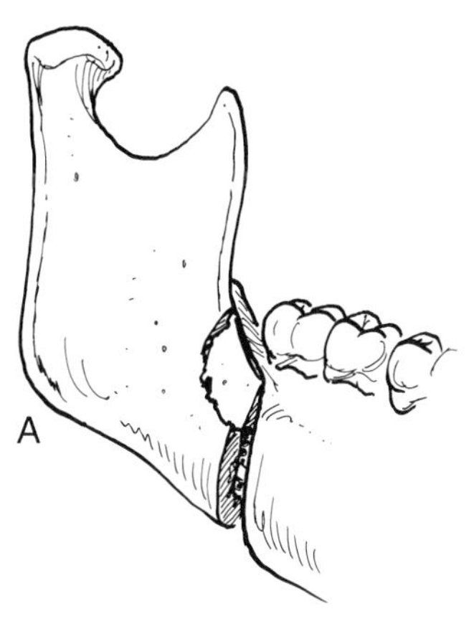

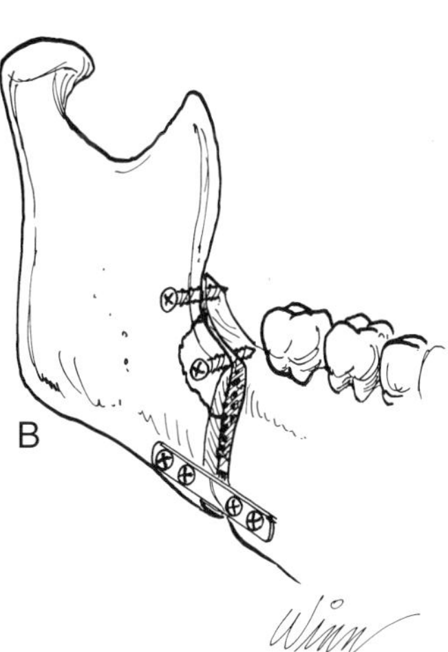

Figure 13–3. *A*, Fracture of anterosuperior aspect of the proximal segment. This fracture decreases the available bone for interfragmentary fixation. *B*, A heavier plate (2.0-mm screws) is used at the inferior border, because the screw fixing the fractured piece does not provide interfragmentary fixation.

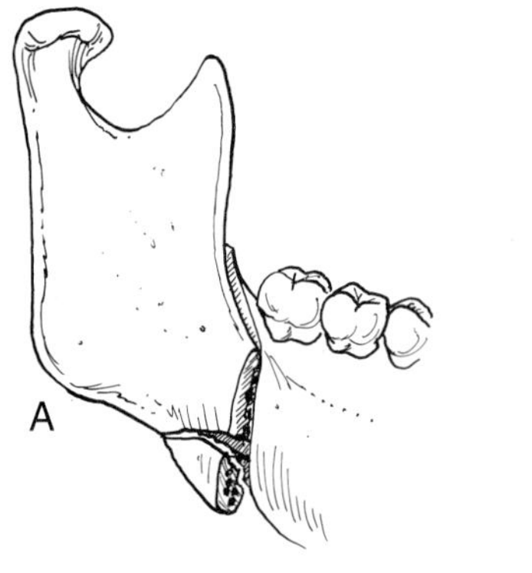

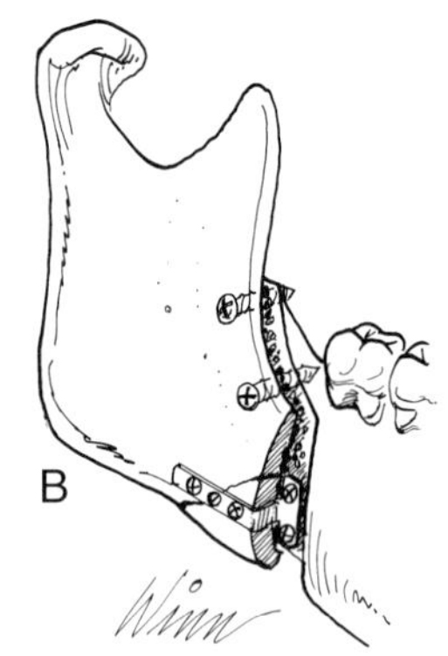

Figure 13–4. *A,* Inferior border fracture limiting the ability to provide fixation that is not in a straight line along the superior border. Straight line placement of more than two screws is to be avoided if possible (see Fig. 13–12). *B,* Inferior border T plate (1.5 to 1.7 mm) plus two bicortical position screws (2.0 mm) at the superior border. The screw passing through the T plate and the fracture segment is a bicortical position screw.

Figure 13–5. *A,* The horizontal ramus fracture is one of the worst unfavorable splits that can occur with the BSSO. The proximal segment containing the condyle and the most distal segment containing the teeth must be fixed together by one continuous device. *B,* A reconstruction plate (2.4 to 2.7 mm) or a Thorpe-type plate is recommended. "Chain-linking" fragments together with a series of short plates is less desirable, because there are many more sites for failure. Additionally, regardless of the amount of bony overlap, the horizontal ramus fracture is the weak link, with a very poor interface between the two edges of the fracture. A tension band is also needed, and the two anteriormost screws are bicortical position screws (2.0 mm).

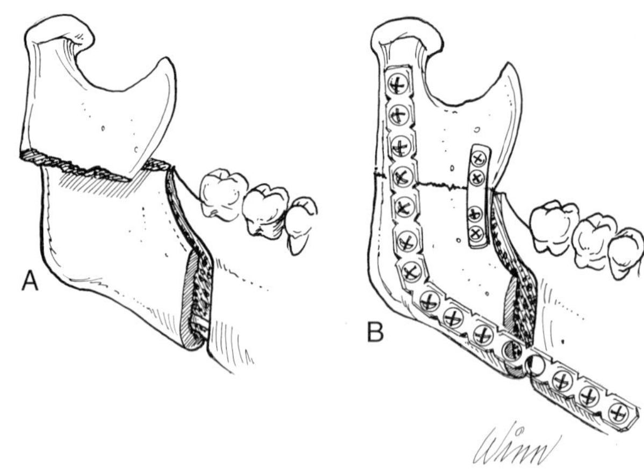

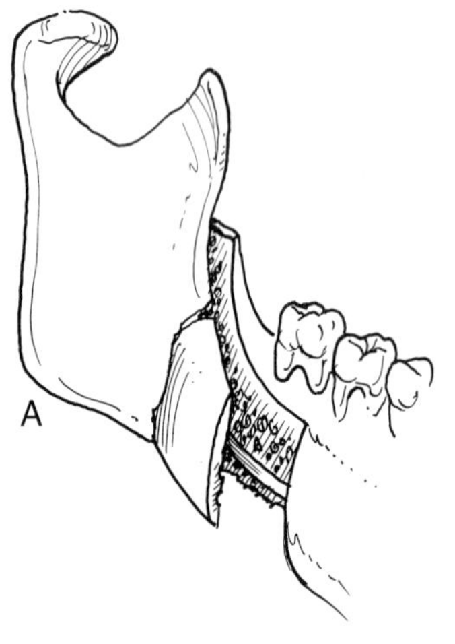

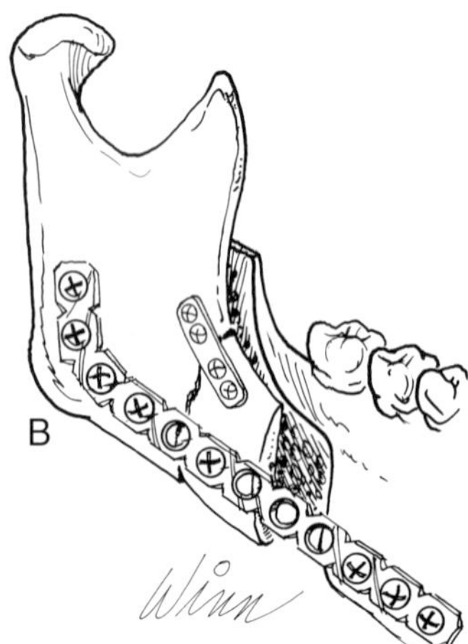

Figure 13–6. *A,* Fracture of a significant part of the proximal fragment can be deceptively difficult to manage successfully. Placing the fragments together using conventional techniques appears adequate, but the surgeon must realize that the only "real" interfragmentary fixation is between the proximal segment with the condyle attached and the distal, tooth-bearing segment. *B,* Therefore, it is recommended here that a rigid reconstruction (2.4 to 2.7 mm) or Thorpe-type plate span the distance between these two segments. The screws in the superior border tension band plate are bicortical position screws (2.0 mm).

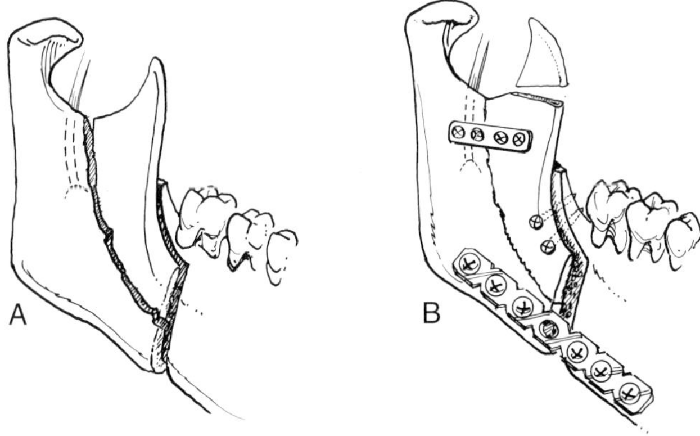

Figure 13–7. *A,* Fracture of the anterior coronoid containing part of the proximal segment is unusual but is problematic when it happens. *B,* The temporalis muscle exerts a strong pull on this segment and should be removed via coronoidectomy or coronoidotomy. Because there is so little contact between the proximal and distal segments, heavy plate (2.4 to 2.7 mm) fixation, as shown in Fig. 13–6, is recommended. The bicortical position screws and the plate on the superior ramus add only minimal interfragmentary stabilization; thus the need for the reconstruction plate.

possible failure point. Some of these segments may be devoid of blood supply. A rigid device, such as a reconstruction plate, should span the distance from condyle segment to distal mandible, and then the additional fragments can be fixed in the appropriate places. It must be realized that, with the loss of orientation between the intact proximal and distal segments, the chances of improper condylar positioning with rigid fixation are increased. In my opinion, however, delayed healing is to be expected in bad splits, especially with advancements, so that nonrigid techniques are likely to result in weak or nonexistent unions that lead to long-term alterations in the gonial angle and skeletal malocclusion. Aggressive rigid fixation of the fragments and early mobilization are strongly recommended.

Postoperative Considerations. Careful observation for evidence of fragment displacement or poor healing is necessary following bad splits. Counterclockwise rotation of a proximal segment is the most common indicator that healing is delayed and mobility of the segments has occurred. Measures should be taken to assess the effects of this problem. If the rotation has not had a major influence on the occlusion, one may opt for no surgical treatment or intermaxillary fixation. If the occlusion has been seriously compromised, reoperation with repositioning and refixation of the segments is necessary. If reoperation is planned, bone grafting should be considered, because poor bone-to-bone contact is to be anticipated.

Additionally, frank non-union or osteomyelitis may occur following a bad split. Fortunately, these complications are rare, although either may lead to major morbidity. Affected patients often end up in academic centers for reconstruction. The lesson to be learned is that a comprehensive, aggressive attempt to fix the problem should be instituted as early as possible in the course of the complication.

Nerve Injury

Prevention. Nerve injuries during BSSO may involve sensory[3–7, 11, 13–15] or motor[3, 10, 16, 17, 29, 30] nerves, although sensory injuries are far more common. The inferior alveolar nerve as it courses through the mandi-

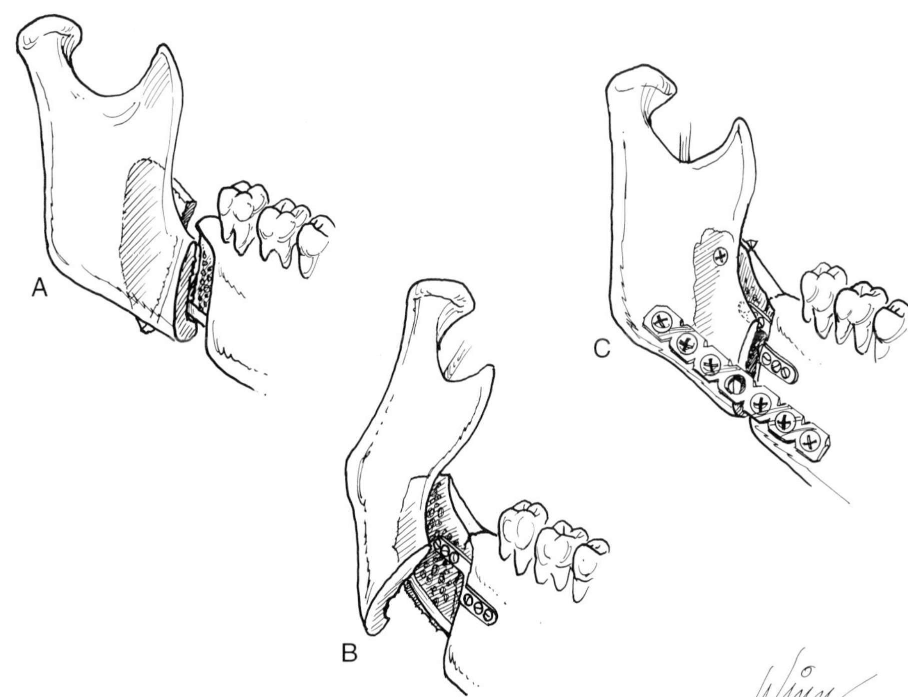

Figure 13–8. *A,* Fractures of the distal segment directly behind the second molar also can be very difficult to fix adequately and are deceiving because there appears to be considerable bony overlap. Fixation of the fractured lingual portion to the proximal segment may appear reassuring but contributes little to the interfragmentary fixation needed to properly stabilize the fracture/osteotomy. *B,* Fixation of the lingual segment to the distal segment can be achieved by adapting a plate (1.7 to 2.0 mm) using monocortical screws. One or two plates may be needed. *C,* As stated previously, however, this process does nothing to establish interfragmentary stabilization, which is instead accomplished with a reconstruction (2.4 to 2.7 mm) or Thorpe-type plate. Bicortical position screws (2.0 mm) may afford additional stability to the fractured lingual segment.

ble is most often damaged.[31] Surgeon-observed intraoperative disruption of nerve continuity is uncommon,[6] but long-term postoperative neurosensory deficit following BSSO is a frequently observed phenomenon.[13, 13]

This section deals only with the issue of operator-observed intraoperative nerve injury. The inferior alveolar nerve is most vulnerable in the more anterior aspect of the split, but it may be damaged anywhere from the pterygomandibular space to the vertical osteotomy anteriorly. The best technique to minimize inferior alveolar nerve injury is described in the section on preventing bad splits. In summary, careful, gradual, controlled splitting under direct vision is recommended (see Fig. 13–1). Additionally, extraction of mandibular third molars at least 9 months prior to sagittal splitting is advisable if possible.

Facial nerve injury can be prevented by simply staying within the periosteal envelope of the mandible throughout the surgical procedure. Penetration of the inferoposterior border during chisel instrumentation could conceivably damage cranial nerve VII. Although it has been suggested that a short split, as opposed to a complete split, may prevent motor nerve injury in large setbacks,[27] there are no data to support this recommendation, nor has it been my experience. A short split is recommended for large setbacks because posterior movement of the distal segment may be obstructed by the styloid process, the mastoid process, or the transverse process of the second cervical vertebra. Whether this movement may potentially damage cranial nerve VII is not known.

Intraoperative Considerations. When the inferior alveolar nerve is visibly damaged or transected completely during BSSO, there are no recommendations in the literature to guide the surgical response. Common sense would dictate that if the nerve is transected and reapproximation without tension on or compromise of the success of the osteotomy is possible, it should be done. If the nerve has been abraded or shredded but is partially intact, the choices are (1) to leave it, excise the entire damaged portion, and graft the defect or (2) to attempt to free both ends, freshen the edges, and perform a direct repair. In order to successfully release enough nerve to accomplish direct repair, the proximal nerve segment has to be removed posteriorly from the bony canal to the mandibular foramen, and most likely, the distal segment must be released to the mental foramen. The likelihood of additional nerve damage during this procedure must be considered. If nerve repair is attempted, the nerve stumps should be freshened and reattached using fine microsurgery sutures and magnification.

Data indicate that there is no correlation between operator-observed nerve injury and postoperative neurosensory changes.[7] This finding suggests that the health of the nerve relative to subsequent function probably cannot be reliably assessed at the time of operation. Therefore, reacting to a perceived nerve injury that does not include complete transection seems ill advised.

As previously stated, to avoid injury to the facial nerve, one must stay within the periosteal envelope during the surgical procedure. Operator-observed facial nerve injury is very unlikely.

Lingual nerve injury has been reported following BSSO, but it is rare and is seldom recognized at the time of surgery.[12] Lingual nerve injury, however, may occur more commonly than has been previously reported.[11] The fundamentals advocated for management of the inferior alveolar nerve apply for the lingual nerve.

Postoperative Considerations. There are few data to guide us in the management of postoperative neurosensory deficits after BSSO. In general, patients with *dysesthesias* should be considered for intervention. There is probably no subjective test that will assist in determining the etiology of the dysesthesia, although a CT scan may help identify nerve compression. In my experience, few dysesthesias have been seen following BSSO. When this problem occurs, however, it is manifest in the early postoperative period. In such cases, inferior alveolar nerve block may assist in localization of the lesion and the possibility of successful surgical management. If nerve block gives profound relief of the dysesthesia for the period of local anesthesia, surgical decompression of the nerve may be helpful in alleviating pain, if not hypesthesia. The patient must be advised regarding the possible need for nerve grafting and the likelihood of success. The lingual nerve should be managed in a fashion similar to that for the inferior alveolar nerve, both intraoperatively and postoperatively.

If postoperative facial paralysis is present, the course of appropriate action is debatable. Evoked electromyography (EEMG) has been advocated as a prognostic test. If the response remains greater than 25% of normal at 5 days postoperatively, the prognosis is good for spontaneous recovery.[32] If the nerve fails to transmit an impulse after 7 days as determined by electroneurography, the prognosis is said to be poor.[32] Therefore, with a good prognosis, observation and supportive therapy are recommended. Such therapy includes management of the eye to prevent drying, through the use of artificial tears and perhaps taping at night. Exercises and transcutaneous electrical nerve stimulation (TENS) have not been shown to be of value in hastening the return of muscle function.

The difficult question is what to do if the tests indicate a poor prognosis. Exploration has been advocated, but good documentation of the benefits or morbidity is lacking.[27] Because it is probably not known where the injury occurred during the procedure and at what location along the nerve, exploration may be a difficult exercise, on the order of hunting for the proverbial needle in a haystack.

Bleeding

Prevention. As in all surgery, the best strategy to prevent bleeding is to obtain a good history of prior bleeding experiences and to apply an excellent knowledge of surgical anatomy. In the absence of a pathologic bleeding history or of a systemic disorder consistent or associated with a coagulopathy, preoperative prothrombin, partial thromboplastin, and bleeding times tests are not indicated.

Intraoperative Considerations. The inferior alveolar artery may be encountered within the bone or in the pterygomandibular space. Usually, hemostasis occurs spontaneously; however, if inferior alveolar artery hemorrhage continues, the vessel should be dissected free from the nerve and ligated rather than cauterized. Also, the masseteric artery may be interrupted in the sigmoid notch. Hemostasis usually occurs spontaneously, but if it does not, direct exposure with cauterization or ligation may be necessary to control hemorrhage.

It is important for the surgeon to stay within the periosteal envelope at all times during the operation to prevent injury to the facial artery and retromandibular vein. Suction drains, elevated head position, and pressure dressings have all been used to decrease postoperative bleeding, swelling, and hematoma formation. Pressure dressings are not recommended here, but bilateral suction drains left in place for a few hours after completion of surgery seem to help decrease hematoma formation and swelling. When reasonable efforts to directly control bleeding have failed, packing with a resorbable material should be attempted. If bleeding is controlled in this way, the wounds may be closed.

Postoperative Considerations. Usually, within 5 to 8 hours postoperatively, the volume of suction drainage decreases significantly. The drains have performed their function of minimizing dead space and evacuating fluid between the bone and soft tissue. If they remain productive or if hematoma is enlarging in spite of the drains, a pressure dressing may be considered with careful observation of the airway. If expansion of the swelling does not respond to these measures within 30 minutes, the patient should be returned to the operating room for exploration, evacuation of hematoma, and achievement of hemostasis.

Proximal Segment Malpositioning

Prevention. Surgery performed on models mounted on a semiadjustable articulator, utilizing a facebow recording, renders information beyond just the planned occlusion. If reference measurements are made on the models corresponding to the vertical and lateral osteotomies, the amount and nature of the movement on each side of the mandible can be documented. The surgeon can then check the relationship of the fragments in the operating room and identify any unplanned or unequal movements. These are most often seen with asymmetries in which the proximal end of the distal fragment shifts mediolaterally (Figs. 13–9 and 13–10) and, perhaps, inferosuperiorly (Fig. 13–11). Preoperative recognition of these complex movements permits development of strategies to deal with proximal segment positioning. Lateral cephalometric tracings do not accurately depict this important information.

Intraoperative Considerations. Discussion of the subject of proximal segment positioning requires differentiation between rigid and nonrigid fixation techniques. The pros and cons of the two are not discussed here; suffice it to say that nonrigid fixation with inferior border wiring works very well with regard to intraoperative proximal segment positioning.[18] Rigid fixation is currently the method used most often, however, and therefore is discussed in greater detail. Multiple methods of condylar positioning, including some that are very complex and cumbersome,[33] have been described. Nevertheless, there is no foolproof method. The most important ingredient is operator experience and "feel." A thorough study of the case preoperatively and a profound understanding of the possible intraoperative interfaces between the proximal and distal segments, along with experience, are the most important factors in achieving proper proximal segment positioning.

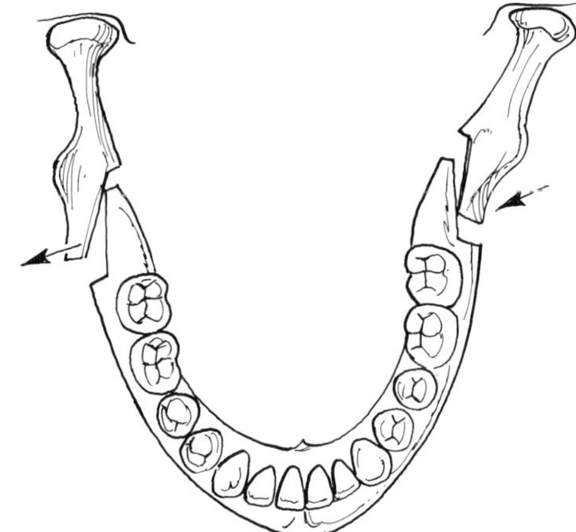

Figure 13–9. An occlusal view of a BSSO in which the distal segment has shifted bodily from left to right, rotating the right proximal segment outward and the left proximal segment inward. Osteoplasty at the most posterior part of the right distal segment may decrease the rotation of the right proximal segment somewhat. Usually, allowing the proximal segment to rotate inward a few degrees is acceptable. The limits of acceptable rotation are not known. If the rotation is judged to be unacceptable, an interpositional graft of bone or hydroxylapatite may be useful.

Aligning the inferior borders in a superoinferior direction is usually the best starting point. In most cases of simple advancement or setback, the inferior borders should be aligned or nearly so. When mandibular movement includes significant clockwise or counterclockwise rotations, mediolateral shifts, or changes in the vertical ramus height (see Fig. 13–11), alignment is more difficult. If the distal segment is to be rotated clockwise more than 3 to 4 degrees to the mandibular plane and the lateral vertical cut of the osteotomy is in the second molar region, the proximal segment would protrude a corresponding amount below the distal segment when fixed, depending on the location of the pivot point around which the distal segment is rotating. Conversely, if counterclockwise rotation is desired (no debate on the advisability of this maneuver is offered), the inferior border of the distal segment would likewise extend below the proximal one (see Fig. 13–11).

Anteroposterior measurements taken at the time of

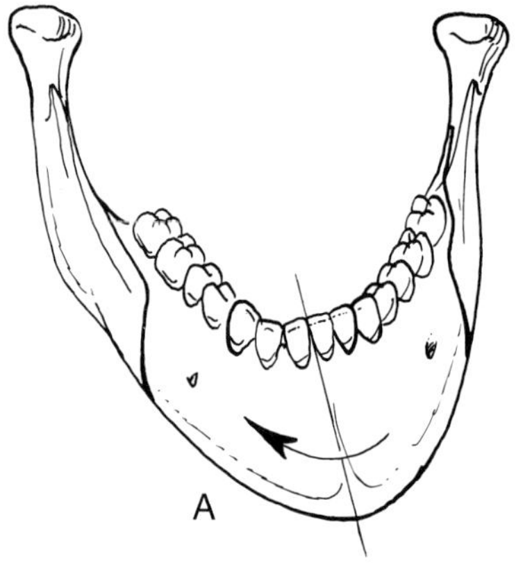

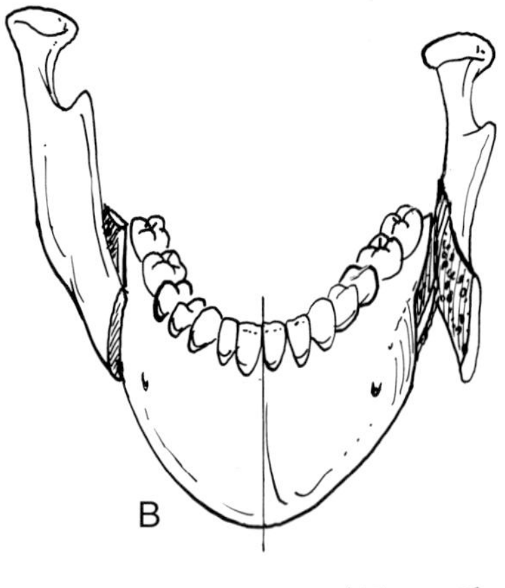

Figure 13–10. *A,* Pivoting of the proximal segment from left to right may give the opposite contact, as seen in Figure 13–9. *B,* In the patient illustrated here, the chin and mandibular midline have shifted to the right, but the posterior end of the distal segment has shifted to the left. Accurate model surgery is the only way to predict these contacts preoperatively. The methods used to manage such situations are shown in Figure 13–9.

model surgery and a gentle "touch" will assist in the correct positioning of the proximal segment. If clockwise or counterclockwise rotations are performed, the superior defect of the vertical osteotomy is different from the inferior one.

The greatest difficulties occur with significant mediolateral moves (see Figs. 13–9 and 13–10). Careful model surgery analysis gives an indication of a lateral shift in the distal segment and also reveals whether that shift is a bodily movement (see Fig. 13–9) or a pivotal one (see Fig. 13–10). If the mandible is pivoting to correct an asymmetry, the analysis should show whether the pivot point is anterior, posterior, or somewhere in between. The important issue is whether the most posterior aspect of the distal segment is moving mediolaterally. If one side is moving bodily to the lateral, the entire proximal segment will be pushed laterally (see Fig. 13–9), but bony contact may or may not be adequate. On the other side, where the distal segment is shifting medially, the proximal segment will follow it by hinging inward, but adequate bony contact usually is preserved (see Fig. 13–9).

If the mandible is pivoting around the anterior teeth, however, the contact between the two segments is only at their most posterior interface on the side of lateral movement (see Fig. 13–10), and on the other side, the contact is at the most anterior aspect of the proximal segment (see Fig. 13–10). Although osteoplasty can be helpful, it may not be possible to eliminate enough bone to facilitate proper bony contact. This is especially true when the premature contact is in the posterior, because the mandibular foramen is close to the posterior border of the distal segment, and only a limited amount of bone can be removed without damage to the nerve. In such cases, an interpositional material such as autologous bone, hydroxylapatite (HA), or allogeneic bone may be inserted.

If a canted occlusal plane is to be corrected, the inferior borders of the proximal and distal segments do not align on both sides (see Fig. 13–11). Whether one side stays aligned while the other changes or they both change in length can be determined only by model surgery preoperatively. If the proximal and distal segments are not at the same vertical level, the

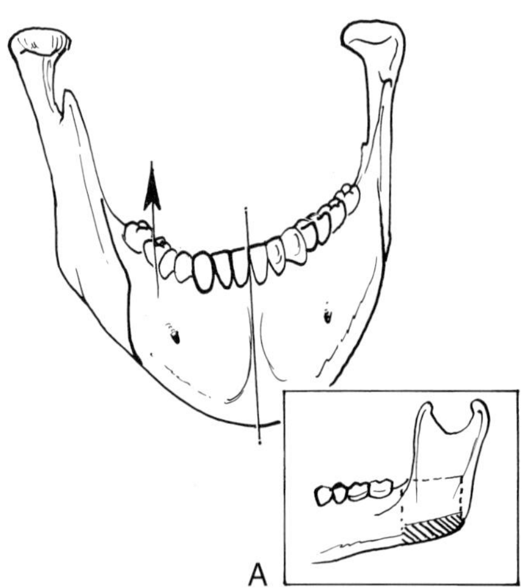

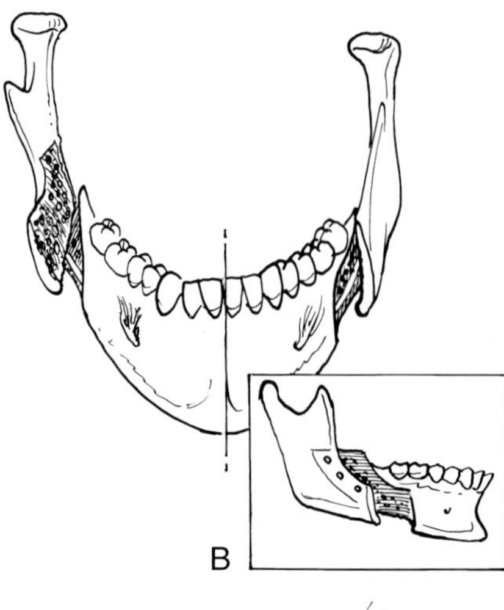

Figure 13–11. *A* and *B,* Illustration of BSSO to correct a canted occlusal plane. Note that the inferior borders are not even, but are parallel. If clockwise or counterclockwise rotation of the segments is planned, the inferior borders would be unparallel accordingly.

inferior borders should be parallel if there is no clockwise or counterclockwise rotation. Finally, secure fixation that does not displace the segments into a different position from what was planned is essential.

Postoperative Considerations. Although panoramic radiographic and cephalographic evaluations should be performed as soon after surgery as is feasible, the most important clue to a shift in proximal segment position is the occlusion. If the proximal segment was fixed in a rotated position and remains there postoperatively, the occlusion may be adequate. If the occlusion is reasonable in spite of a rotated proximal segment, one must decide whether intervention is prudent. Reoperating on the patient with an adequate occlusion in order to correct a radiographically malpositioned proximal segment risks creating a greater problem. The possibility of a cosmetic defect in the antegonial notch area is an added consideration that may influence the decision, although it can be managed later.

A more serious occurrence is shifting of the proximal segment postoperatively (Fig. 13–12). It almost always manifests as an open bite on the opposite side (Fig. 13–12*A*). There may be shifting of the mandibular midline to the affected side. Radiographs usually confirm proximal segment shifting. This complication can occur any time after surgery for several months. In previously uncomplicated cases, if the shifting occurs within the first 3 weeks it is best to intervene as soon as possible. One successful method is to open the wound in the office setting and to place a superior border wire that does not employ the high-low technique but, rather, attempts to align the inferior borders. This commits the patient to a period of intermaxillary fixation for 6 or more weeks. Rigid techniques may be employed but are more invasive.

A more difficult problem occurs when proximal segment shifting is observed after the normal period of healing. This may be either true shifting of segments or remodeling due to weak healing. The choices for management are to deal with it orthodontically or to reoperate with reconstruction and bone grafting. The orthodontist should participate in the decision process. The tendency for long-term shifting to occur is increased with bad splits, because there are more fracture lines to heal and fixation is more difficult. This is the reason for the strong previous recommendation to treat bad splits aggressively.

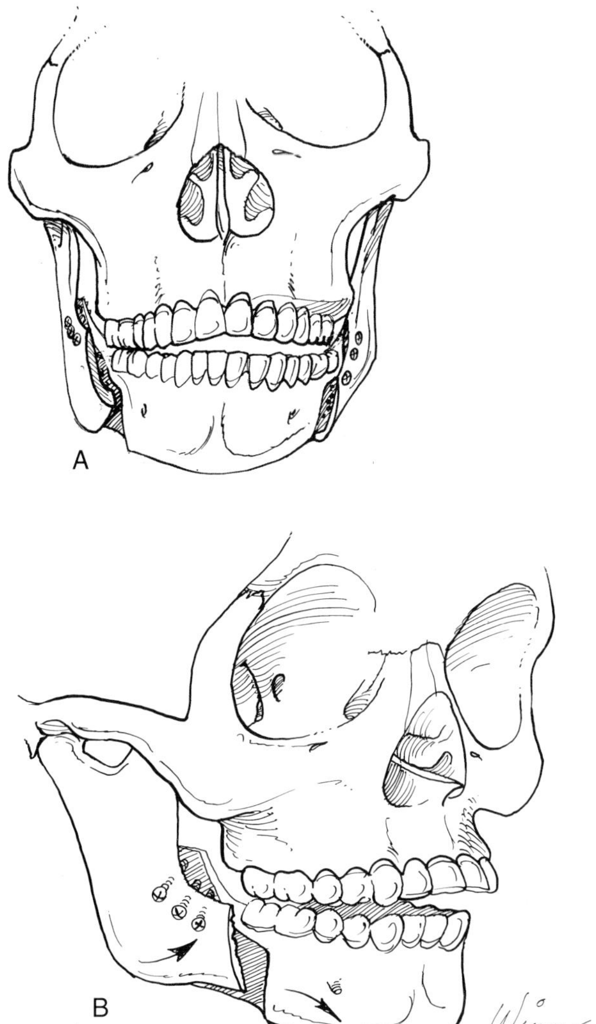

Figure 13–12. *A*, A posterior prematurity in the occlusion that was not present at the end of surgery should alert the surgeon to the probability of shifting at the osteotomy site. Such shifting may happen immediately after surgery or weeks later. Usually, the midline also has shifted to the affected side. *B*, Aggressive examination of the stability of fixation must be performed to identify mobility. The occlusal findings are due to superoanterior shifting of the proximal segment and inferoposterior shifting of the distal segment. (See text for management.)

Condylar Resorption

Prevention. Condylar resorption in nonpatient populations of teenagers and young adults is a known phenomenon.[21] That it occurs following orthognathic and orthodontic procedures may or may not be a coincidence. If a patient is to undergo orthognathic treatment, however, attention must be paid to the radiographic health of the condyles. The management of patients with preexisting condylar resorption and their preoperative preparation is covered elsewhere in this text. Nevertheless, it is becoming increasingly clear that at least one of the causes of long-term relapse is postoperative condylar resorption[21, 22] (Fig. 13–13). The concept of BSSO relapse occurring as a result of condylar malpositioning, osteotomy slippage, and condylar resorption makes a lot of sense.[22] That postoperative condylar resorption occurs is not a question,[19, 23–25, 34] but the etiology is more speculative. Whether compression, disk displacement, or condylar torquing plays a role is not known. Condylar resorption occurs even after maxillary osteotomies.[35] It is clear that postoperative condylar resorption is a disease of white females, because cases in other groups are very rare.[22, 25] High mandibular plane angle has also been implicated in both maxillary[35] and mandibular[25] cases. It is obvious from several perspectives, however, including anatomic studies[36] and common sense, that avascular ne-

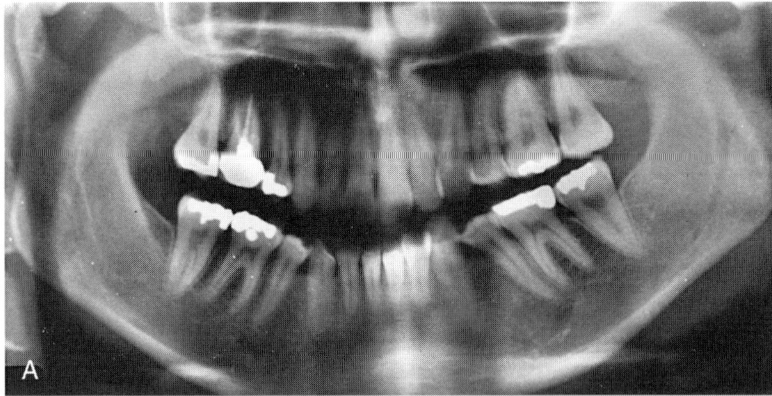

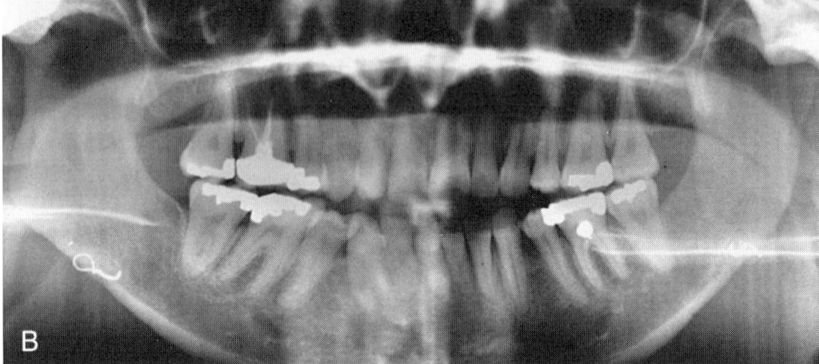

Figure 13–13. *A*, Preoperative panoramic radiograph of a patient who developed a malocclusion secondary to idiopathic condylar resorption. The patient was followed for more than 1 year, and it was determined that resorption had ceased on the basis of a centric relation splint and serial mounted models. BSSO was carried out with inferior border wiring and intermaxillary fixation for 8 weeks. *B*, Panoramic radiograph taken 2 years after BSSO reveals resorption of the other condyle and renewed resorption of the affected condyle.

crosis of the mandibular condyle may not occur.[22] The condylar head receives a rich blood supply from 360 degrees and is probably less likely to undergo devascularization than any other part of the mandible.[36]

Intraoperative Considerations. Inferior border wiring may offer the best protection from postoperative condylar resorption but also may allow more postoperative osteotomy slippage than rigid fixation, thus canceling out the benefit.[19] Superior-border, high-low wiring[4] is distinctly the worst of all options.[19]

Postoperative Considerations. Because little is understood regarding the etiology of condylar resorption, no clear guidelines can be given if it occurs postoperatively. Utilizing a centric relation splint to minimize myofascial pain and stress on the condyles may be beneficial. If significant malocclusion develops owing to condylar resorption, it is unwise to perform another mandibular osteotomy to correct this malocclusion. Maxillary orthognathic surgery may be useful if the resultant position of the mandible is not significantly asymmetric and if it can be determined whether the resorption has arrested. Determination that resorption has ceased is very difficult. Serial mounted models, cephalometric radiographs, and centric relation splints may be useful but are not foolproof. Single photon emission computerized tomography (SPECT) scanning performed at 6-month intervals may demonstrate cessation of resorption.

If maxillary osteotomy alone does not place the maxilla and mandible in appropriate positions, condylar reconstruction is necessary, utilizing the surgeon's method of choice.

Distal Segment Interference in Setbacks

The short split has been advocated to prevent interference with the most posterior part of the distal segment as it is set back.[27, 37] The structures in a position to interfere are the styloid process, mastoid process, and lateral process of C2. An uncontrolled short split is not favored here, because it unduly endangers the mandibular nerve if the split occurs through the canal, as is often described (see Fig. 13–2*A*). If a canal split happens, the nerve has to be pealed out of the proximal segment, undoubtedly inflicting some damage on the nerve.

An alternative is to complete a split posterior to the canal but short of the posterior border. After the split is complete, the surgeon removes the distal segment bone posterior to the mandibular nerve with an oscillating saw similar to the one used for the vertical ramus osteotomy. This is a more controlled method to manage this problem.

Vertical Ramus Osteotomy (VRO)

The VRO is most commonly used for mandibular setbacks. The operation can be completed quicker and with less morbidity than the BSSO but offers less control of the proximal segment.[15, 38] Cases of asymmetry that require large vertical changes between the proximal and distal segments and involve a setback on at least one side may be suitable for VRO (Fig. 13–14) on the long side. For example, a case of hemifacial hyperplasia with severe maxillary canting that requires significant adjustment of the occlusal plane also dic-

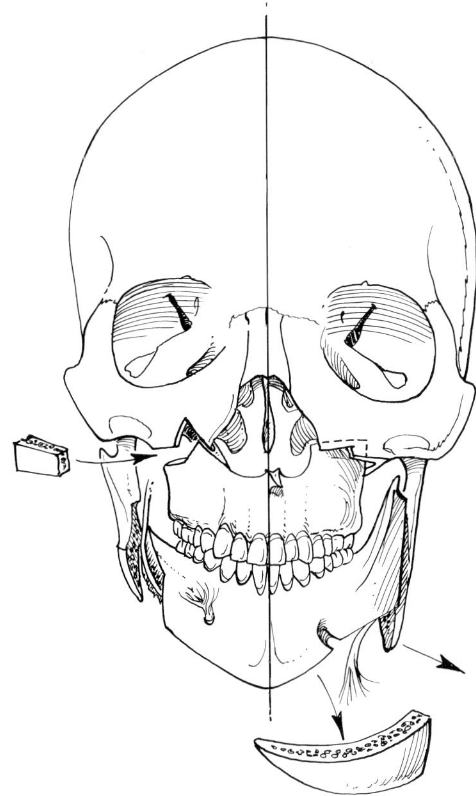

Figure 13–14. In complicated cases of asymmetry, leveling of the maxillary and mandibular occlusal planes may create difficulties in proximal-distal segment compatibility. On the side in which the ramus is shortening vertically, a vertical ramus osteotomy (VRO) may permit better contact than the BSSO; however, the opportunity for rigid fixation is less with the VRO.

tates a shifting of the mandibular rami. On the affected side that requires shortening, BSSO may not afford acceptable bone contact. The VRO is a good choice, because the distal segment is moving posteriorly and superiorly. This movement tends to "seat" the proximal segment, helping to overcome the greatest weakness of the VRO—condylar sag.

The most common complications associated with the VRO are as follows:

- Condylar sag[27, 39–42]
- Bleeding[43]
- Nerve injury[38, 39, 43, 44]
- Inappropriate osteotomy[27, 40, 43]
- Anterior open bite[42, 45]

Prevention of these adverse events and intraoperative and postoperative considerations are discussed here.

Condylar Sag

Prevention. The only preventive measure advocated for avoiding condylar sag is to overcompensate in the presurgical work-up by providing a posterior open bite in the occlusion. An occlusal wafer is built up to fill the space and is left in place during intermaxillary fixation (IMF) and for some time thereafter. The obvious questions are how long to leave the splint in place and what to do with the posterior open bite after splint removal. If the splint is removed before the osteotomy has healed, closure of the open bite may cause movement at the osteotomy site and delayed healing with fibrous union. Conversely, if the osteotomy has healed to a solid bony union, dental elastics used to close the open bite may place excessive stress on the temporomandibular joint. Sequentially reducing the splint while selectively extruding teeth is the safest method for closure of a postoperative posterior open bite.

Intraoperative Considerations. Whether to fix the proximal segment to the distal or not is an issue of surgeon preference. Transoral fixation of the proximal segment is problematic. Maintaining a measure of the medial pterygoid muscle on the proximal segment is offered as a means of minimizing condylar sag.[38]

Postoperative Considerations. Usually, intermaxillary fixation is used for several weeks after VRO. If an overcorrected surgical wafer has been used, it should remain in place during this period and for some time after release to guide the occlusion. The timing of wafer removal is variable. The use of guiding elastics and the timing of re-initiation of orthodontic treatment are also debatable. If postoperative elastics are to be used, however, skeletal wires provide the most stable attachment to the mandible. Use of dental elastics may result in extrusion or displacement of the teeth. If condylar sag has occurred and a skeletal anterior open bite is developing, severe anterior tooth extrusion, especially in the lower arch, is likely if interdental elastic traction is employed.

Bleeding

Prevention. Preventive measures for bleeding during VRO are no different from those described for BSSO.

Intraoperative Considerations. The most likely source of bleeding during VRO is from the masseteric artery as it passes through the sigmoid notch of the ramus.[43] Retraction of the vessel may make it difficult to identify and ligate. This is rarely a problem, but if bleeding from this area cannot be controlled by any other method, packing with a gauze sponge is the first measure. If repeated attempts to remove the packing are unsuccessful, a resorbable packing should be placed, and the operation continued. If the facial artery is injured, it should be isolated, divided, and ligated. Usually, suction drains are not used, but if there is significant oozing, they may prevent postoperative hematoma formation.

Postoperative Considerations. Although very rare, when late bleeding occurs, it usually manifests as an expansile, progressive swelling. A pressure dressing should be placed in combination with intraoral drainage when indicated.

Nerve Injury

Prevention. Sensory nerve injury during the VRO is considerably less likely than with the BSSO,[15, 43] but injury and even transection may occur. Preoperatively, a panoramic radiograph and a cephalograph should be examined to estimate the distance from the posterior border to the lingula, to assist in planning the anteroposterior position of the vertical osteotomy.

Intraoperative Considerations. With use of the information from the preceding radiographic examination, the vertical osteotomy is placed safely behind the mandibular foramen. The inferior alveolar nerve can also be injured if the proximal segment slips medial to the distal segment and then rotates superiorly. Efforts to retrieve the proximal segment from the medial side may injure the nerve. The best prevention is to hold the proximal segment firmly with the retractor during the final stage of the osteotomy and to take care to displace it laterally as it breaks free. An instrument should be placed between the two segments to prevent medial displacement while a portion of the medial pterygoid muscle is elevated from the proximal segment.

Facial nerve injury is unlikely but has been reported during this procedure.[39, 44] Should it occur, the comments made regarding facial nerve injury in the section on BSSO are relevant.

Postoperative Considerations. As with the BSSO, it is recommended that no invasive therapy is appropriate unless a dysesthesia appears, even with significant sensory loss. The likelihood is that significant sensory return will occur over 12 to 18 months via regeneration and recruitment, exceeding what might be expected from interventional nerve surgery.

Inappropriate Osteotomy

Several authors have described a subcondylar osteotomy, including only the condyle and a small portion of the neck, as a *complication* of the VRO.[27, 40, 43] The short osteotomy may result in significant rotation and displacement of the proximal segment (Fig. 13–15). This is a well-known phenomenon but seems to contradict the experience of those who have begun to use the subcondylar osteotomy, described by Ward and associates[46] almost 40 years ago, for TMD treatment.[47] The treatment of TMD is not the subject here, but for orthognathic correction of dentofacial deformities, most surgeons would prefer greater control than this osteotomy provides.

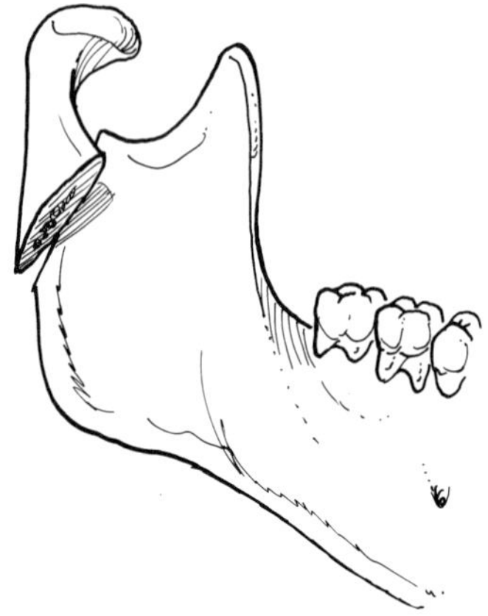

Figure 13–15. Illustration of an inappropriately high VRO that allows anteroinferior displacement of the proximal segment and affords minimal bone-to-bone contact.

Open Bite

Although open bite can occur with any osteotomy, it is more common with the VRO.[42, 45] In contrast to other mandibular osteotomies, the surgeon has the least control over the proximal segments with the VRO technique. Undoubtedly, the most common problem is that the condyle is not seated at the time of surgery and does not spontaneously seat in the postoperative period. If healing between the segments has occurred during intermaxillary fixation (IMF), the muscles of mastication may gradually attempt to reposition the condyles and open the bite anteriorly. "Training elastics" are often recommended, but they must be used with caution unless skeletal wires are present to prevent tooth extrusion and periodontal problems.

Another potential cause of open bite is condylar resorption.[19, 22, 24, 25] This may occur with any mandibular osteotomy. Although avascular necrosis has been suggested as an etiology,[48, 49] there is no evidence that lack of vascularity is involved.[22] The mandibular condyle derives blood supply from its entire circumference rather than from a single or double source like the femoral condyle.[36] Even the most extensive stripping probably would not significantly compromise the vascularity of the condyle. Also, most cases of resorption occur several months to years after operation. On the basis of the timing of the revascularization of autologous bone grafts, it is likely that a proximal segment, however stripped, regains blood supply long before the resorption occurs. Additionally, so few cases show resorption even in the presence of significant stripping that many other factors must be involved. Idiopathic and postorthodontic condylar resorption are also seen in patients similar in age and gender to many of the orthognathic patients. Therefore, it is not clear whether orthognathic surgery has anything at all to do with condylar resorption.

Open bites that are not related to condylar resorption are almost always due to faulty attention to condylar seating at the time of surgery[18, 20] or to slippage at the osteotomy site.[19, 22] This observation is also true for BSSO and other orthognathic procedures.

Body and Symphysis Osteotomies (BASOs)

Osteotomies performed in the mandibular body or symphysis usually pass between teeth. Additionally, they seldom have the amount of bone overlap that ramus procedures do. Those that occur posterior to the mental foramina may endanger the inferior alveolar nerve. If these osteotomies are carried out anterior to the mental foramina, the lower portion of the osteotomy can be split parallel to the long axis of the inferior border,[50] facilitating rigid fixation (Fig. 13–16). If a long axis splitting of the mandible cannot be achieved, usu-

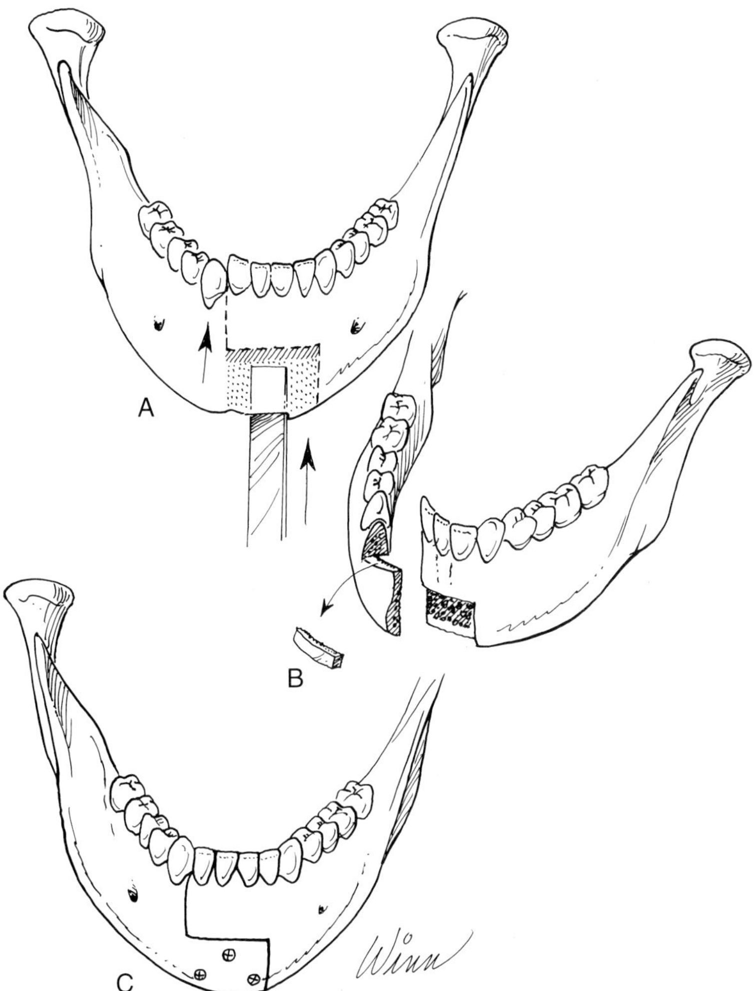

Figure 13–16. *A*, Long axis splitting or step splitting of the mandible for body and symphysis osteotomies (BASOs) affords better bone contact for fixation and healing. Planning the direction of the long axis or step splitting is very important, to avoid the roots of teeth and the inferior alveolar neurovascular bundle. *B*, Appropriate bone removal can be accomplished after splitting has been completed. *C*, If long axis splitting has been performed according to plan, rigid fixation of the segments is often possible, as illustrated here.

ally at least a step rather than a simple straight cut can be placed in the osteotomy, giving greater bone contact.

Segmentation of the entire mandible represents a greater problem than that of the maxilla because of the greater stresses placed on the mandible. Therefore, the risk of malpositioning or nonunion is greater. Fixing the segments with splints is more difficult, because the forces on the mandible may warp the splint while the rigid fixation is being applied.

Body and symphysis osteotomies (BASOs) may be complicated by malpositioning, non-union, periodontal defects, devitalized teeth, and nerve injury.[48]

Malpositioning

Prevention. Careful model surgery and an unyielding surgical wafer are the best defenses against malpositioning of the segment. Accurately mounted models in centric relation are very important, because the proximal segments contain dentoalveolar parts that are not going to be moved. They are tethered to the condyles so that any surgical move other than slight rotation around the condylar pivot point displaces the condyle out of the fossa.

Intraoperative Considerations. Malpositioning is the most common problem associated with osteotomies of the tooth-bearing section of the mandible. As stated previously, the difficulties of positioning the occlusion just right while fixation is applied may be challenging. In contrast to fractures in this region, the segments do not key together. Rigid fixation and techniques to increase bone overlap, such as the long axis splitting[50] (see Fig. 13–16) or step procedure, are recommended. Most importantly, after fixation of the segments, the mandible must be mobilized and rotated around the condyles, with strong emphasis on determining whether the occlusion is correct with the condyles fully seated.

Postoperative Considerations. If the occlusion is incorrect, an early consultation with the orthodontist is necessary to determine whether the case can be salvaged orthodontically. Otherwise, reoperation to properly position the segment is necessary.

Non-Union

Prevention and postoperative management of non-union focus on maximizing bone contact, creating the most idealized occlusal contact to decrease stress forces on the healing bone, and rigid fixation. Reoperation is almost always necessary in the case of a non-union. Bone grafting may also be required.

Periodontal Defects and Devitalized Teeth

Careful surgical technique and proper flap design are the keys to avoiding periodontal problems and devitalized teeth. Periapical radiographs are essential in planning interdental osteotomies. If the root apices are known to be violated, endodontic therapy should be performed as soon as is convenient. If devitalization is suspected, one should follow the teeth clinically for discoloration and radiographically for periapical pathology. Sensory testing is not valid for determining vascular vitality of the teeth.

Nerve Injury

Other than what has already been said about nerve injuries, BASOs require periapical radiographs for evaluation of nerve location. If decortication and relocation of the nerve are planned, there is always some degree of neurosensory loss if the patient is tested carefully. The more handling of the nerve, the greater the risk of sensory loss. Body osteotomies in the bicuspid region may be stepped forward around the mental foramen in many cases, if there is enough space between the apices of the teeth and the roof of the inferior alveolar canal. Otherwise, the neurovascular bundle can be unroofed and moved slightly posterior to permit a step in the osteotomy.

Subapical Segmental Osteotomies (SSOs)

Subapical segmental osteotomies that do not include the inferior border of the mandible may comprise only a few teeth or all of the teeth and the accompanying alveolar bone. If some of the teeth remain in the intact mandible and others are being surgically moved, careful model surgery is once again very important. Problems with non-union are rarely seen, but malpositioning may occur. The occurrence of periodontal defects and devitalized teeth is similar to that described previously for the other mandibular body procedures.

Loss of vascularity, malpositioning, and nerve injury are the most common complications seen with SSOs.[26]

Loss of Vascularity

Prevention. Anterior mandibular segmental osteotomies need only an adequate lingual soft tissue pedicle. Violation of this pedicle may lead to devitalization of the segment. Full labial exposure is safe and generally recommended to facilitate the osteotomies.

Posterior to the mental foramen, the blood supply to the dentoalveolar segments is less dependent on the lingual vascular pedicle. There have been anecdotal reports of vascular compromise and slough when this procedure is performed with only a lingual pedicle.[51] A bipedicle flap design is therefore recommended to avoid this complication (see following discussion).

Intraoperative Considerations. If the loss of blood supply is evident at the time of surgery, it is advisable to return the segment to the original position rather than to stress it more by repositioning it. Furthermore, rigidly fixing the segment to minimize movement and additional stress is important.

Posterior segmental mandibular osteotomies can be safely performed by maintaining bipedicle vascular support. A vertical third molar–like mucoperiosteal incision near the most posterior vertical osteotomy and a horizontal or vertical incision just anterior to the interdental osteotomy give ample exposure. The horizontal osteotomy that connects the two verticals can be performed by tunneling the mucoperiosteum from anterior to posterior. If the neurovascular bundle must be decorticated, the procedure may be done through this approach. Leaving both a lingual and buccal pedicle has proved safe and effective.

Postoperative Considerations. There is no proven method for the management of a devitalized segment other than supportive therapy. Most surgeons would grasp at the straw of hyperbaric oxygenation without hard evidence to prove its value.

Nerve Injury

Prevention. Planning the osteotomies on mounted models and with the aid of appropriate radiographs is the best way to prevent injury to the inferior alveolar nerve.

Intraoperative Considerations. If the inferior alveolar neurovascular bundle must be relocated, a certain amount of neurosensory change is to be expected. If an observed nerve injury occurs, immediate microsurgical repair is recommended.

Postoperative Considerations. Unobserved nerve injuries with resultant neurosensory changes should not be treated surgically unless a significant dysesthesia persists. Hypesthesia rarely can be improved by late attempts at repair.

Genioplasty

Complications most often associated with genioplasty are nerve injury,[52] unaesthetic contours,[26] and ptosis of the soft tissue overlying the bony chin.[53, 54]

Nerve Injury

Some neurosensory loss often occurs after a genioplasty. Usually it is transient, but some hypesthesia may persist. Careful technique to avoid injuring the mental nerves is the only management recommendation (Fig. 13–17), including dissection of the mental nerve to permit adequate retraction to perform the osteotomy.

Asymmetric lower lip function is occasionally seen. Whether this complication represents true motor nerve injury or direct muscle trauma is not clear. Again, careful technique is the best preventive technique.

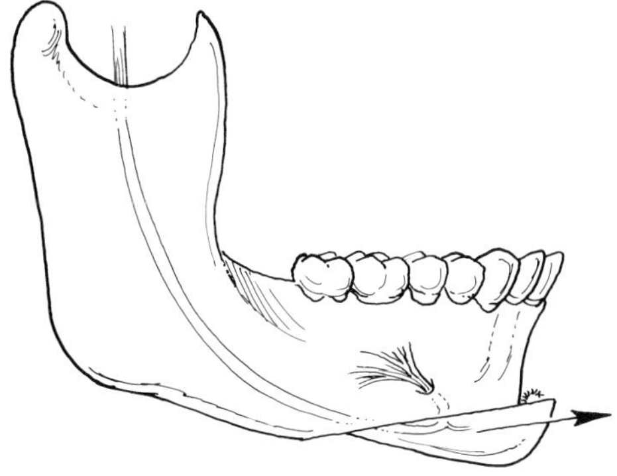

Figure 13–17. The inferior alveolar neurovascular bundle dips inferiorly and anteriorly before exiting the mental foramen. In designing the genioplasty, the surgeon must take this factor into consideration to prevent severance of the neurovascular bundle within the canal. The undesirable approach is shown to demonstrate what *not* to do.

Unaesthetic Contours

The most common undesirable outcome of genioplasty is the keyhole-shaped mandible (Fig. 13–18). This is characterized by indentations on each side of the genioplasty near the most posterior extent of the inferior border cut (Fig. 13–18*B*). It may be prevented by extending the osteotomy as far posteriorly as possible, although such an extension may increase the risk of nerve damage if the dissection is inadequate. Also, the addition of some filler material can be helpful in rounding out the contours of this procedure (Fig. 13–18*D*). Hydroxylapatite crystals mixed with Avitene Hemostat and whole, autologous blood function well as a "grouting" around and above the osteotomies of a genioplasty. Long-term relapse occurs after genioplasty in about 17% of cases.[55]

Ptosis

Ptosis of the soft tissue over the chin may be prevented by the avoiding of excessive subperiosteal stripping, by the reapproximating of the mentalis muscles, by the suturing of the inferior portion of the mentalis muscles to the anterior-superior edge of the distal chin segment, and by the placing of a pressure dressing for 5 days.[53, 54] Treatment, once this complication occurs, is very difficult. Reopening the wound, resuturing the mentalis muscles and periosteum, and placing a pressure dressing for 5 days constitute the best method of management.

Maxillary Procedures

Preoperative Factors That May Adversely Affect Outcomes

Orthodontic preparation, evaluation of maxillary and mandibular midlines and need for mandibular surgery, recognition of *significant* TMD, surgical splint construction, and patient expectations may all adversely affect the outcome of a maxillary orthognathic procedure. Many of the preoperative concerns regarding orthognathic surgery have been addressed in the discussion of mandibular procedures. A few factors, however, are specific to maxillary surgery.

Orthodontic preparation issues specific to the maxilla are arch width incompatibilities, root parallelism, and open bite deformities. The arch width problem has already been discussed. Suffice it to say here that the method of widening the maxilla to achieve arch width compatibility should be decided before orthodontic preparation has begun.[56] Additionally, root parallelism is most important when interdental osteotomies are planned.[57]

One specific instance that requires special planning is the case in which maxillary first bicuspids have been removed at the time of previous nonsurgical orthodontic therapy. This procedure results in very upright maxillary anterior teeth, an obtuse nasolabial angle, and minimal overjet in spite of a severe mandibular retrognathism. It is often desirable to open space between the maxillary canines and second bicuspids and to surgically increase the proclination of the upper anteriors. More space is needed between the roots than between the crowns, because more bone must be removed at the superior extent of the interdental osteotomy than at the alveolar crest to properly procline the anterior teeth.

It is widely accepted that open bites, especially in the anterior region, are difficult to close orthodontically with lasting stability.[57] The attempt is particularly vulnerable to failure in a patient in whom much preoperative orthodontics has been carried out. Evaluation of the preorthodontic models and cephalograms is essential to determine whether tooth extrusion has occurred. If it has, the orthodontic extrusion must be reversed before surgery is performed, to prevent posttreatment open bite.

Another situation that may result in a postoperative open bite is when preoperative orthodontics has left the maxillary molars angled buccally with the palatal cusps lower than the buccal cusps. In such cases, it should be assumed that dental expansion has occurred without skeletal expansion. If this expansion has exceeded the physiologic envelope of stability, the transverse dimension of the maxilla will relapse, probably after all treatment has been completed and the patient is no longer wearing retainers. The transverse relapse would create cuspal interferences resulting in an anterior open bite.

Midline evaluation and assessment of the need for mandibular surgery are even more important, because the maxillary midline is very readily identified by the average person, rendering any discrepancies striking. This issue is most crucial when maxillary surgery is planned *without* mandibular surgery. If mandibular surgery is not to be done, the mandible dictates the maxillary position at the time of surgery. Therefore, not only must the maxillary midline be determined, but the mandibular seated condylar position also must be known. If the mandibular seated position is improperly estimated preoperatively and the surgical wafer is constructed to that position, the resultant maxillary posi-

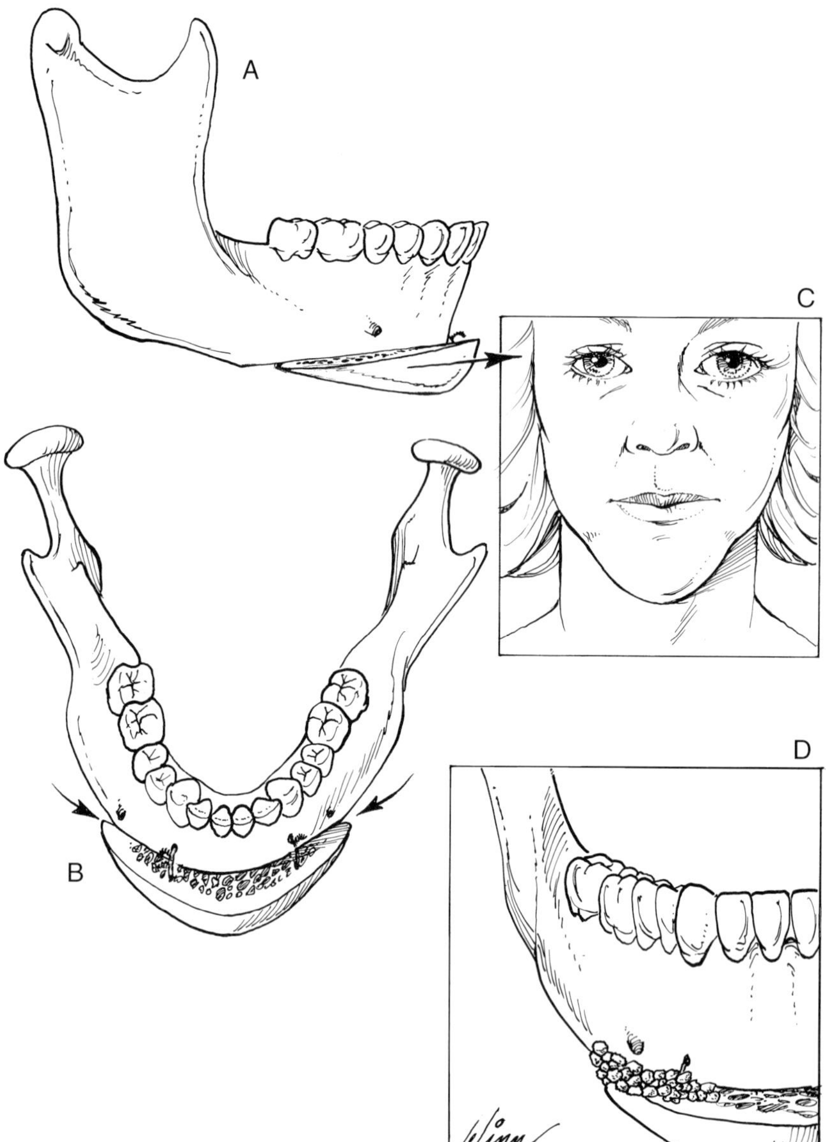

Figure 13–18. *A*, Standard advancement genioplasty provides consistent improvement in the profile. *B*, The indented areas just posterior to the lateral "wings" of the distal segment, however, may lead to contour deficiencies. *C*, After long-term healing (> 6 months), the lateral depressions may become apparent, especially in thin individuals. *D*, Placement of hydroxylapatite crystals mixed with Avitene and blood is useful as "grout" to smooth out contour irregularities.

tion will be incorrect. For example, if the true mandibular position is several millimeters posterior to that of the mounted models and the cephalometric mandibular position, the treatment planning may indicate that the maxilla is going to be placed in an appropriate AP position. Intraoperatively, the surgeon has only the mandibular seated position to use as a landmark for maxillary positioning. Although it may not be possible to fully seat the condyles under general anesthesia in some cases,[58] the surgeon usually can come relatively close to a seated condylar position. If the condyles were not seated at the time the preoperative mounted models were made, the result will be a retropositioned maxilla with poor aesthetics. Likewise, if the true mandibular position is lateral to that recorded on the mounted models and is not recognized as such, single jaw surgery may be inappropriately planned, and the result will produce a deviated maxilla to go with the asymmetric mandible.

Open bites that are to be corrected by maxillary surgery require an assessment of the need for mandibular surgery. In addition to making an accurate assessment of the seated mandibular position, one must realize that the maxilla will be rotating in a clockwise direction as a result of the open bite correction. Therefore, it is possible that the anterior nasal spine may advance and the upper incisors may move posteriorly. Only model surgery with a mechanism for measuring the AP position of both the anterior nasal spine and the upper incisors can provide the operator with the final AP location of the maxillary incisors.

Mounted models in the most accurate centric relation are *essential* to accurate maxillary surgery. The surgical wafer will be the sole determinant of maxillary surgical positioning, and because the wafer is constructed from preoperative mounted models, those models are crucial.

Furthermore, a more intense facial evaluation must

be made prior to maxillary surgery, because the potential negative aesthetic impact of maxillary surgery is greater than with mandibular surgery.[59, 60] Maxillary surgery may change the alar base width, rotation of the nose, width of the upper lip vermilion, nasolabial angle, and profile of the nose. All of these structures must be evaluated and documented preoperatively, even though several of them cannot be satisfactorily managed by the maxillary procedure alone.

Maxillary advancement, superior repositioning, and even inferior repositioning will change most or all of the structures just mentioned. Unfortunately, exactly how to control these changes is not well known. Altering one component favorably often adversely affects another. For example, alar base cinching may minimize widening of the alar bases, at least temporarily, but it will also elevate the nasal tip. The patient with wide alar bases often also has a short, puglike nose. In such a patient, cinching the alar bases may create a very unaesthetic nose from the frontal view. Patients who have short, wide noses and who require maxillary surgery will also need a secondary rhinoplasty, including a procedure to increase projection, decrease rotation, and narrow the alar bases. If the nasal tip is underrotated, however, maxillary surgery may have a very favorable influence on facial aesthetics.

In summary, much has been said and written about control of facial aesthetics during maxillary surgery, but none of the procedures recommended is widely accepted because they have not proved to be consistently effective. Impaction of the maxilla widens the alar bases; cinching the alar bases elevates the nasal tip; V-Y closure of the vestibular incision widens the vermilion medially and narrows it laterally; and no one knows what to do with the depressed oral commissures resulting from large superior maxillary repositioning. The last issue is often the limiting factor in the planning of maxillary impaction for the patient with a "gummy smile." There is much left to be learned about how to control these factors.

Intuitively, maxillary surgery would seem to have a lesser impact on *TMD* than mandibular surgery, and experience probably confirms the impression, especially regarding internal derangement. Condylar resorption has been seen, however, following maxillary surgery alone.[35] Nevertheless, any postoperative malocclusion has the potential to create myofascial pain dysfunction (MPD) or, ultimately, some internal joint problems. This is a good reason to document preoperative TMD status and to attempt to make the patient as comfortable as possible before surgery.

Surgical splints for one-piece maxillary surgery do not differ from other orthognathic surgical splints, but if multiple-piece maxillary surgery is performed, the splint must have cross-arch stabilization, such as a palatal bar. Obviously, this bar must not impinge upon the palatal soft tissue. Additionally, if a surgical splint is to be retained in the mouth postoperatively, it must be constructed so that the mandible can be autorotated into it without prematurity. Otherwise, the occlusion will appear to be incorrect, but the surgeon will not know whether the fault is due to splint prematurities or to the maxillary positioning.

Interestingly, patients and their families are often more intimidated by the concept of maxillary surgery than by that of mandibular surgery. Fortunately, maxillary surgery is not as traumatic to the patient, but the aesthetic considerations mentioned previously (see discussion of midline evaluation) are less controllable. *Patient expectations* may focus unnecessary concern on the acute perioperative period without enough understanding of the intermediate and long-term postoperative outcomes. Conscientious communication with the patient and family assists in minimizing these misconceptions but can never eliminate them altogether.

Intraoperative and Postoperative Complications and Their Prevention

Preventive, intraoperative, and **postoperative** concerns in maxillary operations are combined and categorized according to specific procedures.

Le Fort I Maxillary Osteotomy (LMO)

The Le Fort I osteotomy may be complicated by malpositioning,[61, 62] bleeding,[63–65] perfusion deficiencies,[66, 67] periodontal defects,[68] devitalized teeth,[68] nerve injury,[69–73] ophthalmic[69–72, 74] or nasolacrimal[69, 75–79] injury, oronasal or oroantral fistulas,[80] nasal septal deviations,[59, 69] maxillary sinusitis,[81] unaesthetic soft tissue changes,[59, 60] insufficient bone strength,[61, 62] unfavorable fractures,[82–86] non-union (delayed union),[62] eustachian tube dysfunction, velopharyngeal incompetence, arteriovenous fistulas (carotid cavernous sinus),[87, 88] dysphagia,[89] transverse relapse,[56] and even condylar resorption.[35]

Malpositioning

Prevention. As has already been stated, proper preoperative planning is the only way to ensure accurate positioning of the maxilla. Intraoperative "eyeballing" of proper position is fraught with problems. To ensure an ideal outcome, the surgeon must obtain mounted models with accurate centric relation and an accurate assessment of midlines, and must make an evaluation of the need for mandibular surgery.

Intraoperative Considerations. If one is sure that the preoperative planning has been precisely done, it is not a good idea to deviate from the treatment plan after surgery has begun. Swelling, the nasoendotracheal tube, esophageal stethoscope, and draping make intraoperative assessments hazardous, especially for the inexperienced surgeon. The best advice is to make a sound treatment plan, to double-check it, and to stick with it.

Perhaps the most common cause of malpositioning is an inability to get the mandibular condyles seated while manipulating the two jaws together (Fig. 13–19). Areas of posterior bone prematurities are sometimes difficult to appreciate. The operator must be certain

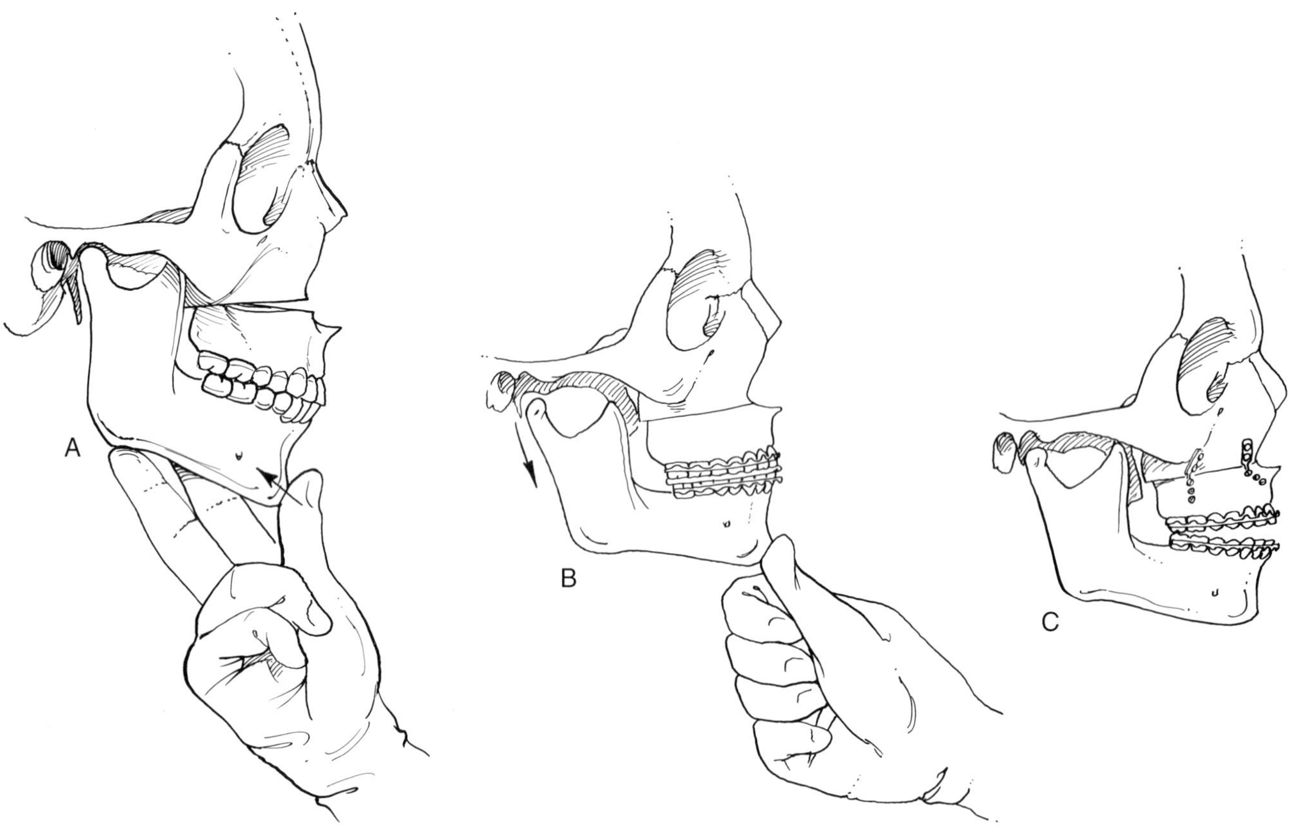

Figure 13–19. *A*, Illustration of the proper method for condylar seating at the time of maxillary positioning prior to fixation. Posterior prematurities are best appreciated with this method. *B*, Pressure on the chin to push the anterior aspect of the maxillary osteotomy together may rotate the condyles inferiorly and posteriorly while maxillary fixation is applied. *C*, Upon release of intermaxillary fixation, the condyles may return to the fossae, and an open bite may appear. Unfortunately, this open bite may not appear immediately, especially if postoperative elastics are used to "guide" the occlusion.

that the condyles are seated first and then the maxillomandibular complex rotated into position until a first contact is felt (Fig. 13–19*A*). Finally, after fixation of the maxilla, the jaws should be unwired, and a critical assessment should be made of the occlusion (Fig. 13–19*C*). If the occlusion is not correct at this point, it will not get better postoperatively.

Postoperative Considerations. Several fixation strategies have been devised to allow postoperative adjustments. The rigid adjustable pin (RAP) system, as described elsewhere in detail,[90] is the only one that permits reasonable three-dimensional adjustability. Other strategies that utilize anterior rigid plates with either wires or adjustable pins posteriorly are addressing the same common problem encountered postoperatively, that of anterior open bite. These systems give the surgeon the opportunity to impact the posterior maxilla a small amount if solid posterior bony contacts have been avoided during the surgery. It is doubtful that the maxilla can be moved through the screws of rigid fixation plates by using interdental elastics; rather, the screws probably just loosen some or the teeth move to an improved occlusion.

Bleeding

Prevention. This discussion is the same as for mandibular procedures.

Intraoperative Considerations. Hypotensive general anesthesia, elevated head position, and vasoconstrictors are all recommended. The anterior and posterior superior alveolar and nasopalatine arteries are all intentionally severed during maxillary surgery. Direct attention to them is required and is not difficult. Much controversy exists regarding the need to preserve the descending palatine arteries to achieve adequate perfusion (see later). From the perspective of hemostasis alone, it seems judicious to ligate them, because they are the leading source of postoperative bleeding.[64] Doing so, however, compromises the blood supply of the maxilla, particularly if a multiple-segment Le Fort I procedure is planned. Once again, staying within the periosteal envelope minimizes bleeding.

If bleeding occurs posterior to the pterygomaxillary osteotomy, packing is the best solution. It may be necessary to leave a resorbable packing material in this area at the completion of the operation. In the extreme circumstance in which bleeding from the maxillary artery or elsewhere cannot be stopped locally, ligation of the external carotid has been suggested.[63] Not enough cases exist to assess the value of this procedure. Intraoperative catheterization with embolization, when available, may be a better solution.

Postoperative Considerations. Elevated head position and control of hypertension are the best immediate measures for postoperative bleeding. If nasal bleeding persists after the first 12 hours, intranasal examination should be performed to determine the source, primarily whether it is anterior or posterior. Packing is the best method of treatment but is only rarely necessary. Cases have been reported in which the patient had to be returned to the operating room for hemostasis.[63–65] One should look for the descending palatine artery first, because it appears to be the most common source of postoperative bleeding.[64]

When postoperative bleeding is not controlled by anterior or posterior nasal packing, an arteriogram should be performed. Embolization of bleeding vessels is the treatment of choice.

Perfusion Deficiencies

Prevention. Generally, prevention of perfusion problems is a matter of adequate planning and preparation. Experience performing maxillary surgery under supervision is essential before one should attempt it alone. Two patient types deserve special comment: patients who have had previous *palatal* surgery (cleft palate) and those who have had previous Le Fort I downfracture.

In patients who have undergone previous palatal surgery, a treatment plan may need to include the maintenance of a labial pedicle if palatal scarring is extensive. Conversely, maxillary downfracture surgery that is to be repeated through the same approach should not encounter compromised blood supply, because the pedicle has been "staged" by the previous procedure, assuming that the palatal pedicle was not damaged by the previous operation. Also, boggy, edematous gingiva that has lost its stippling and is red, rather than pink, is more likely to exhibit poor venous return as maxillary perfusion decreases intraoperatively. Therefore, it is recommended that periodontal evaluation precede surgical intervention in selected cases.

Intraoperative Considerations. Through studies using intraoperative laser Doppler flowmetry, my colleagues and I have revealed that maxillary perfusion as measured at the anterior gingiva declines gradually during the operation.[91] Downfracture and mobilization seem to affect it the most. Ligation, as opposed to preservation, of the descending palatine artery does not show a significant difference in labial gingival perfusion. It is recommended that the surgeon maintain constant vigilance during the operation to assess anterior perfusion. Because downfracture and extreme displacement represent significant stress on the perfusion, occasional relaxation to allow the maxilla to rest passively is recommended to prevent stasis.

No doubt, segmentation is the greatest routine factor associated with compromised perfusion.[92] Segmentation eliminates intrabony perfusion to the anterior segment(s). Also, greater stress is placed on the soft tissue pedicle as the separate segments are repositioned and fixed. Two- and three-piece maxillary osteotomies are routinely done via a circumvestibular incision and downfracture. If a four-piece segmental is planned, or in cases with palatal scarring, an anterior labial soft tissue pedicle is recommended with tunneling to achieve the access for the osteotomies.

If vascular compromise is seen intraoperatively, the operation should be aborted, the maxilla fixed rigidly back into its *original* position, and the incision closed. Splints should be checked to avoid impingement on the soft tissue pedicle.

Postoperative Considerations. If a problem has been seen intraoperatively and the procedure aborted as just described, hyperbaric oxygenation (HBO) may improve the oxygen content of what blood is getting through to the distalmost part of the pedicle. If HBO is to be used, the sooner the better. If poor perfusion is first observed after completion of the procedure, an assessment of the surgical moves should be made to determine whether release of the fixation or removal of a splint might reduce stress on the blood supply. If so, such maneuvers should be accomplished immediately (Fig. 13–20). HBO may also be considered here. It is recognized that there is no scientific documentation to support HBO in such circumstances, but the predicament is so rare and so devastating that any reasonable measure seems worthwhile.

If necrosis occurs, the wound should be managed conservatively with irrigation and oral rinses to maximize oral and wound hygiene (Fig. 13–21). Aggressive removal of hard or soft tissue is not advised.

Periodontal Defects

Prevention. Careful model surgery should alert the surgeon to planned movements that the gingiva may be unable to tolerate. Measurements on the models should be made between the teeth at the level of the cemento-enamel junction and the root apices. The health of the gingiva is examined, and appropriate referrals are sought.

Intraoperative Considerations. In most cases, interdental cuts do not require detachment of the entire interdental papilla. From the horizontal vestibular incision, the periosteum can be tunneled to the crestal bone, and the interdental osteotomy initiated with fine cement spatula osteotomes until they are felt emerging palatally under the mucoperiosteum. If bony defects remain after the segments have been positioned and fixed, bone grafting is recommended. Bone for this purpose can usually be found locally throughout the operative site.

Postoperative Considerations. If periodontal defects occur after surgery, maximum hygiene and good nutrition are all that can be recommended until primary healing has occurred. The patient should be referred to a periodontist.

Devitalized Teeth

Full discussion of this complication can be found in the preceding section on mandibular procedures (see under "Body and Symphysis Osteotomies").

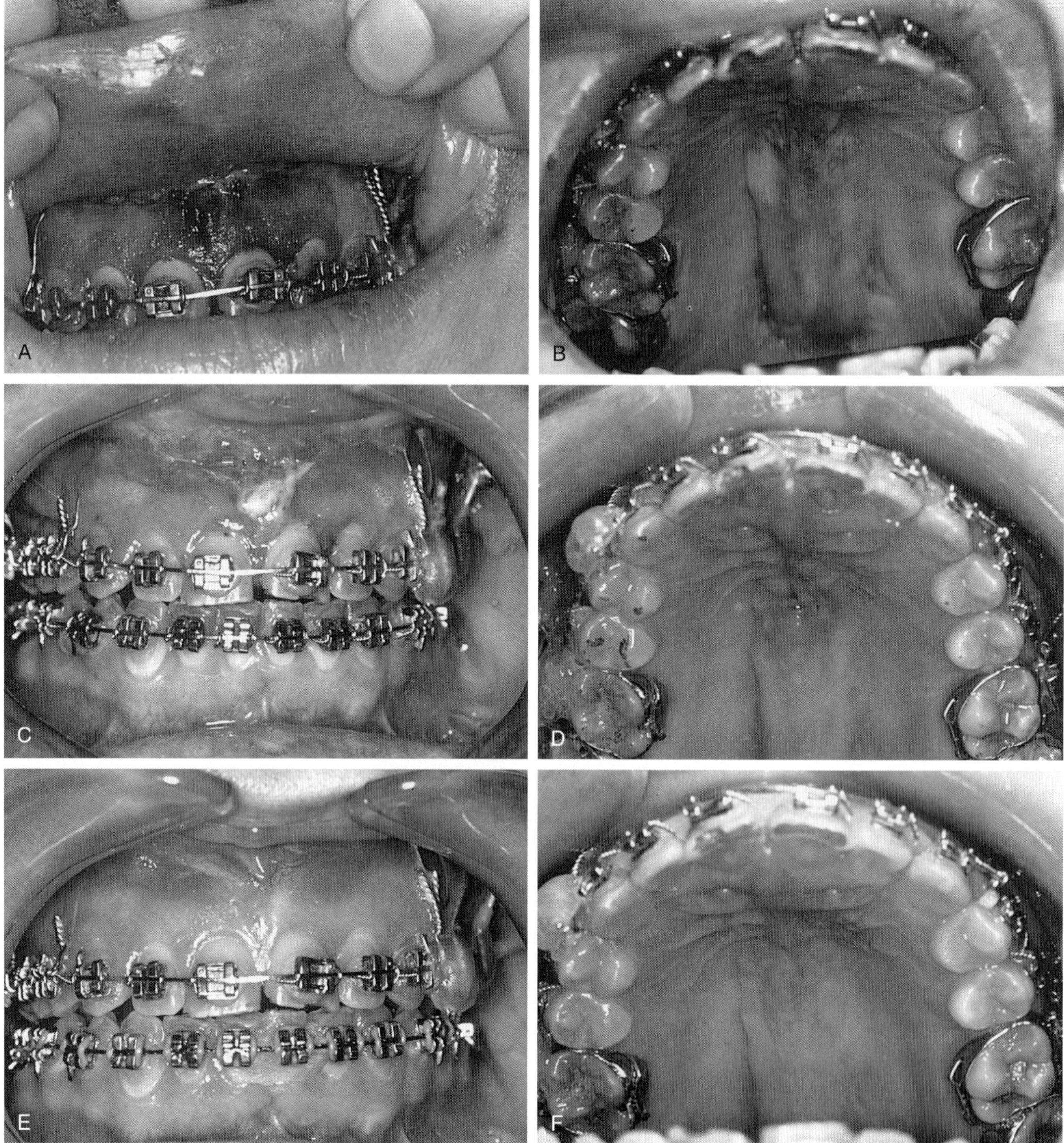

Figure 13–20. *A* and *B*, Labial and occlusal views of a two-piece maxillary osteotomy in which narrowing of the maxilla was achieved. These photographs were taken a few hours postoperatively, just after the occlusal wafer was removed to eliminate potential impingement on the palate. Because perfusion did not improve significantly, hyperbaric oxygenation (HBO) was initiated. *C* and *D*, Labial and occlusal views after 12 HBO treatments for more than 7 days. No further treatment was performed. *E* and *F*, Labial and occlusal views at 2 months postoperatively. It is not known whether HBO influenced the outcome in this case.

Nerve Injury

Prevention. Nerve injuries in maxillary downfracture osteotomies can be divided into sensory, motor, secretory motor, and special sensory (optic nerve) injuries. Prevention, as always, consists of careful planning and a profound knowledge of the anatomy of the operative field.

Intraoperative Considerations. Neurosensory changes that occur commonly in the immediate postoperative period are the result of traction on the infraorbital nerves and direct trauma to the anterior, middle, and posterior superior alveolar, nasopalatine, and descending palatine nerves. Careful retraction of the infraorbital nerves is the best measure to prevent excessive postoperative paresthesia of the facial soft tissues. No comprehensive studies have been conducted on the long-term persistence of neurosensory changes of the facial skin following maxillary orthognathic surgery. Interestingly, whether the nerves are divided or preserved seems to make little difference. Sensation to the gingiva, teeth, and palate returns to acceptable levels in nearly all patients, with a quarter of the patients exhibiting objective hypesthesia.[73] In my experience, except for the nasopalatine distribution, sensation to the remainder of the palate invariably returns regardless of the management of the descending palatine nerve. In addition to the nasopalatine area, the skin at the alar base occasionally remains hypesthetic.

Intraoperative observation of motor nerve injuries to cranial nerves III and VI is very unlikely, because these injuries are probably due either to unfavorable fracture of the naso-orbital-ethmoid bones or to hematoma formation in or about the orbit. It is also unlikely that injuries to the secretory fibers of the nasociliary branch of V_1 or cranial nerve II will be seen at the time of surgery. Paying careful attention to the details of the osteotomy lines, so that unexpected fractures do not occur, is the best means of preventing nerve injuries.

Postoperative Considerations. There is no indication that anything can or should be done for routine postoperative neurosensory deficits except for reassurance of the patient. If infraorbital dysesthesia were to occur, exploration and decompression might be considered. Cases of abducens nerve (CN VI) palsy have been reported, all of which resolved after surgery.[69–71] Oculomotor nerve (CN III) injury has also occurred and resolved in the postoperative period.[69, 72] Obviously, supportive therapy and ophthalmic consultation are in order. Blindness (CN II) has been reported in at least three instances.[69] In one case, multiple sphenoid and middle cranial fossa fractures were seen on postoperative CT scans, and nothing was observed on the CT scans in the other two cases. Retrobular hematoma was blamed for the other two cases.[69] The blindness resolved in one of the normal CT cases but did not in the other, nor did it resolve in the multiple fracture case. Finally, several cases of xerophthalmia have been seen, which may be due to injury to the secretory fibers of CN V_1.[69] Supportive therapy is recommended until lacrimation returns.

Ophthalmic and Nasolacrimal Injuries

In addition to the ophthalmic nerve injuries mentioned earlier, a few other reports have been made regarding ocular injury, unilateral tonic pupil,[74] and nasolacrimal disruptions.[69, 75–79] The case of unilateral tonic pupil resolved within 1 year except for a slight accommodation defect.[74] Most of the epiphora seen after maxillary osteotomy resolves within a few weeks, but occasionally it does not. Epiphora seems to be more common with high Le Fort osteotomies.[77, 78] The etiology has been cited as disruption of the nasolacrimal duct[69, 75, 76] and nasal septal deviation.[69] Dacryocystorhinostomy or, in cases of nasal septal deviation, septorhinoplasty has been occasionally necessary.[69] Determination of the etiology is very important before treatment is recommended.

Oronasal and Oroantral Fistulas

Prevention. Preoperative model surgery reveals the amount of expansion to be expected at the time of maxillary osteotomy. Large expansions (> 8 mm) increase the risk of soft tissue breakdown as well as relapse. In selected cases requiring very large expansions, it may be wiser to treat the patient with a bilateral crossbite in the posterior occlusion. Usually, a suitable functional occlusion can be achieved, and the

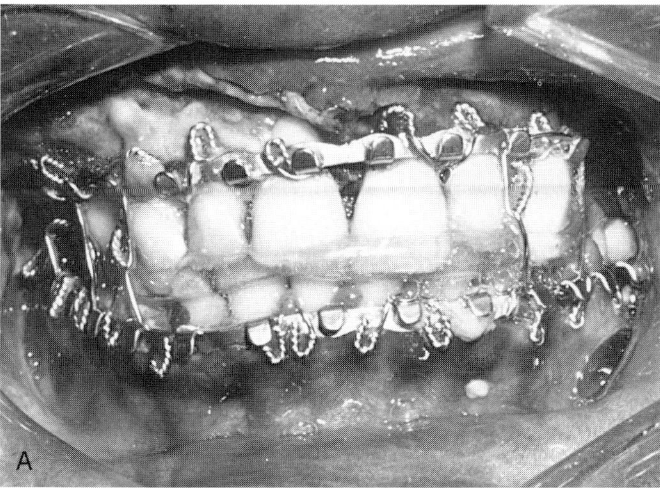

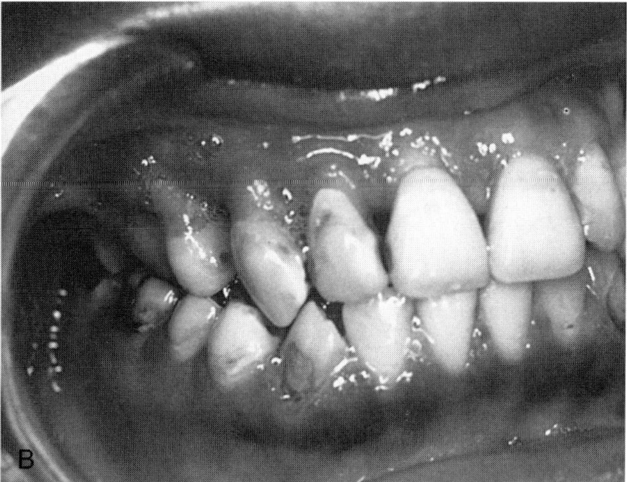

Figure 13–21. *A*, Immediate postoperative view of right anterior maxillary segment following four-piece maxillary osteotomy. Twenty HBO treatments were carried out over 10 days. *B*, View of the same area 6 months postoperatively. Gingival recession is noted with exposed roots. Gingival grafting was performed later. The value of HBO is not known in this case.

expansion will be at least 6 to 8 mm less. Oronasal fistulas are more common than oroantral fistulas, probably because of the greater tension placed on the palatal mucosa as the maxilla is widened.[80]

Intraoperative Considerations. The palatal mucosa may be torn at the time of surgery or may break down later as a result of wound tension. In either case, maintenance of an intact nasal mucosa is the best way to prevent development of a fistula. If a tear occurs in the palatal mucosa, closure should be attempted only if it can be done without tension. If the tear cannot be closed without tension, the nasal mucosa should be inspected and sutured, if necessary, and the potential for placing some bone in the area should be considered. Also, a barrier, such as Gore-Tex, or a dressing (Xeroform) can be placed over the defect. The barrier is eventually exfoliated but may assist in hygiene and separation of the oral and nasal cavities.

Postoperative Considerations. Routine instructions against nose blowing should be given. Also, decongestants, nasal sprays, and possibly antibiotics may be utilized. If an oronasal fistula persists after healing, conscientious hygiene and maintenance of sinus and upper respiratory health often allow spontaneous closure. If not, operative closure may be necessary, depending on the location. Bone grafting is rarely necessary unless the defect is very large. An obturator may be useful to maintain nasal or sinus health while awaiting complete maxillary healing. Oroantral fistulas, although rare, should be treated in the same manner intraoperatively and postoperatively.

Nasal Septal Deviation

Prevention. Preoperative evaluation of nasal symmetry is very important, not only in treatment planning but also in documentation of the existing condition. Deviation of the nasal septum secondary to maxillary osteotomy has been associated with nasolacrimal obstruction,[69] increased airway resistance, and aesthetic complaints.[80] Assuming that the nose is straight preoperatively, it is important to take measures necessary to prevent septal buckling intraoperatively.

Intraoperative Considerations. From posterior to the nasopalatine foramen to the leading edge of the anterior nasal spine (ANS), the septal crest of the maxilla must be reduced more than expected to avoid upward pressure on the nasal septal cartilage.[93] Between the ANS and the nasopalatine foramen, the maxillary bone rises superiorly and then falls (Fig. 13–22). The septal cartilage follows this arc. Therefore, if the maxilla is to be repositioned anteriorly even without any impaction, the highest point on the maxillary septal crest of bone contacts the septal cartilage with pressure and causes it to buckle or deviate. If sufficient bone and cartilage have been removed in the area of the ANS after the maxilla has been fixed rigidly, one should be able to pass a periosteal elevator between the maxillary septal crest and the septal cartilage without resistance.[93]

Finally, to avoid displacement of the septum in the recovery phase, a hole should be drilled through the

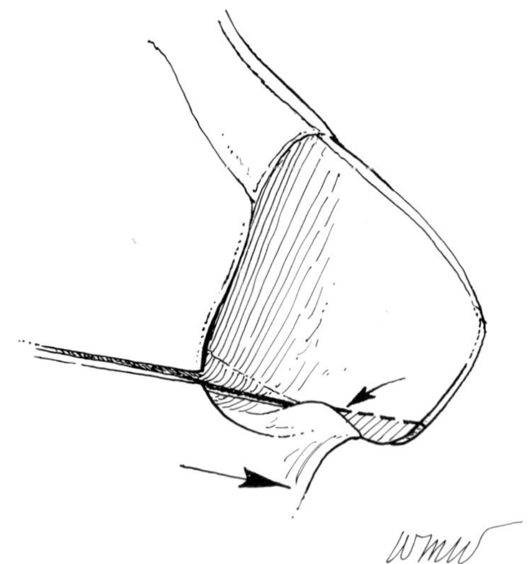

Figure 13–22. The septal crest of the maxilla rises from the tip of the anterior nasal spine (ANS) to a more superior level before falling inferiorly in the posterior region. The septal cartilage follows this undulating course. Therefore, there is septal cartilage over the ANS that will be buckled by the most prominent part of the maxilla as it is advanced, even if the maxilla is not superiorly repositioned.

ANS, and the septum attached to the ANS with a heavy resorbable suture. The perichondrium should be included in the suturing to prevent the cartilage from tearing through.[93] Numerous postanesthesia events, such as nasal extubation, nasal airway placement, suctioning, and vomiting, cannot displace the septum when it is fixed this way.

Postoperative Considerations. If the septum has not been fixed and is seen to be deviated, it should be treated at the earliest possible moment in the recovery room, patient room, or office. If one is sure that sufficient bone and cartilage were removed at the time of surgery, repositioning can be done at the bedside. Local anesthesia and manual manipulation are adequate. Stabilization with packing is usually not necessary. If insufficient tissue has been removed, however, a septoplasty must be performed.

Maxillary Sinusitis

Prevention. Although it is possible for maxillary sinusitis to develop postoperatively, more sinusitis is cured by maxillary osteotomy than created by it.[81] If the patient has a history of sinusitis preoperatively, the usual medical treatments should be employed, such as decongestants, antihistamines, nasal spray, and possibly antibiotics, to provide the best surgical environment possible.

Intraoperative Considerations. Removal of infected or polypoid tissue discovered in the maxillary sinus at the time of maxillary osteotomy is recommended. Otherwise, the antral mucosa should be left intact. Also, avoidance of septal deviation and superolateral crushing of the inferior turbinate ensures adequate drainage of the maxillary sinus postoperatively.

Postoperative Considerations. Decongestants with

antihistamines and occasional nasal spray are helpful during the early postoperative phase. The purpose of the antihistamines in the postoperative mix is not so much for treatment of allergic swelling but to offset the sympathomimetic effects of the decongestant. Many postoperative patients have trouble sleeping, and decongestants alone may exacerbate this complaint. Sinus complaints that persist after 8 weeks should be investigated in the usual clinical and radiographic manner.

Unaesthetic Soft Tissue Changes

This topic has been discussed previously in the consideration of preoperative factors in maxillary surgery. In addition to adequate informed consent and a detailed explanation of expected outcomes, it should be explained to the patient that postoperative procedures may be needed to achieve the desired results. Septorhinoplasty and Weir procedures are the most commonly useful operations to enhance the negative outcomes of maxillary orthognathic surgery.[59, 60] It is most helpful to identify the possible need for these procedures preoperatively and to incorporate them into the treatment plan.

"Down-turned" or unsupported oral commissures result most commonly from excessive superior repositioning of the maxilla. This latter result often occurs because the inexperienced surgeon plans the operation on the basis of the relationship of the central incisors to the upper lip clinically and on the basis of the relaxed lateral cephalogram. The position of the canines relative to the upper lip and the drape of the upper lip is ignored. The surgeon should avoid excessive impaction of the maxilla, because it produces one of the worst aesthetic outcomes we see in orthognathic surgery. Periosteal suturing to reestablish support for the elevators of the upper lip (levator anguli oris, nasalis and incisive muscles) prior to closure of the mucosal incision may be helpful in limiting this unpleasant outcome.

The V-Y closure technique has not been rewarding in our experience, as it robs Peter to pay Paul. Increased midline vermilion is achieved at the expense of lateral vermilion narrowing. It is possible to minimize vermilion narrowing by keeping the anterior aspect of the mucoperiosteal incision close to the mucogingival junction, suturing the periosteum, and closing the mucosa with small bites.

Insufficient Bone Strength

Prevention. According to the experience of many, very thin anterior maxillary bone can be predicted in cases of vertical maxillary excess[61, 62] and in all skeletal open bite cases. The lack of functional stresses over a lifetime renders the buttresses and piriform rims less than substantial.

Intraoperative Considerations. For the most part, rigid fixation techniques have decreased the significance of this problem. The RAP system is especially valuable in managing poor bone-to-bone contact after maxillary osteotomy,[90] not only because it does not require solid bone on the inferior side of the osteotomy but also because one can utilize solid bone at a great distance from the osteotomy. Rigid plating systems are also helpful in stabilizing maxillas that do not have adequate[62] bone contact. In addition to rigid fixation, bone grafting may be useful in cases with poor bone contact or strength.

Postoperative Considerations. Superior shifting of the maxilla postoperatively indicates a breakdown in the fixation system if rigid fixation has been used and poor bony stops if wire fixation has been used. In either case, the occlusion and aesthetics must be reevaluated and a decision made as to whether reoperation is needed.

Unfavorable Fractures

Several unusual fractures have occurred with maxillary osteotomies, including complete vomer avulsion,[85] pterygoid plate fracture,[82–84, 86] sphenoid bone fracture,[69] and middle cranial fossa fracture.[69, 84] Most have been discussed previously. One issue worthy of discussion here is the need for ideal splitting between the maxillary tuberosity and the pterygoid plates. Bad splits here have been considered a complication by some,[64, 65, 71] but others have shown, in studies of large groups of patients, that avoidance of a chisel in the pterygomaxillary fissure does not increase the number of pterygoid plate fractures or increase the incidence of complications.[84] In fact, CT studies indicate that pterygoid plate fractures occur in 85% of cases regardless of whether a chisel is used.[84, 86] Completion of all of the other osteotomies and avoidance of excessive force are probably most important in reducing the incidence of unfavorable fractures.

Non-Union (Delayed Union)

Non-union and delayed union were relatively common complications of maxillary surgery prior to rigid fixation.[62] Currently, extended periods of postoperative maxillary mobility are rare but still possible. With rigid fixation, the most likely cause of delayed union is a traumatic occlusion. The situation in which some of the teeth contact upon closure before the rest places an unbalanced force on the maxilla, and if the bony healing has not progressed to the strength capable of resisting this force, maxillary mobility occurs. If this movement is habitual, a fibrous union develops, and delayed healing results. Furthermore, if maxillary mobility persists for several weeks, vertical bone resorption may occur, causing foreshortening of the maxillary height.

Whether a postoperative wafer is used or not, the occlusion must be monitored carefully for several weeks to ensure that the maxilla is not being mobilized. If maxillary mobility is observed, measures must be taken to eliminate it. Mobility is usually not seen within the first 6 to 10 weeks because of rigid fixation; therefore, if mobility surfaces later, one can assume that the fixation is no longer holding the maxilla. To avoid reoperating on the maxilla, it is suggested that occlusal management be considered. A consultation with the treating orthodontist and construction of a splint to equalize the occlusal forces on the maxilla until solidification has occurred are recommended. Use of a splint to equalize postoperative occlusion is appropriate when the orthodontist and surgeon agree that the traumatic occlusion is salvageable by orthodontic means.

Eustachian Tube Dysfunction

Blockage of the middle ear is common following any nasoendotracheal intubation but particularly so after maxillary osteotomy. In addition to the irritation of the endotracheal tube, the palatal muscles have been traumatized and displaced by the osteotomy. Therefore, many patients complain of fullness in the ears, decreased hearing acuity, and pain. Postoperative decongestants, nasal sprays, and reassurance guide patients through this phase. In the weeks following surgery, the tympanic membranes (TMs) should be examined routinely to detect fluid behind them, and appropriate treatment initiated if needed.

Velopharyngeal Incompetence

Although velopharyngeal incompetence (VPI) probably occurs to a minor degree after every maxillary osteotomy,[94] it has been most commonly documented following maxillary advancement in patients with cleft palate.[94, 95] For other patients, no special considerations are recommended. Patients who have undergone previous palatal surgery should have a speech evaluation preoperatively. The surgeon and speech pathologist should discuss the level of compensation that the patient has already achieved, so that a projection of the long-term result can be estimated. If the patient is fully compensated with adequate velopharyngeal function, it is most likely that no significant VPI will develop postoperatively; however, if the patient's velopharyngeal function is considered "borderline" preoperatively, surgically induced symptomatic VPI may occur.[94] Such patients should be advised that a pharyngeal flap may be necessary later to restore adequate velopharyngeal competence. It should be noted that labiodental speech is improved with maxillary advancement, representing a significant speech benefit in spite of the potential for VPI.[95]

If the patient has an intact pharyngeal flap and a maxillary advancement is planned, not only should VPI be evaluated, but taking down the flap should be considered. During the maxillary advancement, if the flap restricts maxillary advancement, it should be released, and plans should be made for renewing it later, after the maxillary osteotomy has healed. All of these issues should be discussed with the patient and family preoperatively.

Arteriovenous Fistulas

Arteriovenous (AV) fistulas, including carotid–cavernous sinus fistulas, have occurred following maxillary osteotomy.[87, 88] Because so little is known about the etiology and mechanism, only careful osteotomy technique can be recommended. Unexpected peripheral neurologic signs and symptoms, especially ophthalmic, should be carefully and quickly investigated.

Dysphagia

One case of complete dysphagia has been reported after maxillary advancement and mandibular setback.[89] After 8 weeks without resolution, myotomy of the cricopharyngeus muscle was performed and seemed to alleviate the problem. It is not known whether this problem was secondary to the maxillary advancement, the mandibular setback, or both.

Transverse Relapse

Significant transverse relapse after multiple-piece maxillary osteotomy for widening has been observed for many years.[56] Careful studies consistently show this phenomenon to be more prevalent than commonly thought. Transverse relapse is a latent problem, because the effects do not show up until the patient has finished with orthodontic appliances and retainers. When transverse relapse occurs, it may appear as an anterior open bite and an AP rotation of the mandible downward and backward, simulating mandibular relapse. Because bone grafting and rigid fixation do not seem to make a difference, perhaps an alternative strategy should be considered. Surgically rapid palatal expansion (SRPE) has been shown to be quite stable.[96, 97] SRPE does not, however, address vertical problems but seems to be significantly stable compared with multiple-piece maxillary osteotomy for transverse widening. Perhaps it should be considered even when multiple-piece osteotomies are to be performed later for vertical discrepancies.

Condylar Resorption

Condylar resorption has been reported after maxillary osteotomy;[35] however, it is doubtful that the surgery had anything to do with the condylar changes. Numerous authors have identified the group at risk for condylar resorption regardless of the osteotomy. That group comprises white females with high mandibular plane angles and mandibular retrognathism.[23, 24, 35]

Anterior Maxillary Segmental Osteotomy (AMSO)

The AMSO is subject to nearly all of the complications discussed for the Le Fort I osteotomy; the issues discussed previously are not reiterated here. Over the last 20 years, the necessity for AMSO has radically declined owing to the advancements in orthodontic-orthognathic preparation. A few considerations deserve mention here, however.

Difficulties seen with the AMSO depend to a certain degree on which of the techniques are employed, because access greatly influences the potential for complications. The more difficult the access, the greater the risks of a poor outcome. In cases that require a clockwise rotation of the anterior maxilla, access to the most medioposterior aspect of the anterior maxillary segment may inhibit proper bone removal or increase the risk of devascularization. In anterior maxillary segmental surgery, planning is the most important element. The surgeon must think through the operation and anticipate the most difficult parts. In choosing the flap design, access to the most challenging areas must be envisioned and planned. Basically, there are three possible flap designs for AMSO, with a few variations.[93] The anterior maxilla can be pedicled on the palate,[98] the labia,[99] or both. The palatal pedicle seems to offer the best perfusion, but an anterior labial pedicle is acceptable if the soft tissue is carefully maintained.[100] If bicuspids are to be extracted and the palatal mucoperiosteum used as the sole vascular source, one must take care not to crimp the palatal mucosa at the time of setback. Using the palatal mucosa as the pedicle for this move is ill advised anyway, because the palatal tissue obstructs access to the most critical area of bony obstruction—the medial palate.

If vascular compromise is seen postoperatively, removal of the splint should be considered to alleviate compression and stress on the pedicle. If rigid fixation has not been used, removal of the splint will come at the cost of instability of the segment. If the splint is removed, a new fixation system should be constructed to minimize tension on the soft tissue. Hyperbaric oxygenation may be considered as described previously.

Posterior Maxillary Segmental Osteotomy (PMSO)

Relapse is not now a significant issue with PMSO; however, in the infancy of orthognathic surgery, relapse of PMSO was found to be excessive.[101] The disparity here is explained by the different techniques studied. Subsequently, procedures have been developed that offer excellent stability.[102] Not only are the techniques a factor, but so is the preoperative planning. Because it is not known how these cases were prepared for surgery, a surgeon's own past experience is the only guide. PMSOs do not relapse interiorly, especially if rigidly fixed. If open bites develop postoperatively, the most likely explanation is that the mandibular condyles were not seated at the time of posterior maxillary segmental positioning and fixation. Thus, the posterior segments were not impacted enough, and postoperatively, when the condyles seated, the open bite was revealed. This explanation is highly likely, because placing these segments appropriately using the mandible as the known reference is tricky when the anterior maxilla has not been mobilized. Many areas of bony interferences may obscure the desired posterior maxillary location.

Before scheduling a bilateral PMSO, one should reconsider a Le Fort I osteotomy in three pieces as an option that is much less difficult, more controllable, and more predictable. Unilateral PMSO makes sense because it usually is done for prosthetic reasons, and a certain amount of latitude is permissible before dental restoration.

Surgical Rapid Palatal Expansion (SRPE)

Few procedures I have performed have been as free of serious complications as the SRPE.[96, 97] The procedure as described elsewhere renders predictable results with minimal complications.[96] A few problems have been encountered, however, when this procedure is performed in an outpatient setting. Both hemimaxillas must be fully mobilized to facilitate symmetric expansion. The segments must not be overexpanded, however, or the interdental tissue between the central incisors may be compromised, resulting in a loss of papillary contour. If the interdental papilla between the central appears compromised in the early postoperative period, the expansion appliance should be backed down a few notches.

Nasal bleeding is not uncommon in the early postoperative period but should cease within 12 hours. If bleeding persists beyond this time, the intranasal structures should be examined and a posterior nasal pack considered.

References

1. Jacobs JD, Sinclair PM: Principles of orthodontic mechanics in orthognathic surgery cases. Am J Orthod 1983;84:399.
2. Bell WH, Jacobs JD: Tridimensional planning for surgical/orthodontic treatment of mandibular excess. Am J Orthod 1981;80:263.
3. Behrman SJ: Complications of sagittal osteotomy of the mandibular ramus. J Oral Surg 1972;30:544.
4. Epker BN, Wolford LM: Modified sagittal ramus osteotomy. *In* Epker BN, Wolford LM (eds): Dentofacial Deformities: Surgical-Orthodontic Correction. St Louis, CV Mosby, 1980, p 66.
5. MacIntosh RB: Experience with the sagittal osteotomy of the mandibular ramus: A 13-year review. J Maxillofac Surg 1981;8:151.
6. Turvey T: Intraoperative complications of sagittal osteotomy of the mandibular ramus: Incidence and management. J Oral Maxillofac Surg 1985;43:504.
7. Cunningham LL, Tiner BD, Clark GM, et al: Surgeon's assessment of nerve damage vs patient's report of neurosensory deficit. J Dent Res 1995;74:1159.
8. Martis CS: Complications after mandibular sagittal split osteotomy. J Oral Maxillofac Surg 1984;42:101.
9. Naples RJ, Van Sickles JE, Jones DJ: Long-term neurosensory deficits associated with bilateral sagittal split osteotomy versus inverted "L" osteotomy. Oral Surg 1994;77:318.
10. Piecuch JF, Lewis RA: Facial nerve injury as a complication of sagittal split ramus osteotomy. J Oral Maxillofac Surg 1982;40:309.
11. Schalit CJ, Jacks SC, Turvey TA, Zuniga JR: Incidence of lingual nerve injury following bilateral sagittal split osteotomies. J Dent Res 1995;74:1158.
12. Schendel SA, Epker BN: Results after mandibular advancement surgery: An analysis of 87 cases. J Oral Surg 1980;38:265.
13. Walter JM, Gregg JM: Analysis of postsurgical neurologic alterations in the trigeminal nerve. J Oral Surg 1979;37:410.
14. White RP, Peters PB, Costich ER, et al: Evaluation of sagittal split ramus osteotomy in 17 patients. J Oral Surg 1969;27:851.
15. Zaytoun HS, Phillips C, Terry BC: Long-term neurosensory deficits following transoral vertical ramus and sagittal split osteotomies for mandibular prognathism. J Oral Maxillofac Surg 1986;44:193.
16. De Vries K, De Vries PP, Hovinga J, Van den Akker HP: Facial palsy after sagittal split osteotomies. J Craniomaxillofac Surg 1993;21:50.

17. Dendy RA: Facial nerve paralysis following sagittal split mandibular osteotomy: A case report. Br J Oral Surg 1973;11:101.
18. Singer RS, Bays RA: A comparison between superior and inferior border wiring techniques in sagittal split ramus osteotomy. J Oral Maxillofac Surg 1985;43:444.
19. Arnett GW, Tamborello JA, Rathbone JA: Temporomandibular joint ramifications of orthognathic surgery. *In* Bell WH (ed): Modern Practice in Orthognathic and Reconstructive Surgery. Philadelphia, WB Saunders, 1992.
20. Dennis S, Rebellato G: Postoperative condylar movement: A kinematic center of rotation study. J Dent Res 1995;74:1614.
21. Arnett GW, Tamborello JA: Progressive class II development: Female idiopathic condylar resorption. Oral Maxillofac Surg Clin North Am 1990;2:699.
22. Arnett GW: A redefinition of bilateral sagittal osteotomy (BSO) advancement relapse. Am J Orthod Dentofac Orthop 1993;104:506.
23. Kerstens HC, Tuinzing DB, Goldong RP, van der Kwast WA: Condylar atrophy and osteoarthrosis after bimaxillary surgery. Oral Surg 1990;69:274.
24. Merkx MAW, Van Damme PA: Condylar resorption after orthognathic surgery: Evaluation of treatment in 8 patients. J Craniomaxillofac Surg 1994;22:53.
25. Moore KE, Gooris PJJ, Stoelinga PJW: The contributing role of condylar resorption to skeletal relapse following mandibular advancement surgery. J Oral Maxillofac Surg 1991;49:448.
26. O'Ryan F: Complications of orthognathic surgery. Oral Maxillofac Surg Clin North Am 1990;2:593.
27. Van Sickels JE, Tucker MR: Prevention and management of complications in orthognathic surgery. *In* Peterson LJ (ed): Principles of Oral and Maxillofacial Surgery. Philadelphia, JB Lippincott, 1992, p 1465.
28. Bays RA: Arthrotomy and orthognathic surgery for TMD. *In* Kraus SL (ed): Temporomandibular Disorders, ed 2. New York, Churchhill Livingstone, 1994, p 237.
29. Kline SN: Electrical testing for injuries of the seventh nerve. J Oral Surg 1975;33:215.
30. Karabouta-Voulgarpoulou I, Martis C: Facial paresis following sagittal split osteotomy. Oral Surg 1984;57:600.
31. Rachel J, Ellis E, Fonseca RJ: The anatomical location of the mandibular canal: Its relationship to the sagittal ramus osteotomy. Int J Adult Orthod Orthogn Surg 1988;1:37.
32. Blumenthal F, May M: Electrodiagnosis. *In* May M (ed): The Facial Nerve. New York, Thieme, 1986, p 1.
33. Bays RA, Fisher KL: Evaluation of condylar position and rigid fixation of sagittal split osteotomies. [Abstract.] American Association of Oral and Maxillofacial Surgeons, Anaheim, CA, 1987.
34. Crawford JG, Stoelinga PJW, Blijdorp PA, Brouns JJA: Stability after reoperation for progressive condylar resorption after orthognathic surgery: Report of seven cases. J Oral Maxillofac Surg 1994;52:460.
35. De Mol van Otterloo JJ, Dorenbos J, Tuinzing DB, van der Kwast WAM: TMJ performance and behavior in patients more than 6 years after Le Fort I osteotomy. Br J Oral Maxillofac Surg 1993;31:83.
36. Boyer CC, Williams TW, Stevens FW: Blood supply of the temporomandibular joint. J Dent Res 1964;43:224.
37. Hunsuck EE: Modified intraoral sagittal splitting technique for correction of mandibular prognathism. J Oral Surg 1968;26:250.
38. Hall HD, McKenna SJ: Further refinement and evaluation of intraoral vertical ramus osteotomy. J Oral Maxillofac Surg 1987;45:684.
39. Egyedi P, Houwing M, Julen E: The oblique subcondylar osteotomy: Report of results of 100 cases. J Oral Surg 1981;39:871.
40. O'Ryan F: Complications of orthognathic surgery. I: Mandibular surgery. Sel Read Oral Maxillofac Surg 1989;1:1.
41. Sinn DP, Ghali GE: Management of intraoperative complications in orthognathic surgery. Oral Maxillofac Surg Clin North Am 1990;2:869.
42. Eckerdal O, Sund G, Astrand P: Skeletal remodeling in the temporomandibular joint after oblique sliding osteotomy of the mandibular rami. Int J Oral Maxillofac Surg 1986;15:233.
43. Tuinzing DB, Greebe RB: Complications related to the intraoral vertical ramus osteotomy. Int J Oral Surg 1985;14:319.
44. Guralnick W, Kelly JP: Palsy of the facial nerve after intraoral oblique osteotomies of the mandible. J Oral Surg 1979;37:743.
45. Hall HD, Chase DC, Payor LG: Evaluation and refinement of the intraoral vertical subcondylar osteotomy. J Oral Surg 1975;33:333.
46. Ward TG, Smith DG, Sommar M: Condylotomy for mandibular joints. Br Dent J 1957;103:147.
47. Nickerson JW, Veaco NS: Condylotomy in surgery of the temporomandibular joint. Oral Maxillofac Surg Clin North Am 1989;1:303.
48. Piper MA: Microscopic disc preservation surgery of the temporomandibular joint. Oral Maxillofac Clin North Am 1989;1:279.
49. Schellhas KP, Pollei SR, Wilkes CH: Pediatric internal derangements of the temporomandibular joint: Effect on facial development. Am J Orthod Dentofac Orthop 1993;104:51.
50. Hale RG, Timmis DP, Bays RA: A new mandibulotomy technique for the dentate patient. Plast Reconstr Surg 1991;87:362.
51. Epker BN: Vascular considerations in orthognathic surgery. I: Mandibular osteotomies. Oral Surg 1984;57:472.
52. Lindquist CC, Obeid G: Complications of genioplasty done alone or in combination with sagittal split-ramus osteotomy. Oral Surg 1988;66:13.
53. Park HS, Ellis E, Fonseca RJ: A retrospective study of advancement genioplasty. Oral Surg 1989;67:481.
54. Rubens BC, West RA: Ptosis of the chin and lip incompetence: Consequences of lost mentalis muscle support. J Oral Maxillofac Surg 1989;47:359.
55. Polido WD, Bell WH: Long-term osseous and soft tissue changes after large chin advancements. J Craniomaxillofac Surg 1993;21:54.
56. Bell WH, Jacobs JD, Quejada JG: Simultaneous repositioning of the maxilla, mandible and chin. Am J Orthod 1986;89:28.
57. Sinclair P, Thomas PM, Tucker MR: Common complications in orthognathic surgery: Etiology and management. In Bell W (ed): Modern Practice in Orthognathic and Reconstructive Surgery. Philadelphia, WB Saunders, 1992, p 48.
58. McMillen B: Border movements on the human mandible. J Prosthet Dent 1972;27:524.
59. O'Ryan F, Schendel S: Nasal anatomy and maxillary surgery. II: Unfavorable nasolabial esthetics following the Le Fort I osteotomy. Int J Adult Orthod Orthogna Surg 1989;4:75.
60. Schendel SA, Williamson LW: Muscle reorientation following superior repositioning of the maxilla. J Oral Maxillofac Surg 1983;41:235.
61. Frost ED, Koutnic AW: Alternative stabilization of the maxilla during simultaneous jaw mobilization procedures. Oral Surg 1983;56:125.
62. Schendel SA, Eisenfeld J, Bell WH, et al: Superior repositioning of the maxilla: Stability and soft-tissue osseous relations. Am J Orthod 1976;70:663.
63. Lanigan D, Hey J, West R: Major vascular complications of orthognathic surgery: Hemorrhage associated with Le Fort I osteotomies. J Oral Maxillofac Surg 1991;48:561.
64. Lanigan DT, West RA: Management of postoperative hemorrhage following the Le Fort I maxillary osteotomy. J Oral Maxillofac Surg 1984;42:367.
65. Newhouse R, Schow S, Kraut R, et al: Life-threatening hemorrhage from a Le Fort I osteotomy. J Oral Maxillofac Surg 1982;40:117.
66. Parnes EI, Becker ML: Necrosis of the anterior maxilla following osteotomy. Oral Surg 1972;33:326.
67. Westwood RM, Tilson HB: Complications associated with maxillary osteotomies. J Oral Surg 1975;33:104.
68. Vedtofte P, Nattestad A: Pulp sensibility and pulp necrosis after Le Fort I osteotomy. J Craniomaxillofac Surg 1989;17:167.
69. Lanigan DT, Romanchuk MD, Olson CK: Ophthalmic complications associated with orthognathic surgery. J Oral Maxillofac Surg 1993;51:480.
70. Reiner S, Willoughby JH: Transient abducent nerve palsy following a Le Fort I maxillary osteotomy: Report of a case. J Oral Maxillofac Surg 1988;46:699.
71. Watts PG: Unilateral abducent nerve palsy: A rare complication following a Le Fort I maxillary osteotomy. Br J Oral Maxillofac Surg 1984;22:212.
72. Carr RJ, Gilbert P: Isolated partial third nerve palsy following Le Fort I maxillary osteotomy in a patient with cleft lip and palate. Br J Oral Maxillofac Surg 1986;24:206.

73. De Jongh M, Barnard D, Birnie D: Sensory nerve morbidity following Le Fort I osteotomy. J Maxillofac Surg 1986;14:10.
74. Sirikumara M, Sugar AW: Adie's pupil following Le Fort I maxillary osteotomy: A complication or coincidence? Br J Oral Maxillofac Surg 1990;28:306.
75. Tomasetti BJ, Broutsas M, Gormley M, et al: Lack of tearing after Le Fort osteotomy. Br J Oral Maxillofac Surg 1976;34:1095.
76. Shoshani Y, Samet N, Ardekian L, Taicher S: Nasolacrimal duct injury after Le Fort I osteotomy. J Oral Maxillofac Surg 1994;52:406.
77. Keller EE, Sather AH: Quadrangular Le Fort I osteotomy: Surgical technique and review of 54 patients. J Oral Maxillofac Surg 1990;48:2.
78. Freihofer HPM, Brouns JJH: Midface movements. Oral Maxillofac Surg Clin North Am 1990;2:761.
79. Demas PN, Sotereanos GC: Incidence of nasolacrimal injury and turbinectomy associated atrophic rhinitis with Le Fort I osteotomies. J Craniomaxillofac Surg 1989;17:116.
80. Sher MR: Treatment of oral-antral-nasal fistula after anterior maxillary osteotomy. J Oral Surg 1980;38:212.
81. Bell CS, Thrash WJ, Zysset MK: Incidence of maxillary sinusitis following Le Fort I maxillary osteotomy. J Oral Maxillofac Surg 1986;44:100.
82. Wikkeling O, Koppendraaier J: In vitro studies on lines of osteotomy in the pterygoid region. J Maxillofac Surg 1973;1:209.
83. Robinson P, Hendy C: Pterygoid plate fractures caused by the Le Fort I osteotomy. Br J Oral Maxillofac Surg 1986;24:198.
84. Precious DS, Goodday RH, Bourget L, Skulsky FG: Pterygoid plate fracture in Le Fort I osteotomy with and without pterygoid chisel: A computed tomography scan evaluation of 58 patients. J Oral Maxillofac Surg 1993;51:151.
85. Smith KS, Heggie AAC: Vomero-sphenoidal dysarticulation during the Le Fort I maxillary osteotomy: Report of case. J Oral Maxillofac Surg 1995;53:465.
86. Renick B, Symington JM: Postoperative computed tomography study of pterygomaxillary separation during the Le Fort I osteotomy. J Oral Maxillofac Surg 1991;49:1051.
87. Habal M: A carotid cavernous sinus fistula after maxillary osteotomy. Plast Reconstr Surg 1986;77:981.
88. Lanigan DT, Hey JH, West RA: False aneurysms and arteriovenous fistulas following orthognathic surgery. J Oral Maxillofac Surg 1991;49:571.
89. Gaukroger MC: Dysphagia following bimaxillary osteotomy. Br J Oral Maxillofac Surg 1993;31:189.
90. Bays RA: Maxillary osteotomies utilizing the rigid adjustable pin (RAP) system: A review of 31 clinical cases. Int J Adult Orthod Orthognath Surg 1986;1:275.
91. Dodson TB, Neuenschwander MC, Bays RA: Intraoperative measurement of maxillary blood flow during Le Fort I osteotomy [abstract]. J Oral Maxillofac Surg 1993;58:138.
92. Lanigan D, Hey J, West RA: Aseptic necrosis of the maxilla: Report of 36 cases. J Oral Maxillofac Surg 1990;48:142.
93. Bays RA, Timmis DP: Techniques for maxillary orthognathic surgery. *In* Peterson L (ed): Principles of Oral and Maxillofacial Surgery. Philadelphia, JB Lippincott, 1991, p 1349.
94. Witzel MA: The effects of Le Fort I osteotomy with maxillary movement on articulation, resonance and velopharyngeal function. Cleft Palate J 1989;26:199.
95. Schwarz C, Gruner E: Logopaedic findings following advancement of the maxilla. J Maxillofac Surg 1976;4:40.
96. Bays RA, Greco J: Surgically assisted rapid palatal expansion: An outpatient technique with long-term stability. J Oral Maxillofac Surg 1992;50:110.
97. Kuo PC, Will LA: Surgical orthodontic treatment of maxillary constriction. Oral Maxillofac Surg Clin North Am 1990;4:751.
98. Wassmund M: Lehrbuch der probleschen Chirurgie des Mundes und der Keifer. Leipzig, Meusser, 1935.
99. Wunderer S: Erfahrungen mit der operatiren Behandlung hochgradiger Prognathien. Dtsch Zahn Mund Keiferheilkd 1963;39:451.
100. Nelson RL, Path MG, Ogle RG, et al: Quantitation of blood flow after anterior maxillary osteotomy: Investigation of three surgical approaches. J Oral Surg 1978;36:106.
101. Schuchardt K: Experiences with the surgical treatment of deformities of the jaws: Prognathia, micrognathia and open bite. *In* Wallace AB (ed): International Society of Plastic Surgeons. London, E&S Livingstone, 1959.
102. Bell WH: Correction of skeletal type anterior open bite. J Oral Surg 1971;29:706.

Chapter 14
COMPLICATIONS ASSOCIATED WITH THE USE OF RIGID INTERNAL FIXATION IN MAXILLOFACIAL SURGERY

by

David H. Perrott

Introduction

Rigid internal fixation (RIF) is routinely used in the treatment of maxillofacial trauma,[1–13] maxillofacial reconstructive,[14–19] and craniofacial[20–23] procedures. The advantages of RIF include stability, immediate function, and improved results. The procedure, however, is highly technique sensitive with little room for error. Complications range from minor infections to total system failure. Although hardware failure can occur, the vast majority of complications can be attributed to operator error. Therefore, the surgeon must have a thorough understanding of biomechanical principles and RIF surgical skills to minimize complications.

The Subjects Discussed in This Chapter Are:

- General complications
  - Metal sensitivity
  - Screw failure
  - Plate fracture
  - Stress shielding
  - Tooth injury
  - Hardware removal secondary to plate extrusion, tissue discoloration, or cold sensitivity
  - Diagnostic limitations imposed by RIF
- Complications of mandibular RIF procedures
  - Fracture treatment
  - Mandibular orthognathic surgery
  - Mandibular surgical defect stabilization and reconstruction
- Complications of midface and craniofacial RIF procedures
  - Fracture treatment
  - Orthognathic and craniofacial surgery

General Complications

Many complications associated with RIF are common to mandibular and midface-craniofacial procedures. These general complications are presented, and their treatment is discussed first.

Metal Sensitivity

A variety of metals have been used to manufacture surgical implants. At present, the three primary metals used are stainless steel, Vitallium (Howmedica Inc., Rutherford, NJ), and titanium. Chromium, cobalt, and nickel, all components of stainless steel and Vitallium, appear to cause an allergic response in a very small number of people. Sensitivity to other metal alloys (aluminum and molybdenum) and pure titanium is very rare and may not even exist.[24, 25]

Symptoms of implant metal sensitivity, generally localized to the implant area, are eczema, erythema, and vesicles of the overlying skin or mucosa.[26] These symptoms usually occur 3 to 6 months after placement and should not be confused with other immune responses due to infection. Routine preoperative intracutaneous testing is not recommended, because it could sensitize patients to the metallic elements.[27] A history of previous metal sensitivity (e.g., jewelry), however, is predictive for implant sensitivity.

The role of metal sensitivity in prosthesis failure has been studied by several investigators.[28–31] There seems to be little evidence to support a direct correlation between metal sensitivity and prosthesis loosening. It does appear, however, that loosening of the prosthesis and subsequent metal fretting may produce a cutaneous sensitivity.

Treatment for metal sensitivity is implant removal. Prevention may be difficult, especially when treatment requires the use of a metal implant. Because it appears that there are no sensitivities to titanium, however, the use of implants constructed with titanium is recommended for those patients with a history of metal sensitivities.

Screw Failure

Failure of a screw to hold within the bone may occur at the time of insertion or postoperatively. Screw failure

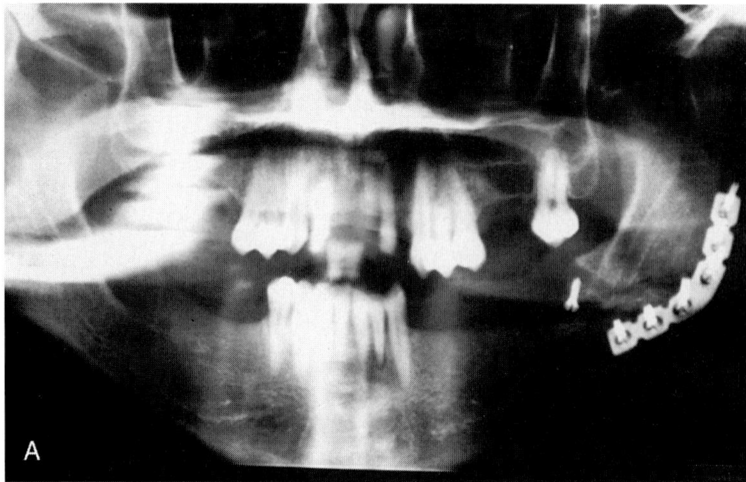

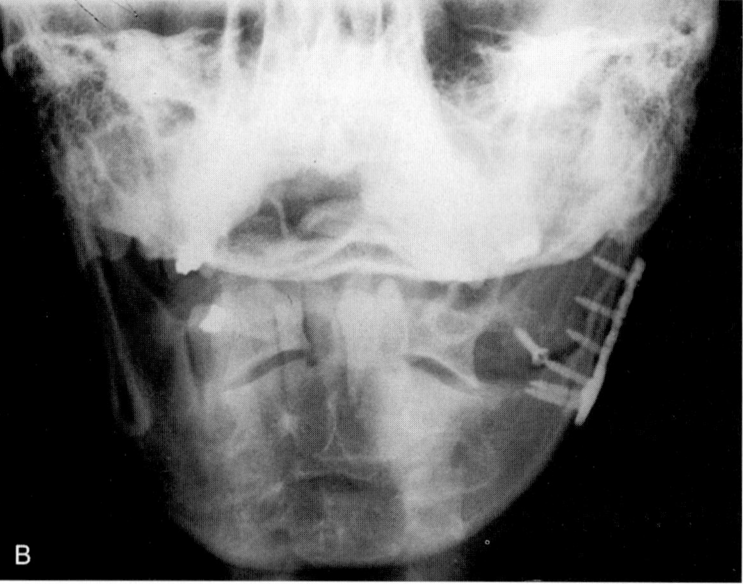

Figure 14–1. Panoramic radiograph (*A*) and PA radiograph (*B*) demonstrating lag screw failure secondary to countersink drill hole being placed into cancellous bone, which resulted in the screw's pulling through cortical bone.

during insertion can be attributed to any of six factors: (1) improper hole size or screw diameter (2) incomplete tapping of the hole (if required), (3) improper hole placement (too close to fracture or osteotomy sites), (4) poor bone quality (5) improper screw alignment (cross-thread), or (6) excessive insertional torque resulting in screw fracture.

When a screw fails during placement, it must be removed and replaced with a larger emergency screw[32] or a new screw hole must be placed in a different position. Failure to address a loose screw almost certainly produces a postoperative complication. All of the causes of screw failure at insertion can be prevented by following good RIF surgical principles and techniques.

Postoperative screw failure may be the result of functional forces exceeding the load capabilities of the screw, metal stress fatigue, or failure of the surgeon to recognize screw failure at placement. It has been reported that a screw loosens in 1% to 5% of patients undergoing immediate stabilization of mandibular defects with or without bony reconstruction (Fig. 14–1).[14–17]

Usually, fracture mobility or the presence of an infection is a good indicator of screw failure. Treatment is removal of the screw and restabilization of the bony segments. Postoperative screw failure can be prevented by properly positioning and placing the correct size and number of screws and carefully evaluating all screws during placement. Long-term bridging of a bony defect with a plate appears to be directly related to screw loosening. Therefore, some have advocated the use of the titanium hollow screw reconstruction plate (THORP) system (Synthes Maxillofacial, Paoli, PA).[15, 17] This system's design allows for rigid fixation of the head of the screw to the plate, avoiding unphysiologic loads to the bone underneath the plate. In addition, use of a titanium, plasma-coated, perforated hollow screw enables the development of direct bone-titanium contact as well as the ingrowth of bone into the lumen and perforations. Results indicate that the design does prevent screw loosening over long-term use.[15, 17]

Plate Fracture

Plate fracture is an uncommon complication associated with the use of rigid fixation techniques. Today's fixation hardware has been tested for adequate strength in appropriate clinical situations. The incidence of plate fracture ranges from zero to 10% when a plate is used long-term to bridge a bony defect.[13–16, 33–34] The incidence of plate fracture following other maxillofacial procedures is difficult to determine because it is seldom reported. The incidence is low because sufficient bony union occurs before long-term functional stresses produce a plate fracture.

Plate fracture can be attributed to surgeon error in judgment or technique to metal failure. The surgeon must understand bone biomechanics in choosing the proper-size plate for rigid fixation. Large functional forces upon a very small plate result in either screw or plate fracture (Fig. 14–2). In addition, the surgeon must not overbend the plate at the time of placement. Numerous bends prior to placement can induce metal fatigue, thereby leading to fracture upon functional loading.

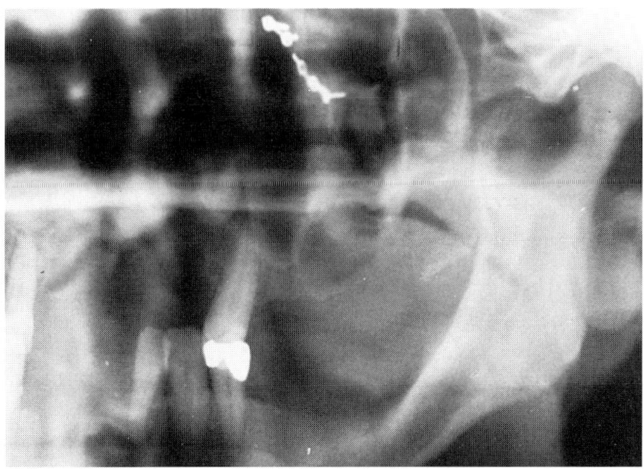

Figure 14–2. Improper selection of plate size, resulting in fracture. (Courtesy of Dr. John Bradick.)

Treatment for plate fracture is replacement if rigid fixation is still required. If a bony union has occurred, the plate may be left in place unless problems develop.

Stress Shielding

A potential complication of RIF is the possibility that plates will absorb the functional stress on the bone, resulting in a disuse osteoporosis termed "stress shielding" (Fig. 14–3). Protection from stress occurs if the RIF system has a higher modulus of elasticity than the bone to which it is attached.[35] In addition, periosteal compromise during implant placement may also

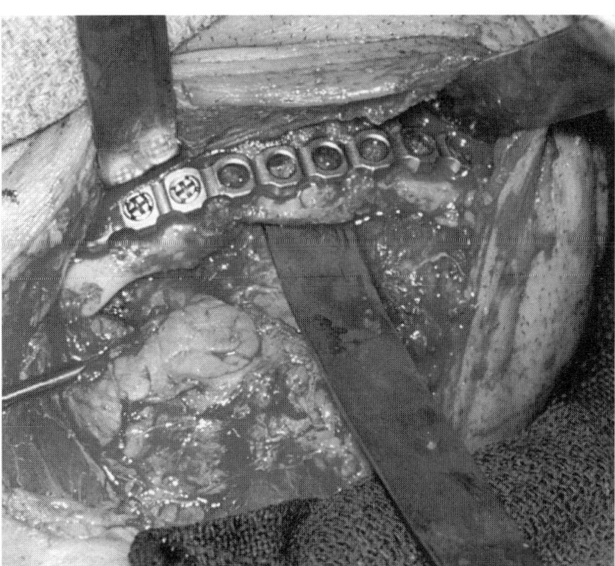

Figure 15–3. Bony osteoporosis under plate following bone graft.

promote osteoporosis, thus contributing to stress shielding.[36]

For the maxillofacial surgeon, stress shielding appears to be of concern in the use of RIF in mandibular continuity defects reconstructed with bone.[37–40] The need for and timing of bone plate removal following grafting procedures remains controversial. Recommendations for timing of plate removal range, however, from 6 months to 1 year.[41]

Plate designs using a limited bone contact appear to reduce postoperative circulatory compromise,[42] and this concept has been applied to maxillofacial rigid fixation devices. No studies, however, have been completed that indicate a reduction in stress shielding after the use of mandibular reconstruction techniques. Study of other variables in both in vitro and in vivo models is needed to better understand this potential clinical complication in maxillofacial surgery.

Tooth Injury

Injury to a tooth or a developing tooth bud can occur during placement of screws.[42, 43] In a laboratory setting, Assael[42] found the incidence of tooth injury to be 7%. Generally, tooth injury is identified on postoperative radiographs. Treatment may consist of observation or screw removal. Following screw removal, the erupted tooth may require no treatment, endodontic therapy, or extraction if pain or infection develops. The unerupted tooth many require orthodontically assisted eruption or extraction. Prevention of this complication is achieved by careful screw placement, removal of third molars in sagittal split osteotomy sites, and, as indicated, the smallest-diameter screw (Fig. 14–4).

Hardware Removal Secondary to Plate Extrusion, Tissue Discoloration, or Cold Sensitivity

Hardware removal itself may not be a complication of RIF, but the indications for removal may be. Screw failure, metal sensitivity, plate fracture, stress shielding, and tooth injury have previously been addressed. Additional indications for removal of hardware are plate extrusion,[44] plate palpation,[11, 45] tissue discoloration,[25, 46, 47, 48] cold sensitivity,[48, 49] infection,[8, 11, 13, 25, 36, 42–48, 50] plate exposure,[13, 44, 46, 50] and nerve hyperesthesia.[42, 46, 50] Many of these problems will be eliminated when fully resorbable plates are developed.

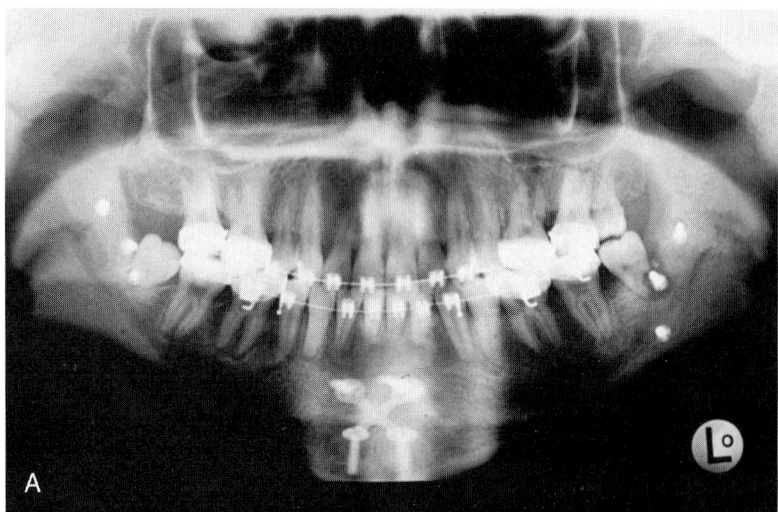

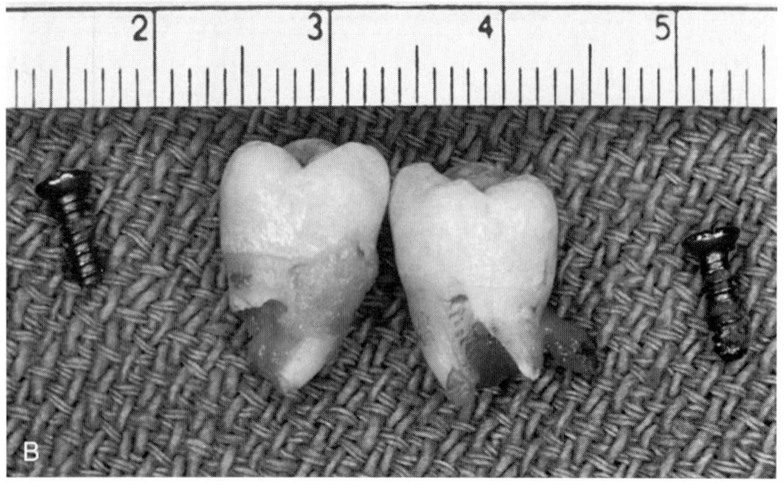

Figure 14–4. A 19-year-old female treated with bilateral mandibular sagittal split osteotomies and genioplasty stabilized with RIF. *A*, Panoramic radiograph illustrating screw placement into third molars. *B*, Removed screws and injured third molars.

Plate extrusion is very uncommon, is usually associated with infection, and requires plate removal. It is prevented by utilizing sound RIF techniques.

Occasionally, plates and screws become visible through the skin or are palpable by the patient. The incidence of plate palpation that requires removal is very uncommon following mandibular procedures. The incidence of plate palpation following midface/craniofacial procedures, however, ranges from 2.8% to 6%.[11, 45] and is most common in very thin individuals or when thick plates have been used.

Microsystems (1.0-mm screw diameter or smaller) are best suited for use in frontal sinus and nasoethmoid region, where the overlying skin is thin. In the region of the infraorbital rim or frontozygomatic suture, either paired microplates or plates using screws 1.3 mm or less are recommended. Miniplate systems using screws 1.5 mm or less should be reserved for the zygomaticomaxillary and nasomaxillary buttress, where vertical loads are greater and the skin is thicker. Similar rules should be followed in orthognathic procedures (Fig. 14–5).

Careful layered closure of skin incisions overlying the hardware should be performed. If the patient complains of these symptoms, plate removal is required after bone healing has occurred.

The incidence of clinically significant tissue discoloration ranges from zero to 7.6%.[46] Microscopic visible pigmentation, however, has been documented in 71.8% of patients following miniplate placement.[48] Pigmentation can be attributed to corrosion from fretting between the screws and plates. Unless the patient complains of the discoloration, the clinical significance of these findings remains unknown. Tissue sensitivity may result, however, from the release of chromium, nickel, and cobalt from stainless steel and Vitallium metals. If any of these symptoms should occur, plate removal is recommended.

Cold sensitivity is seldom reported as a reason for hardware removal. Large plates, thin overlying tissues, and climate contribute to this problem. Treatment is hardware removal. Prevention is achieved by utilizing an appropriate plate size and obtaining adequate tissue coverage.

Complications associated with infections, plate exposure, and nerve hyperesthesia are addressed in the discussion of mandibular and midface/craniofacial complications.

Diagnostic Limitations Imposed by RIF

In the past, large (thickness and length) implant devices were utilized for maxillofacial procedures. This raised concern with regard to postoperative computed tomography (CT) and magnetic resonance imaging (MRI) scans.[51, 52]

Fiala and associates[51] studied CT artifacts produced by maxillofacial RIF devices. In the bone and soft tissue window settings, the severity of the "starburst" artifact was found to be related to the physical size of the implant. Also, the severity was greatest with Vitallium metals and least with titanium metals. These investigators recommended that in areas where postoperative CT imaging is important, the surgeon should use the smallest appropriate size of titanium implants.

In a study evaluating MRI artifacts, Fiala and colleagues[52] found that titanium hardware produced the least amount of "black-hole" artifact. Vitallium and stainless steel devices of similar size produced significantly more artifacts. No heating or magnification deflections were seen with any of the metals, however. In conclusion, these investigators recommended the use of titanium hardware in areas where postoperative MRI scans were needed.

With today's modern titanium hardware devices, previous concerns about imaging are no longer serious issues. The ultimate answer, however, is fully resorbable implants.

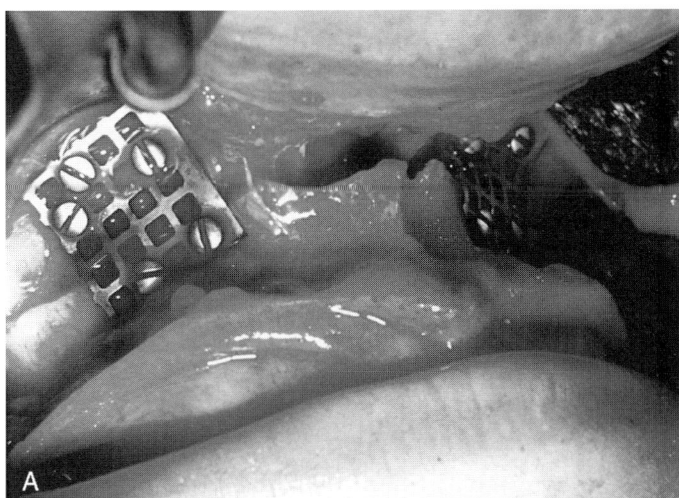

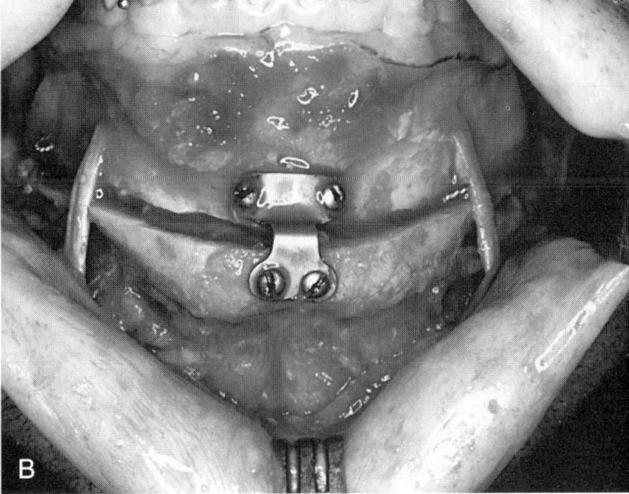

Figure 14–5. Orthognathic procedures using large implants palpated by the patient. *A*, Mesh used to stabilize Le Fort I osteotomy. Note the screw head above the mesh. *B*, Genioplasty stabilized with plate and screws.

Complications of Mandibular RIF Procedures

The rate of complications associated with the use of RIF in mandibular procedures ranges from 6.1% to 24%.[1–11, 36, 42, 46, 47, 50, 53–56] Iizuka and associates[56] attributed this high complication rate to surgeon inexperience. Using the mandibular fracture model, Kearns and colleagues[57] retrospectively evaluated two 24-month patient care periods separated by an intervening 12-month period. The major difference between the two time periods was an increase in operator experience. Results of the study demonstrated a downward trend in the complication rate as surgeon experience increased. The trend was not statistically significant, however. These investigators concluded that mandibular RIF complication rate is probably multifactorial but that technical problems still remain an important source of complications.

There are unique complications associated with the use of RIF in mandibular fractures, orthognathic surgery, and reconstructive procedures. Therefore, this section is divided into discussions of these three categories of surgery for clarity and completeness.

Mandibular Fracture Treatment

Complications of RIF for mandibular fracture are infections (soft tissue or bone), wound dehiscence with plate exposure, malocclusion (minimal and severe), non-union, nerve dysfunction (inferior alveolar and facial nerve), and hypertrophic scar formation. Of these complications, postoperative infection is potentially the most serious.

Infections

Infections following the use of RIF to treat mandibular fractures can be subdivided as soft tissue infections without involvement of bone and RIF implants and infections involving the bone and RIF implants. It is important that the surgeon clearly delineate soft tissue infections from bone and implant infections.

The incidence of soft tissue infection ranges from 1% to 8.6%.[9, 10, 46, 50, 57] These infections usually occur within 14 days of the operation. In addition, careful radiographic and clinical examinations reveal that both the plate and the fracture are stable. Treatment of soft tissue infections includes incision and drainage, appropriate wound care, culture and sensitivity testing, and antibiotics. If the infection does not demonstrate signs of improvement within 7 days, one must consider a bone or plate infection. Prevention of soft tissue complications includes treatment of the initial injury within 24 hours, appropriate use of drains, and good surgical techniques.

Bone and plate infections are more common (1.0% to 17.6%) and much more serious.[1, 5, 6, 9, 10, 42, 46, 50, 54–56] Clinical findings are local and distant signs of infection (i.e., swelling, drainage, lymphadenopathy), fracture mobility, pain, malocclusion, and wound dehiscence. Radiographic signs include displacement of the plate or screw, displacement of the fracture, and bony changes indicative of infection (Fig. 14–6). Radionuclide scans, bone cultures, and microscopic examination can assist in the diagnosis of osteomyelitis.[18]

Historically, maxillomandibular fixation (MMF) and external fixation devices have been the preferred method to immobilize infected fractures. Internal fixation was not used, because placement of wire or other foreign material into contaminated wounds was thought to be contraindicated. RIF with plates or screws was not used for contaminated or infected fractures, because the metal was thought to induce a foreign body reaction and possibly harbor bacteria.

Further research and greater experience in the use of RIF have demonstrated that infections resolve and infected fractures heal with plates and screws in the wound, provided that the hardware remains rigidly fixed. Koury and associates[18] and Koury and Ellis[58] confirmed the successful use of plates in the presence of infections. In the first study, the protocol used to treat mandibular osteomyelitis is as follows:

1. Incision and drainage.
2. Bone and soft tissue cultures.
3. Administration of appropriate antibiotics.
4. Débridement of any necrotic bone.
5. Reduction and rigid stabilization of the fracture; if a previously placed plate is stable, the plate is maintained, and loose screws are replaced.
6. The use of suction drains.
7. If necessary, bony reconstruction 6 to 12 months following treatment.

The most common causes of bone and plate infections are fracture instability, hardware (screw and plate) failure, and patient noncompliance. Fracture instability is usually the result of operator error. The surgeon must understand mandibular tension and compression properties to determine the type of fixation to be placed. In addition, the surgeon must properly execute fracture reduction and compression, selection of plate size and number of screws, plate and screw placement, and rigid fixation of the bony segments. Violations of these principles results in a potentially serious bone or plate infection (Fig. 14–7).[36] Hardware failure is uncommon and has been previously discussed.

Finally, the surgeon must carefully evaluate the patient's ability to comply with the chosen treatment plan. This issue is very important when the fracture is not rigidly fixed with plates or screws, thus requiring a period of MMF. Failure to comply with MMF may result in an infection.[4, 9, 10, 43, 46]

Wound Dehiscence with Plate Exposure

Wound dehiscence with or without implant exposure is a rare complication of RIF. Proper placement of incisions away from the gingival margin, tension-free closure, and use of antibiotics generally result in adequate tissue healing.

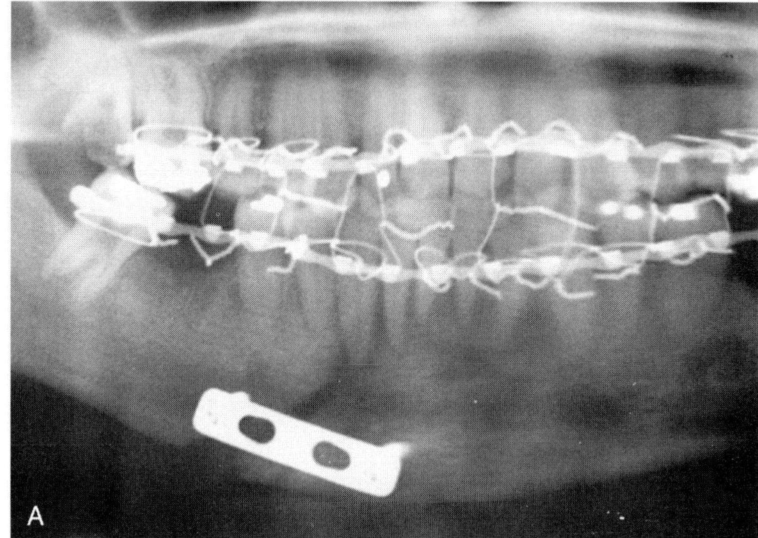

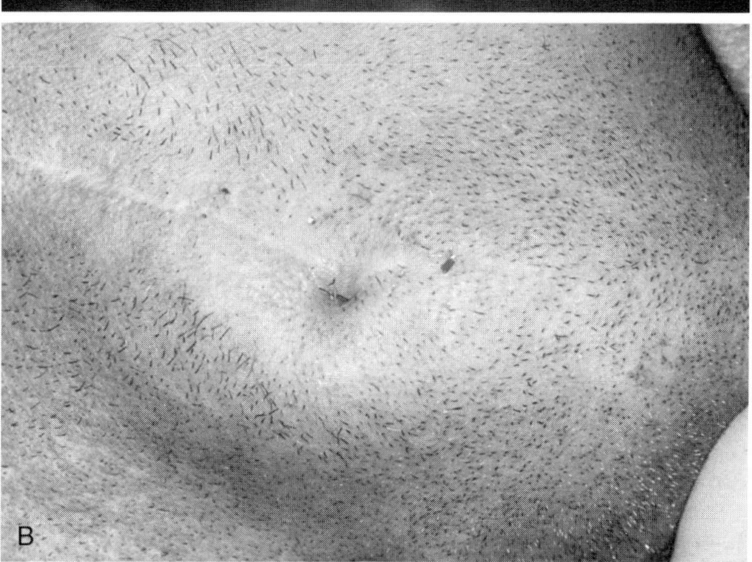

Figure 14–6. Mandibular fracture treated with inadequate stabilization resulting in osteomyelitis and draining fistula. *A,* Panoramic radiograph demonstrating osteomyelitis. *B,* Extraoral fistula.

When dehiscence does occur, the surgeon must be first carefully evaluate fracture stability. If the fracture is stable and good wound management is practiced, the wound closes by second intention. The wound must be kept clean with irrigation several times a day. The use of Xeroform gauze (Sherwood Medical, St. Louis, MO) for extraoral wound breakdown or Peridex (Procter and Gamble, Cincinnati, OH) for intraoral wound breakdown is recommended (Fig. 14–8). The temptation to primarily close a dehisced wound or to advance a flap in the area of RIF hardware should not be followed. If wound closure over the plate does not occur, the hardware can be removed as soon as bony union has occurred.

Malocclusion

Malocclusion has been reported in 3.6% to 14% of patients with mandibular fractures treated by RIF.[1, 46, 50, 55] Minor occlusal discrepancies can be treated with selective occlusal adjustments. An operation is required, however, to address major occlusal problems. Removal of the RIF hardware and re-fracture of the bone site(s) or the use of selected osteotomies is required to treat major occlusal discrepancies.

Occlusal complications can be attributed to surgical error. Failure to recognize all mandibular fractures often contributes to postoperative malocclusion. Undiagnosed condylar fractures, especially in conjunction with a symphyseal fracture, may produce widening of the posterior mandible as RIF hardware is placed.

Failure to obtain intraoperative MMF allows occlusal displacement during fracture reduction. The use of arch bars with wire MMF is the only method to achieve occlusal stability. Elastics and Ivy loops provide insufficient stability. In severely comminuted mandibular fractures or alveolar fractures, acrylic occlusal splints are often required. Also, lingual splints are helpful when symphyseal fractures occur in conjunction with other mandibular fractures, such as bilateral, severely displaced, condylar fractures.

Improper reduction of the fracture also produces a severe malocclusion. Various reduction instruments are available and should be utilized to achieve proper reduction.

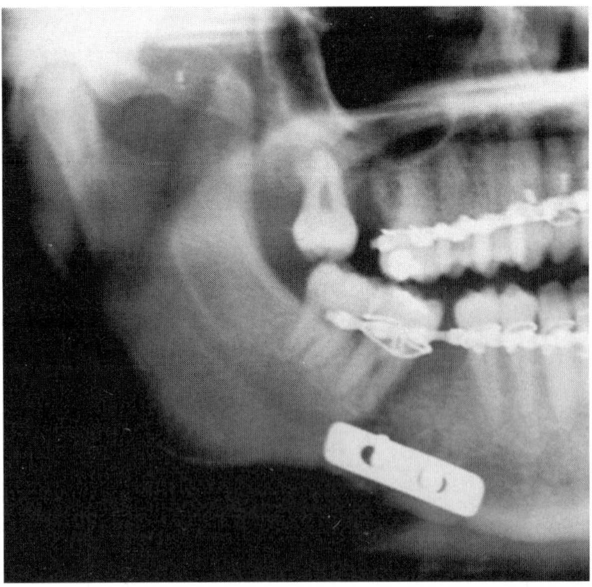

Figure 14–7. Radiograph illustrating improper selection of plate size and placement of screw through fracture site resulting in infection.

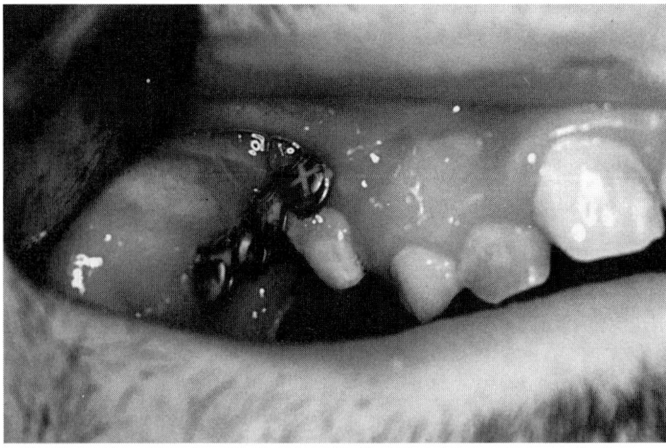

Figure 14–8. Exposed maxillary plate. The plate, if not loose, can remain until the bone heals. (Courtesy of Dr. John Bradick.)

The plate-screw complex is stronger than methods used to achieve MMF. Therefore, as an improperly bent plate is secured, the fracture is displaced and the teeth are pulled from their proper occlusal relationship. To prevent this complication, it is essential that all hardware be well adapted to the fracture and the occlusion verified intraoperatively (Fig. 14–9).

Non-Union

Non-union of mandibular fractures treated with RIF in reported to occur in 1% to 3% of cases.[1, 4, 8, 46] Fracture instability is the sole reason for the development of a non-union. The etiology of fracture instability and its treatment have been addressed previously.

Nerve Dysfunction

The marginal mandibular branch of the facial nerve and the inferior alveolar nerve (V_3) are at risk for potential injury during treatment of mandibular fractures with RIF. An extraoral approach is often used to reduce and stabilize mandibular fractures, thereby risking injury to the marginal mandibular branch of the facial nerve. The incidence of postoperative facial nerve palsy (FNP) ranges from 2% to 16%.[1, 7, 8, 55] Good surgical dissection and adequate incision length to accommodate the plate reduce the incidence of FNP. It is important to note that this complication is transient in all studies.

V_3 nerve injury can occur at the time of fracture, reduction, or screw placement. Therefore, the exact etiology is often difficult to determine. Nevertheless, Iizuka and Lindqvist,[55] prospectively evaluating 121 mandibular fractures, found the nerve dysfunction rate to be 53.1% preoperatively and 76.1% postoperatively, thus indicating intraoperative injury. Treatment of this complication consists of hardware removal with possi-

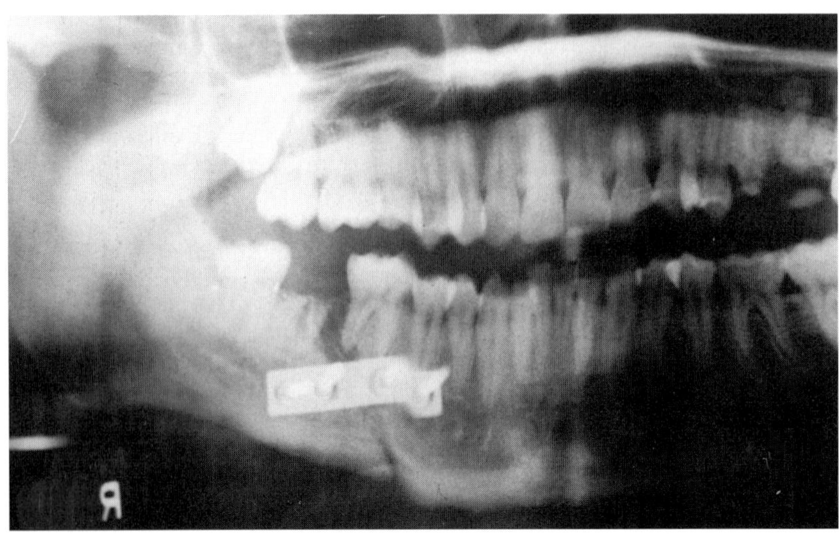

Figure 14–9. Panoramic radiograph illustrating poorly reduced fracture and improperly bent plate leading to malocclusion and malunion.

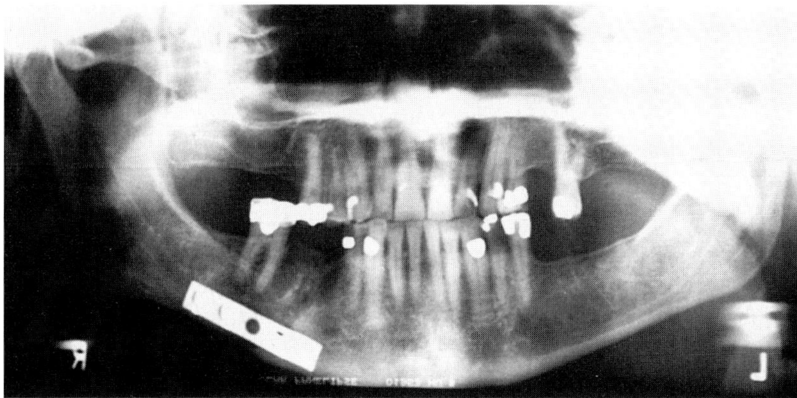

Figure 14–10. Panoramic radiograph showing screw placement into inferior alveolar canal resulting in anesthesia. (Courtesy of Dr. Michael Koury.)

ble microneurosurgical nerve repair. Gentle fracture reduction and careful screw placement can minimize the chances of this complication (Fig. 14–10).

Scar Hypertrophy

Many mandibular fractures that require an open reduction can be approached through an intraoral incision. Until improved intraoral fracture stabilization and RIF techniques are developed, however, many mandibular fractures must be treated through extraoral incisions.[55] Iizuka and Lindqvist[55] found that extraoral hypertrophic scars developed in 6% of young patients requiring open reduction with RIF.

An extraoral incision with a resultant scar is not unique to RIF techniques, although incision placement and size are different. In standard fixation techniques, only a small area of the fracture needs to be exposed. To apply the RIF hardware, a larger incision is required to expose more of the mandible. Therefore, it is critical that the incision be properly placed to avoid marginal mandibular nerve injury and to best camouflage the incision (Fig. 14–11). In planning the incision site, the surgeon must properly diagnosis the location and type of fracture. Some fractures may require a larger incision to enable proper placement of the RIF hardware.

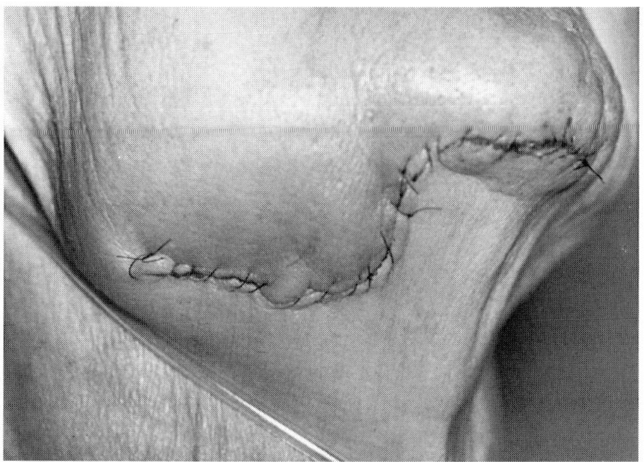

Figure 14–11. Poor incision design secondary to extension of the incision to place the plate.

Finally, the surgeon must use good soft tissue techniques to avoid unsightly postoperative scars.

Mandibular Orthognathic Surgery

Many issues related to the use of RIF in mandibular orthognathic surgery (i. e., hardware palpation and removal, tooth injury) have been discussed previously. Other complication issues, such as condylar position and stability, are discussed in other chapters.

Infection and Non-Union

Little information exists in the literature comparing infection or non-union rates in RIF and standard stabilization techniques in mandibular orthognathic procedures. Most surgeons believe, however, that there is no difference. When 150 RIF cases were compared with 120 wire fixation cases at the University of North Carolina, the infection rate in mandibular osteotomies was 9% for RIF and 3% for wire fixation.[59] No difference in wound dehiscence was found in the two groups. One non-union occurred in a patient treated with wire fixation. In summary, it appears that the complications seen with RIF are similar to those seen with non-RIF techniques, provided that sound RIF surgical principles are followed.

Nerve Injury

Neurosensory alterations affecting the distribution of the inferior alveolar nerve or lingual nerve after mandibular orthognathic surgery are well documented.[60–62] The surgical technique in orthognathic surgery has a profound influence on the incidence of neurosensory injuries, making comparison between wire and RIF techniques very difficult.

Paulus and Steinhauser[63] evaluated two groups of patients who had undergone bilateral sagittal split osteotomy (BSSO) 2 years previously. They found that 57% of patients treated with screw osteosynthesis for BSSO and 50% of those with wires had neurosensory dysfunction. These rates were based upon subjective findings, however. Jones and Wolford[64] used intraoperative somatosensory evoked potentials during BSSO in a group of patients stabilized with RIF to evaluate nerve injury. They found that mean amplitude peaks were significant during retraction to complete the medial bone split. Placement of 2-mm bicortical screws did not have any effect, however, upon evoked potentials. Nishioka and associates[65] evaluated 21 patients following BSSO stabilized with RIF. When evaluated with two alternative forced testing techniques with light touch sensory response, 45.2% of the inferior alveolar nerves tested demonstrated decreased response postoperatively. Comparing these results with those in the literature, these investigators concluded that BSSO with RIF does not cause a higher incidence of nerve injury than non-RIF techniques.[65]

Although these studies are inconclusive, I do not believe that there is a higher incidence of inferior alveolar nerve injury with RIF. Many surgeons no longer use lag screws or lag screw technique to stabilize the osteotomy site. Many believe that compression of segments can cause nerve injury and therefore use positional screws or miniplates for stabilization.[65] There are no studies to confirm this hypothesis, but conceptually, it appears valid. Most agree that if a surgeon uses good RIF techniques, the nerve complication rate of RIF should be similar to that of non-RIF techniques.

Lingual nerve injuries following BSSO procedures have been reported. Hegtvedt and Zuniga[66] reported a lingual nerve injury as a complication of RIF following BSSO. They found the cause was most likely the application of bicortical screws for RIF. In the past, little consideration has been given to protecting the lingual nerve through the use of a lingual retractor during BSSO procedures. When using RIF, however, the surgeon must protect tissues containing the lingual nerve and minimize the distance of penetration beyond the mandibular lingual plate when drilling the hole and placing the screw.

Mandibular Surgical Defect Stabilization and Reconstruction

RIF is routinely used for stabilization of mandibular surgical defects secondary to bony resection. Plates and screws provide stable bridging of the defect, thus allowing mandibular function. Despite significant advances in RIF, complication rates following mandibular resection continue to range from 5.6% to 50%.[13–17, 25, 36] The complications associated with the use of RIF are infection, wound dehiscence with plate exposure, effects on radiation therapy, hardware failure, and stress shielding. Hardware failure and stress shielding have been discussed previously.

Infection

As with mandibular fractures, infections can be classified as either soft tissue without involvement of the bone plate and screws or infection of the bone plate and screws. Lindqvist and colleagues[34] evaluated 34 patients undergoing oncologic mandibular surgery in whom RIF was used to stabilize the defect. These investigators found that 14% of the patients required plate removal owing to chronic infections and fistulae. In a study evaluating 64 patients undergoing similar procedures, Gullane[67] did not remove any plates because of infection, although 6% of the patients did develop minor soft tissue infections that were treated conservatively.

It does appear that the incidence of infections in patients undergoing mandibular resections, with or without bone grafts, is greater than that in patients undergoing RIF for mandibular fractures. This increase is probably due to a larger operation, the use of bone grafts and myocutaneous flaps, and irradiation. In general, the treatment of infections is similar to that described for mandibular fractures. If the patient has been treated with irradiation, however, treatment of an infection must be aggressive to prevent even greater complications (i.e., osteoradionecrosis). Adherence to good surgical and RIF principles is the best way to avoid infections.

Wound Dehiscence with Plate Exposure

Wound dehiscence with plate exposure is the most common complication following mandibular resection. The incidence of early wound dehiscence averages 15%,[13, 16, 33] with many causative factors. Flap ischemia, necrosis, and dehiscence can be potentiated by systemic vascular disease, infection, pedicle compression, and excessive tension on the suture line. Relative to RIF, plate overcontouring and inadequate flap coverage of the plate may contribute to wound dehiscence with plate exposure.

Treatment depends on the size of the dehiscence and exposure and the quality of surrounding tissue. Small wound breakdown can be managed conservatively without the need for plate removal. Large wound dehiscence, in the presence of irradiated tissue, however, may require closure with a flap or removal of the plate. Finally, affected patients must be carefully monitored for late wound dehiscence and plate exposure. Freitag and colleagues[16] reported late wound dehiscence and plate exposure 20 months following the operation.

Effects on Radiation Therapy

In the past, there was considerable controversy over the advisability of placing RIF hardware in patients who also must undergo radiation therapy to the same area. The plate does cause radiation dose perturbations, causing an increase in the radiation dose at the entrance side of the metal and a decrease at the exit side. In one study, the absorbed dose was enhanced 29% to 36% adjacent to metal trays.[68]

In an attempt to resolve this controversy, Gullane[67] developed a radiation dosimetric model using both stainless steel and titanium implants. He found that when a parallel pair of beams was used, an excess dose of irradiation for the lowest-energy colbalt 60 is 13%, for 6 mV it is 15%, and for 18 mV it is 20%. The excess tissue dose, for both stainless steel and titanium plates, extends for about 0.2 mm for cobalt 60, for 1.1 mm at 6 mV, and for 25 mm at 18 mV. Gullane[67] concluded that patients with plates can be treated safely with postoperative irradiation using either cobalt 60 or 6-mV energy.

Complications of Midface and Craniofacial RIF Procedures

Fracture Treatment

Complications following treatment of midface fractures include malocclusion and infection. Plate exposure and palpation have been previously discussed.

Malocclusion

Postoperative malocclusion is probably the most common complication of the use of RIF in midface trauma. Stoll and Schilli[69] reported a major malocclusion rate of 9.7%, whereas Stanley and Funk[12] reported a 14% incidence. Minor occlusal discrepancy was noted in 24% of the patients studied by Jensen and colleagues.[11]

Malocclusion complications are hard to evaluate, because the injuries are so varied that it is difficult to adjust the case mix to make valid comparisons or conclusions. Stable MMF using arch bars prior to open reduction and fixation of the fracture is required, however. The plates must be adequately adapted to prevent segment rotation, and the mandibular condyles must be properly seated in the fossae to prevent a postoperative malocclusion.[12] If these principles are adhered to, good postoperative occlusion can be achieved. A more detailed discussion of these problems is presented in Chapter 10.

Infection

The infection rate following open reduction with RIF of midface fractures appears to be minimal. Infections are often associated with small fragments of bone or bone grafts.[70] Successful treatment consists of incision and drainage, removal of any necrotic tissue, and antibiotics. Plate or screw removal is necessary only if mobility is present.

Orthognathic and Craniofacial Surgery

Infection

The majority of complications associated with RIF in orthognathic and craniofacial surgery are similar to those previously discussed. Infection rates for the plates and screws have not been reported. It is my opinion, however, that the rate is extremely low. The causes of malocclusion are similar to those seen in trauma. Poor plate adaptation is probably the leading cause of malocclusion in RIF.

Palpable Plates

Palpable plates are probably the most common postoperative orthognathic or craniofacial RIF complications. As was previously discussed, thin patients with large plates are the major cause. The use of miniplates and microplates has reduced the incidence of this complication.

Growth Restriction

An area of major concern is the effect of RIF on craniofacial growth. Although no long-term clinical results are available because of the short time that such fixation technology has been available, a growing body of experimental evidence indicates that some degree of bone growth restriction occurs after the placement of bone plates on the developing cranium.[71, 72] The amount and location of this restriction vary. Eppley and colleagues[73] and Mooney and associates[74] have reported that the cranium does have regional bone compensatory mechanisms. In addition, Yaremchuck and coworkers[75] found that the degree of growth restriction increases with the amount of fixation hardware.

Because these results indicate that RIF does restrict craniofacial growth, removal of the fixation hardware soon after healing of the osteotomy site should be considered in the very young patient. Until further definitive results are obtained, the surgeon must carefully consider timing, extent, and fixation techniques when planning craniofacial surgery.

Conclusion

In this chapter, the complications common in maxillofacial surgery using RIF have been discussed. Most complications can be attributed to operator error; seldom is RIF hardware the source. Because RIF is an unforgiving system, the surgeon must fully understand and follow established surgical and RIF principles. Patients will benefit with immediate function and improved long-term results.

References

1. Dodson TB, Perrott DH, Kaban LB, et al: Fixation of mandibular fractures: A comparative analysis of rigid internal fixation and standard fixation techniques. J Oral Maxillofac Surg 1990;48:362.
2. Prein J, Kellam RM: Rigid internal fixation of mandibular fractures—basics of AO technique. Otolaryngol Clin North Am 1987;20:441.
3. Levine PA: AO compression plating technique for treating fractures of the edentulous mandible. Otolaryngol Clin North Am 1987;20:437.
4. Worthington P, Champy M: Monocortical miniplate osteosynthesis. Otolaryngol Clin North Am 1987;20:607.
5. Thaller SR, Reavie D, Daniller A: Rigid internal fixation with miniplates and screws: A cost-effective technique for treating mandible fractures? Ann Plast Surg 1990;24:469.
6. Smith BR, Johnson JV: Rigid fixation of comminuted mandibular fractures. J Oral Maxillofac Surg 1993;51:1320.
7. Iizuka T, Lindqvist C: Rigid internal fixation of mandibular fractures: An analysis of 270 fractures treated using the AO/ASIF method. Int J Oral Maxillofac Surg 1992;21:65.
8. Anderson T, Alpert B: Experience with rigid fixation of mandibular fractures and immediate function. J Oral Maxillofac Surg 1992;50:555.
9. Ellis E, Ghali GE: Lag screw fixation of anterior mandibular fractures. J Oral Maxillofac Surg 1991;49:13.

10. Ellis E, Ghali GE: Lag screw fixation of mandibular angle fractures. J Oral Maxillofac Surg 1991;49:234.
11. Jensen J, Sindet-Petersen S, Christensen L: Rigid fixation in reconstruction of craniofacial fractures. J Oral Maxillofac Surg 1992;50:550.
12. Stanley RB, Funk GF: Rigid internal fixation for fractures involving tooth-bearing maxillary segments. Arch Otolaryngol Head Neck Surg 1988;114:1295.
13. Davidson MJ, Gullane PJ: Prosthetic plate mandibular reconstruction. Otolaryngol Clin North Am 1991;24:1419.
14. Murphy JB: Follow-up report of immediate stabilization of mandibular surgical defects after tumor resection. Oral Surg Oral Med Oral Pathol 1991;72:646.
15. Vuillemin T, Raveh J, Sutter F: Mandibular reconstruction with the titanium hollow screw reconstruction plate (THORP) system: Evaluation of 62 cases. Plast Reconstr Surg 1988;82:804.
16. Freitag V, Hell B, Fischer H: Experience with AO reconstruction plates after partial mandibular resection involving its continuity. J Craniomaxillofac Surg 1991;19:191.
17. Gullane PJ, Holmes H: Mandibular reconstruction: New concepts. Arch Otolaryngol Head Neck Surg 1986;112:714.
18. Koury ME, Perrott DH, Kaban LB: The use of rigid internal fixation in mandibular fractures complicated by osteomyelitis. J Oral Maxillofac Surg 1994;52:1114.
19. Luhr HG: A micro-plate system for cranio-maxillofacial skeletal fixation. J Craniomaxillofac Surg 1988;1:35.
20. Ardary WC, Tracy DJ, Brownridge GW, et al: Comparative evaluation of screw configuration on the stability of the sagittal split osteotomy. Oral Surg Oral Med Oral Pathol 1988;68:125.
21. Perrott DH, Lu YF, Pogrel MA, et al: Stability of sagittal split osteotomies: A comparison of three stabilization techniques. Oral Surg Oral Med Oral Pathol 1994;78:696.
22. Rosen HM: Miniplate fixation of Le Fort I osteotomies. Plast Reconstr Surg 1986;78:748.
23. Tucker MR, Ochs MW: Basic concepts of rigid internal fixation: Mechanical considerations and instrumentation overview. *In* Tucker ML, Terry BC, White RP, Van Sickels JE (eds): Rigid Fixation For Maxillofacial Surgery, Philadelphia, JB Lippincott, 1991, p 51.
24. Cramers M, Lucht U: Metal sensitivity in patients treated for tibial fractures with plates of stainless steel. Acta Orthop Scand 1977;48:245.
25. Merle C, Vigan M, Devred D, et al: Generalized eczema from vitallium osteosynthesis material. Contact Dermatitis 1992;27:257.
26. Lewin J, Lindgren U, Wahlberg JE: Screw fixation in bone of guinea pigs sensitized to nickel and cobalt. Acta Orthop Scand 1982;53:672.
27. Merritt K, Mayor MB, Brown SA: Metal allergy and implants: Concepts and clinical significance. *In* Uhthoff HK (ed): Current Concepts of Internal Fixation of Fractures. New York, Springer-Verlag, 1980, p 165.
28. Kubba R, Taylor JS, Marks KE: Cutaneous complications of orthopedic implants. Arch Dermatol 1981;117:554.
29. Webley M, Kates A, Snaith ML: Metal sensitivity in patients with a hinge arthroplasty of the knee. Ann Rheum Dis 1980;39:476.
30. Evans EM, Freeman MA, Miller AJ, Vernon-Roberts B: Metal sensitivity as a course of bone necrosis and loosening of the prosthesis in total joint replacement. J Bone Joint Surg Br 1974;56:626.
31. Rooker GD, Wilkinson JD: Metal sensitivity in patients undergoing hip replacement: A prospective study. J Bone Joint Surg Br 1980;62:502.
32. Bahr W: Comparison of torque measurement between cortical screws and emergency replacement screws in the cadaver mandible. J Oral Maxillofac Surg 1992;50:45.
33. McCann KJ, Irish JC, Gullane PJ, et al: Complications associated with rigid fixation of mandibulotomies. J Otolaryngol 1994; 23:210.
34. Lindqvist C, Soderholm A, Laine P, et al: Rigid reconstruction plates for immediate reconstruction following mandibular resection for malignant tumors. J Oral Maxillofac Surg 1992;50:1158.
35. Moyen BJL, Lahey PJ, Weinburg MS, et al: Effects on intact femurs of dogs of the application and removal of metal plates. J Bone Joint Surg Am 1978;60:940.
36. Janes GC, Collpy DM, Price R, et al: Bone density after rigid fixation of tibial fractures. J Bone Joint Surg Br 1993;75:914.
37. Assael L: Complications of rigid internal fixation of the facial skeleton. Oral Maxillofac Surg Clin North Am 1990;3:615.
38. Alexander R, Theodus L: Fracture of the bone-grafted mandible secondary to stress shielding. J Oral Maxillofac Surg 1993;51:695.
39. Throckmorton GS, Ellis E, Winkler AJ, et al: Bone strain following application of a rigid bone plate: An in vitro study in human mandibles. J Oral Maxillofac Surg 1992;50:1066.
40. Kennedy MC, Tucker MR, Lester GE et al: Stress shielding effect of rigid internal fixation plates on mandibular bone grafts. Int J Oral Maxillofac Surg 1989;18:307.
41. Ochs MW, Tucker ML, White RP Jr: Biologic concepts of rigid internal fixation. *In* Tucker ML, Terry BC, White RP, Van Sickels JF (eds): Rigid Fixation for Maxillofacial Surgery. Philadelphia, JB Lippincott, 1991, p78.
42. Assael L: Evaluation of rigid internal fixation of mandible fractures performed in the teaching laboratory. J Oral Maxillofac Surg 1993;51:1315.
43. Nixon F, Lowery MN: Failed eruption of the permanent canine following open reduction of a mandibular fracture in a child. Br Dent J 1990;168:204.
44. Macleod PRS, Bainton R: Extrusion of a microplate: An unusual complication of osteosynthesis. J Craniomaxillofac Surg 1992;20:303.
45. Llewelyn J, Sugar A: Lag screws in sagittal osteotomies: Should they be removed? Br J Oral Maxillofac Surg 1992;30:83.
46. Naeamura S, Takenoshita Y, Oka M: Complications of miniplate osteosynthesis for mandibular fractures. J Oral Maxillofac Surg 1994;52:233.
47. Rahn B: Theoretical considerations in rigid fixation of facial bones. Clin Plast Surg 1989;16:21.
48. Rosenberg A, Gratz KW, Sailer HF: Should titanium miniplates be removed after bone healing is complete? Int J Oral Maxillofac Surg 1993;22:185.
49. Kellman RM, Schilli W: Plate fixation of fractures of the mid and upper face. Otolaryngol Clin North Am 1987;20:559.
50. Zachariades N, Papademetriou I, Rallis G: Complications associated with rigid internal fixation of facial bone fractures. J Oral Maxillofac Surg 1993;51:273.
51. Fiala TGS, Novelline RA, Yaremchuk MJ: Comparison of CT imaging artifacts from craniomaxillofacial internal fixation devices. Plast Reconstr Surg 1993;92:1227.
52. Fiala TGS, Paige KT, Davis TL, et al: Comparison of artifact from craniomaxillofacial internal fixation devices: Magnetic resonance imaging. Plast Reconstr Surg 1994;93:725.
53. Kroon FMH, Mathisson M, Cordey JR, et al: The use of miniplates in mandibular fractures. J Craniomaxillofac Surg 1991;19:199.
54. Stone I, Dodson TB, Bays RA: Risk factors for infection following operative treatment of mandibular fractures. Plast Reconstr Surg 1993;91:64.
55. Iizuka T, Lindqvist C: Rigid internal fixation in the angular region of the mandible: An analysis of factors contributing to different complications. Plast Reconstr Surg 1993;91:265.
56. Iizuka T, Lindqvist C, Hallihainen D, et al: Infection after rigid internal fixation of mandibular fractures: A clinical and radiographic study. J Oral Maxillofac Surg 1991;49:585.
57. Kearns GJ, Perrott DH, Kaban LB: Rigid fixation of mandibular fractures: Does operator experience reduce complications? J Oral Maxillofac Surg 1994;52:226.
58. Koury M, Ellis E: Rigid internal fixation of infected mandibular fractures. J Oral Maxillofac Surg 1993;50:434.
59. Tucker MR, Frost DE, Terry BC: Mandibular surgery. *In* Tucker MR, Terry BC, White RF, Van Sickels JE (eds): Rigid Fixation For Maxillofacial Surgery, Philadelphia, JB Lippincott, 1991, p 286.
60. McDow CD, Ellis E, Fonseca EE, Upston LG: Comparison of neurosensory deficits following bilateral sagittal and vertical ramus osteotomies. J Oral Maxillofac Surg 1988;46:751.
61. Zaytoun HS Jr, Phillips C, Terry BC: Long-term neurosensory deficits following transoral vertical ramus and sagittal split osteotomies for mandibular prognathism. J Oral Maxillofac Surg 1986;44:193.
62. Walter JM, Gregg JM: Analysis of postsurgical neurologic alteration in the trigeminal nerve. J Oral Maxillofac Surg 1979;37:410.
63. Paulus GW, Steinhauser EW: A comparison study of wire osteosynthesis versus bone screws in the treatment of mandibular prognathism. Oral Surg Oral Med Oral Pathol 1982;54:607.

64. Jones DL, Wolford LM: Intraoperative monitoring of trigeminal evoked potentials during sagittal split osteotomies. J Oral Maxillofac Surg 1988;46:119.
65. Nishioka G, Zysset MK, Van Sickels JE: Neurosensory disturbance with rigid fixation of the bilateral sagittal split osteotomy. J Oral Maxillofac Surg 1987;45:20.
66. Hegtvedt AK, Zuniga JR: Lingual nerve injury as a complication of rigid fixation of the sagittal ramus osteotomy: Report of a case. J Oral Maxillofac Surg 1990;48:647.
67. Gullane PJ: Primary mandibular reconstruction: Analysis of 64 cases and evaluation of interface radiation dosimetry on bridging plates. Laryngoscope 1991;101:1.
68. Schwartz HC, Wollin MS, Leake DL, Kagan AR: Interface radiation dosimetry in mandibular reconstruction. Arch Otolaryngol 1979;105:203.
69. Stoll P, Schilli W: Primary reconstruction with A-O mini-plates after severe craniomaxillofacial trauma. J Craniomaxillofac Surg 1988;16:18.
70. Klotch DW, Gilliland R: Internal fixation vs. conventional therapy in midface fractures. J Trauma 1987;27:1136.
71. Lin KY, Bartlett SP, Yaremchuk MJ, et al: An experimental study on the effect of rigid fixation on the developing craniofacial skeleton. Plast Reconstr Surg 1991;87:229.
72. Marschall MA, Chidyllo SA, Figueroa AA, et al: Long-term effects of rigid fixation on the growing craniomaxillofacial skeleton. J Craniofac Surg 1991;2:63.
73. Eppley BL, Platis JM, Sadove AM: Experimental effects of bone plating in infancy on craniomaxillofacial skeletal growth. Cleft Palate Craniofac J 1993;30:165.
74. Mooney MP, Losken HW, Siegel MI, et al: Plate fixation of the premaxillary suture and compensatory midfacial growth changes in the rabbit. J Craniofac Surg 1992;3:197.
75. Yaremchuk MJ, Fiala GS, Barker F, et al: The effects of rigid fixation on craniofacial growth of rhesus monkeys. Plast Reconstr Surg 1994;93:1.

Chapter 15
COMPLICATIONS OF FACIAL COSMETIC SURGERY

by

John R. Werther

Introduction

Complications are distressing to the patient as well as to the surgeon. This is particularly true in facial cosmetic surgery. The only sure way to avoid surgical complication is to avoid operation. Many potential complications can be prevented by careful assessment of the patient before surgery. Medical history, socioeconomic factors, and psychologic profile of the patient are important considerations. Operating on a patient with vague complaints or ill-defined goals carries the potential for trouble in the postoperative period. It is necessary for the patient to articulate the problem and for the surgeon to understand the patient's view of the deformity and the reason for having surgery. Patients with unrealistic expectations, those who ascribe major deformity to minor anatomic abnormality, and those suffering from body dysmorphic syndrome[1] should be considered with caution. Unhappy patients have even been known to kill the surgeon who performed the cosmetic surgery.[2] Because of the crucial importance of the face, the surgeon must be cognizant of the psychologic makeup of the patient; the reader is referred to the works of Goin and Goin,[3] Gifford,[4] and Wright[5, 6] for extensive discussions of this complex topic. The patient must understand what can be reasonably achieved with surgery and, importantly, what cannot. Richard Webster noted that "when you tell a patient about a complication before surgery, it is considered informed consent. When you tell them about it afterward, it is considered an excuse."

When surgical complications occur, they are best managed early in an aggressive manner. Empathetic support and close supervision by the physician (not just the staff), direct acknowledgment of the problem, and a clear-cut plan of action are indicated.[7, 7] Patients are much less likely to institute legal action if they perceive that the doctor cares about their problem.[8] Frequent office visits and referral to other specialists, if necessary, can help ensure that problems are identified early and appropriately managed. Complete, accurate records and photographs help document the problem and are useful to the surgeon who will critically evaluate the results when reconstructing the events that occurred. It is said that good judgment comes from experience with bad judgment. Our mistakes and untoward outcomes after surgery, no matter how unfortunate, represent an excellent—in some cases unparalleled—learning opportunity.

THE SUBJECTS DISCUSSED IN THIS CHAPTER ARE:

Genioplasty

Alloplastic or osseous genioplasty is commonly performed in conjunction with orthognathic or rhinoplastic surgery to improve overall facial balance and proportion and to improve cervical contour. Selected patients with sleep apnea are also well served by advancement genioplasty. The popularity of alloplastic chin implants relates, in part, to the facts that alloplastic genioplasty is faster and technically easier to perform and that many cosmetic surgeons are not trained in osseous genioplasty. Alloplastic materials may be used in cases of mild to moderate chin hypoplasia but are contraindicated when the chin is vertically deficient or asymmetric. With osseous genioplasty, horizontal and vertical changes in chin position are relatively easy to achieve. The asymmetric chin, however, is often associated with other facial asymmetry, and correction of the combined deformity is more difficult.

Problems common to alloplastic and osseous genioplasty include infection, hematoma, nerve injury, bone resorption, and unfavorable external appearance.[9–19] Alloplast-specific complications are extrusion, malposition or migration, erosion into tooth roots with pulpal necrosis and devitalization, and a less predictable soft tissue response (1:0.6) compared with osseous advancement genioplasty (1:0.8–0.9).[9, 10, 17, 18] These problems appear to be independent of the incision used (transoral versus transcutaneous) for access to the bony chin and of whether the implant is placed in a subperiosteal or supraperiosteal pocket.[19, 20]

Nerve Injury

One of the most common complications after mentoplasty is neurosensory deficit.[21, 22] Patients commonly have cutaneous hypesthesia in the area that is surgically undermined, as a byproduct of the dissection. Injury to the mental nerve is more troublesome to the patient. In a retrospective analysis of 76 patients undergoing mentoplasty, Guyuron and Raszewski[17] observed that 19 of 27 patients (70%) undergoing osseous genioplasty, and 15 of 32 patients (47%) undergoing alloplastic genioplasty had neurosensory deficits after surgery. The majority of the sensory deficits were temporary, but 7% and 9% of patients, respectively, were noted to have long-term abnormal sensation. Nishioka and associates[21] analyzed 15 patients undergoing osseous genioplasty and found that all but one patient had a temporary neuropraxia after surgery. The patient who still had a moderate deficit at 26 months believed that it did not adversely affect her quality of life.

Careful study of the preoperative radiographs, direct visualization and retractor protection of the nerve, and placement of the osteotomy at least 5 mm inferior to the mental foramen can help decrease, but not entirely eliminate, mental nerve injury. Frank discussion about the possibility of nerve injury with the patient before surgery and careful monitoring of nerve function after surgery are indicated.

Bone Resorption

Modeling of bone occurs after virtually all genioplasty procedures, whether alloplastic or osseous.[11–14] Polido and colleagues[24] and Precious and associates[25] have documented the long-term changes that occur after advancement osseous genioplasty. The sharply demarcated edges of the osteotomy site soften with time. There is an area of bone deposition along the labial surface of the mandible superior to the osteotomy site, and resorption at the anterosuperior aspect of the advanced osseous segment. These changes tend to be clinically minor and are not externally visible.

In contrast, bone changes after alloplastic augmentation are universally resorptive in nature. Beginning in the 1960s, surgeons noticed resorption of the underlying buccal plate in the area of pogonion in up to 85% of patients with alloplastic chin implants.[12–14] Guyuron and Raszewski[17] documented bone resorption of 0.5 to 2.0 mm at 1 year in all patients undergoing alloplastic chin augmentation, as measured by lateral cephalometric radiograph. Common to this and other studies in patients with bone resorption after alloplastic augmentation is that the soft tissue profile typically remains unchanged despite bone loss. Pediatric patients undergoing alloplastic or osseous genioplasty tend to have more significant bone resorption than adults. Peled and associates[23] followed 50 children with Down syndrome who were treated with alloplastic facial augmentation to improve facial appearance. Of the 12 subperiosteal chin implants placed, 75% showed bone resorption underneath the implant. When the implants were removed, the bone modeled to the level of the preoperative contour.

The patient shown in Figure 15–1 had undergone multiple previous operations, including alloplastic chin augmentation. Resorption of the anterior mandible underneath the implant can be seen on the lateral cephalometric radiograph (Fig. 15–1*A*). The patient underwent maxillary osteotomy for open-bite correction and removal of the chin implant with immediate advancement genioplasty for improved facial balance (Fig. 15–1*B*).

Infection

Infection can occur after transoral or transcutaneous access is made to the bony chin during surgery. The risk of infection after genioplasty is approximately 2% to 6%.[15, 17] Higher rates of infection have been reported when alloplastic implants or fillers are used, when the chin button is completely degloved of its soft tissue for large advancement,[26] and when the chin is multiply segmented for maximal advancement. Whereas the submental approach can be completed in a sterile fashion, transoral incisions are at least clean-contaminated; thus, prophylactic antibiotics are indicated.[27] Localized infection after surgery may respond to antibiotics and local measures. If an alloplastic implant is persistently or progressively infected, however, or if it becomes exposed, it must be removed. Typically, an infected osseous genioplasty site breaks down with opening of

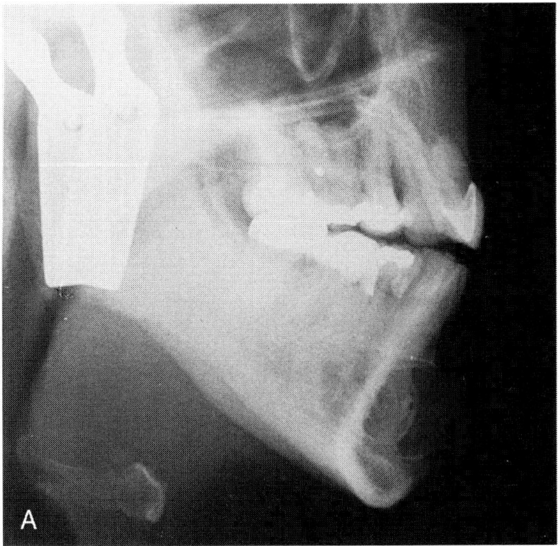

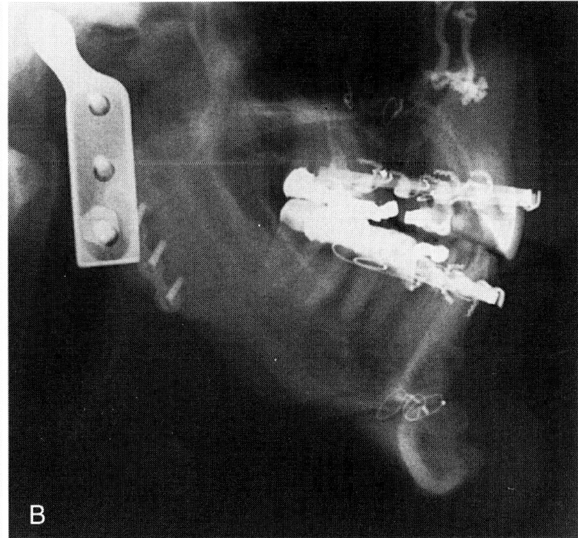

Figure 15–1. *A,* Patient had undergone multiple previous operations, including chin augmentation with a soft silicone implant. Substantial resorption of the bone is evident. The incisor root tips are not involved. *B,* Twenty-four hours after Le Fort I osteotomy to close open bite and transoral implant removal with immediate advancement genioplasty.

both the mucosal and musculoperiosteal layers. Obvious necrotic material should be removed, and the area packed open to allow for resolution of the infection. Often the hardware does not need to be removed. The wound typically heals well by secondary intention.

The patient shown in Figure 15–2 had juvenile rheumatoid arthritis with severe mandibular and chin deficiency but an acceptable occlusion (Fig. 15–2*A*). She elected to have only a genioplasty, and underwent a two-step genioplasty for maximal advancement (Fig. 15–2*B*). The vascular supply to the middle segment of bone was exceeded, and the wound became infected, ultimately necessitating débridement of the necrotic bone segment and removal of all hardware. On radiographs, there appeared to be near-total loss of the bony chin (Fig. 15–2*C*). Interestingly, 2 years after surgery, marked bone regeneration had occurred, and the soft tissue profile was maintained to a greater extent than would have been anticipated (Fig. 15–2*D*).

Hematoma

The vast majority of patients with bleeding disorders can be diagnosed by history and physical examination. Routine preoperative screening tests are not recommended if the history and physical examination are negative.[28, 29] Patients should avoid aspirin and related compounds for at least 2 weeks prior to surgery. Although bleeding with hematoma formation after genioplasty is uncommon, persistent oozing after osseous genioplasty can occur. If excessive oozing is noted during surgery, a closed-suction drain should be considered. If a hematoma forms after surgery, it is rarely large enough to require formal drainage. Patients should be warned before surgery that bruising may occur after genioplasty and can extend onto the neck and anterior chest wall.

Unfavorable External Appearance

Isolated advancement of the chin in patients with horizontal mandibular deficiency as well as microgenia rarely (if ever) achieves a cosmetic result as good as can be obtained by simultaneous mandibular and chin advancement. The classic example of this is the class II deep bite patient with a prominent mentolabial fold and marginally acceptable vertical chin length. Even if the chin is vertically lengthened or the osteotomy site augmented in such a patient,[30, 31] lip support is unchanged, and the overall appearance is suboptimal when isolated genioplasty is performed.

The patient shown in Figure 15–3 opted to be treated by maxillary premolar extraction and nonsurgical maxillary retraction orthodontics (Fig. 15–3*A*). Genioplasty was recommended to improve the facial profile. The genioplasty segment was advanced along an inclined plane, shortening the vertical dimension of the chin, creating a prominent chin button, and accentuating the mentolabial fold (Fig. 15–3*B*).

A better solution to the problem of mandibular and chin deficiency is to simultaneously advance the mandible and the chin. The chin osteotomy can be designed more horizontally, so that the chin does not shorten with advancement, as shown in Figure 15–4. The vertical dimension of the chin should be checked during surgery, and if undesirable shortening is noted, interpositional material can be used to insure correct position and lengthen the osteotomy segment. A mortise technique[30] or bone plates are helpful for appropriate three-dimensional positioning of the chin segment.

If malposition of the chin is noted in the first 2 to 3 days after sliding genioplasty, it may be adjusted in the clinic using local anesthesia or intravenous sedation. The wound is easily opened, and problematic bleeding is rarely encountered. The fixation can be

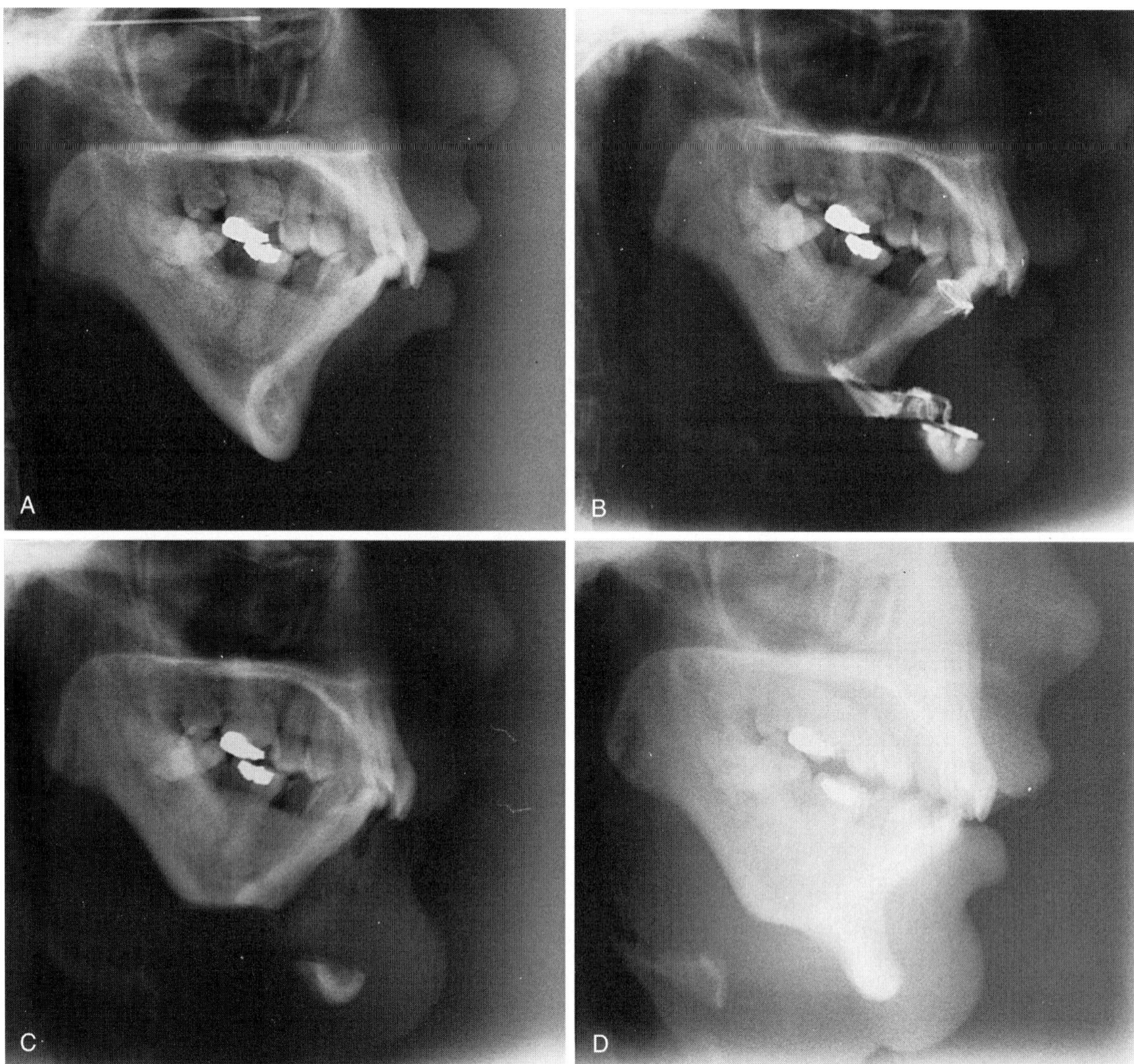

Figure 15–2. *A*, Patient with juvenile rheumatoid arthritis as well as severe mandibular and chin deficiency. *B*, Twenty-four hours after two-step advancement genioplasty. *C*, Six weeks after surgery, the wound became infected and completely broke down, exposing the middle bony segment, which was necrotic. This bone and all the hardware were removed. There is no obvious support for the bony chin. *D*, Twenty-six months after surgery. Bone continuity has been reestablished through healing. There is definite improvement in bone and soft tissue contour compared with before surgery. (*A* to *D* courtesy of H. David Hall, DMD, MD.)

loosened and the segments adjusted and then retightened to achieve the desired result.

Chin ptosis and lip incompetence caused by malposition of the mentalis muscle after osseous and alloplastic genioplasty have been described.[32, 33] Zide and McCarthy[34] suggest three main causes for this problem: (1) inferior displacement of the mentalis origin, (2) elongation and redraping after reduction genioplasty or removal of large alloplastic implants, and (3) deficiency of the mentalis muscle after partial or total resection. Treatment depends on whether the problem is primarily osseous, muscular, or a combination of the two. When the oral route is used to access the chin, a generous cuff of mentalis muscle should be left attached to the mandible above and below the implant or osteotomy site. Resuspension of the mentalis muscle at the end of the operation, utilizing atraumatic needles to avoid laceration of the musculoperiosteal layer, is recommended. Once all sutures are placed and checked for adequacy, they can be tied securely. If insufficient muscle remains above the implant or osteotomy site, the inferior mentalis muscle can be resuspended to sutures placed in transosseous fashion and tied on the lingual surface mandible.[33–36]

Silicone implants are the most common alloplastic materials used for chin augmentation. As in other areas of the body, they develop a capsule. If capsular contraction occurs, malposition, asymmetry, and contour abnormality may result. This process is rare and unpredictable. Cohen and associates[36] described chin dis-

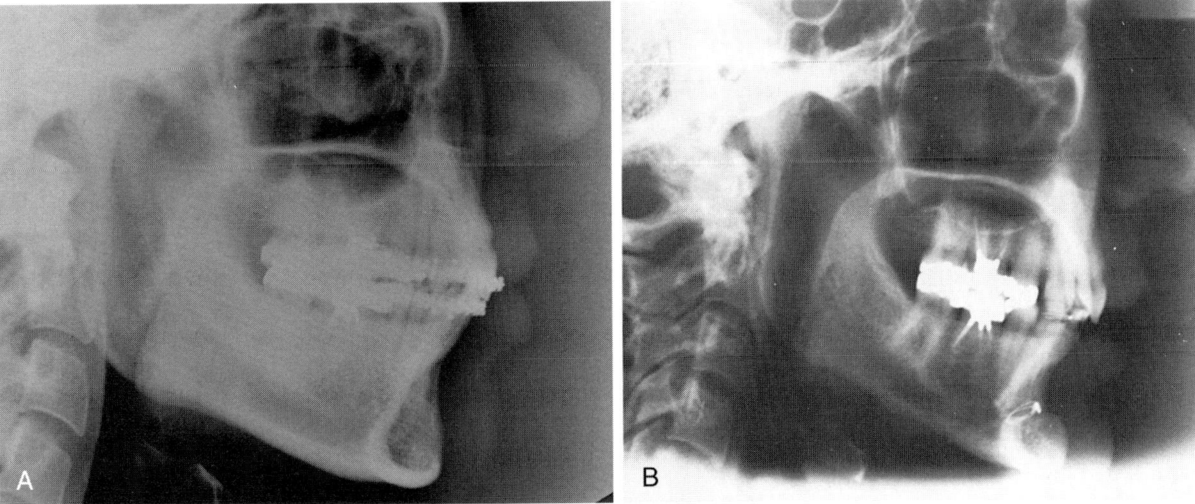

Figure 15–3. *A,* Patient has mild, relative chin deficiency following non-surgical orthodontics. Vertical height of the chin is marginally acceptable. *B,* Two years after advancement genioplasty. The chin was advanced along an inclined plane, resulting in an unfavorable shortening of the chin as well as accentuation of the mentolabial fold.

figurement following removal of transorally placed alloplastic chin implants in a series of ten female patients. The deformities included chin ptosis and soft tissue dimpling seen on repose or animation. Lateral cephalometric radiographs revealed bone resorption and blunting of the pogonion in seven of the ten patients. Because the late deformity was found to be nearly uncorrectable, Cohen and associates[36] recommended immediate osseous genioplasty at the time of implant removal as the best chance to achieve a satisfactory result.

Malar Augmentation

Like genioplasty, malar augmentation can be achieved by osteotomy or alloplastic implant. The vast majority of malar augmentations performed in the United States are done with alloplastic materials, including silicone, Proplast, polyethylene, and hydroxyapatite. The complications of alloplastic malar augmentation are similar to those seen with genioplasty. They include infection, extrusion, asymmetry, numbness, bone resorption, malposition, capsular contracture, undercorrection, overcorrection, hematoma, pain, and pulpal necrosis.[10, 22, 37–41] In contrast to genioplasty, achieving a satisfactory and symmetric result in malar augmentation is difficult for even the most experienced surgeon.

Extraction of buccal fat pads and removal of posterior teeth, alone or in combination with malar augmentation to create "a hollow" inferior to the malar eminence, should be avoided. Destruction of underlying

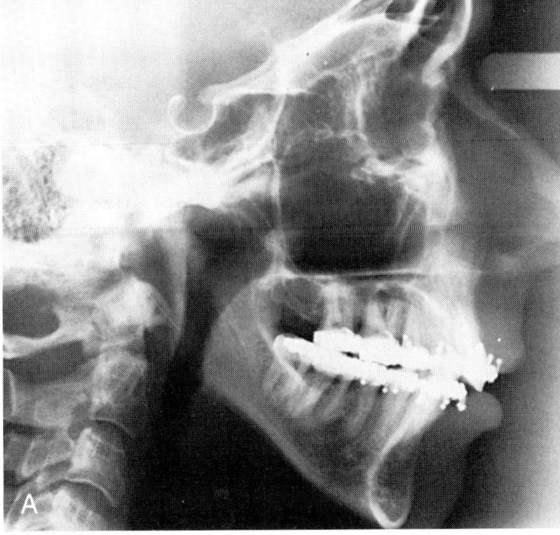

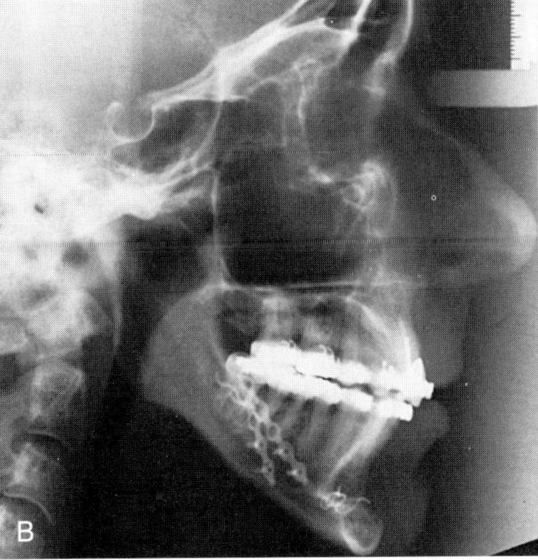

Figure 15–4. *A,* Patient with mandibular and chin horizontal deficiency. *B,* Eight months after surgery. Simultaneous mandibular and chin advancement has resulted in improved lip and chin position. The slope of the osteotomy is nearly horizontal to avoid vertical shortening of the chin.

bony anatomy, in combination with expected loss of facial fat during the aging process, will ultimately lead to a skeletonized look that is difficult to reconstruct.

Rhinoplasty

Rhinoplasty is generally considered the most difficult facial cosmetic operation to master because of the complexity and the multiple different component aspects of the operation as well as the potentially capricious nature of the healing process. A satisfactory result at 1 year may evolve unfavorably over the subsequent 10 to 20 years. Patient satisfaction is the *sine qua non* of success in rhinoplasty. Patients can be quite happy with a result that is unsatisfactory in the eyes of the surgeon. It is incumbent upon other surgeons who see the patient after rhinoplasty not to be critical of the work of the previous surgeon.[42] The second surgeon does not have the benefit of seeing the original deformity and may not appreciate the technical difficulty encountered during the first operation. Further, the unpredictable nature of the healing process is beyond the control of the operating surgeon. As in all surgical endeavors, the key to achieving a good result in primary or revision rhinoplasty lies in making the correct diagnosis.

Serious and Life-threatening Complications

Fortunately, life-threatening or highly morbid complications, including intracranial events, necrotizing fasciitis, blindness, and death after rhinoplasty, are rare.[43–54] A combination of hypertension and cocaine-induced intracranial hemorrhage was thought to be causal in a report of two cases of stroke after nasoseptal surgery.[50] Most intracranial complications are traumatic in origin and follow manipulation of the skull base in nasal and sinus surgery.[43, 45, 46] When deviated segments of the perpendicular plate of the ethmoid or vomer are to be removed during septorhinoplasty, a scissor or back-action forcep should be used to first create the desired horizontal fracture plane. If the entire ethmoid is rocked to create the fracture, a crack in the cribriform plate can occur, leading to cerebrospinal fluid (CSF) leak, pneumocephalus, and intracranial infection as well as damage to adjacent intracranial vasculature. If a CSF leak is noted intraoperatively, immediate neurosurgical consultation should be obtained. Exploration and temporalis fascia patch reconstruction of the dural defect may be indicated. Most CSF leaks noted after surgery resolve spontaneously in about 2 weeks if the patient is treated with bed rest and head elevation. Lumbar drainage or surgical exploration may be necessary for persistent leaks.

Blindness following nasal surgery has been attributed to mechanical trauma to the optic nerve after osteotomy, intranasal steroid injection, and retrograde flow of an intraarterial local anesthetic, which causes occlusion of the central retinal artery with loss of optic nerve function.[46, 47, 49, 52, 53]

Hemorrhage

The incidence of excessive bleeding following septorhinoplasty is approximately 2% to 4%, but can be as high as 10% when simultaneous turbinate surgery is performed.[44–46] The anterior ethmoid and sphenopalatine vessels are usually involved. Patients should be carefully screened before surgery and advised to avoid all platelet-altering medications, including aspirin and vitamin E.[57] One of the primary concerns with intranasal bleeding is that an unrecognized and untreated septal hematoma can lead to saddle nose deformity. Treatment of epistaxis depends on the location and size of the bleeding source. Progressive management may involve direct intranasal cauterization, anterior nasal packing, or nasal balloon tamponade.[44–46] Persistent bleeding, in some cases, may require transantral ligation of the sphenopalatine artery, ligation of the anterior or posterior ethmoid artery, or, possibly, angiography and embolization.[46, 58, 59]

Infection

Infection is uncommon after rhinoplasty, occurring in less than 3% of cases.[44, 45, 55, 60] Devastating infection, such as toxic shock syndrome,[46, 61–63] cavernous sinus thrombosis, and brain abscess, has been described.[64, 65] An argument for antibiotic prophylaxis in nasal surgery can be made on the basis that the nose is a contaminated field. Prospective studies, however, have failed to demonstrate a decrease in incidence of infection after nasal surgery when prophylactic antibiotics were used.[66] Furthermore, prophylactic antibiotics do not eliminate the risk of toxic shock syndrome in susceptible individuals. Although many surgeons use prophylactic antibiotics for cosmetic and reconstructive rhinoplasty, the issue is controversial.[67, 68] Meyers[69] has recommended antibiotic use in the following circumstances: (1) active infection at the operative site, (2) nasal packing used for more than 24 hours, (3) the presence of hematoma, (4) use of alloplastic implants, and (5) immunocompromised or immunosuppressed host.

Nasal Obstruction

Nasal obstruction following cosmetic rhinoplasty has been reported in up to 10% of cases and has largely been attributed to mismanagement of the nasal septum, untreated inferior turbinate hypertrophy, and damage to the nasal valve.[70, 71] Complete evaluation of the airway before revision surgery is critical to success. Direct visualization of the septum and turbinate before and after nasal decongestion can offer clues to differentiate between structural and mucosal or allergic causes of nasal obstruction. Improved or normal nasal breathing after decongestion is consistent with mucosal or allergic obstruction. The Cottle and cotton-tipped swab tests are simple, easy, inexpensive, and clinically useful tests of nasal valve collapse. The Cottle test involves pulling the cheek laterally away from the nose to assess the vestibular component of the nasal valve (nostril,

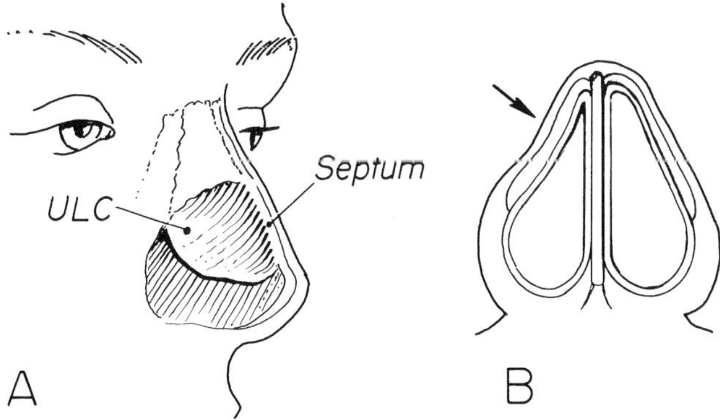

Figure 15–5. *A* and *B*, The upper lateral cartilage (*ULC*) can collapse on the septum, decreasing the nasal valve angle and causing increased resistance to breathing.

upper lateral cartilage, and alar rim) for obstruction (Fig. 15–5). The cotton-tipped swab test is performed by placing a cotton applicator (Q-Tip) beneath the upper lateral cartilage and elevating it supero-laterally to increase the nasal valve angle. If this maneuver improves ipsilateral nasal breathing, a spreader graft may be indicated to reverse nasal valve collapse (Fig. 15–6).

A cotton applicator can also be used to elevate the caudal margin of the alar cartilage to assess alar collapse and to determine whether alar batten or lateral crural strut grafts are indicated. If the caudal aspect of the upper lateral cartilage is insufficiently trimmed during reduction rhinoplasty, the "scroll" area can impinge on the nasal valve. It can be reduced directly through an intercartilaginous incision.[72, 73] Excessive narrowing of the nasal bones during surgery can also lead to nasal airway obstruction, particularly if the osteotomies are performed below the level of the inferior turbinate. If excessive narrowing has occurred, out-fracture of the bones in combination with stenting grafts to maintain the space may be necessary.[72]

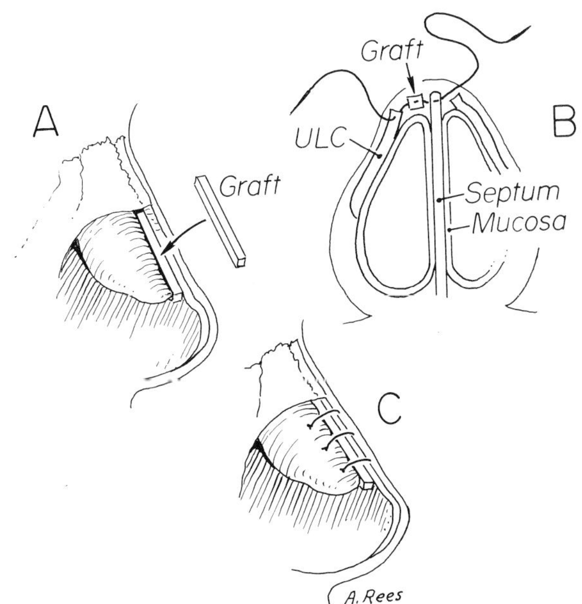

Figure 15–6. *A*, A spreader graft is placed between the upper lateral cartilage (*ULC*) and septum to stent open the nasal valve and improve nasal airway obstruction. *B*, The graft is ideally placed in an intramucosal position and secured with suture to the ULC and septum. *C*, Three sutures help secure the graft and prevent inadvertent displacement.

Dorsal Deformities

Polly beak deformity, saddle nose deformity, overcorrection, undercorrection, asymmetry, and dorsal irregularity are the most common dorsal complications seen after rhinoplasty. The position of the dorsal profile should be carefully discussed with the patient before surgery. Computer-aided video imaging is particularly helpful in this discussion as a communication aid, because it allows the patient and doctor to come to a visual "understanding" about what can and cannot be achieved by surgery.

Polly Beak Deformity

Supratip fullness or rounding that occurs following rhinoplasty is known as the "polly beak" deformity (Fig. 15–7). The causes of polly beak deformity, which are numerous, include inadequate dorsal septal reduction, excessive dorsal septal reduction, loss of tip support, and postoperative scarring.[74–76] Correction of this complex problem requires accurate diagnosis.

If the tip cartilages are fully exposed through a delivery technique and a transfixion incision is also used, tip support may be lost. At the end of surgery, the tip should be elevated above the dorsum–superior septum angle, and all tip support structures should be reconstructed. Despite these precautions, as the tip settles to a stable position during the healing process, the dorsum may become relatively higher than the tip, resulting in a polly beak. Correction should be directed at lowering the dorsum to the appropriate height while maintaining or increasing support of the nasal tip.

The ability of the soft tissues to redrape over the reduced nasal skeleton is finite. If the dorsal cartilage is excessively reduced and the soft tissues cannot adequately redrape, a polly beak can result. In this case, nasal reconstruction (augmentation) of the dorsum and tip area would be indicated.

Patients with thick, oily skin are at particular risk for unpredictable scarring and supratip fullness in the nasal tip region after surgery. Options for preventive management during primary rhinoplasty are defatting of the tip region to improve skin redraping, dome suture techniques, and medial crural I-beam fixation to increase tip definition and projection. Tip cartilage grafts may also be indicated. The supratip region should be carefully taped at the conclusion of the operation to help eliminate dead space. Careful steroid injection into the supratip region to control scar formation after surgery may also be considered.

Saddle Nose Deformity

The saddle nose deformity, an inward bowing of the cartilaginous or bony dorsum, is most commonly seen

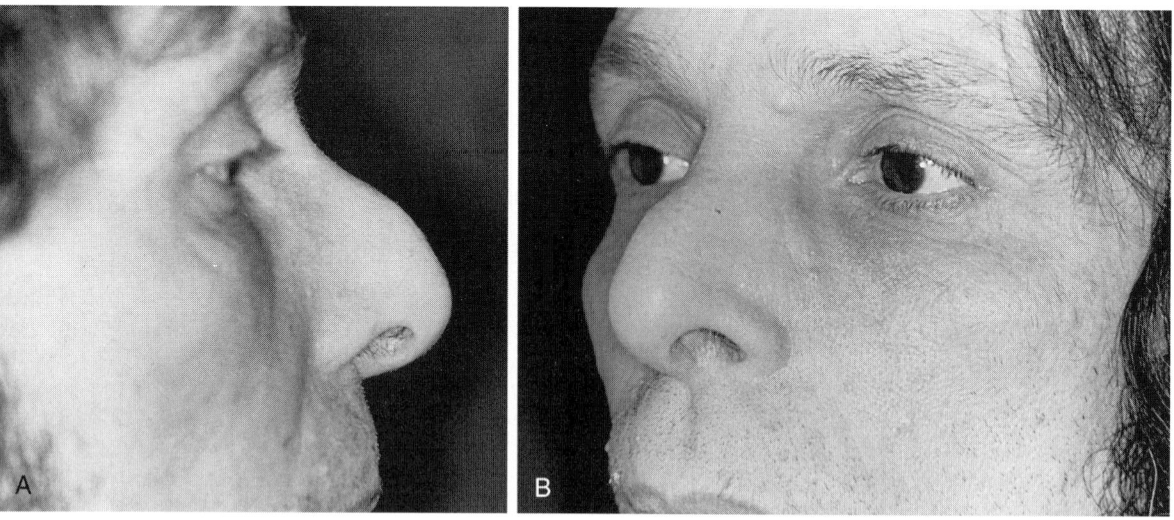

Figure 15–7. *A* and *B,* An example of polly beak deformity, which resulted from a lack of tip support. The patient underwent rhinoplasty in 1969 consisting of complete transfixion incision and tip cartilage modification via the delivery technique.

after nasal trauma but can occur after cosmetic rhinoplasty if the dorsum is overreduced.[60, 77, 78] Septal hematoma or septal infection may lead to chondromalacia with loss of dorsal support. If simultaneous septoplasty and dorsal reduction rhinoplasty are performed, the procedures should be sequenced appropriately. Specifically, the dorsal reduction should precede the septal work such that a 1.0-cm to 1.5-cm dorsal and caudal strut of cartilage remains at the completion of the combined procedures to prevent dorsal settling.

Reconstruction of the saddle nose deformity depends on the degree of deformity. Autogenous materials to rebuild dorsal structure are preferred.[78] For mild to moderate dorsal deformity, single or stacked septal or ear cartilage grafts work nicely. When severe dorsal deficiency is present, rib or bone grafts are necessary.[79] Rib cartilage provides abundant material for reconstruction, is resistant to infection even with subsequent trauma, and has been shown to remain viable for decades.[80] Even if the graft is carved carefully to balance intrinsic tensile forces, however, it can warp over time and cause external deformity.[81] Bone grafts work best for deformity in the upper third of the nose. The aesthetic disadvantage to using bone grafts to reconstruct the entire dorsum is that the nose looks and feels like a bone graft. Further, the grafts undergo variable resorption over time, even if harvested from the cranium and rigidly fixed.[79]

Undercorrection and Asymmetry

In rhinoplasty in a male, it is better to err on the side of undercorrection and relative dorsal convexity (Fig. 15–8) than to produce a concave "ski slope" effect. It is easier to refine an inadequately lowered dorsum than to rebuild one that is overreduced.

Asymmetry of the dorsum after surgery usually results from unrecognized, preexisting structural deviation. The crooked nose, particularly deformity in the middle third of the nose, is notoriously difficult to correct. Leveling the nasal pyramid with osteotomy and attention to septal position during surgery can improve, but often not completely correct, underlying structural deformity. Therefore, camouflage dorsal grafts are usually necessary to achieve a maximal aesthetic outcome.[82, 83]

Rocker Deformity

The thickness of the frontal process of the maxilla and the nasal bones increases markedly in the region of the radix, superior to the medial canthus. If the lateral osteotomy is carried into this thick bone, the twist motion of the osteotome in the medial direction frequently leads to a greenstick fracture. The transverse cephalic and medial osteotomies, if they occur, will be incomplete and will "rock": Superior pressure will cause inferolateral movement of the nasal bone complex, and vice versa.[84] This can also occur if the medial osteotomy is carried too high into the radix.[85] The rocker deformity is prevented by keeping the lateral osteotomy within the thinner bone, below the radix. Clinically, this positioning correlates with the level of the medial canthi. Alternatives to manage the rocker deformity include the use of the shatter-fracture osteotome or a percutaneous osteotomy to create the appropriate fracture lines.

Open Roof Deformity

When the dorsum is reduced, a gap is created between the bony septum and the lateral bones. Nasal osteotomies are used to close this gap and recreate the dorsal confluence of bone. If the osteotomies become greenstick fractures or are incompletely mobilized, a visible three wall defect, known as the *open roof deformity,* may result (Fig. 15–9). It may lead to a visible external deformity. In addition, patients may complain

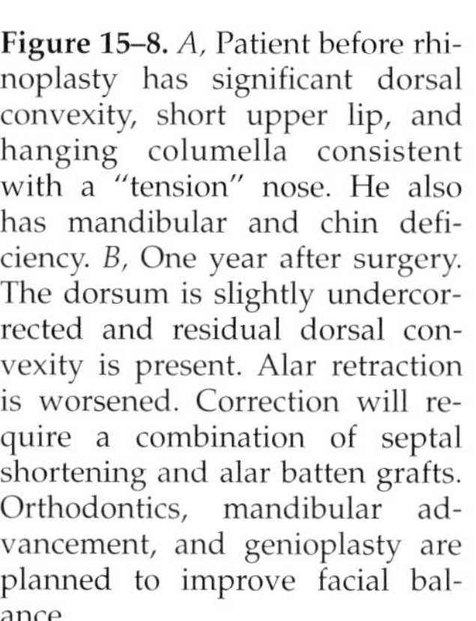

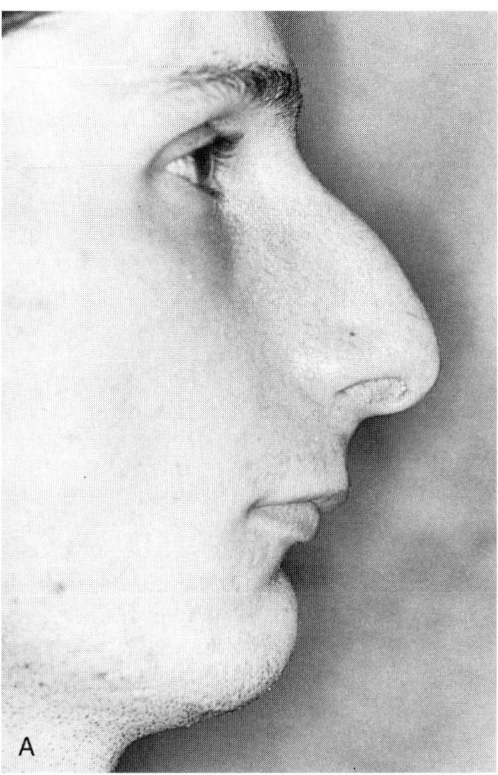

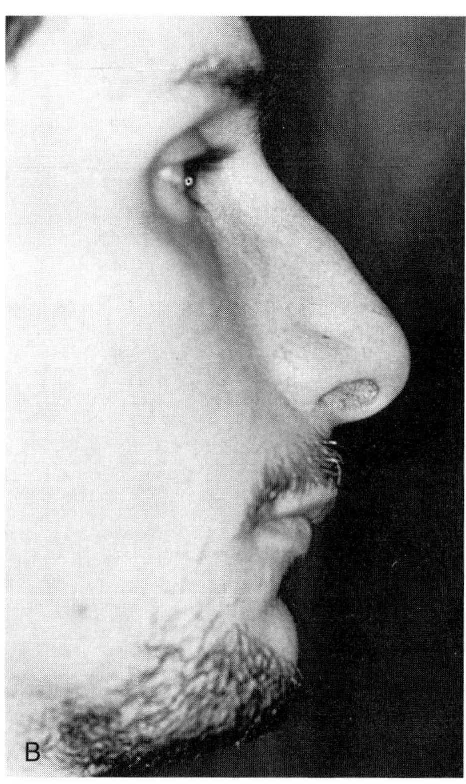

Figure 15–8. *A,* Patient before rhinoplasty has significant dorsal convexity, short upper lip, and hanging columella consistent with a "tension" nose. He also has mandibular and chin deficiency. *B,* One year after surgery. The dorsum is slightly undercorrected and residual dorsal convexity is present. Alar retraction is worsened. Correction will require a combination of septal shortening and alar batten grafts. Orthodontics, mandibular advancement, and genioplasty are planned to improve facial balance.

of exaggerated cold sensitivity in the area. The open roof deformity is prevented by confirming that the nasal bones are fully mobilized during surgery. If this step alone is inadequate, a dorsal graft may be necessary. When a very large hump is removed, lateral osteotomies alone may be insufficient to recreate the dorsum. Skoog[86] has described using the modified resected nasal bone as a free graft to cover the deformity.

Dorsal Irregularity

At the end of surgery, the nose should be checked to see that (1) the rhinion is the highest point and the superior septal angle the lowest point on the dorsum, (2) fragments of bone and cartilage have been removed, and (3) the area is smooth. Despite these precautions, patients commonly complain of palpable (but not visible) dorsal irregularity. A number of materials, including temporalis fascia[87] and polyglactin mesh,[88] can be used as a covering blanket to smooth out and minimize the problem of dorsal irregularity.

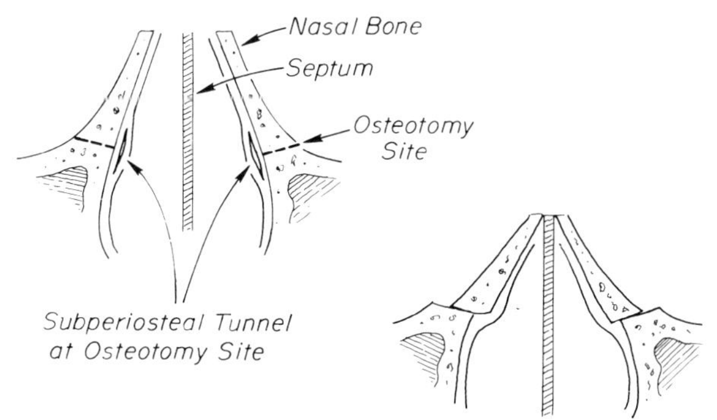

Figure 15–9. When the bony dorsum is reduced, an open roof deformity results. This is managed by performing lateral osteotomies through a narrow, subperiosteal pocket to mobilize the bones medially and recreate dorsal confluence.

Nasal Tip Deformity

Surgery of the nasal tip is generally considered the most difficult aspect of rhinoplasty to master. Revision rhinoplasty is most commonly performed to correct nasal tip deformity, in part because minor asymmetry of the nasal tip can be quite noticeable, may not manifest until years after surgery, and may lead to functional deformity. The rate of revision rhinoplasty varies between 5% and 18%, depending on the surgeon and the criteria used for revision.[55, 75, 89, 90]

There is no perfect approach or technique to manage the nasal tip, and each method involves tradeoffs. The transcartilaginous approach should be used with caution, because the residual cartilage is not directly seen, and asymmetry may result. Progressive tip narrowing may be achieved, in increasing order of complexity and irreversibility, with complete strip, dome suture, and dome interruption techniques.[91–97] Although dome division generally allows for greater tip alteration, it is also more unpredictable in the long term. Despite careful reapproximation of the cut cartilage edges, slippage can occur during the healing process, leading to asymmetry, knuckling, and bossa formation. Suturing an overlay bolster of cartilage on top of the dome division site may help lessen this problem. Excessive removal of tip cartilage can lead to decreased nasal tip projection, tip ptosis, an unaesthetically pinched tip, and alar collapse with airway obstruction (Fig. 15–10). This error can be prevented by leaving a residual alar cartilage strip of 5 to 7 mm. Removal of cartilage beyond 15 to 17 mm lateral to the dome does not materially increase tip definition and can lead to alar pinching and collapse.

The open rhinoplasty approach affords superior visualization of the osseocartilaginous nasal structures and is indicated in cases of severe asymmetry as well as posttraumatic and cleft nasal deformities. In addition to the more prolonged tip swelling associated with the open approach, unfavorable scarring of the transcolumellar incision may occur (Fig. 15–11), especially in patients with thick, oily skin.[98] A carefully executed incision closed with eversion sutures under loupe magnification can help diminish this problem. The patient should be warned before surgery that scar revision with dermabrasion may be necessary after surgery.

Blepharoplasty

Blepharoplasty is the most commonly performed facial cosmetic surgical procedure in the United States. Complications associated with this procedure vary from minor aesthetic deformity to sight-threatening injury. Careful diagnosis and patient management are crucial to avoiding problems in eyelid surgery. Prior to surgery, all patients should be evaluated for visual acuity, lid laxity, lid and brow ptosis, levator function, and lid crease asymmetry. Tear production, visual field testing, and formal ophthalmologic examination may be indicated in selected patients.

Blindness

Blindness after blepharoplasty is the most feared complication. It is estimated to occur in approximately 0.04% of all cosmetic eyelid operations.[99–105] To date, more than 75 cases of partial or complete blindness after blepharoplasty have been reported.[106, 107] A number of mechanisms have been postulated to account for blindness. The most commonly accepted etiology is intraorbital hemorrhage resulting from vascular trauma secondary to excessive traction on the orbital fat pads. Increased intraorbital pressure may lead to either ischemic optic neuropathy or central retinal artery occlusion and result in progressive loss of vision.

The surgeon performing blepharoplasty must have a protocol in place for dealing with blindness after surgery. Timely management is crucial, because the retina can tolerate only about 90 minutes of vascular occlusion before severe visual impairment results.[108] Severe orbital pain, loss of vision, increased intraocular pressure, proptosis, and ophthalmoplegia are consistent with impending blindness. The patient should be carefully examined. An emergency ophthalmology consultation should be obtained, but initial evaluation and treatment should not be delayed. The goal of treatment is to decompress the orbit.

If visual acuity is intact and there is no evidence of active bleeding, gentle use of ice packs, head elevation, and frequent orbital checks constitute sufficient treatment. If active bleeding is present, sutures should be removed and the area explored. Medical decompression can be started with intravenous acetazolamide and mannitol. Surgical intervention, including lateral canthotomy with cantholysis, orbitotomy, and anterior chamber paracentesis, may be necessary.

Dry-Eye Syndrome

A history of dry-eye symptoms, such as burning, tearing, and a rough, gritty feeling, in a patient with an abnormal periocular physical examination, are more accurate than tests of tear production and tear film breakup time in identifying a patient likely to suffer from dry-eye symptoms after blepharoplasty.[109] Man-

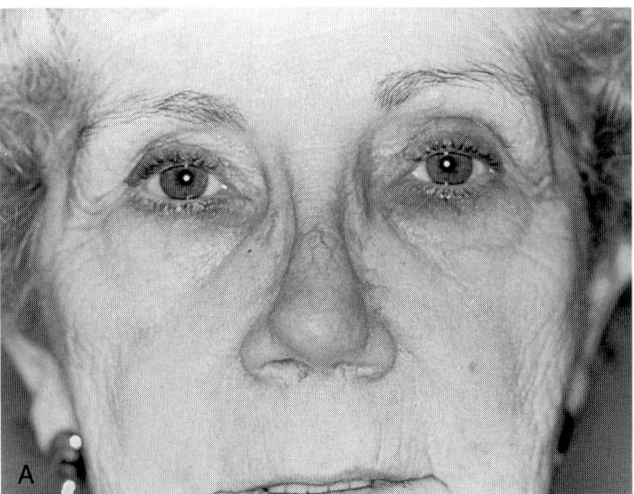

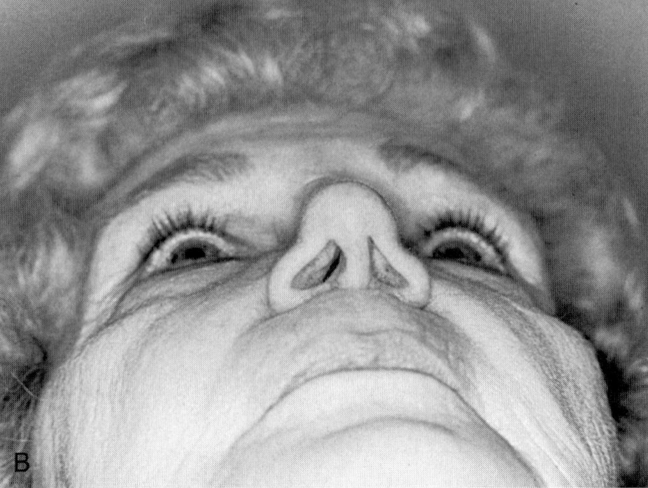

Figure 15–10. *A* and *B*, Patient has a markedly pinched dorsum and alar collapse with near-total airway obstruction following three previous rhinoplasty procedures.

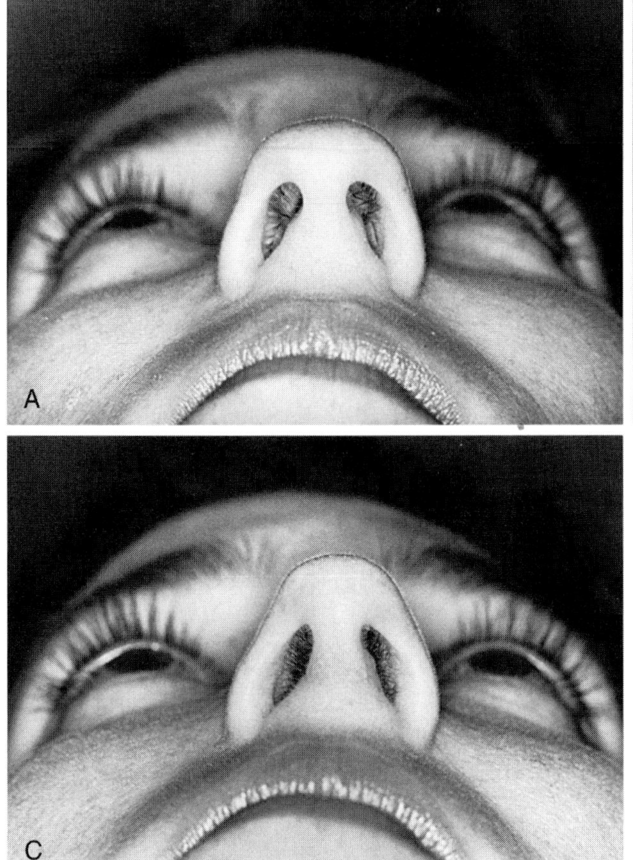

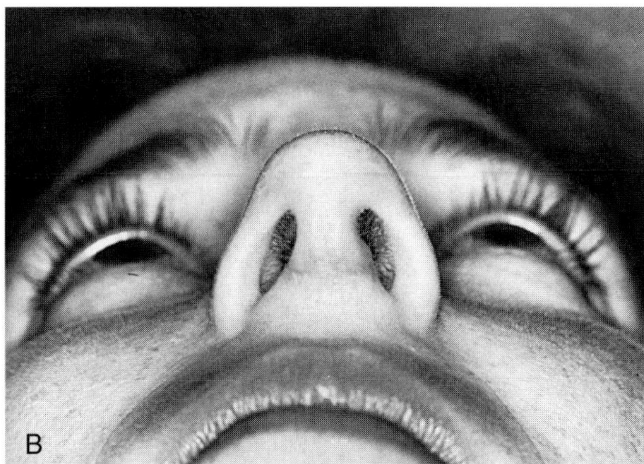

Figure 15–11. *A*, Wide, boxy nasal tip before surgery. *B*, Two weeks after rhinoplasty: The transcolumellar incision is swollen and erythematous. *C*, Six months after surgery: A persistent step in the right lateral columella is noted. Dermabrasion is planned.

agement of this problem is controversial. Although most workers recommend either conservative surgery or no surgery at all, Vold and associates[110] noted that 87% of patients with dermatochalasis and dry-eye symptoms had symptomatic improvement following upper lid blepharoplasty. These researchers propose that compensatory chronic brow elevation, an impaired blink mechanism, and evaporation of the tear film leading to a dry ocular surface in these patients are reversed by blepharoplasty and account for the improvement after surgery.

Lid Malposition

Malposition of the eyelid is the most common complication seen after lower lid blepharoplasty.[111–116] It can range from canthal rounding and increased scleral "show" to frank ectropion. The primary risk factor is laxity of the lower eyelid. If the lid can be horizontally distracted away from the globe more than 7 mm (eyelid distraction test; Fig. 15–12), or if the lid takes more than 1 second to resume its position against the globe when vertically pulled down (snap test; Fig. 15–13), significant eyelid laxity is present. Lateral canthal tightening procedures can be combined with either cutaneous or transconjunctival blepharoplasty to restore proper lid support. Malposition noted after surgery often responds to massage, lid taping, and intralesional corticosteroid injection. If these measures are unsuccessful, the cicatricial scar must be released and the canthus resuspended. In patients in whom the lid is vertically short, a full-thickness skin graft may be necessary. Vertical lid shortening can be prevented or mini-

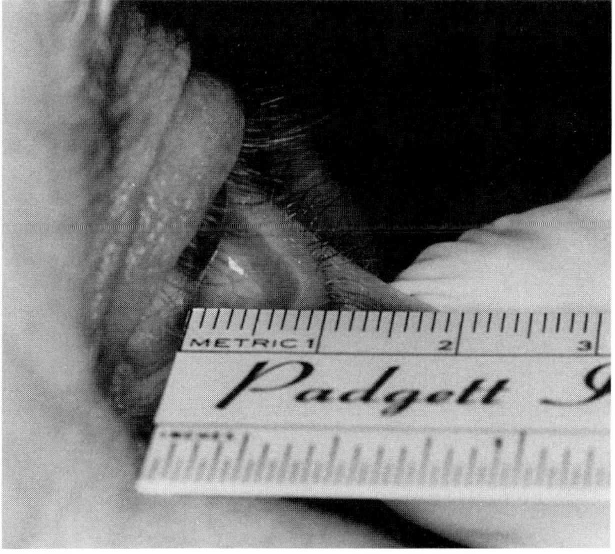

Figure 15–12. Eyelid distraction test. If the lower lid can be distracted more than 7 mm away from the globe, significant lid laxity is present.

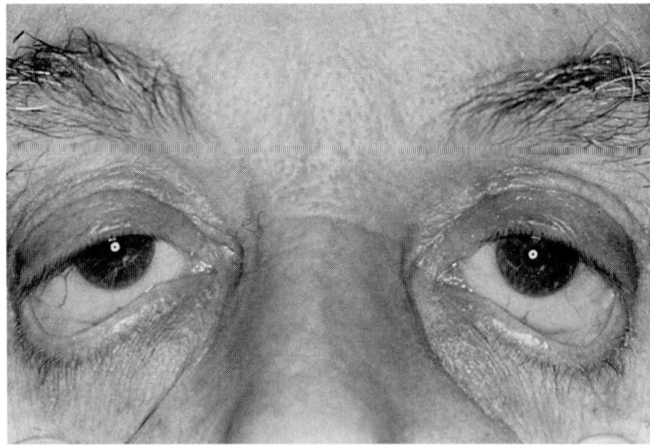

Figure 15–13. The snap test is performed by pulling down on the lower eyelid skin as illustrated. The patient is instructed not to blink when the skin is released. If the lid fails to return to the globe within 1 second, significant laxity exists.

mized by judicious excision of skin during cutaneous lower lid blepharoplasty.

Ptosis

The diagnosis and management of ptosis is complex but important in evaluating and treating patients who desire cosmetic blepharoplasty.[107, 117] History and documentation of the lid abnormality are helpful in determining the type of ptosis present and the appropriate treatment. The heights of the lid crease and of the vertical palpebral fissure, function of the upper eyelid levator muscle, and light reflex margin distance are sensitive indicators of ptosis. The patient should be examined in all fields of gaze. In acquired ptosis, the abnormal lid remains ptotic in all positions of gaze. In congenital ptosis, the ptotic lid is higher than the normal, opposing lid in downgaze. Levator muscle function is assessed by measuring the movement of the upper lid from extreme downgaze to extreme upgaze while the brow and forehead are held in the neutral position. This distance is normally at least 15 mm. If the lid moves less than 10 mm, significant levator muscle dysfunction is suggested. Elderly patients with a high or absent lid crease and a thin upper lid may have levator muscle attenuation or disinsertion. If disinsertion is confirmed intraoperatively or if the levator muscle is cut during surgery, it should be repaired.[118] Lid edema, hematoma, and supratarsal fixation can lead to temporary ptosis after surgery. A delay of 3 to 6 months is recommended for patients in whom ptosis is noted after surgery, to allow for spontaneous resolution before treatment is considered.

Patients undergoing blepharoplasty should be assessed for concomitant eyebrow ptosis.[119, 120] Unless the position of the brow is addressed, excision of skin and muscle during blepharoplasty worsens an uncorrected ptotic brow by pulling it further inferiorly.

Prolapsed Lacrimal Gland

There are two fat pads in the upper eyelid, the medial and the central. A prolapsed lacrimal gland in the lateral aspect of the upper lid may be mistaken for a fat pad. The gland is deeper in color and significantly more textured than a fat pad. The gland is divided into the medial palpebral portion and the lateral orbital portion by the levator aponeurosis. The orbital component of the lacrimal gland accounts for the majority of tear production, and its inadvertent removal can lead to significant dry-eye symptoms. If the lacrimal gland is prolapsed, it should be carefully identified and resuspended within the orbit by means of a double-armed permanent or slowly resorbable suture.[117, 118, 121, 122]

Lagophthalmos

At the conclusion of upper lid blepharoplasty, there should be a gap of 1 to 2 mm between the upper and lower lids. Over time, this gap typically closes on its own as the lid skin stretches. If excessive skin is removed during surgery and the patient is unable to close the eye, drying of the ocular surface with corneal ulceration can occur, particularly if the Bell phenomenon is absent or diminished.[107, 123] Patients with significant lagophthalmos noted after surgery should be treated with lubricating drops or ointment, manual lid massage, and possibly a bubble eye patch at night. If the lagophthalmos does not resolve, it may be necessary to reconstruct the lid with a full-thickness skin graft. Donor sites for such a graft include the contralateral upper lid and the retroauricular, preauricular, or supraclavicular skin. The cosmetic result of full-thickness skin graft reconstruction of the upper lid is almost universally inferior to that of cosmetic blepharoplasty. It is easier to leave a little excess skin, which can be revised at a secondary surgery, than to take too much and necessitate eyelid reconstruction.

Diplopia

Temporary diplopia after blepharoplasty is usually attributed to wound reaction, edema, or resolving hematoma.[107, 124, 125] Direct injury to the extraocular muscles can occur. The inferior and superior oblique muscles, which lie relatively superficially within the orbit, are the two muscles most commonly involved in diplopia. The inferior oblique muscle lies between the central and medial fat pads of the lower lid and is at risk in both cutaneous and transconjunctival blepharoplasty.[126] Accurate identification during surgery is the most effective means of prevention. The superior oblique muscle can be injured during cautery control of bleeding of the nasal fat pad of the upper lid.[127] Direct visualization of the bleeding points and bipolar or battery cautery can help minimize this problem.[128] If persistent strabismus results, referral to an ophthalmology consultant is recommended.

Face-Lift

Face-lift procedures can be performed for isolated regions of the face, such as the forehead and brow, or can be combined to treat the entire face and neck. The larger the operation and the more areas treated, the greater the risk of complications. A number of more complex face-lift techniques have been promulgated by various surgeons to improve results achieved with conventional methods.[129–132] Although the early data suggest that these procedures are associated with minimal complications, long-term results remain to be seen. The most common complications associated with face-lift surgery are hematoma, nerve injury, skin slough, alopecia, and infection.[133–137]

Hematoma

Hematoma is the most common complication of face-lift surgery, occurring in up to 15% of cases. The incidence of bleeding requiring surgical attention is approximately 4%.[133, 136, 138, 139] Risk factors for hematoma are preexisting hypertension, aspirin ingestion within 2 weeks of surgery, male sex, general anesthesia, and vomiting after surgery.[139–143] Most hematomas occur within the first 24 hours. Prevention of hematoma can be aided by the tumescent anesthetic technique[144, 145] and meticulous intraoperative hemostasis obtained with the patient at his or her normal resting blood pressure.[139] The use of suction drains may be helpful to prevent hematoma formation.[146] The patient should avoid lifting heavy objects or turning the head sharply for at least 2 weeks after surgery to minimize the risk of injuring fragile healing blood vessels.

Patients and caregivers should be instructed in the warning signs of hematoma and instructed to call the doctor immediately if they occur. Sudden onset of swelling or pain, especially if unilateral, suggest hematoma formation. Because it greatly increases the risk of necrosis of the overlying flap, hematoma represents a true emergency. The patient should be seen, dressings removed, and the area examined. If drains are present, they should be assessed for patency. If a small hematoma is present, it may be possible to aspirate the area or place a percutaneous drain. If a moderate hematoma is encountered, it can sometimes be drained by opening some of the skin sutures and rolling the flap manually to express the hematoma. A liposuction cannula may also be introduced through the wound opening to remove the blood. A large hematoma, however, requires exploration and evacuation. Whether this procedure is done in the emergency room with sedation or in the operating room using general anesthesia depends on the extent of the hematoma as well as on the patient's and surgeon's preference. In most cases of early hematoma, a single bleeding vessel is not found. This is in contrast to the late hematoma that develops because of isolated superficial temporal vessel bleeding. Goldwyn[147] recommends direct ligation of the superficial temporal vessels if they cause bleeding during face-lift surgery as the best chance to prevent subsequent hematoma.

In addition to vascular compromise and slough of the overlying skin, hematoma can cause compression nerve injury, infection, and skin pigmentation changes. In some cases, the skin color changes may be permanent. Further, delayed recovery after surgery is usually noted for the patient who has had a significant hematoma.

In the patient shown in Figure 15–14, a small hematoma is seen in the retroauricular region. This swelling was noted 24 hours after surgery and could not be aspirated because it had coagulated. The swelling resolved with gentle massage. Mottled hyperpigmentation was noted in this same area for several months after surgery but faded spontaneously.

Nerve Injury

Most patients have variable, temporary cutaneous anesthesia of the skin in the areas that were undermined during surgery. The most common sensory nerve trunk injured in face-lift surgery is the greater auricular nerve.[133, 136, 148, 149] This nerve emerges from the posterior aspect of the sternocleidomastoid (SCM) muscle and lies just deep to the SCM fascia. The greater auricular nerve is most vulnerable to injury where it crosses over the SCM muscle (Fig. 15–15). If the nerve is injured or severed, the patient may complain of a woody numbness or, worse, a burning dysesthesia of the preauricular region and inferior half of the ear. Injury to the greater auricular nerve can be prevented by maintaining flap depth superficial to the SCM fascia. Sutures in the superficial musculoaponeurotic system (SMAS) layer at the anterior border aspect of the SCM muscle do not

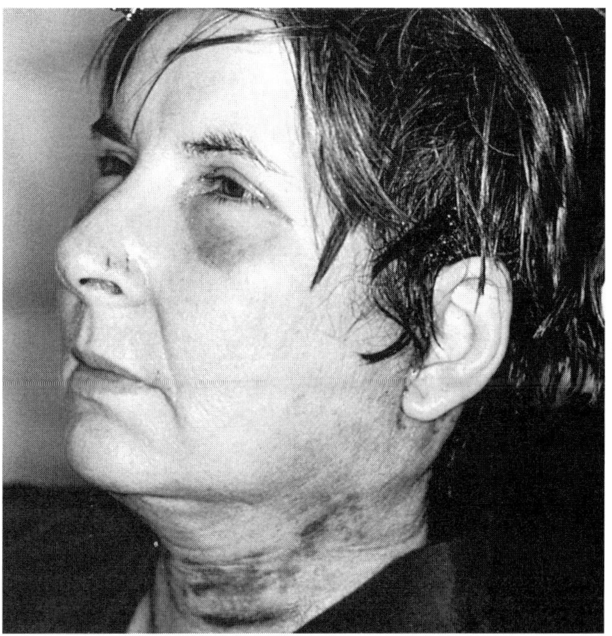

Figure 15–14. Twenty-four hours after cervicofacial rhytidectomy, upper and lower blepharoplasty, and alar batten grafts to the nose. Swelling and ecchymosis of the neck are evident. A hematoma was noted in the retro- and infra-auricular region but could not be aspirated because it had coagulated. The area resolved spontaneously.

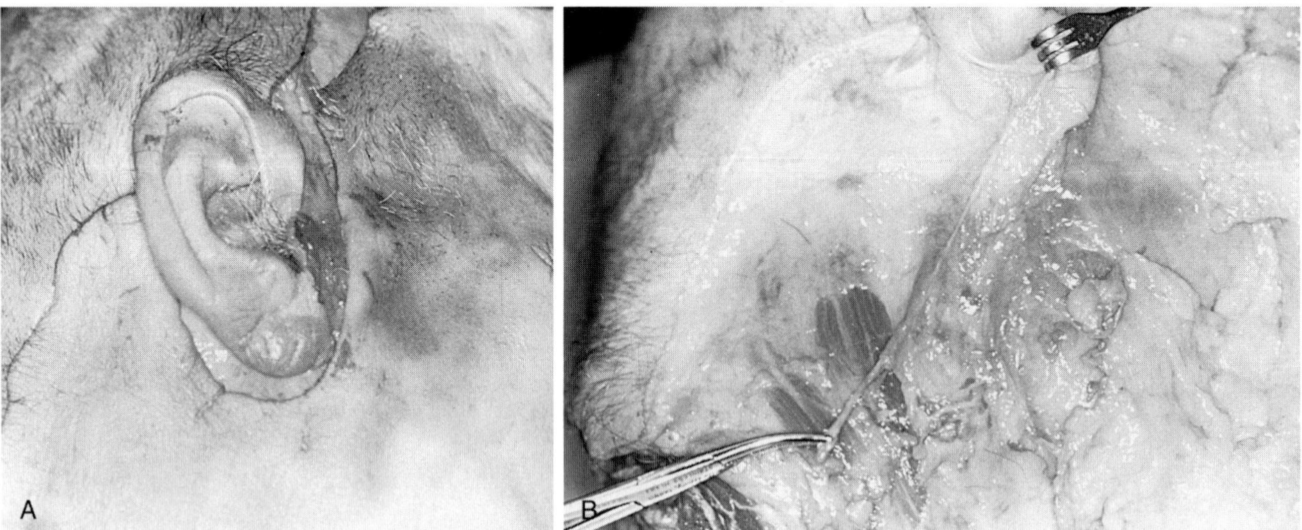

Figure 15–15. *A,* Fresh cadaver specimen with skin flap incised. *B,* Fresh cadaver specimen demonstrating path of the greater auricular nerve. The retractor is on the posterior aspect of the lobule of the ear. The hemostat is on the greater auricular nerve as it emerges from the posterior aspect of the sternocleidomastoid muscle (SCM). Muscle fibers of the SCM can clearly be seen underlying the nerve.

entrap the nerve.[150] If the fascia is violated and SCM fibers are clearly seen exposed during the course of the surgery, the wound should be explored to verify the location of the greater auricular nerve. If cut it should be repaired under loupe or microscopic magnification. Hypesthesia of the greater auricular nerve noted after surgery may resolve spontaneously over 3 to 6 months. If the patient has dysesthesia or a Tinel sign, suggesting neuroma formation, reexploration with nerve repair and grafting may be necessary.[152]

Injury to the facial nerve during face-lift surgery is uncommon, occurring in 0.1% to 2.6% of patients.[133, 135, 136, 153] The branches most likely to be injured are the frontal branch and the marginal mandibular branch.[153–156] Fortunately, most facial nerve weakness is temporary.

As the frontal branch of the temporal nerve courses superiorly, it switches from a relatively deep to a quite superficial position where it crosses the zygomatic arch.[157] Pitanguy and Ramos[154] have described the path of the nerve. It courses on a line extending from 0.5 cm inferior to the tragus to 1.5 cm superior and lateral to the eyebrow. Dissection in the temporal hairline is subgaleal to avoid injury to the hair follicles. As the dissection proceeds anteriorly, an abrupt transition from the subgaleal to the subcutaneous plane must be made at the margin of the hairline to avoid injury to the frontal branch of the facial nerve.

The marginal mandibular nerve lies deep to the platysma. It may be injured directly during extended sub-SMAS dissection or may become caught in a suture during SMAS suspension. If transection is noted during surgery, the nerve should be repaired. If facial paralysis occurs after surgery, the patient should be followed closely and advised that nerve exploration and repair may be necessary.

Infection

Despite a contaminated field, the incidence of infection following face-lift surgery is quite low, typically less than 1%.[133, 135, 157] The use of antibiotics in face-lift surgery is controversial. No controlled clinical trials exist. If antibiotics are used, a cephalosporin to cover gram-positive organisms is suggested. In a series of 6,166 consecutive face-lift patients 11 required hospital re-admission and treatment for infection following surgery.[157] Infection in the first week after surgery involved either staphylococcal or streptococcal organisms. Late infection was more likely to be contaminated with gram-negative bacteria.

Skin Slough

The face-lift is a rotation-advancement flap, and typically, the skin is inset with some degree of tension. The later modifications of the face-lift, including the deep plane and composite lift, attempt to transfer the vector of tension from the skin flap to the underlying musculature.[130, 132] Risk factors for skin slough include hematoma, excessive flap tension, and smoking.[136, 139, 158–160] The most common area of necrosis is the retroauricular skin over the mastoid. Fortunately, even full-thickness skin loss in this area can heal with an acceptable result through careful wound cleansing and management. Once wound contraction has occurred, the scar can be evaluated and, if necessary, excised and revised.

Hairline Changes

The most common hair-associated complications after face-lift surgery are alopecia, elevation of the temporal hairline, and alteration of the retroauricular hairline.[161, 162] Loss of hair can result from direct injury to the hair follicle or excessive wound tension. Techniques to minimize hair loss include making scalp incisions parallel to the hair follicles and carefully coagulating bleeding areas in the scalp flap.[163] "Tension alopecia" can be decreased by ensuring adequate deep support of the wound and avoiding excess tension at the skin closure site. Persistent alopecia may necessitate excision of the bald area with primary closure or a local scalp flap.

If the temporal incision is carried vertically within the hairline, posterior and superior advancement of the flap elevates the preauricular tuft of hair, possibly leading to an unnatural appearance. This complication can be prevented by designing the temporal incision to preserve a portion of the preauricular hair. Proper incision design in a secondary face-lift allows an elevated hairline to be advanced inferomedially to reconstruct the preauricular tuft.

The placement of the preauricular incision is very important in the male face-lift patient.[164, 165] If an endaural incision is made and bearded skin is advanced over the tragus, an abnormal appearance may result even when careful depilation is carried out. This complication can be avoided by placing the incision in the preauricular crease and leaving the tragus untouched.

A stair-step deformity can occur in the retroauricular hairline if the cervical flap is rotated superiorly and the hairline above and below the incision site is not carefully reapproximated. The chances of such an occurrence can be minimized by carrying the retroauricular incision horizontally into the hairline, excising a triangular wedge of tissue (with the base at the hairline and the apex within the scalp), and then reapproximating the hairline as the first step in tailoring the cervical skin flap.[166, 167]

References

1. Phillips, KA: Body dysmorphic disorder: The distress of imagined ugliness. Am J Psychiatry 1991;148:1138.
2. Wright MR: The male aesthetic patient. Arch Orolaryngol Head Neck Surg 1987;113:724.
3. Goin JM, Goin MK: Psychological screening of the rhinoplasty patient. *In* Goin JM, Goin MK (eds): Changing the Body: Psychological Effects of Plastic Surgery. Baltimore, Williams & Wilkins, 1981, p 137.
4. Gifford S: Cosmetic surgery and personality change: A review of some clinical observations. *In* Goldwyn RM (ed): The Unfavorable Result in Plastic Surgery: Avoidance and Treatment, ed 2, vol I. Boston, Little, Brown, 1984, p 21.
5. Wright MR, Wright WK: A psychological study of patients undergoing cosmetic surgery. Arch Otolaryngol Head Neck Surg 1973;101:145.
6. Wright MR: How to recognize and control the problem patient. J Dermatol Surg Oncol 1984;10:389.
7. Wright MR: Management of patient dissatisfaction with results of cosmetic procedures. Arch Otolaryngol Head Neck Surg 1980;106:466.
8. Hickson GB, Clayton EW, Entman SS, et al: Obstetricians' prior malpractice experience and patients' satisfaction with care. JAMA 1994;272:1583.
9. Snyder GB: Augmentation mentoplasty. *In* Goldwyn RM (ed): The Unfavorable Result in Plastic Surgery: Avoidance and Treatment, ed 2, vol II. Boston, Little, Brown, 1984, p 651.
10. Terino ED: Chin and malar augmentation. *In* Peck GC (ed): Complications and Problems in Aesthetic Plastic Surgery. New York, Gower Medical Publishing, 1992, p 6.1.
11. Bell WH: Correction of the contour-deficient chin. J Oral Surg 1969;27:110.
12. Robinson M, Schuken R: Bone resorption under plastic chin implants. J Oral Surg 1969;27:116.
13. Robinson M: Bone resorption under plastic chin implants: Follow-up of a preliminary report. Arch Otolaryngol 1972;95:30.
14. Friedland JA, Coccaro PJ, Converse JM: Retrospective cephalometric analysis of mandibular bone absorption under silicone rubber chin implants. Plast Reconstr Surg 1976;57:144.
15. Dann JJ, Epker BM: Proplast genioplasty: A retrospective study with treatment recommendations. Angle Orthod 1977;47:173.
16. Binder WJ, Kamer FM, Parkes ML: Mentoplasty—a clinical analysis of alloplastic implants. Laryngoscope 1981;91:383.
17. Guyuron B, Raszewski RL: A critical comparison of osteoplastic and alloplastic augmentation genioplasty. Aesthetic Plast Surg 1990;14:199.
18. McDonnell JP, McNeill RW, West RA: Advancement genioplasty: A retrospective cephalometric analysis of osseous and soft tissue changes. J Oral Surg 1977;35:640.
19. Webster RC: Chin augmentation: Subperiosteal and supraperiosteal implants. Aesthetic Plast Surg 1977;1:149.
20. Scaccia FJ, Allphin AL, Stepnick DW: Complications of augmentation mentoplasty: A review of 11,095 cases. Am J Cosmetic Surg 1993;10:189.
21. Nishioka GJ, Mason M, Van Sickels JE: Neurosensory disturbance associated with the anterior mandibular horizontal osteotomy. J Oral Maxillofac Surg 1988;46:107.
22. Lindquist CC, Obeid G: Complications of genioplasty done alone or in combination with sagittal split-ramus osteotomy. Oral Surg Oral Med Oral Pathol 1988;66:13.
23. Peled IJ, Wexler MR, Ticher S, et al: Mandibular resorption from silicone chin implants in children. J Oral Maxillofac Surg 1986;44:346.
24. Polido WD, Regis LD, Bell WH: Bone resorption, stability, and soft-tissue changes following large chin advancements. J Oral Maxillofac Surg 1991;49:251.
25. Precious DS, Armstrong JE, Morais D: Anatomic placement of fixation devices in genioplasty. Oral Surg Oral Med Oral Pathol 1992;73:2.
26. Mercuri LG, Laskin DM: Avascular necrosis after anterior horizontal augmentation genioplasty. J Oral Surg 1977;35:296.
27. Peterson LJ: Antibiotic prophylaxis against wound infections in oral and maxillofacial surgery. J Oral Maxillofac Surg 1990; 48:617.
28. Rappaport SI: Preoperative hemostatic evaluation: Which tests if any? Blood 1983;61:229.
29. Rohrer MJ, Michelotti MC, Nahrwold DL: A prospective evaluation of the efficacy of preoperative coagulation testing. Ann Surg 1988;208:554.
30. Wolford LM, Bates JD: Surgical modification for the correction of chin deformities. Oral Surg Oral Med Oral Pathol 1988;66:279.
31. Hintz CS: Alloplastic graft for cosmetic improvement of the accentuated mental crease. Am J Cosmetic Surg 1993;10:197.
32. Rubens BC, West RA: Ptosis of the chin and lip incompetence: Consequences of lost mentalis muscle support. J Oral Maxillofac Surg 1989;47:359.
33. Brennan GH, Giammanco PF: The ptotic chin syndrome corrected by mentoplasty. Ann Plast Surg 1987;18:200.
34. Zide BM, McCarthy J: The mentalis muscle: An essential component of chin and lower lip position. Plast Reconstr Surg 1989;83:413.
35. Wolfe SA: Chin advancement as an aid in correction of deformities of the mental and submental regions. Plast Reconstr Surg 1981;67:624.
36. Cohen SR, Mardach OL, Kawamoto HK Jr: Chin disfigurement following removal of alloplastic chin implants. Plast Reconstr Surg 1991;88:62.
37. Wilkinson TS: Complications in aesthetic malar augmentation. Plast Reconstr Surg 1983;71:643.
38. Courtiss E: Complication in aesthetic malar augmentation—discussion. Plast Reconstr Surg 1983;71:648.
39. Kent JN, Westfall RL, Carlton DM: Chin and zygomaticomaxillary augmentation with Proplast: Long-term follow-up. J Oral Surg 1981;39:912.
40. Whitaker LA: Aesthetic augmentation of the malar midface structures. Plast Reconstr Surg 1987;80:387.
41. Szachowicz TE, Kriden RWH: Adjunctive measures to rhinoplasty. Otolaryngol Clin North AM 1987;20:895.
42. Webster RC, Smith RC: Malpractice from the viewpoint of the

plastic surgeon. *In* Goldwyn RM (ed): The Unfavorable Result in Plastic Surgery: Avoidance and Treatment, ed 2, vol II. Boston, Little, Brown, 1984, p 1103.
43. Lawson W, Kessler S, Biller HF: Unusual and fatal complications of rhinoplasty. Arch Otolaryngol Head Neck Surg 1983;109:164.
44. Teichgraeber JF, Riley WB, Parks DH: Nasal surgery complications. Plast Reconstr Surg 1990;85:527.
45. Teichgraeber JF, Russo RC: Treatment of nasal surgery complications. Ann Plast Surg 1993;30:80.
46. Maniglia AJ: Fatal and major complications secondary to nasal and sinus surgery. Laryngoscope 1989;99:276.
47. Castillo GD: Management of blindness in the practice of cosmetic surgery. Otolaryngol Head Neck Surg 1989;100:559.
48. Moscona R, Ullmann Y, Peled I: Necrotizing periorbital cellulitis following septorhinoplasty. Aesthetic Plast Surg 1991;15:187.
49. Lacy GM, Conway H: Recovery after meningitis with convulsions and paralysis following rhinoplasty: Cause for pause. Plast Reconstr Surg 1965;36:254.
50. Marshall DR, Slattery PG: Intracranial complications of rhinoplasty. Br J Plast Surg 1983;36:342.
51. Hallock GG, Trier WC: Cerebrospinal fluid rhinorrhea following rhinoplasty. Plast Reconstr Surg 1983;71:109.
52. Cheney ML, Blair PA: Blindness as a complication of rhinoplasty. Arch Otolaryngol Head Neck Surg 1987;113:768.
53. Byers B: Blindness secondary to steroid injection into the nasal turbinates. Arch Ophthalmol 1979;97:79.
54. Caleel RT, Eubanks RL Jr, Shaenboen MJ: Intracranial hemorrhage associated with medical use of cocaine: Case reports. Am J Cosmetic Surg 1992;9:85.
55. Klabunde EH, Falces E: Incidence of complications in cosmetic rhinoplasties. Plast Reconstr Surg 1964;34:192.
56. Goldwyn RM: Unexpected bleeding after selective nasal surgery. Ann Plast Surg 1979;2:201.
57. Churukian MM, Zemplenyi J, Steiner M, et al: Post-rhinoplasty epistaxis. Role of vitamin E? Arch Otolaryngol Head Neck Surg 1988;114:748.
58. DeFillip GJ, Rubinstein M, Drake A, et al: The role of angiography and embolization in the management of recurrent epistaxis. Arch Otolaryngol Head Neck Surg 1988;99:597.
59. Breda SD, Choi IS, Persky MS, et al: Embolization in the treatment of epistaxis after failure of internal maxillary artery ligation. Laryngoscope 1989;99:809.
60. Holt GR, Garner ET, McLarey D: Postoperative sequelae and complications of rhinoplasty. Otolaryngol Clin North Am 1987;20:853.
61. Thomas SW, Baird IM, Frazier RD: Toxic shock syndrome following submucous resection and rhinoplasty. JAMA 1982; 247:2402.
62. Jacobson JA, Kasworm EM: Toxic shock syndrome after nasal surgery. Arch Otolaryngol Head Neck Surg 1986;112:329.
63. Fairbanks DNF: Complications of nasal packing. Otolaryngol Head Neck Surg 1986;94:412.
64. Casaubon JN, Dion MA, Labrisseau A: Septic cavernous sinus thrombosis after rhinoplasty. Plast Reconstr Surg 1977;59:119.
65. Maniglia AJ, Goodwin J, Arnold JE, et al: Intracranial abscesses secondary to nasal, sinus and orbital infection in adults and children. Arch Otolaryngol Head Neck Surg 1989;15:1424.
66. Eschelman LT, Schleunig AJ, Brummett RE: Prophylactic antibiotics on otolaryngologic surgery: A double-blind study. Trans Am Acad Ophthalmol Otolaryngol 1971;75:387.
67. Slavin SA, Rees TD, Guy CL, et al: An investigation of bacteremia during rhinoplasty. Plast Reconstr Surg 1983;71:196.
68. Jacobson JA, Stevens MH, Kasworm EM: Evaluation of single-dose cefazolin prophylaxis for toxic shock syndrome. Arch Otolaryngol Head Neck Surg 1988;114:326.
69. Meyers AD: Prophylactic antibiotics in nasal surgery. Arch Otolaryngol Head Neck Surg 1990;116:1125.
70. Beekhuis GJ: Nasal obstruction after rhinoplasty: Etiology and techniques for correction. Laryngoscope 1976;86:540.
71. Sachs ME: Post-rhinoplastic nasal obstruction. Otolaryngol Clin North Am 1989;22:319.
72. Kasperbauer JL, Kern EB: Nasal valve physiology: Implications in nasal surgery. Otolaryngol Clin North Am 1987;20:699.
73. Goode R: Surgery of the incompetent nasal valve. Laryngoscope 1985;95:546.
74. Beekhuis GJ, Colton JJ: Soft tissue "polly beak" deformity: Avoidance and management. Am J Cosmetic Surg 1985;21.
75. Kamer FM, McQuown SA: Revision rhinoplasty: Analysis and treatment. Arch Otolaryngol Head Neck Surg 1988;114:257.
76. Tardy ME, Kron TK, Younger R, et al: The cartilaginous polly-beak: Etiology, prevention and treatment. Facial Plast Surg 1989;6:113.
77. Stuzin JM, Kawamoto HK: Saddle nose deformity. Clin Plast Surg 1988;15:88.
78. Tardy ME, Schwartz M, Parras G: Saddle nose deformity: Autogenous graft repair. Facial Plast Surg 1989;6:121.
79. Posnick JC, Seagle MB, Armstrong D: Nasal reconstruction with full-thickness cranial bone grafts and rigid internal fixation through a coronal incision. Plast Reconstr Surg 1990;86:894.
80. Horton CE, Matthews MS: Nasal reconstruction with autologous rib cartilage: A 43-year follow-up. Plast Reconstr Surg 1992;89:131.
81. Gibson T, Davis WB: The distortion of autogenous cartilage grafts: Its cause and prevention. Br J Plast Surg 1958;10:257.
82. Larabee WF: Open rhinoplasty and the upper third of the nose. Facial Plast Surg Clin North Am 1993;1:23.
83. Constantian MB: An algorithm for correcting the asymmetrical nose. Plast Reconstr Surg 1989;83:801.
84. Anderson JR, Ries WR: Rhinoplasty: Emphasizing the External Approach. New York, Thieme, 1986, p 98.
85. McKinney P, Cunningham BL: Rhinoplasty. New York, Churchill Livingstone, 1989, p 62.
86. Skoog T: A method of hump reduction. Arch Otolaryngol 1966;83:283.
87. Baker TM, Courtiss EH: Temporalis fascia grafts in open secondary rhinoplasty. Plast Reconstr Surg 1994;93:802.
88. Gilmore J: Use of Vicryl mesh in prevention of post-rhinoplasty dorsal irregularities. Ann Plast Surg 1989;22:105.
89. Tardy ME, Cheng EY, Jernstrom V: Misadventures in nasal tip surgery. Otolaryngol Clin North Am 1987;20:797.
90. McKinney P, Cook JQ: A critical evaluation of 200 rhinoplasties. Ann Plast Surg 1981;7:357.
91. McCollough EG, Mangat DS: Systematic approach to the nasal tip in rhinoplasty. Arch Otolaryngol 1981;107:12.
92. Anderson JR: A reasoned approach to nasal base surgery. Arch Otolaryngol 1984;110:349.
93. Gunter JP: Tip rhinoplasty: A personal approach. Facial Plast Surg 1987;4:263.
94. Tardy ME, Patt BS, Walter MA: Transdomal suture refinement of the nasal tip: Long-term outcomes. Facial Plast Surg 1993;9:275.
95. Tardy ME, Walter MA, Patt BS: The overprojecting nose: Anatomic component analysis and repair. Facial Plast Surg 1993;9:306.
96. Peck CG: Techniques in Aesthetic Rhinoplasty. New York, Gower Medical Publishers, 1990, p 18.
97. Tebbetts JB: Shaping and positioning the nasal tip without structural disruption: A new, systematic approach. Plast Reconstr Surg 1994;94:61.
98. Hoffman JF, Cook TA: Complications of rhinoplasty. *In* Eisele DW (ed): Complications in Head and Neck Surgery. St Louis, Mosby–Year Book, 1993, p 555.
99. Jafek BW, Kreiger AE, Morledge D: Blindness following blepharoplasty. Arch Otolaryngol 1973;98:366.
100. Hartley JH, Lester JC, Schatten WE: Acute retrobulbar hemorrhage during elective blepharoplasty. Plast Reconstr Surg 1973;52:8.
101. Moser MH, DiPirro E, McCoy F: Sudden blindness following blepharoplasty. Plast Reconstr Surg 1973;51:364.
102. Putterman AM: Temporary blindness after cosmetic blepharoplasty. Am J Ophthalmol 1975;80:1081.
103. Heinze JB, Heuston JT: Blindness after blepharoplasty: Mechanism and early reversal. Plast Reconstr Surg 1978;61:347.
104. Rafaty FM: Transient total blindness during cosmetic blepharoplasty: Case report and discussion. Ann Plast Surg 1979;3:373.
105. Anderson RL, Edwards JJ: Bilateral visual loss after blepharoplasty. Ann Plast Surg 1980;5:288.
106. Callahan MA: Prevention of blindness after blepharoplasty. Ophthalmology 1983;90:1047.
107. Lowry JC, Bartley GB: Complications of blepharoplasty. Surv Ophthalmol 1994;38:327.

108. Hayreh SS, Kolder AG, Weingeist TA: A central retinal artery occlusion and retinal tolerance time. Ophthlamology 1980;87:75.
109. McKinney P, Zulkowski ML: The value of tear film breakup and Schirmer's tests in preoperative blepharoplasty evaluation. Plast Reconstr Surg 1989;84:572.
110. Vold SD, Carroll RP, Nelson JD: Dermatochalasis and dry eye. Am J Ophthalmol 1993;115:216.
111. Edgerton MT: Causes and prevention of lower lid ectropion following blepharoplasty. Plast Reconstr Surg 1972;49:367.
112. Rees TD: Correction of ectropion resulting from blepharoplasty. Plast Reconstr Surg 1972;50:1.
113. Hamako CM, Baylis HI: Lower eyelid retraction after blepharoplasty. Am J Ophthalmol 1980;89:517.
114. Tenzel RR: Complications of blepharoplasty: Orbital hematoma, ectropion, and scleral show. Clin Plast Surg 1981;8:797.
115. McCord CD, Shore JW: Avoidance of complications in lower lid blepharoplasty. Ophthalmology 1983;90:1039.
116. McCord CD: Complications of orbital surgery. Otolaryngol Clin North Am 1988;21:183.
117. Hornblass A: Ptosis and pseudoptosis and blepharoplasty. Clin Plast Surg 1981;8:811.
118. Baylis HI, Sutcliffe T, Fett DR: Levatory injury during blepharoplasty. Arch Ophthalmol 1984;102:570.
119. McKinney P, Rossie RD, Zukowski ML: Criteria for the forehead lift. Aesthetic Plast Surg 1991;15:141.
120. Matarasso A, Terino EO: Forehead-brow rhytidoplasty: Reassessing the goals. Plast Reconstr Surg 1994;93:1378.
121. Smith B, Petrelli R: Surgical repair of prolapsed lacrimal glands. Arch Ophthalmol 1978;96:1132.
122. Beer GM, Kompatscher P: A new technique for treatment of lacrimal gland prolapse in blepharoplasty. Aesthetic Plast Surg 1994;18:65.
123. Tiliff NT, Iwamoto M: Complications of blepharoplasty. *In* Eisele DW (ed): Complications in Head and Neck Surgery. St Louis, Mosby–Year Book, 1993, p 471.
124. Hayworth RS, Lisman RD, Muchnick RS, et al: Diplopia following blepharoplasty. Ann Ophthalmol 1984;16:448.
125. Harley RD, Nelson LB, Flanagan JC, et al: Ocular motility disturbances following blepharoplasty. Arch Ophthalmol 1986;104:542.
126. Baylis HI, Long JA, Groth MJ: Transconjunctival lower eyelid blepharoplasty. Ophthalmology 1989;96:1027.
127. Wesley RW, Pollard ZF, McCord CD: Superior oblique paresis after blepharoplasty. Plast Reconstr Surg 1980;66:283.
128. Kaye BL: Two helpful technical aids in blepharoplasty. Plast Reconstr Surg 1983;71:714.
129. Psillakis JM: Subperiosteal approach as an improved concept for correction of the aging face. Plast Reconstr Surg 1988;82:383.
130. Hamra ST: The deep-plane rhytidectomy. Plast Reconstr Surg 1990;86:53.
131. Ramirez OM, Maillard GF, Musolas A, et al: The extended subperiosteal lift: A definitive soft tissue remodeling for facial rejuvenation. Plast Reconstr Surg 1991;88:227.
132. Hamra ST: Composite rhytidectomy. Plast Reconstr Surg 1992;90:1.
133. Baker TJ, Gordon GL: Complications of rhytidectomy. Plast Reconstr Surg 1967;40:31.
134. Lemmon ML, Hamra ST: Skoog rhytidectomy: A 5-year experience with 577 patients. Plast Reconstr Surg 1980;65:283.
135. Baker DC: Complications of cervicofacial rhytidectomy. Clin Plast Surg 1983;10:543.
136. Owsley JQ Jr: The unfavorable result following face and neck lift. *In* Goldwyn RM (ed): The Unfavorable Result in Plastic Surgery: Avoidance and Treatment, ed 2, vol II. Boston, Little, Brown, 1984, p 591.
137. Duffy MJ, Friedland JA: The superficial-plane rhytidectomy revisited. Plast Reconstr Surg 1994;93:1392.
138. Rees TD, Lee YC, Coburn RJ: Expanding hematoma after rhytidectomy. Plast Reconstr Surg 1973;51:149.
139. Rees TD, Barone CM, Valuri FA, et al: Hematomas requiring surgical evacuation following face lift surgery. Plast Reconstr Surg 1994;93:1185.
140. Berner RE, Morain WD, Noe JM: Postoperative hypertension as an etiologic factor in hematoma after rhytidectomy. Plast Reconstr Surg 1976;57:314.
141. Mara JE, Baker JL: Hypertension and haematomas: Prophylaxis with Apresoline. Br J Plast Surg 1977;30:169.
142. Straith RE, Raju D, Hipps C: The study of hematomas in 500 consecutive face lifts. Plast Reconstr Surg 1977;59:694.
143. Rose FA, Wiemer DR: Platelet coagulopathy secondary to topical salicylate use. Ann Plast Surg 1983;11:340.
144. Klein JA: The tumescent technique for liposuction surgery. Am J Cosmetic Surg 1987;4:263.
145. Schoen SA, Taylor CO, Owsley TG: Tumescent technique in cervicofacial rhytidectomy. J Oral Maxillofac Surg 1994;52:344.
146. Huang TT, Blackwell SJ, Lewis SR: Routine use of suction drain in facial rhytidectomy. Ann Plast Surg 1987;18:30.
147. Goldwyn RM: Late bleeding after rhytidectomy from injury to the superficial temporal vessels. Plast Reconstr Surg 1991;88:433.
148. Lewin ML, Tsur H: Injuries of the great auricular nerve in rhytidectomy. Aesthetic Plast Surg 1978;1:409.
149. Pitanguy I, Ceravolo MP, Degand M: Nerve injuries during rhytidectomy: Considerations after 3203 cases. Aesthetic Plast Surg 1980;4:257.
150. McKinney P, Katrana DJ: Prevention of injury to the great auricular nerve during rhytidectomy. Plast Reconstr Surg 1980;66:675.
151. McKinney P, Gottlieb J: The relationship of the great auricular nerve to the superficial musculoaponeurotic system. Ann Plast Surg 1985;14:310.
152. Manstein CH, Manstein G: Bilateral neuromata of great auricular nerve 8 years following face lift. Plast Reconstr Surg 1985;76:937.
153. Baker DC, Conley J: Avoiding facial nerve injuries in rhytidectomy. Plast Reconstr Surg 1979;64:781.
154. Pitanguy I, Ramos AS: The frontal branch of the facial nerve: The importance of its variations in face lifting. Plast Reconstr Surg 1966;38:352.
155. Robbins TH: The protection of the frontal branch of the facial nerve in face lift surgery. Br J Plast Surg 1981;34:95.
156. Dingman RO, Grabb WC: Surgical anatomy of the mandibular ramus of the facial nerve based on dissection of 100 facial halves. Plast Reconstr Surg 1962;29:266.
157. Stuzin JM, Wagstrom L, Kawamoto HK, et al: Anatomy of the frontal branch of the facial nerve: The significance of the temporal fat pad. Plast Reconstr Surg 1989;83:265.
158. LeRoy JL Jr, Rees TD, Nolan WB III: Infections requiring hospital readmission following face lift surgery: Incidence and sequelae. Plast Reconstr Surg 1994;93:533.
159. Rees TD, Liverett DM, Guy CL: The effect of cigarette smoking on skin flap survival in the face lift patient. Plast Reconstr Surg 1984;73:911.
160. Riefkihl R, Wolfe JA, Cox EB, et al: Association between cutaneous occlusive vascular disease, cigarette smoking, and skin slough after rhytidectomy. Plast Reconstr Surg 1986;77:592.
161. Mulliken JB, Healey NA: Pathogenesis of skin flap necrosis from an underlying hematoma. Plast Reconstr Surg 1979;63:540.
162. Vecchione TR: Treatment of temporal scalp wound separation in the rhytidectomy patient. Plast Reconstr Surg 1984;73:837.
163. Ellenbogen R: Avoiding visual tipoffs to facelift surgery: A trouble-shooting guide. Clin Plast Surg 1992;19:447.
164. Parkes ML, Kamer FM, Bassilios MI: Treatment of alopecia in temporal region following rhytidectomy procedures. Laryngoscope 1977;87:1011.
165. Baker DC, Aston SJ, Guy CL, et al: The male rhytidectomy. Plast Reconstr Surg 1977;60:514.
166. Webster RC, Fanous N, Smith RC: Male and female face-lift incisions. Arch Otolaryngol 1982;108:299.
167. Peterson RA: Facelift: Inconspicuous scars about the ears. Clin Plast Surg 1992;19:425.

Section 3
The Long-Term Unfavorable Result

Chapter 16
THE LONG-TERM UNFAVORABLE RESULT IN ORTHOGNATHIC SURGERY I

Mandibular, Maxillary, and Combined Deformities

by

Douglas P. Sinn
G. E. Ghali

Introduction

The paramount goal of orthognathic and reconstructive maxillofacial surgery is to establish or reestablish a functional dental skeletal complex. As our understanding of the relationship between hard and soft tissues continues to grow, a concomitant goal has become the achievement of optimal soft tissue aesthetics. Both surgeon and orthodontist must fully understand the soft tissue responses to the planned surgical corrections if they are to avoid unfavorable aesthetic outcomes.[1,2] Additionally, long-term condylar occlusal, bite force, and neurosensory unfavorable outcomes are reviewed.

THE SUBJECTS DISCUSSED IN THIS CHAPTER ARE:

- Unfavorable aesthetic outcomes
  Maxillary skeletal surgery
  Mandibular skeletal surgery
- Unfavorable occlusal outcomes
- Neurosensory complications
- Unfavorable functional outcomes
  Mandibular hypomobility and TMJ dysfunction
  Compromised bite force

Unfavorable Aesthetic Outcomes

Maxillary Skeletal Surgery

In maxillary surgery, inaccurate transference of the planned treatment from the model surgery or cephalometric tracings to the operating room may result in unfavorable aesthetic outcomes. Unfavorable outcomes are also related to poor surgical execution and technique. Some of the more common technical errors related to maxillary surgery are (1) failure to remove posterior osseous interferences, (2) loss of vertical stops with overimpaction, (3) inadequate management of the anterior nasal spine, pyriform aperture, and/or nasal septum, (4) failure to control alar base width, and (5) improper closure of the circumvestibular incision.

Secondary soft tissue changes associated with maxillary surgery are similar to those found in the aging face.[3–5] These alterations include alar base widening,[3–7] thinning of the upper lip with loss of visible vermilion,[3–8] and downsloping of the commissures of the mouth.[3–7] Wolford and coworkers[1, 9] have postulated the following three etiological factors contributing to unfavorable post-orthognathic surgery soft tissue changes: (1) elevation of paranasal soft tissues without adequate reattachment, (2) increased osseous support in advancements, and (3) postoperative edema.

Upper Lip and Nose

Many surgeons have emphasized the importance of repositioning and reattaching the muscles that are detached during periosteal stripping for the Le Fort I osteotomy.[6, 9, 10] If left unattached, these muscles shorten and retract laterally, causing alar base flaring and upper lip thinning. One may also observe the apparent loss of visible vermilion from inclusion of excessive amounts of soft tissue during closure or an inappropriately high vestibular incision.[9]

Waite[11] has noted that the alar base widening often seen in association with maxillary surgery may be desirable in patients with vertical maxillary excess and narrow alar bases. Therefore, it is of extreme importance to assess the alar base width preoperatively, as these changes become undesirable in patients whose alar bases are wide before surgery.

The length and amount of exposed upper lip vermilion can essentially remain unchanged when the maxillary vestibular incision is closed utilizing a V–Y closure.[6] At the completion of the Le Fort I osteotomy, the upper lip vermilion is undermined with scissors; the vertical length of the V–Y closure is generally 20 to 30 mm (Fig. 16–1).[12] In 1983, Schendel and Williamson[10] discussed the regional anatomy of the perinasal musculature and described a technique for repositioning the nasolabial tissues in conjunction with a V–Y closure. Utilizing this technique for closure of maxillary ad-

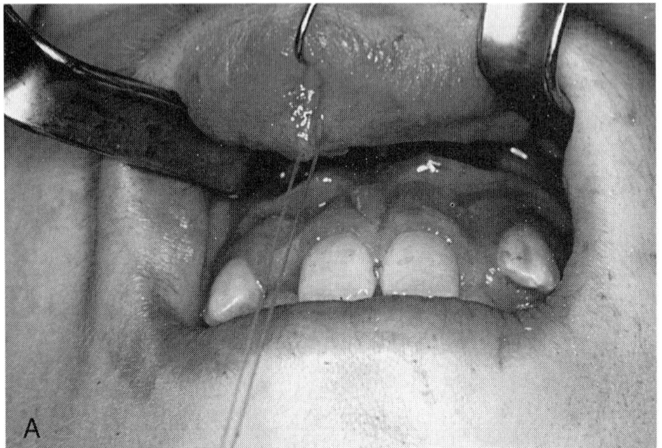

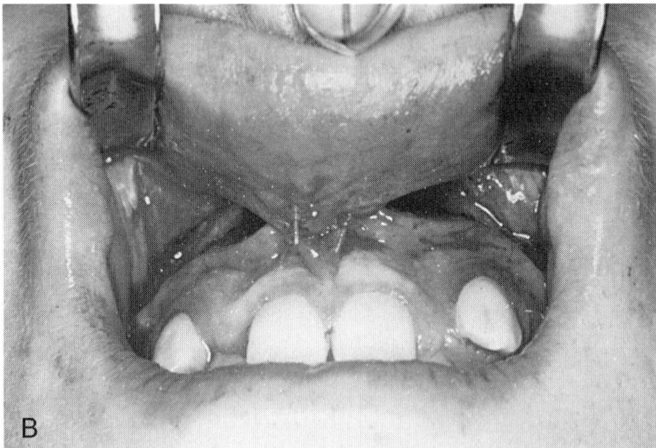

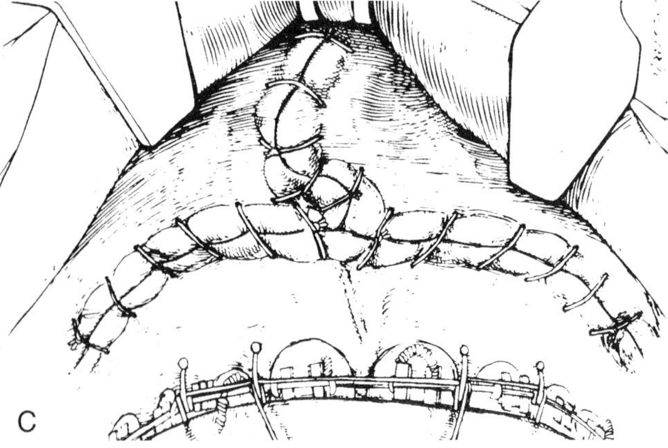

Figure 16–1. Technique for V–Y mucosal closure of Le Fort I incision. *A* demonstrates labial closure (vertical limb of "Y") prior to anchorage to alveolar mucosa *(B)*. *C* graphically depicts completed V–Y closure. (From Bell W (ed): Modern Practice in Orthognathic and Reconstructive Surgery. Philadelphia, WB Saunders, 1992, p 312.)

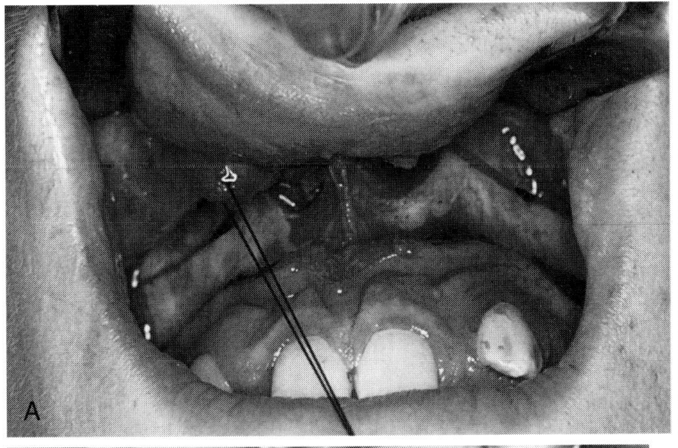

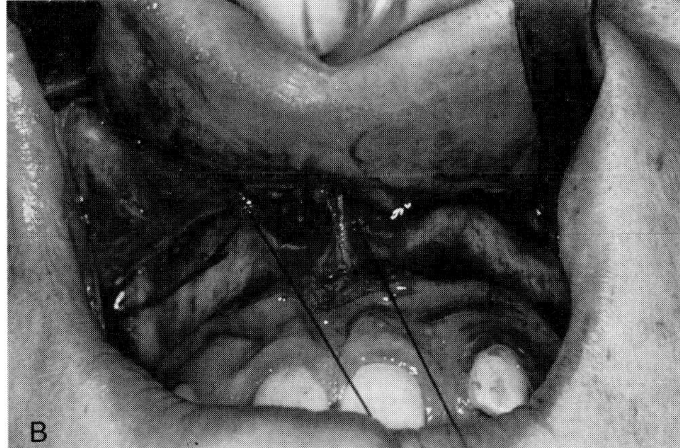

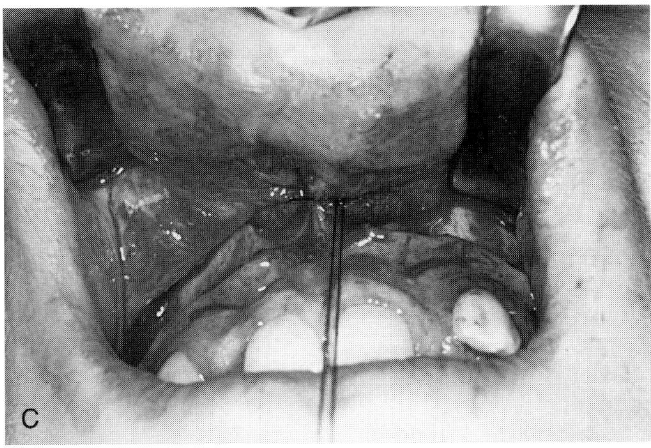

Figure 16–2. Technique for maxillary alar cinch suture. Alar base tissues are identified within the vestibular incision and individually secured on the right and left sides with permanent 2–0 suture material *(A, B)*. Suture is passed through a bur hole placed in the region of the anterior nasal spine and tightened to achieve the desired alar width *(C)*.

vancements, Carlotti and associates[6] were able to maintain preoperative lip form and length with a near one-to-one ratio of labial soft tissue advancement.

Whenever it is desirable to prevent widening of the alar base or to narrow it, a bilateral alar cinch is performed with maxillary surgery (Fig. 16–2).[13] Rarely, alar base widening may occur as a consequence of total maxillary surgery. We choose to manage such a case via a simple lateral nostril sill excision or Weir procedure with undermining and reapproximation (Fig. 16–3). Others have recommended secondary rhinoplasty for the correction of alar base widening and flattening of the upper lip in their patients following maxillary surgery.[14]

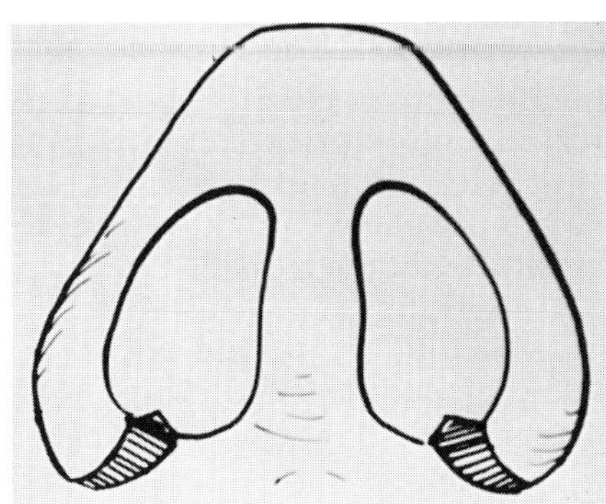

Figure 16–3. Technique for alar base reduction utilizing a modified Weir excision.

Additionally, inadequate removal of the inferior aspect of the cartilaginous nasal septum with resultant septal deviation or its excessive removal with resultant nasal tip droop may occur during maxillary surgery. The precise removal of specific amounts of cartilaginous septum should be accomplished at the termination of all maxillary surgery. When increased nasal tip projection is desired, minimal septal cartilage is removed, just enough to prevent septal deviation. On the other hand, when the nasal tip is overprojected, a small amount of the septum is removed such that it just falls short of the repositioned maxilla. Care should be taken to inspect the position of the septum prior to final stabilization of the maxilla, and also to inspect it again after nasal tubes are removed. If the septum was in the midline at the termination of surgery, but is found to be deviated after removal of the endotracheal tube, it should be straightened manually.

When the preceding considerations are not taken into account during the primary procedure, and complications result, the situation is best managed via a septorhinoplasty. If the problem is excessive nasal septal deviation or nasal tip elevation, an endonasal submucous septoplasty should be accomplished as soon as possible. The goal is to remove, via an intranasal transfixation incision, a specific amount of the caudal cartilaginous nasal septum. When excessive septum

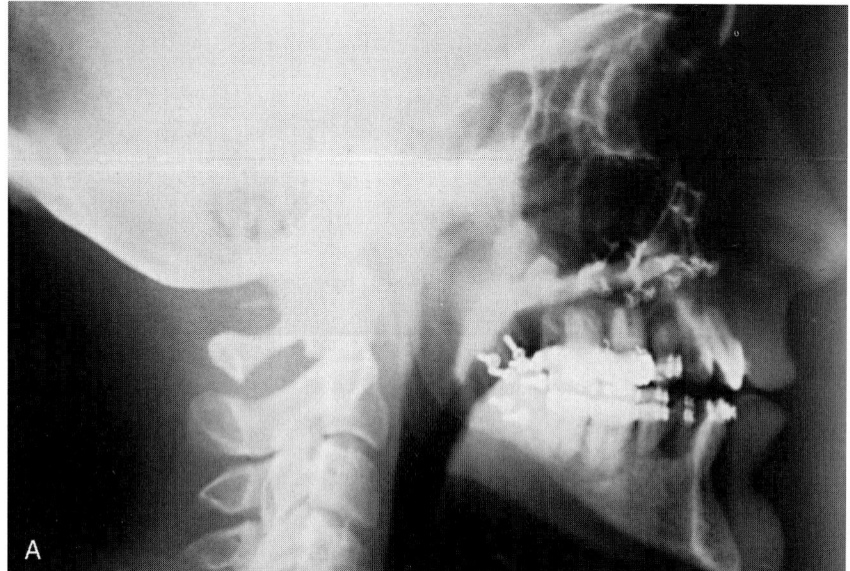

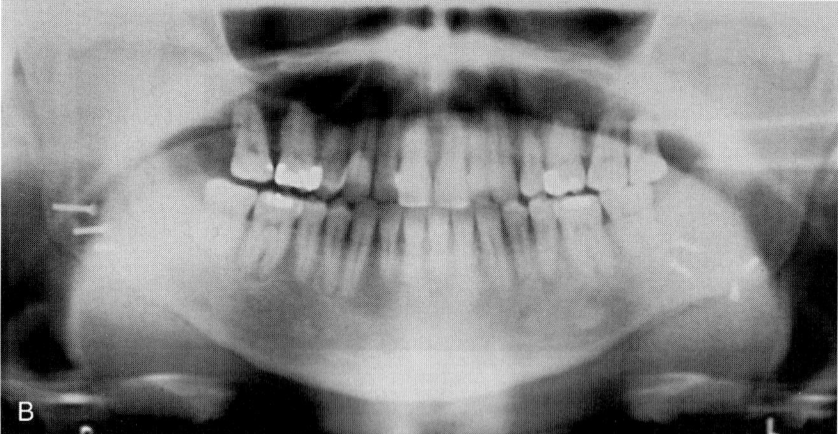

Figure 16–4. Cephalometric *(A)* and panographic, radiographic *(B)* appearance after proximal segment rotation with the loss of mandibular angle and antegonial notch anatomy.

has been removed, however, as evidenced by nasal tip droop, a delayed rhinoplasty should be considered after allowing 4 to 6 months for maxillary healing. The goal is usually accomplished via a combination of lower lateral cartilage repositioning, columellar strut placement, and tip grafting.

Exposure of Incisors

The maxillary central incisor is the keystone to vertical positioning of the maxilla during orthognathic surgery. Inadequate reduction of the exposed maxillary incisor and excessive reduction of the exposed maxillary incisor are the two vertical extremes inherent in maxillary orthognathic surgery. Inadequate reduction of exposed maxillary incisors is usually not of as great a significance, because the patient experiences a surgical change to a more positive appearance. Depending on the extent of exposure and patient desires, a secondary operation may not be necessary.

Of more significance, relative to unfavorable aesthetics, is excessive reduction of the exposed maxillary central incisors. Patients exhibiting vertical maxillary excess who undergo excessive vertical maxillary repositioning typically develop an edentulous appearance. This is a negative surgical change that requires early reoperation and the placement of autogenous bone grafts for vertical support.

Mandibular Skeletal Surgery

Poor proximal segment control and failure to reapproximate the mentalis muscle after genioplasty are the two most common errors committed during mandibular orthognathic surgery that result in unfavorable aesthetics.[12, 15–18] The use of rigid fixation techniques over the past decade has introduced additional variables that may affect the aesthetic outcome of orthognathic surgery. Rigid fixation techniques are known to be less forgiving than wiring techniques and may result in postoperative asymmetries.[19–21] Postoperative relapse may progressively result in unfavorable aesthetics and is related to poor technique, preoperative orthodontic compensations, continued patient growth, and condylar remodeling.[12, 22–25]

Submental-Neck Region and Gonial Angle

The careful assessment of the patient's cervical-mental region is of paramount importance, particularly in the planning of a mandibular setback procedure.[12, 26] In patients with ill-defined cervical-mental proportions or short submental lengths, mandibular setback surgery predictably worsens the conditions, resulting in a "double-chin" appearance. This unfavorable aesthetic result can be minimized by incorporating a concomitant advancement genioplasty and/or a submental liposuction procedure.

Inadequate stabilization of the mandibular segments or failure to properly reposition the segments prior to stabilization may result in proximal segment rotation with the loss of gonial angle definition. The unfavorable aesthetic appearance secondary to loss of gonial angle definition is best evaluated from the profile view (Fig. 16–4). When loss of gonial angle definition follows mandibular surgery, options for correction are (1) reoperation with repositioning of the segments if the complication is diagnosed in the first 3 weeks postoperatively, and (2) augmentation via autogenous or alloplastic materials if the complication was not treated in the early phase of bone healing (Fig. 16–5).

LaBanc and coworkers[27] address the problem of the more severe, long-standing situation in which the proximal segment rotation is associated with mandibular dysfunction as well as unfavorable facial aesthetics. They state that the resulting mandibular anatomy is usually not conductive to predictably recreating a sagittal slit and recommend a transfacial approach with bone grafting and bone plate stabilization.

Lower Lip and Chin

In the lower lip, ptosis is the most common unfavorable aesthetic problem associated with mandibular

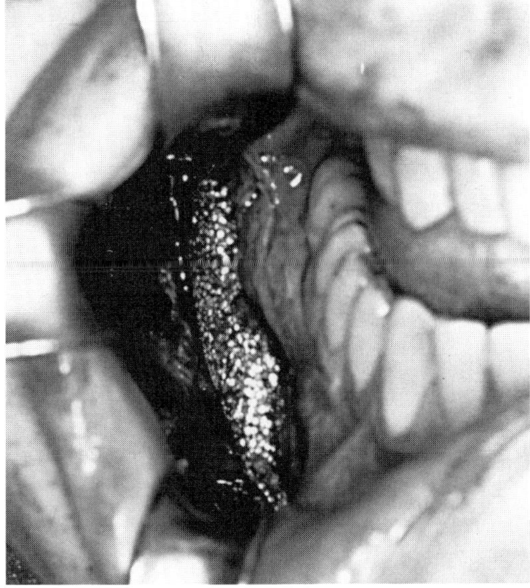

Figure 16–5. Placement of alloplast to treat unfavorable gonial and definition secondary to poor proximal segment position.

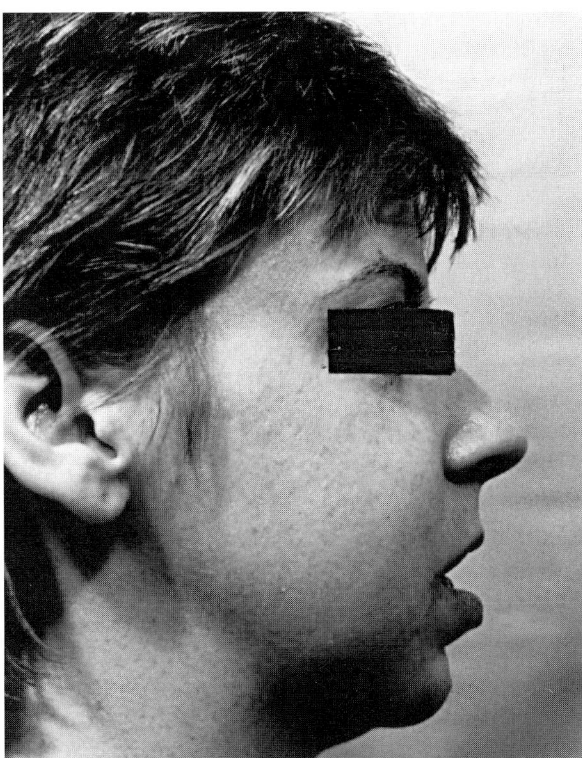

Figure 16–6. Clinical appearance of patient with lip ptosis secondary to lack of mentalis muscle approximation after genioplasty.

symphysis surgery (Fig. 16–6). Lower lip ptosis is predictable after complete degloving of the symphysis without proper mentalis muscle reapproximation. Prevention of lower lip ptosis is achieved by preservation of at least 1 cm of inferior border chin attachment and primary reapproximation of the mentalis muscles.[12] When this complication is recognized in the immediate postoperative phase, the chin is reopened, the muscles are reattached, and the chin is taped for 3 to 4 days. In the event of delayed reconstruction, we prefer to deglove the symphysis completely and dissect free the mentalis muscles. With slowly absorbable suture, the mentalis muscles are tagged and resuspended to the canine teeth bilaterally. Additionally, the chin is taped during the initial healing phase.

In evaluating the soft tissue changes associated with advancement genioplasty, Gallagher and coworkers[28] detailed factors that may compromise the results of chin surgery. They noted the following contributions to poor genioplasty results: incorrect planning, vestibular scarring, excessive detachment of soft tissue from the chin, suprahyoid myotomy, improper closure of the soft tissue incision, hematoma formation, genial remodeling, and excessive bone resorption.

Chin ptosis, or "witch's chin," is the most common unaesthetic complication in the chin if one excludes problems associated with improper treatment planning.[29] Chin ptosis results from either a degloving dissection in the symphysis region or lack of reattachment of the mentalis muscle at the time of surgery. This leads to inferior tissue prolapse, causing excess interlabial incompetence, lower tooth exposure, and redundant submental tissue.[30, 31] Prevention of these problems is easier than their secondary correction.

Unfavorable Occlusal Outcomes

Some minor malocclusions after orthognathic surgery, particularly those that are of little or no functional or aesthetic consequence, are often acceptble to both patient and surgeon. When unfavorable postoperative occlusion is first identified, the surgeon and orthodontist must jointly assess the problem and concur on the treatment options. In addition to a clinical occlusal evaluation, all orthognathic surgery patients should receive an immediate postoperative cephalometric radiograph. The preoperative predication tracing should be superimposed onto this radiograph to evaluate the occlusal result cephalometrically.

For the purpose of this discussion, only those unfavorable occlusal outcomes that manifest in the late (months to years) postoperative period are considered. Classically, postoperative occlusal probles are categorized as anteroposterior, vertical, or transverse.[12, 32] Idiopathic condylar resorption and unfavorable growth are the two most common causes of unfavorable long-term anteroposterior malocclusions.[12, 32] As the term applies, the exact etiology of idiopathic condylar resorption is unknown, and multiple investigators have speculated as to its cause.[33, 34] Idiopathic condylar resorption typically produces a gradual and late relapse after orthognathic surgery, with the development of a class II open bite malocclusion (Fig. 16–7).[35, 36] For proper documentation of condylar resorption, sequential cephalometric and tomographic radiographs should be obtained at 6-month intervals. The classic cephalometric findings after sagittal split osteotomies are slowly progressive B-point posterior movement with migration of the screws or wires toward the glenoid fossa.[33] In our experience, the malocclusion can be managed with maxillary surgery only after B-point stability has been established via sequential radiographs. Other options are condylar reconstruction to reestablish vertical dimension and sagittal split osteotomies of the mandibular ramus to correct anteroposterior and vertical problems.

Epker and Fish[12] describe the late unfavorable occlu-

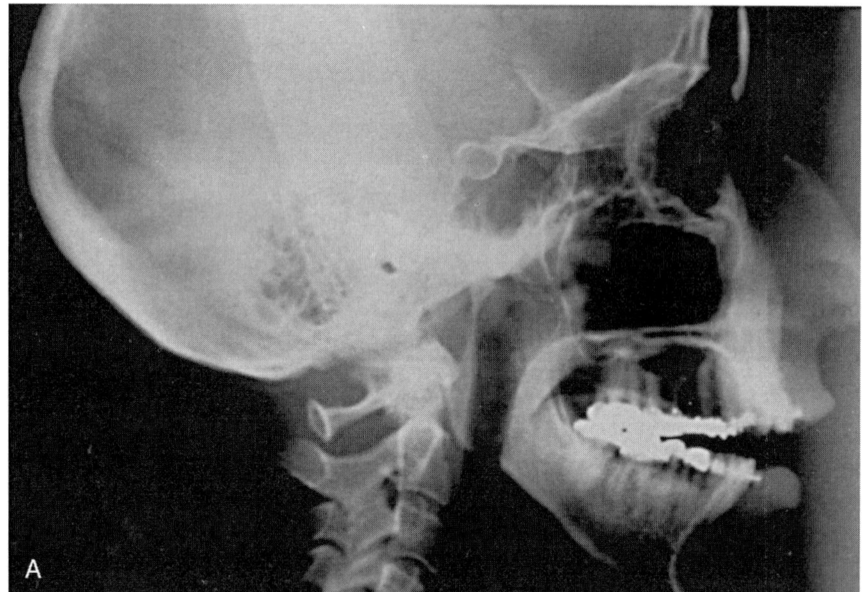

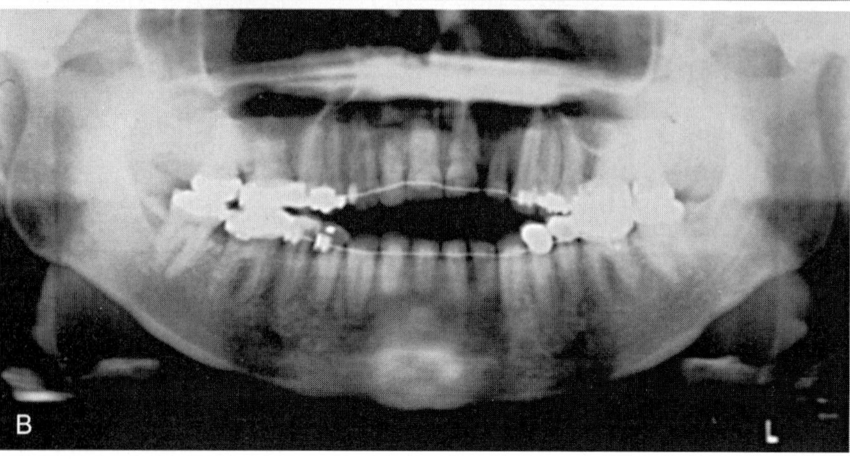

Figure 16–7. *A* and *B*, Radiographic appearance of facial skeleton with open bite and clockwise rotation of mandible secondary to idiopathic condylar resorption.

sal outcomes that develop secondary to disproportionate cranial base–maxillary–mandibular growth.[12] They recommend obtaining serial cephalometric radiographs and delaying definitive orthognathic surgery until growth has ceased.

Unfavorable long-term malocclusions in the vertical plane are classified as posterior or anterior open bites. Most posterior and anterior open bites are evident in the immediate or early postoperative period and are not discussed here. In some instances, maxillary or mandibular incisor teeth may become extruded during presurgical orthodontics. This event produces an unstable condition, with the development of an anterior open bite manifesting months to years after surgery; correction usually requires reoperation after the removal of orthodontic compensations.

Unfavorable transverse malocclusions may result from orthodontic relapse, skeletal relapse, a combination of the two, or poorly adapted rigid fixation appliance.[12, 32] These problems often require reoperation followed by long-term orthodontic retention to salvage the occlusion. In some cases, minor transverse discrepancies may be tolerated.

Neurosensory Complications

By virtue of the proximity of orthognathic surgery to the peripheral branches of the trigeminal and facial nerves, neurologic disturbances are not uncommon. Many surgeons have studied the incidence and severity of neurosensory complications after orthognathic surgery.[21, 37–56] In general, most such injuries result in favorable outcomes, although great variability in nerve dysfunction is reported. The key to managing neurosensory disturbances involves serial examinations to monitor the magnitude of the deficit and the outcome of regeneration. The clinical neurosensory examination consists of five basic tests used to assess touch, pain, and thermal sensitivity.[56, 57] In our protocol in patients exhibiting neurosensory deficits, such tests are administered immediately postoperatively, at 1 month, 3 months, and 6 months following surgery and then every 6 months or until sensation is recovered.

Although all orthognathic procedures have been examined for the potential of neurosensory dysfunction, the sagittal split ramus osteotomy (SSRO) of the mandible has been studied the most. The general consensus is that the SSRO has the greatest propensity to produce such neurosensory deficits, with reported rates ranging from as high as 85% to as low as 20%.[37–57] Transient neurologic disturbances of the lower lip and chin are common after SSRO of the mandible. Although this deficit may disappear within a few months, it may persist indefinitely. In 1978, Peppersack and Chausse[47] reported on the long-term follow-up of the sagittal splitting technique for correction of mandibular prognathism. Some of the patients in their study described the return of sensation as occurring as long as 4 years postoperatively; in our opinion, this is the exception rather than the rule.

Neurosensory dysfunction following vertical ramus osteotomies of the mandible has been studied by several investigators.[42, 50–53] The most consistent finding is an overall lower incidence of neurologic dysfunction compared with the SSRO of the mandible. There still exists, however, a wide variability in the reported incidence of deficits, ranging from 50% to 0%.[46, 53] Neurosensory dysfunction associated with genioplasty procedures has also been noted to be less prevalent than that reported for the sagittal split procedure.[37, 38] Nishioka and coworkers[38] evaluated 15 patients treated with genioplasties and detected only 1 nerve of 30 tested with a neurosensory deficit 26 months postoperatively; the remaining had complete recovery. Neurosensory deficits after Le Fort I osteotomy of the maxilla have not been widely investigated or reported in the literature; most studies focus on alterations in intraoral sensation or tooth vitality.[54, 55] The only investigation that prospectively evaluated the cutaneous recovery patterns following the most commonly performed orthognathic surgical procedures in 22 patients was published in 1990.[56] In this study, the SSRO group had the highest percentage of sites with immediate postsurgical neurosensory deficits (67% to 72%), followed by the Le Fort I osteotomy (50% to 58%), genioplasty (6% to 27%), and intraoral vertical osteotomy groups (11% to 18%). Most importantly, over the 6-month recovery period, each surgical group approached preoperative levels of sensation at variable rates, with the Le Fort group recovering the fastest (96% within 3 months) and the SSRO group the slowest (90% within 6 months). Interestingly, in none of the studied surgical groups was a statistically significant correlation evident between the severity of the initial neurosensory deficit and length of time to complete recovery.

If the inferior alveolar nerve is transected, immediate microneurosurgical repair in an epineural fashion is the recommendation.[58, 59] Neuropraxia-type injuries generally show almost complete recovery within 1 month postoperatively. For axonotmesis-type injuries, one would expect recovery to take several months. In these injuries, neurosensory examinations are serially performed utilizing the preceding protocol, and surgery is delayed as long as sensibility is improving. If the anesthesia persists for more than 1 month or there is no improvement in cutaneous sensibility, surgical exploration should be done. Paresthesias usually do not benefit from surgical exploration. On the other hand, painful nerve injuries that persist for more than 1 month without evidence of subsiding generally warrant surgical exploration.

Unfavorable Functional Outcomes

Unfavorable functional outcomes are divided into mandibular hypomobility, temporomandibular joint (TM) dysfunction, and compromised bite force. For the purposes of this discussion, mandibular hypomobility and TMJ dysfunction are considered jointly. Multiple investigators have reported these unfavorable functional outcomes for both the intraoral vertical ramus osteotomy[60–69] and SSRO[48, 61, 62, 70–78] of the mandible.

Mandibular Hypomobility and Temporomandibular Joint Dysfunction

In 1983, O'Ryan and Epker[71] evaluated 10 patients at least 2 years after they had undergone sagittal split osteotomies for mandibular advancement; they found a mean interincisal opening of just over 42 mm. In their comparison of preoperative with postoperative mandibular range of motion in a prospective manner, Aragon and colleagues[72] found that maximum interincisal opening went from a preoperative value of 56.7 mm to 39.9 mm after mandibular advancement via SSRO followed by 6 weeks of intermaxillary fixation. Boyd and coworkers[62] evaluating recovery of mandibular mobility following orthognathic surgery, found a functional return to normal within 3 months postoperatively. In this study of mandibular advancement patients stabilized with rigid screw fixation without intermaxillary fixation, the nearly normal interincisal preoperative opening (50.7 mm) was maintained postoperatively (46.7 mm).

With mandibular setback procedures utilizing the SSRO, there also is a tendency, although lesser, toward postoperative mandibular hypomobility. In 1987, Stacy[74] studied the recovery of opening following SSRO for mandibular prognathism. In this study, 40 patients were evaluated, and 95% demonstrated normal vertical mandibular function 6 to 9 months postoperatively. In 1988, Ellis and coworkers[75] compared stimulated bite force after mandibular advancement utilizing nonrigid and rigid fixation. They theorized that counterclockwise proximal segment rotation results in shortening of the pterygomasseteric and temporalis muscles. These findings, in combination with a period of intermaxillary fixation, predispose to muscle atrophy and eventual mandibular hypomobility.

Limited mandibular range of motion following orthognathic surgery can have extracapsular or intracapsular causes. Extracapsular problems are low-intensity, dull aches that are diffuse and not always aggravated by mandibular movements. Intracapsular problems, however, are generally sharp pains localized to the temporomandibular joints and aggravated by mandibular movements.

Regardless of the etiology, physical therapy should be recommended for all orthognathic surgery patients. In our experience, the technique best suited for most orthognathic surgery patients is the one described by Epker and Fish,[12] involving a combination of isotonic and isometric exercises, which the patient practices in front of a mirror for 15 minutes four times a day. Prior to the planned surgical procedure, the patient is allowed an opportunity to practice in the office in front of a mirror and is shown the preoperative maximal interincisal opening. The patient is then instructed that this opening should be regained within 1 month postoperatively; if it is not achieved within 1 month, diagnostic evaluation is started to search for intracapsular versus extracapsular etiologies. The diagnostic evaluation consists of a careful history, palpation of muscles and temporomandibular joints, an intraoral examination, and imaging studies. According to the literature, possible etiologies of mandibular hypomobility include intracapsular ankylosis, anterior disk displacements, noncompliance with postoperative physiotherapy, psychogenic factors, masticatory muscle discomfort, excessive scarring, and muscle contracture.[56, 61, 69, 73, 74] For each of these etiologies (except ankylosis), nonoperative measures should be tried initially, followed by surgical intervention in the most severe or unresponsive cases.

Many investigators have found unfavorable changes in the temporomandibular joint following SSRO of the mandible.[24, 71, 78] Overall, these unfavorable changes ranged from surface erosions and sclerosis to ankylosis to complete atrophy of the condyles. As previously discussed in the section on unfavorable occlusal outcomes, most cases of postsurgical condylar resorption occur 18 to 30 months postoperatively and present as relapse into a class II open-bite malocclusion. Mandibular hypomobility secondary to disk malpositioning should initially be managed via jaw manipulation, splint therapy, and joint lavage. In the most severe or unresponsive cases, arthrotomy with disk repositioning or plication should be accomplished. Obviously, true TMJ ankylosis should be managed with arthrotomy followed by aggressive physiotherapy. Several investigators have evaluated the effect of the vertical ramus osteotomy on the temporomandibular joints.[64–68] All studies evaluated condylar–proximal segment positioning as well as skeletal remodeling, but none critically evaluated temporomandibular joint function clinically. Overall, the incidence of TMJ dysfunction following the SSRO with rigid fixation or the intraoral vertical ramus osteotomy is low.[43, 80, 81]

Compromised Bite Force

Dechow and Carlson[76] studied the occlusal force after advancement of the mandible in the adult rhesus monkey. They consistently detected a reduction in masticatory bite force for up to 1 year after SSRO in combination with 6 weeks of intermaxillary fixation for mandibular advancement. Two years later, Ellis collaborated with the same investigators[75] and found that bite force was reduced postoperatively in primates regardless of whether intermaxillary fixation was utilized or not. Although the intermaxillary group had a greater degree of early postoperative reduction in bite force, the two groups showed comparable reductions in bite force at the ninth postoperative week. Some surgeons have published variable results relative to postoperative bite force changes. In a study by Proffit and associates,[77] some patients demonstrated increases in bite force one year postoperatively, but others had decreases in bite force following SSRO for mandibular advancement.

Summary

The majority of late postoperative complications are optimally avoided by meticulous treatment planning. In general, complications can be anticipated on the basis of preoperative clinical and radiographic findings. As a general rule, complications in the postoperative phase of orthognathic surgery are best managed prior to bony healing if possible.

References

1. Guymon M, Crosby DR, Wolford LM: The alar base cinch suture to control nasal width in maxillary osteotomies. Int J Adult Orthod Orthogn Surg 1988;3:89.
2. Sakima T, Sachdeva R: Soft tissue response to Le Fort I maxillary impaction surgery. Int J Adult Orthod Orthogn Surg 1987;4:221.
3. O'Ryan F, Schendel S: Nasal anatomy and maxillary surgery. I: Esthetic and anatomic principles. Int J Adult Orthod Orthogn Surg 1989;4:27.
4. O'Ryan F, Schendel S: Nasal anatomy and maxillary surgery. II: Unfavorable nasolabial esthetics following the Le Fort I osteotomy. Int J Adult Orthod Orthogn Surg 1989;4:75.
5. O'Ryan F, Schendel S, Carlotti A: Nasal anatomy and maxillary surgery. III: Surgical techniques for correction of nasal deformities in patients undergoing maxillary surgery. Int J Adult Orthod Orthogn Surg 1989;4:157.
6. Carlotti A, Aschaffensburg P, Schendel S: Facial changes associated with surgical advancement of the lip and maxilla. J Oral Maxillofac Surg 1986;44:593.
7. Schendel S, Delaire J: Facial muscles: Form, function, and reconstruction in dentofacial deformities. *In* Bell WH, Proffit WR, White RP (eds): Surgical Correction of Dentofacial Deformities. Philadelphia, WB Saunders, 1980, pp 259–280.
8. Tomlak D, Piecuch J, Weinstein S: Morphologic analysis of upper lip area following maxillary osteotomy via the tunneling approach. Am J Orthod 1984;85:488.
9. Wolford L: Discussion of Rosen H: Lip-nasal aesthetics following Le Fort I osteotomy. Plast Reconstr Surg 1988;81:180.
10. Schendel S, Williamson L: Muscle reorientation following superior repositioning of the maxilla. J Oral Maxillofac Surg 1983;41:235.
11. Waite P: Simultaneous orthognathic surgery and rhinoplasty. Oral Maxillofac Surg Clin North Am 1990;2:339.
12. Epker B, Fish L: Definitive immediate presurgical planning. *In* Dentofacial Deformities: Integrated Orthodontic and Surgical Correction, vol 1. St Louis, CV Mosby, 1986, pp 103–127.
13. Collins P, Epker B: The alar cinch: A technique for prevention of alar base flaring secondary to maxillary surgery: Oral Surg Oral Med Oral Pathol 1982;53:549.
14. Bell W, McBride K: Correction of the long face syndrome by Le Fort I osteotomy. Oral Surg Oral Med Oral Pathol 1977;44:493.
15. Jonsson E, Svartz K, Welander U: Mandibular rami osteotomies and their effect on the gonial angle. Int J Oral Surg 1981;10:168.
16. Rubens B, West R: Ptosis of the chin and lip incompetence: Consequences of lost mentalis muscle support. J Oral Maxillofac Surg 1989;47:359.
17. Wylie G, Epker B: Control of the condylar–proximal mandibular segments after sagittal split osteotomy to advance the mandible. Oral Surg Oral Med Oral Pathol 1986;62:613.
18. Ellis E: Condylar positioning devices for orthognathic surgery: Are they necessary? J Oral Maxillofac Surg 1994;52:536.
19. Buckley M, Tulloch J, White R, et al: Complications of orthognathic surgery: A comparison between wire fixation and rigid fixation. Int J Adult Orthod Orthogn Surg 1989;4:69.
20. Turvey T, Hall F: Intraoral self-threading screw fixation for sagittal osteotomies: Early experiences. Int J Adult Orthod Orthogn Surg 1986;1:243.
21. Schendel S, Epker B: Results after mandibular advancement surgery: An analysis of 87 cases. J Oral Surg 1980;38:265.
22. Ive J, McNeill R, West R: Mandibular advancement: Skeletal and dental changes during fixation. J Oral Surg 1977;35:881.
23. McNeill R, Hooley J, Sundberg R: Skeletal relapse during intermaxillary fixation. J Oral Surg 1973;31:212.
24. Phillips R, Bell W: Atrophy of mandibular condyles after sagittal ramus split osteotomy: Report of case. J Oral Surg 1978;36:45.
25. Sesenna E, Raffaini M: Bilateral condylar atrophy after combined osteotomy for correction of mandibular retrusion. J Maxillofac Surg 1985;13:263.
26. Betts N, Fonseca R: Soft tissue changes associated with orthognathic surgery. *In* Bell W (ed): Modern Practice in Orthognathic and Reconstructive Surgery. Philadelphia, WB Saunders, 1992, pp 2170–2209.
27. La Banc J, Epker B, Jones D, et al: Nerve sharing by an interpositional sural nerve graft between the great auricular and inferior alveolar nerve to restore lower lip sensation. J Oral Maxillofac Surg 1987;45:621.
28. Gallagher D, Bell W, Storum K: Soft tissue changes associated with advancement genioplasty performed concomitantly with superior repositioning of the maxilla. J Oral Maxillofac Surg 1984;42:238.
29. Bell W, Brammer J, McBride K, et al: Reduction genioplasty: Surgical techniques and soft tissue changes. Oral Surg Oral Med Oral Pathol 1981;51:471.
30. Bell W, Gallagher D: The versatility of genioplasty using a broad pedicle. J Oral Maxillofac Surg 1983;41:763.
31. Scheideman G, Legan H, Bell W: Soft tissue changes with combined mandibular setback and advancement genioplasty. J Oral Surg 1981;39:505.
32. Sinclair P, Thomas P, Tucker M: Common complications in orthognathic surgery: Etiology and management. *In* Bell W (ed): Modern Practice in Orthognathic and Reconstructive Surgery. Philadelphia, WB Saunders, 1992, pp 49–82.
33. Arnett G, Tamborello J, Rathbone J: Temporomandibular joint ramifications of orthognathic surgery. *In* Bell W (ed): Modern Practice in Orthognathic and Reconstructive Surgery. Philadelphia, WB Saunders, 1992, pp 523–591.
34. Arnett G, Tamborello J: Progressive class II development: Female idiopathic condylar resorption. Oral Maxillofac Surg Clin 1990;2:699.
35. Doyle M: Stability and complication in 50 consecutively treated surgical-orthodontic patients: A retrospective longitudinal analysis from private practice. Int J Adult Orthod Orthogn Surg 1986;1:23.
36. Worms F: Posttreatment stability and esthetics of orthognathic surgery. Angle Orthod 1980;50:251.
37. Lindquist C, Obeid G: Complications of genioplasty done alone or in combination with sagittal split-ramus osteotomy. Oral Surg Oral Med Oral Pathol 1988;66:12.
38. Nishioka G, Mason M, Van Sickels J: Neurosensory disturbance associated with the anterior mandibular horizontal osteotomy. J Oral Maxillofac Surg 1988;46:107.
39. Nishioka G, Zysset M, Van Sickels J: Neurosensory disturbance with rigid fixation of the bilateral sagittal split osteotomy. J Oral Maxillofac Surg 1987;45:20.
40. Campbell R, Shamaskin R, Harkins S: Assessment of recovery from injury to inferior alveolar and mental nerves. Oral Surg Oral Med Oral Pathol 1987;64:519.
41. Coghlan K, Irvine G: Neurological damage after sagittal split osteotomy. Int J Oral Maxillofac Surg 1986;15:369.
42. Zaytoun H, Phillips C, Terry B: Long-term neurosensory deficits following transoral vertical ramus and sagittal split osteotomies for mandibular prognathism. J Oral Maxillofac Surg 1986;44:193.
43. Paulus G, Steinhauser E: A comparative study of wire osteosynthesis versus bone screws in the treatment of mandibular prognathism. Oral Surg Oral Med Oral Pathol 1982;54:2.
44. Brusati R, Fiamminghi L, Sesenna E, et al: Functional disturbances of the inferior alveolar nerve after sagittal osteotomy of the mandibular ramus: Operating technique for prevention. J Maxillofac Surg 1981;9:123.
45. MacIntosh R: Experience with the sagittal osteotomy of the mandibular ramus: A 13 year review. J Maxillofac Surg 1981;8:151.
46. Walter J, Gregg J: Analysis of postsurgical neurologic alteration in the trigeminal nerve. J Oral Surg 1979;37:410.
47. Peppersack W, Chausse J: Long term follow-up of the sagittal splitting technique for correction of mandibular prognathism. J Maxillofac Surg 1978;6:117.
48. Freihofer H, Petresevic D: Late results after advancing the mandible by sagittal splitting of the rami. J Maxillofac Surg 1975;3:250.
49. Behrman S: Complications of sagittal osteotomy of the mandibular ramus. J Oral Surg 1972;30:554.
50. Hall H, McKenna S: Further refinement and evaluation of intraoral vertical ramus osteotomy. J Oral Maxillofac Surg 1987; 45:684.

51. Tuinzing D, Greebe R: Complications related to the intraoral vertical ramus osteotomy. Int J Oral Surg 1985;14:319.
52. Hall H, Chase D, Payor L: Evaluation and refinement of the intraoral vertical subcondylar osteotomy. J Oral Surg 1975;33:333.
53. Massey G, Chase D, Thomas P, et al: Intraoral oblique osteotomy of the mandibular ramus. J Oral Surg 1974;32:755.
54. Kahnberg K, Engstrom H: Recovery of maxillary sinus and tooth sensibility after Le Fort I osteotomy. Br J Oral Maxillofac Surg 1987;25:68.
55. de Jongh M, Barnard D, Birnie D: Sensory nerve morbidity following Le Fort I osteotomy. J Maxillofac Surg 1986;14:10.
56. Karas N, Boyd S, Sinn D: Recovery of neurosensory function following orthognathic surgery. J Oral Maxillofac Surg 1990; 48:124.
57. Ghali G, Epker B: Clinical neurosensory testing: Practical applications. J Oral Maxillofac Surg 1989;47:1074.
58. Bell W, Proffitt W, White R: Surgical Correction of Dentofacial Deformities. Philadelphia, WB Saunders, 1980; pp 248–680, 854–916.
59. Sinn D, Ghali G: Management of intraoperative complications in orthognathic surgery. Oral Maxillofac Surg Clin 1990;2:869.
60. Quinn P, Wedell D: Complications from intraoral vertical subsigmoid osteotomy: Review of literature and report of two cases. Int J Adult Orthod Orthogn Surg 1988;4:189.
61. Storum K, Bell W: Hypomobility after maxillary and mandibular osteotomies. Oral Surg Oral Med Oral Pathol 1984;57:7.
62. Boyd S, Karas N, Sinn D: Recovery of mandibular mobility following orthognathic surgery. J Oral Maxillofac Surg 1991; 49:924.
63. Astrand P, Ridell A: Positional changes of the mandible and the upper and lower anterior teeth after oblique sliding osteotomy of the mandibular rami. Scand J Plast Reconstr Surg 1973;7:120.
64. Hollender L, Ridell A: Radiography of the temporomandibular joint after oblique sliding osteotomy of the mandibular rami. Scand J Dent Res 1974;82:466.
65. Wisth P, Tornes K: Radiographic changes in the temporomandibular joint subsequent to vertical ramus osteotomy. Int J Oral Surg 1975;4:242.
66. Sund G, Eckerdal O, Astrand P: Changes in the temporomandibular joint after oblique sliding osteotomy of the mandibular rami. J Maxillofac Surg 1973;11:87.
67. Eckerdal O, Sund G, Astrand P: Skeletal remodelling in the temporomandibular joint after oblique sliding osteotomy of the mandibular rami. Int J Oral Maxillofac Surg 1986;15:233.
68. Weinberg S, Craft J: Unilateral atrophy of the mandibular condyle after closed subcondylar osteotomy for correction of mandibular prognathism. J Oral Surg 1980;38:366.
69. Troyer S: Ankylosis of the coronoid process of the mandible to the zygomatic arch subsequent to the surgical correction of prognathism. J Hosp Dent Pract 1971;5:19.
70. White R, Peters P, Costich E, Page H: Evaluation of sagittal split ramus osteotomy in 17 patients. J Oral Surg 1969;27:851.
71. O'Ryan F, Epker B: Surgical orthodontics and the temporomandibular joint. II. Mandibular advancement via modified sagittal split ramus osteotomies. Am J Orthod 1983;83:408.
72. Aragon S, Van Sickels J, Dolwick M, et al: The effects of orthognathic surgery on mandibular range of motion. J Oral Maxillofac Surg 1985;43:938.
73. Edlund J, Hansson T, Petersson A, Willmar K: Sagittal splitting of the mandibular ramus. Scand J Plast Reconstr Surg 1979;13:437.
74. Stacy G: Recovery of oral opening following sagittal ramus osteotomy for mandibular prognathism. J Oral Maxillofac Surg 1987;45:487.
75. Ellis E, Dechow P, Carlson D: A comparison of stimulated bite force after mandibular advancement using rigid and nonrigid fixation. J Oral Maxillofac Surg 1988;46:26.
76. Dechow P, Carlson D: Occlusal force after mandibular advancement in adult rhesus monkeys. J Oral Maxillofac Surg 1986; 44:887.
77. Proffitt W, Turvey T, Fields H, Phillips C: The effect of orthognathic surgery on occlusal force. J Oral Maxillofac Surg 1989;47:457.
78. Worms F, Spiedel T, Brevis R: Post-treatment stability and esthetics of orthognathic surgery. Angle Orthod 1980;50:251.
79. Nitzan D, Dolwick M: Temporomandibular joint fibrous ankylosis following orthognathic surgery: Report of eight cases. Int J Adult Orthod Orthogen Surg 1989;4:7.
80. Nickerson J, Veaco N: Condylotomy in surgery of the temporomandibular joint. Oral Maxillofac Surg Clin North Am 1989;1:2, 303.
81. Spitzer W, Steinhauser E: Condylar position following ramus osteotomy and functional osteosynthesis: A clinical function analytic and computer tomographic study. Int J Oral Maxillofac Surg 1987;16:257.

Chapter 17
THE LONG-TERM UNFAVORABLE RESULT IN ORTHOGNATHIC SURGERY II

Injury to the Temporomandibular Joint and Trigeminal Nerve

by

G. William Arnett
Stephen Milam

Introduction

Both temporomandibular joint (TMJ) and trigeminal nerve injury may be associated with orthognathic surgery. These problems are normal and generally self-correcting side effects of orthognathic surgery. When these injuries are persistent and do not resolve, patients and doctors may be dissatisfied with the treatment outcome.

THE SUBJECTS DISCUSSED IN THIS CHAPTER ARE:

Injuries to the Temporomandibular Joint

Condylar resorption is a late temporomandibular (TMJ) complication associated with orthognathic surgery. If the resorption is significant, the distance from condylion to the lower incisors shortens, resulting in a class II dental relationship. Surgical compression of the condyles and systemic factors affecting the response of the condyles to the surgical compression are responsible for condylar resorption and late mandibular relapse.

Compression of the mandibular condyle stimulates direct resorptive remodeling at the site of injury owing to local tissue disruption and impaired cellular functions. Additionally, the entire mandibular condyle can undergo a remodeling change as a result of a number of systemic factors that are not yet fully understood.

TMJ Compression Related to Treatment

Any mechanical stress provokes molecular, soft tissue, and osseous adaptive remodeling responses in the normal temporomandibular joint. All forms of mechanical TMJ stress can elicit several different molecular events that may decrease the tissue volume of the articular surfaces. Tissue volume decrease, when significant, may alter the occlusion toward a class II relationship.

Molecular Changes

Excessive or prolonged mechanical stress leads to molecular changes. At the molecular level, change is marked by early, characteristic, and multiple simultaneous events that end in cell death and decreased tissue volume. First, excessive mechanical stress leads to direct physical cellular disruption in affected tissues, leading to cell death. Excessive or prolonged mechanical loading of articular tissues of the temporomandibular joint may also adversely affect nutrient supply to local cell populations. Impedance of regional blood flow may additionally lead to ischemic reperfusion injury and temporomandibular joint resorption. There is evidence that free radicals, reactive molecules that can destroy tissue and alter cell functions, are produced in excessively loaded joints as the end-products of ischemic reperfusion injury.[1–3] Concurrently, neurogenic inflammation and increased sympathetic tone may contribute to net tissue loss following biomechanical stresses to the temporomandibular joint.

Soft Tissues

Soft tissues of the temporomandibular joint typically undergo a rapid physical transformation when subjected to chronic or excessive mechanical forces. Isberg and Isacsson[4] observed a flattening of the posterior band of the articular disk with changes in its collagen fiber orientation when the mandibular condyle was displaced posteriorly for a period of 5 weeks. Furstman[5] created unstable occlusion in rats by adding vertical occlusal interferences unilaterally. This manipulation led to greater deposition of fibrous connective tissue and osteoid matrix on the articular surface of the glenoid fossa. In addition, an increased thickness and disorientation of collagen fibers of the articular disk were observed.

Osseous Remodeling Responses

Ultimately, joint soft tissue changes may contribute to osseous remodeling or destruction. Multiple studies have assessed the osseous changes associated with condylar compression.[6–16] These studies have shown consistent osseous resorption of the postglenoid spine and posterior condylar surface when the condyle is posteriorized and compressed in the glenoid fossa. Similarly, Arnett and colleagues[7] have demonstrated morphologic changes of the mandibular condyle associated with posteriorization and medial or lateral torquing during orthognathic surgery.

Surgical Joint Compression

Posterior B-point relapse can occur at only two anatomic locations after bilateral sagittal split osteotomies (BSSO) for mandibular advancement: the osteotomy site and the temporomandibular joint (TMJ). B-point relapse occurs at (1) the osteotomy site through slippage,[6–8, 17] (2) the temporomandibular joint through condylar sag,[6–8, 17–24] and (3) the temporomandibular joint through morphologic change.[6–9, 25–29] Osteotomy slippage and condylar sag cause relapse during osteotomy healing. Morphologic TMJ change occurs between 9 and 18 months postoperatively.

Osteotomy slippage, condylar sag, and condylar compression are the primary sources of early and late B-point relapse associated with mandibular advancement using a BSSO procedure. This statement can be applied to other mandibular ramus surgical procedures.

Osteotomy Slippage

Osteotomy slippage occurs before osteotomy union in response to paramandibular connective tissue (PMCT) stretch, which produces a force that pulls the tooth-bearing fragment posteriorly after advancement. The PMCT consists of skin,[17] subcutaneous tissue,[17] muscle,[17, 30–36] and periosteum.[17] When stretched, these tissues are under tension, forming a vector that pulls the tooth-bearing fragment toward its presurgical position. Counteracting the PMCT vector are (1) osteosynthesis hardware, such as bicortical screws, superior border wires, inferior border wires, circummandibular wires, or plates with unicortical screws, (2) skeletal suspension,[37, 38] and (3) the condyle, if seated in the glenoid fossa.[6]

Condylar Sag

True condylar sag is an immediate postoperative position of the condyle such that it does not contact the glenoid fossa anteriorly, posteriorly, medially, or laterally; is inferiorly positioned; and does not support B point.[6] It is most often associated with wire osteosynthesis. During the first 8 postoperative weeks, the sagging condyle returns to the preoperative glenoid fossa position.[6-8, 21, 22, 24, 39, 40] The magnitude of B-point relapse with condylar sag depends on the effectiveness of skeletal suspension and intermaxillary fixation (IMF) holding the tooth-bearing fragment in the advanced position while the condyle reseats.

Morphologic TMJ Change

Surgical loading occurs as either posterior, medial, or lateral condylar compression.

Posterior condylar compression is the result of changing the condyle to a more posterior position during the surgical procedure (Figs. 17–1 and 17–2). The condyles and retrodiscal tissues are compressed against the posterior fossa wall. In response to compression, remodeling of the joint structures (which causes B-point relapse)[6-9] may start 9 to 18 months after surgery. As remodeling occurs, the condyle seats superiorly, resulting in B-point and dental relapse over the long term (Figs. 17–1 and 17–2). This compression-resorption cycle is identical to that seen in multiple animal studies, in which posteriorization leads to resorption.[6-16]

Medial or lateral compression can also cause TMJ remodeling and produce late B-point and dental relapse.[6-9] When the tooth-bearing fragment is advanced, a first contact point develops between the condylar-bearing and tooth-bearing fragments (Figs. 17–3 and 17–4). If clamping or bicortical screws close the gap between segments, condylar torquing results. As the gap is closed, rotation occurs at the first contact point, and the condyle torques to the medial or lateral aspect of the fossa, creating compression. Condylar torque is commonly associated with clamp stabilization of the proximal and distal fragments followed by application of bicortical screws.[41-46] Avoiding osteotomy gap closure minimizes potential condylar torquing.

The condyles can be displaced posteriorly, medially, or laterally into a compressive position by either the surgeon or the hardware. The *surgeon* influences the postoperative condyle position by both the direction of seating[6-9, 47] and the intensity of the force he or she applies to the seating.[6] It is apparent that the condyle does not go to the uppermost position in the fossa merely because the surgeon pushes the condyle toward the fossa.[6-9] If the direction and intensity of force displace the condyle, long-term relapse at the B point can occur.[6-9] This B-point relapse can be related to changes in the disk thickness and condylar length as a result of surgeon-induced injury during the surgical procedure.

The *hardware*—inferior border wires, superior border wires, bicortical screws (clamping), unicortical screws and plates—applied to immobilize the tooth-bearing fragment relative to the condylar fragment is capable of distorting condyle position in all three planes of space. The hardware should be used to hold the condyle passively in the position in which the surgeon places it, not as a propulsion system to push the condyle into the fossa. Late relapse of the B point can occur as a result of damage to the disk and condyle during surgery[6-9] and can be related to hardware-induced condyle positioning errors at surgery.

Factors that Affect the Condylar Response to Compression

The tissue response to treatment compression may be variable and largely depends on systemic factors.

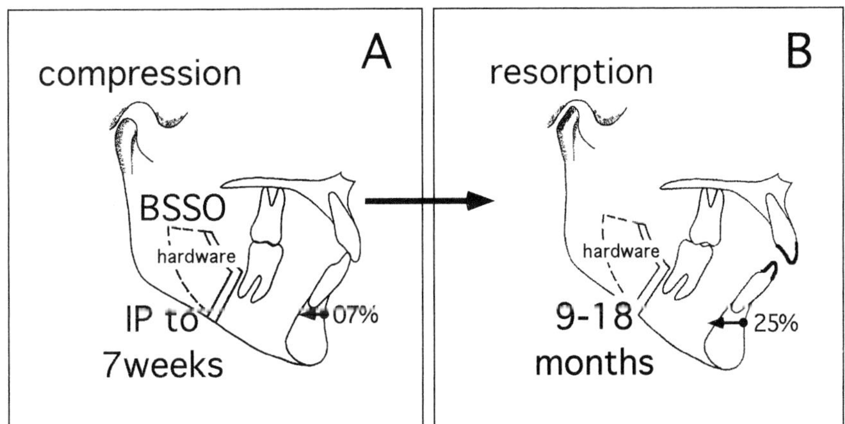

Figure 17–1. Bilateral sagittal osteotomy. *A,* Intraoperative posterior condylar position change is depicted. The surgeon and/or hardware can produce changes in condyle position. Excellent early stability (7% relapse) occurs when B point is supported by the condyle compressed on the posterior fossa wall. *BSSO,* bilateral sagittal split osteotomy; *IP,* immediate postoperation. *B,* Intraoperative condyle compression leads to late condylar morphologic change and associated B point relapse (25%). Skeletal relapse may not cause bite relapse when orthodontic dental movements are able to compensate. (*From* Arnett GW, Tamborello JA, Rathbone JA: Temporomandibular joint ramifications of orthognathic surgery. *In* Bell WH (ed): Modern Practice in Orthognathic and Reconstructive Surgery. Philadelphia, WB Saunders, 1992; pp 523–593.)

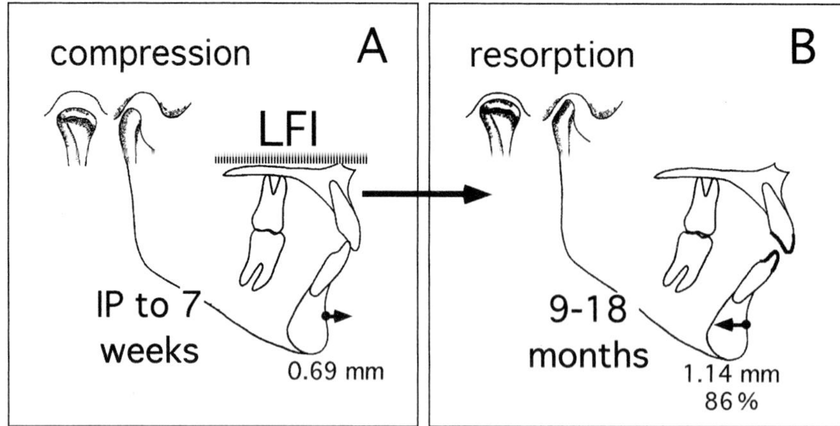

Figure 17–2. Le Fort I. *A,* Intraoperative posterior condylar position change is depicted. The surgeon and/or hardware can produce changes in condyle position. By the seventh week, B point actually rebounds anteriorly (0.69 mm) as the condyle moves anteriorly from the posterior compressed position. *IP,* immediate postoperation; *LFI,* Le Fort I. *B,* Late B point relapse occurs as posterior condylar resorption progresses. Condyle remodeling is due to the compression placed on the TMJ during surgery. Eighty-six percent of patients undergoing Le Fort I procedures had late posterior B point relapse of the mandible (1.14 mm). (*From* Arnett GW, Tamborello JA, Rathbone JA: Temporomandibular joint ramifications of orthognathic surgery. *In* Bell WH (ed): Modern Practice in Orthognathic and Reconstructive Surgery. Philadelphia, WB Saunders, 1992, pp 523–593.)

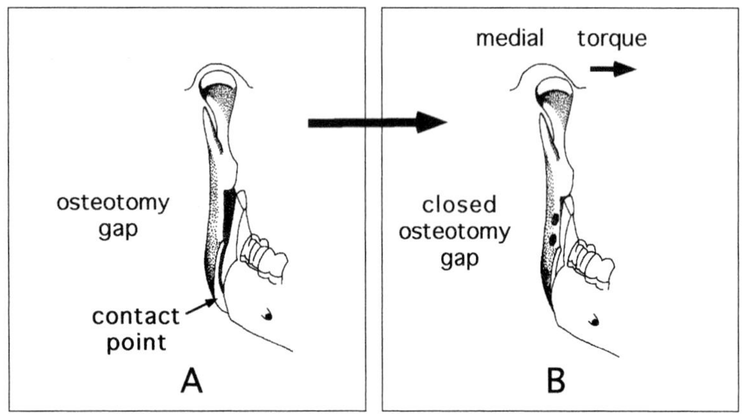

Figure 17–3. Medial torque. *A,* The right mandible is depicted after sagittal osteotomy advancement with the teeth in intermaxillary fixation. A first contact point develops between the condylar and tooth-bearing fragments. The osteotomy gap is the space formed between the fragments with the condyle seated at first contact. *B,* Medial torque occurs when clamping and/or bicortical screw placement closes the osteotomy gap. When the gap closes, the condylar fragment rotates on the first contact point, torquing the condyle medially.

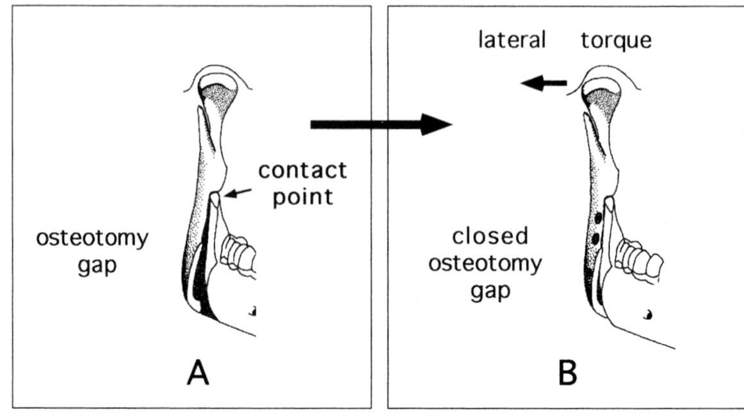

Figure 17–4. Lateral torque. *A,* The right mandible is depicted after sagittal osteotomy advancement with the teeth in intermaxillary fixation. A first contact point develops between the condylar and tooth-bearing fragments. The osteotomy gap is the space formed between the fragments with the condyle seated at first contact. *B,* Lateral torque occurs when clamping and/or bicortical screw placement closes the osteotomy gap. When the gap closes, the condylar fragment rotates on the first contact point, torquing the condyle laterally.

Therefore, one patient may exhibit signs and symptoms of aggressive dysfunctional remodeling (i.e., condylysis), whereas another, given a similar physical insult to the joint, may be capable of adapting to the changing mechanical stress with functional remodeling.

The effects of mechanical compression are influenced by the magnitude and duration of compression as well as to coexisting hidden factors. Systemic factors are age, systemic illness, hormones, internal derangements, parafunction, macrotrauma, unstable occlusion, genetic predisposition, emotional stress, nutritional status, and drugs.

Age

Condylysis, as reported in the literature, is a disease of the second and third decades.[7, 8, 48] The factors accounting for this disorder are not understood, but aggressive remodeling (condylysis, progressive condylar resorption, idiopathic condylar resorption) is reported only at these ages. Additionally, and at the opposite pole, advancing age undoubtedly reduces the host adaptive capacity.[48–50] Accordingly, the response of articular tissues of the temporomandibular joint to mechanical stress may be less than optimal in the aged population. Nevertheless, the aged population is not reported as experiencing aggressive condylar resorption.

Systemic Illness

Autoimmune diseases have been associated with condylar resorption in numerous publications.[48, 51–56] Hyperparathyroidism may also adversely affect temporomandibular joint remodeling.[48, 57]

Hormones

Sex hormones (estrogen and prolactin) are increasingly associated with aggressive condylar resorption. Arnett and Tamborello[7] reported on 10 female patients with idiopathic condylar resorption. Forty other cases (all in female patients) of severe condylar resorption (condylysis) have been reported in the literature.[25, 58–64] These clinical experiences indicate that some females may be predisposed to dysfunctional remodeling of the temporomandibular joint in response to loading associated with occlusal treatment. This female preponderance of dysfunctional remodeling of the temporomandibular joint suggests a potential role of sex hormones as modulators of this response.

Abubaker and colleagues[65] studied human temporomandibular joints for estrogen and progesterone receptors using an immunohistochemical method. They found that 72% of symptomatic females and only 14% of asymptomatic females had immunodetectable estrogen receptors in tissue specimens obtained from their temporomandibular joints. These findings suggest that symptomatic females may have different responses to estrogen levels, based on available target receptors within the temporomandibular joint. It is conceivable that prolactin may mediate some effects that have previously been attributed to estrogen. Prolactin probably contributes to the accelerated condylysis that has been observed in some pregnant females.

Corticosteroids have been reported as causing joint resorption.[48, 66, 67] It is conceivable that changes in corticosteroid levels may, in some individuals, initiate mandibular condyle resorption and attendant progressive class II occlusion.

Internal Derangement

When internal derangement and morphologic alteration occur concurrently, the internal derangement may produce condylar morphologic change by compression. In this scenario, impaired translation of the mandibular condyle may be attributed to a physical obstruction of condylar movement by the displaced articular disk. The obstruction produces compressive forces that are imparted to contacting structures of the joint. Therefore, internal derangement may produce condylar remodeling by contributing to compressive loading of the articular tissues. This concept may be supported by multiple studies that have shown that condylar remodeling is more likely to be associated with anterior disk displacement without reduction (ADNR) than with anterior disc displacement with reduction (ADR).[59, 68–71]

Alternatively, deBont and Stegenga[72] have proposed that articular disk displacements result from, and are not the cause of, degenerative changes affecting the temporomandibular joint. These investigators speculate that decreased joint lubrication leading to changes in the structure of the articular surfaces (irregularities) may increase frictional forces between the mandibular condyle, temporal bone, and articular disk, thus pulling the disk forward with translatory movements. The net result of these adverse changes in the biomechanics of the joint leads to articular disk displacement. The decrease in lubrication and resulting surface irregularity may be the products of molecular-level changes. Physical disruption of cells,[73] impaired cellular function,[75] impeded regional blood flow,[1–3] and release of inflammatory peptides[75–81] may lead to decreases in lubrication.

Internal derangement (anterior disk displacement) and increased condylar intramedullary pressure have been theorized to produce avascular necrosis (AVN) of the mandibular condyle.[82–85] First, advocates of the internal derangement theory argue that the dependent blood supply to the mandibular condyle enters anteriorly near the attachment of the lateral pterygoid muscles and that the anteriorly displaced disk occludes the artery, causing avascular necrosis.[82–85] Boyer and colleagues[86] studied the blood supply to the TMJ, however, and found an extensive vascular plexus that receives blood vessels most prominently from the posterior aspect of the mandibular condyle, directly contradicting the anterior dependent artery concept. Additionally, there is no evidence to support the notion that an anteriorly displaced articular disk can occlude the anterior blood supply to the TMJ. Second, it is theorized that multiple factors increase the condylar intramedullary pressure, preventing arterial inflow or venous outflow and thus leading to avascular necrosis. This theory is unsubstantiated by animal or clinical research.

Parafunction

Parafunction may produce compression that is capable of initiating condylar resorption[9, 61, 87–91] or enhancing resorption caused by other factors that initiate this process. It is likely that these forces contribute to condylar resorption by at least two mechanisms. First, direct biomechanical stress can disrupt the integrity of articular tissue and inhibit important systemic functions of affected cell populations. Second, it is possible that tissue damage resulting from excessive loading of the temporomandibular joint is secondary to an ischemia-reperfusion injury.[92] Increased intracapsular pressures occur with bruxism.[93] These intracapsular pressures exceed the capillary perfusion pressure and can therefore impair blood flow to intracapsular tissues, leading to ischemia. Cell populations in ischemic tissues adjust their metabolic pathways to accommodate lower oxygen tensions. When blood flow is reestablished in the joint (i.e., through reduced intracapsular pressure following relaxation of jaw muscles), oxygen tension rapidly rises in affected tissues. Cells with altered metabolic pathways still functioning generate free radicals under this condition. Parafunction increases intracapsular pressures,[93] inhibits capillary perfusion, and, thus, creates an ischemia-reperfusion injury with attendant loss of temporomandibular tissue volume, leading to mandibular retrusion.

Macrotrauma

Macrotrauma may also promote condylar resorption.[6–9, 62] Macrotrauma consists of one episode (compression or stretch) of large-magnitude force that is transmitted to articular structures of the temporomandibular joint. The mechanism of delayed condylar resorption secondary to macrotrauma is not understood. Condylar resorption can be the result of physical injury or impairment of cellular functions. Reflex sympathetic dystrophy (RSD) may be associated with delayed macrotrauma resorption.[9]

Unstable Occlusion

Unstable occlusion may contribute to condylar resorption via compression. Two forms of occlusion exist independent of Angle classification, stable and unstable. A stable occlusion does not deflect the condyle position during muscular interdigitation of the dentition (regardless of Angle classification). An unstable occlusion produces compressive deflection of the condyle during muscular interdigitation of the teeth (regardless of Angle classification). Multiple animal studies have shown the correlation between unstable occlusion and TMJ change.[4, 5, 9–16, 94–96]

According to this definition, class I occlusion with condylar compression is an unstable occlusion (Figs. 17–5 and 17–6). Correction (by orthodontics, orthognathic surgery, prosthetics) of occlusal discrepancies to a class I dental relationship, if associated with joint compression, can lead to condylar resorption. This was demonstrated in the study by Arnett and colleagues,[7] in which class I occlusions with joint compression led to late condylar resorption.

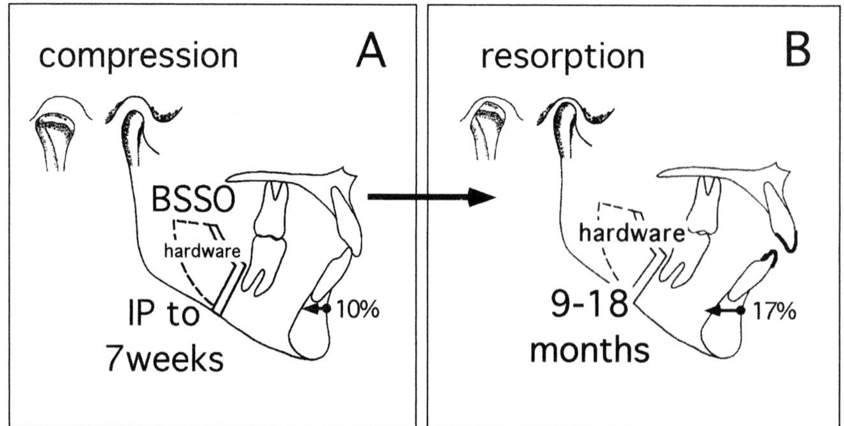

Figure 17–5. *A,* Intraoperative lateral condylar position change is depicted. The surgeon and/or hardware (force and direction) have changed the condyle position to the lateral rim of the glenoid fossa. Good early stability (10% relapse) occurs because the laterally compressed condyle supports B point. *BSSO,* bilateral sagittal split osteotomy; *IP,* immediate postoperation. *B,* Late B point relapse (17%) occurs secondary to condylar morphologic change. Morphologic change occurs because of the lateral compression that was applied at surgery. Skeletal relapse does not cause bite relapse if dental compensations occur via orthodontic tooth movements. (*From* Arnett GW, Tamborello JA, Rathbone JA: Temporomandibular joint ramifications of orthognathic surgery. *In* Bell WH (ed): Modern Practice in Orthognathic and Reconstructive Surgery. Philadelphia, WB Saunders, 1992, pp 523–593.)

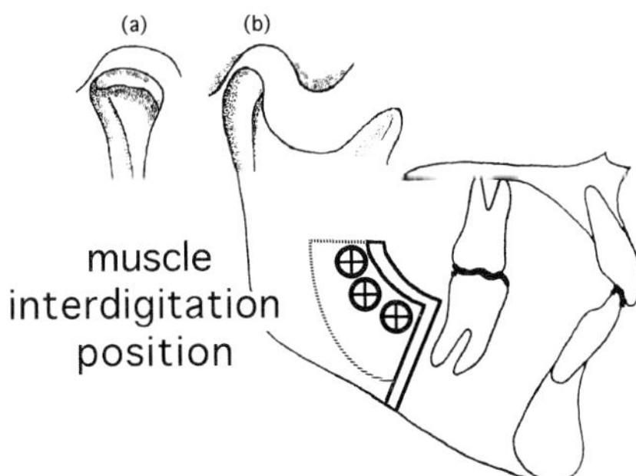

Figure 17–6. A bilateral postoperative sagittal osteotomy is depicted. The condyle was surgically misplaced laterally (a) and posteriorly (b) when the bite was corrected to class I occlusion. Under muscle force, the teeth are interdigitated into class I occlusion, deflecting and compressing the condyle posteriorly and laterally. Condylar morphologic change may occur in response to condylar compression. By definition, this class I example, which compresses the joints, is an unstable occlusion.

Other Factors

Genetic predisposition, emotional stress, nutritional status, and drug use are capable of influencing mechanical stresses. In particular, emotional stress greatly influences mechanical stress via parafunction.

Conclusion

The etiology of condylar remodeling is clearly multifactorial, as shown in Figure 17–7. The extent of remodeling is based upon the interaction of three groups of factors: (1) mechanical stresses, (2) circulating systemic factors, and (3) basic adaptive capacity factors. Functional remodeling is characterized by focal adaptation of the articular structures of the temporomandibular joint in response to focal mechanical stress(es).[97, 98]

Other factors, such as age, hormonal status, and the presence of systemic disease, can accentuate the focal effects of compression on the total condyle. When the magnitude or duration of mechanical stress is extreme, total condylar remodeling can occur without the presence of additional factors.

Injuries to the Trigeminal Nerve

Trigeminal nerve injury may occur during orthognathic surgery as a result of excessive retraction of soft tissues (mental or mandibular foramen), transection of the nerve branch during the osteotomy cuts, excessive stretching of the nerve during positioning of the bone segments, or compression of the nerve with fixation of the bony segments. Clinical investigations have revealed sensory disturbances in more than 80% of patients undergoing bilateral sagittal split osteotomies.[99, 100] Abnormal sensations may persist for more than a year in 4% to 20% of such patients.[100, 101] In rare instances, unpleasant or painful sensations may result from these iatrogenic injuries.

Determining a Prognosis for Normal Sensory Recovery

Depending on the extent of the injury, a damaged trigeminal neuron undergoes a variety of metabolic responses, ranging from cell death to healing (regeneration). Variables that may affect neuronal responses to injury are the site of the injury (i.e., proximal or distal), type of injury (i.e., stretch, crush, transection, avulsion), and host factors (i.e., systemic disease, nutritional deficiencies, drugs) (Table 17–1).

Site of Injury

When a neuron is injured, (i.e., axonal disruption), a series of molecular events leading to either neuronal death or regeneration of the damaged axon is initiated. Apparently, the closer an injury is to the neuron's nucleus (proximal injury), the more likely the injured neuron is to die. If this assumption is correct, a neuronal injury produced at the level of the mandibular foramen should have a poorer prognosis for recovery than an injury of similar type and magnitude produced at the level of the mental foramen. Accordingly, aggressive medial retraction in the area of the lingula may be associated with prolonged and possibly permanent inferior alveolar nerve injury.[101a]

Type of Injury

A trigeminal nerve branch may be crushed, compressed, stretched, torn, or transected during orthognathic surgery. In addition to the proximal versus distal location of injury, the prognosis for normal neuronal regeneration (normal sensation) following injury depends primarily on the integrity of the affected axons and surrounding nonneural tissues after injury. *Crush* injuries (between proximal and distal fragments) typically produce minimal disruption in the physical integrity of the affected nerve. Thus, sensory recovery following a crush injury is typically faster and more complete than after a transection injury.[102] In contrast, a *stretch* injury (stretching the osteotomy site) may produce extensive damage if the injury results in the

Table 17–1. Three Variables Affecting Nerve Regeneration Following Injury

Site of Injury	Host Factors	Type of Injury
Proximal	Systemic illness	Stretch/avulsion
Distal	Diabetes mellitus	Transection
	Multiple sclerosis	Compression/crush
	Collagen vascular disease	
	Malabsorption disease	
	Alcoholism	
	Neurotoxic drugs	
	ETOH	
	Colchicine	
	Age	
	Nerve regeneration	

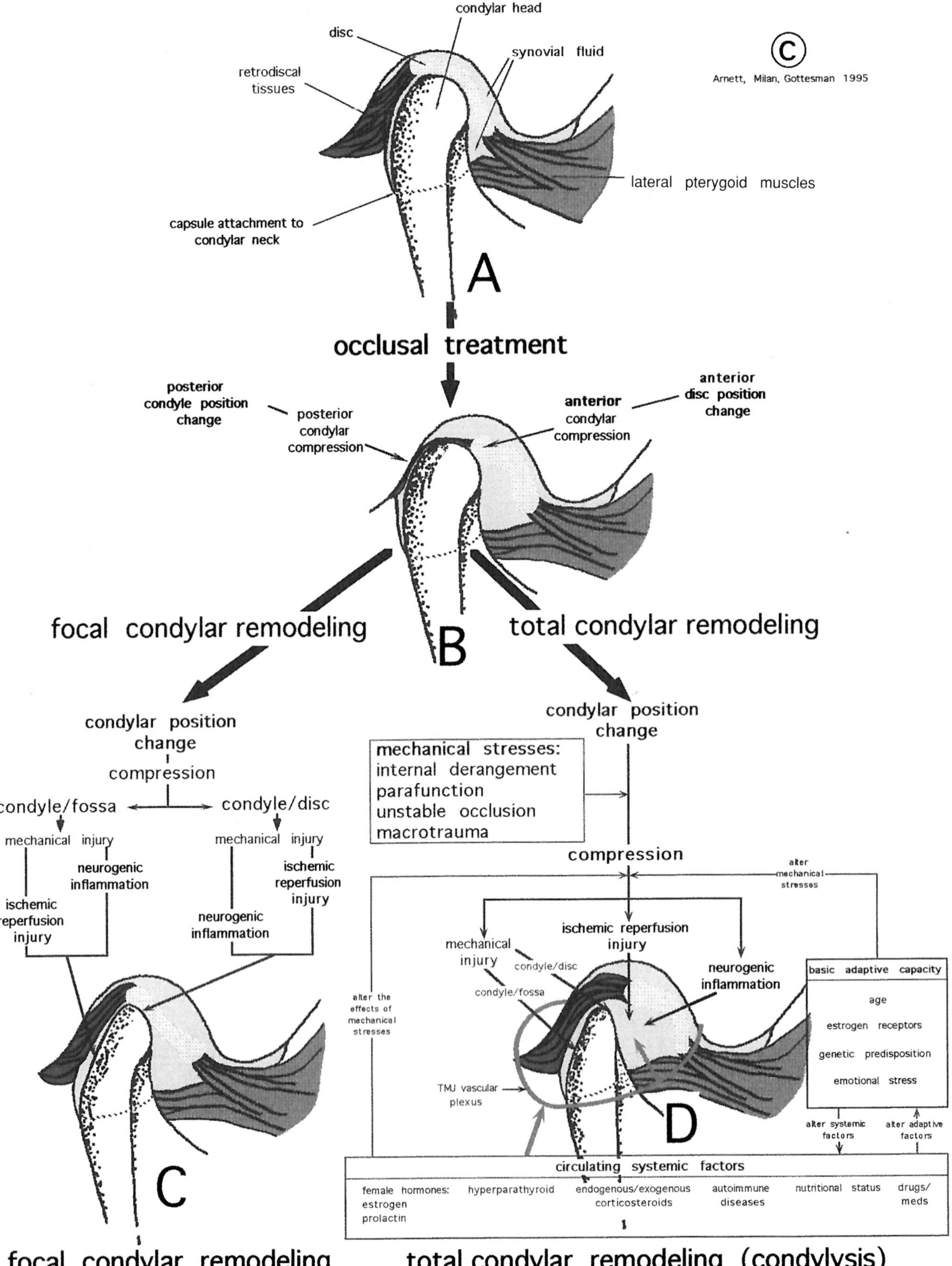

Figure 17–7 *See legend on opposite page*

tearing of axons. The region involved in this type of injury may extend far beyond the point at which force is applied to the nerve. Generally speaking, a poor prognosis for complete sensory recovery is associated with injuries affecting more than a 3-cm length of nerve.[103]

Host Factors

Host factors may also contribute to the ultimate outcome of a trigeminal nerve injury. For example, diabetes mellitus and alcoholism are common causes of peripheral neuropathy. It is conceivable that certain systemic illnesses may impair normal regenerative processes following trigeminal nerve injury. Because nutritional status may influence healing after a nerve injury, gastrointestinal disorders associated with malabsorption may also adversely affect neuronal regeneration after injury. It is also conceivable that certain collagen vascular diseases (e.g., rheumatoid arthritis, scleroderma, polyarthritis) may compromise the healing of both neural and nonneural tissues, leading to incomplete regeneration of injured trigeminal nerve. Finally, aging may also reduce the prognosis for sensory recovery after trigeminal nerve injury. With aging, nonneural cell populations that are believed to be important in the regenerative process are reduced. With these considerations in mind, one may anticipate a relatively good prognosis for complete neurosensory recovery in a young, healthy patient who sustains a crush injury to a distal branch (e.g., mental nerve) of the trigeminal nerve. In contrast, a relatively poor prognosis for complete neurosensory recovery should be anticipated in a middle-aged adult with collagen vascular disease who sustains a transection of the mandibular nerve at the level of the mandibular foramen.

Surgical Intervention for Trigeminal Nerve Injuries

Biologic Considerations

Typically, a trigeminal nerve injury is viewed simply as an injury to a group of neurons (or their axons). In order to fully understand the significance of a particular injury, however, one should remember that the trigeminal nerve is a complex tissue. It is composed of multiple cell types, including neurons, fibroblasts, endothelial cells, and Schwann cells. Physical disruption of this complex tissue evokes responses from all involved cell populations. Harmonious interactions among these cells may be critical to the repair process. Therefore, nerve regeneration following injury results from a dependent, sequenced cascade of cellular and molecular events. The assumption that these events are sequenced (i.e., event B will not precede event A) and dependent (i.e., event B will not occur if event A does not occur) is clinically relevant, for it implies that any therapeutic intervention, including surgical repair, must be appropriately timed to optimize the outcome. Furthermore, any intervention that disrupts the normal sequence of biologic events associated with nerve regeneration may significantly compromise the ultimate outcome of this process.

Timing of Surgical Repairs

On the basis of our current knowledge of the early molecular event underlying nerve regeneration, an optimum time for nerve repair has been estimated to be 2 to 3 weeks after injury.[104] It is during this time frame that nonneural tissues have become sufficiently reorganized to support the extension of the regenerating unit of the damaged nerve. Furthermore, concentrations of neurotropic factors (i.e., neurite-promoting factors) dra-

---

Figure 17–7. The possible morphologic effects of occlusal treatment compression on the TMJ. *A,* Normal joint anatomy. The disk rests over the condyle with the posterior band situated directly behind the apex of the condylar head. Occlusal treatment (orthognathic surgery, orthodontics, prosthetics) may cause a change in normal joint structure relationships. Treatment of the bite may move the condyle medially, laterally, or posteriorly, thereby mechanically stressing the hard and soft tissue components of the joint. The net effect of treatment loading on joint morphology depends on the presence of additional agents—mechanical stress factors, circulating systemic factors, and basic host adaptation factors.

B, Treatment-generated posterior condylar position change with associated compression. Anterior displacement of the meniscus may occur as a secondary effect of posterior condyle displacement. In this example, compression occurs posteriorly because of condyle position change and anteriorly because of disc dislocation. Anterior compression occurs when the condyle translates forward in an attempt to open against the closed lock.

C, Mechanical compression creates *focal condylar remodeling* at the site(s) of load. Mechanical remodeling is usually functional; the occlusion is not altered. Any source of mechanical compression causes remodeling via three mechanisms: direct mechanical injury to cell populations, ischemic reperfusion injury, and neurogenic inflammation.

D, Treatment (mechanical) compression may lead to *total condylar remodeling* when the compression is prolonged and severe or other conditions occur concurrently. Other forms of mechanical compression, such as parafunction, unstable occlusion, and internal derangement, can accentuate the effects of treatment compression and cause gross condylar and occlusal alteration. Systemic factors also accentuate the extent of remodeling caused by mechanical compression of the TMJ. Estrogen, prolactin, corticosteroids, hyperparathyroid, antibodies associated with collagen vascular diseases, nutritional disorders, and drugs circulate to the TMJ. When present, these systemic factors may exaggerate focal compressive remodeling to total condylar resorption. Basic host adaptive capacity factors such as age (second to third decade), TMJ estrogen receptors, emotional stress, genetic predisposition, and nutritional disorders are capable of modifying the degree of remodeling secondary to mechanical stresses and systemic factors.

Mechanical stress, systemic factors, and basic host adaptation lead to the accumulation of chemical irritants (cytotoxins, cGRP, sub P, etc.) in the synovial fluid. These irritants reduce the size of the entire condyle contained within the joint space, thus decreasing the condylion to lower incisor distance, which in turn leads to mandibular retrusion with or without open bite.

matically increase 10 to 21 days after injury.[105] These factors, along with specific extracellular matrix molecules such as laminin, fibronectin, and collagen, appear to be necessary for direction of the regeneration unit to the distal target site.

For several reasons, however, it may not be feasible or advisable to attempt surgical repair of a suspected trigeminal nerve injury 2 to 3 weeks after injury. An observed nerve transection injury should be repaired immediately. In lieu of microscopic repair, simple reapproximation without tension should be performed. This simple procedure is often sufficient to enable adequate regeneration to occur. Following repair, baseline neurosensory tests should be obtained and periodically reassessed for signs of return of sensory function.

Perhaps the most valid reason for delaying repair of an unobserved nerve injury is based on consideration of the possibility that the injury was a low-grade (e.g., crush) injury that has high potential for spontaneous recovery. Although the literature supports the view that neurosensory recovery is better for nerve repairs performed within 3 to 6 months of injury, clinical experiences indicate that some neurosensory recovery can be gained from trigeminal nerve repairs performed 1 to 2 years after injury. Therefore, if a patient experiences a neurosensory deficit following orthognathic surgery and a trigeminal nerve injury is not observed at surgery, it is prudent to monitor the patient repeatedly in the postoperative period with appropriate neurosensory testing for signs of neurosensory recovery. If the deficit is problematic and if signs of recovery are not evident within 3 to 6 months, consideration should be given to surgical exploration and nerve repair.

Managing Posttraumatic Trigeminal Dysesthesias

Abnormal, unpleasant sensations (i.e., dysesthesias) may also result from trigeminal nerve injury.[106, 107] These unpleasant or painful sensations may be generated spontaneously or evoked by innocuous stimuli, such as facial movements and light touch. With time, the unpleasant sensations may become increasingly distressful to many patients. Under chronic conditions, some patients with chronic dysesthesias may become debilitated by the perception that the sensations are increasing in frequency and intensity.

The mechanisms of the genesis of trigeminal dysesthesias are unknown but may involve (1) ectopic impulse generation and ephapsis (cross-talk between adjacent axons) in a segment of injured trigeminal nerve that is demyelinated (segmental demyelination), (2) aberrant CNS sensitivity or reorganization from partial or total loss of sensory innervation in a trigeminal dermatome (deafferentation), (3) abnormal expression of neurotransmitter receptors at axon terminals of damaged neurons (e.g., sympathetically maintained pain, neuromas), and (4) neuroma formation.

Several nonsurgical remedies have been suggested for management of these dysesthesias (Table 17–2). The success of a particular treatment, either nonsurgical or surgical, depends on the pathophysiologic process(es) underlying the dysesthesias. In general, a poor prognosis is associated with deafferentation. The resultant CNS reorganization believed to be associated with deafferentation appears to perpetuate chronic pain in some unfortunate individuals. This condition is typically refractory to conventional therapies. Segmental demyelination or neuroma may, however, be treated successfully with surgical repair, depending on the location and extent of the derangement. Unfortunately, at present, there are no diagnostic tests that can reliably differentiate these neuropathies. Pain evoked by palpation or percussion (Tinel sign) or pain relief from a local anesthetic administration may indicate a focal lesion or neuroma affecting a branch of the trigeminal nerve, but these tests do not exclude the possibility of

Table 17–2. Pharmacologic Management of Trigeminal Dysesthesias

Agent(s)	Dosage	Mechanism	Comments
Antidepressants			
Amitryptyline	25–100 mg q HS	Mixed NE-serotonin-anticholinergic mechanisms	Electric shock–like or burning pain
Desipramine	25–100 mg q HS	NE mechanisms	Electric shock–like or burning pain
Doxepin	25–100 mg q HS	Mixed NE-serotonin	Electric shock–like or burning pain
Anticonvulsants			
Carbamazepine	200–1200 mg qd	Facilitates activation of inhibitory pathways in CNS; inhibits Na^+ influx	Electric shock–like pain
Phenytoin	300–600 mg qd	Inhibits Na^+ and Ca^{++} influx	Electric shock–like pain
Baclofen	30–60 mg qd	GABA agonist	Electric shock–like or burning pain
Clonazepam	1.5–20 mg qd	GABA agonist	Electric shock–like pain
Sympatholytics			
Phentolamine (IV)	25–50 mg IV	$alpha_1$-Adrenergic block	Burning pain
Prazocin	2–20 mg qd	$alpha_1$-Adrenergic block	Burning pain
Phenoxybenzamine	20–120 mg qd	$alpha_1$-Adrenergic block	Burning pain
Clonidine	0.1–0.3 mg qd Transdermal	$alpha_2$-Adrenergic agonist	Burning pain
Others			
Local anesthetics	Local or IV	Na^+ channel blockers	Electric shock–like or burning pain
Mexiletine	150–200 mg bid	Na^+ channel blockers	Electric shock–like or burning pain
Opiates	Scheduled regimen	Opiate agonists	Refractory pain
Glucocorticoids	Perineural injection	Inhibits ectopic discharge	Electric shock–like pain, neuroma

centrally mediated pain (i.e., deafferentation). Conceptually, pain from deafferentation may also be evoked by peripheral stimulation via CNS hyperexcitability or receptive field expansion. Deafferentation pain may also be reduced by peripheral local anesthetic administration (by blocking afferent impulses from the affected region).

Some dysesthesias may be identified on the basis of specific clinical findings. For example, sympathetically maintained pain (SMP) is believed to result from an abnormal expression of functional alpha$_1$-adrenergic receptors at axonal terminals of sensory neurons.[107a] The typical burning pain described by patients suffering from SMP may be alleviated by a systemic administration of alpha$_1$-adrenergic blockers, such as phentolamine.[108] Burning pain relieved by the administration of alpha$_1$-adrenergic blockers is diagnostic for SMP.

Future Therapies for Trigeminal Nerve Injuries

The regenerating neuron develops multiple axoplasmic sprouts at the site of its damaged axon within 24 hours of injury. These sprouts eventually become ensheated by Schwann cells and are collectively known as the regenerating unit of the damaged neurons.[103, 109] The regenerating unit advances distally guided by both chemical signals (i.e., neurotrophic factors) from the surrounding environment and by adhesion to specific extracellular matrix molecules, such as laminin, fibronectin, and collagens, that are located in the pathway. In some cases, such as that observed in the primate facial nerve regeneration model, the regenerating unit may advance over 8-cm distances, successfully reaching its target organ.[103] Later studies have shown, however, that even though axonal advancement may extend relatively large distances, the quality of this regenerative effort is poor if the traversed span is greater than 3 cm.[103] The efficiency of regeneration over lengthy distances may be improved if a conduit is provided to guide the advancing regenerating unit and to protect it from impingement by surrounding tissues. Several materials have been used as conduits to support nerve regeneration, including autogenous nerve grafts, autogenous vein grafts, allogenic nerve grafts with immunosuppression, and bioresorbable materials.[103]

Several molecules have been identified that may positively influence nerve regeneration after injury. Extracellular matrix molecules, such as laminin, collagen, fibronectin, and proteoglycans, are important for guidance of the advancing regenerating unit of damaged nerve through adjacent tissues. These important molecules have been, or are currently being, tested for use to enhance trigeminal nerve regeneration following injury. Several important neurotropic molecules have been discovered that may be used to stimulate regeneration in injured nerve; application of these substances has been reviewed.[110] It is likely that as our understanding of the molecular requirements for optimum nerve regeneration grows, novel biomaterials will be developed that will significantly improve the regenerative capacity of damaged trigeminal nerve.

References

1. McCord JM: Oxygen-derived free radicals in postischemic tissue injury. N Engl J Med 1985;312:159–163.
2. Blake DR, Unsworth J, Outhwaite JM, Morris CJ: Hypoxic-reperfusion injury in the inflamed human joint. Lancet 1989;1:288–293.
3. Henrotin Y, Deby DG, Deby C, et al: Active oxygen species, articular inflammation and cartilage damage. EXS 1992;62:308–322.
4. Isberg AM, Isacsson G: Tissue reactions of the temporomandibular joint following retrusive guidance of the mandible. J Craniomand Pract 1986;4:143–148.
5. Furstman L: The effect of loss of occlusion upon the temporomandibular joint. Am J Orthod 1965;51:245–261.
6. Arnett GW, Tamborello JA, Rathbone JA: Temporomandibular joint ramifications of orthognathic surgery. *In* Bell WH (ed): Modern Practice in Orthognathic and Reconstructive Surgery. Philadelphia, WB Saunders, 1992, pp 523–593.
7. Arnett GW, Tamborello JA: Progressive class II development—female idiopathic condylar resorption. Oral Maxillofac Clin North Am 1990;2:699–716.
8. Arnett GW: A redefinition of bilateral sagittal osteotomy (BSO) advancement relapse. Am J Orthod Dentofacial Orthop 1993;104:506–515.
9. Arnett GW, Milam SB, Gottesman L: Progressive mandibular retrusion—idiopathic condylar resorption. Part I: Am J Orthod Dentofac Orthop in press.
10. Janzen EK, Bluher JA: The cephalometric, anatomic and histological changes in *Macaca mulatta* after application of a continuous acting retraction force in the mandible. Am J Orthod 1965;51:823–855.
11. Ramfjord SP, Hiniker JJ: Distal placement of the mandible in adult rhesus monkeys. J Prosthet Dent 1966;16:491–502.
12. Adams CD, Merkle MC, Norwick KW, et al: Dentofacial remodeling produced by intermaxillary forces in *Macaca mulatta*. Arch Oral Biol 1972;17:1519–1535.
13. Joho J-P: The effects of extraoral low-pull traction of the mandibular dentition of *Macaca mulatta*. Am J Orthod 1973;64:555–577.
14. Shimozuma K: Effects of vertical forces on the dentofacial complex of *Macaca irus*. Nippon Kyosei Shika Gakkai Zasshi 1982;41:413–449.
15. Asano T: The effects of mandibular retrusive force on the growing rat mandible. Am J Orthod 1986;90:464.
16. Ellis E III, Hinton RJ: Histologic examination of the temporomandibular joint after mandibular advancement with and without rigid fixation: An experimental investigation in adult *Macaca mulatta*. J Oral Maxillofac Surg 1991;49:1316–1327.
17. Epker BN, Wessberg GA: Mechanisms of early skeletal relapse following surgical advancement of the mandible. Br J Oral Surg 1982;20:175–182.
18. Epker BN, Wolford LM, Fish LC: Mandibular deficiency syndrome: II. Surgical considerations for mandibular advancement. Oral Surg Oral Med Oral Path 1978;45(3):349–363.
19. Freihofer HPM Jr, Petresevic D: Late results after advancing the mandible by sagittal splitting of the rami. J Maxillofac Surg 1975;3:250–257.
20. Isaacson RJ, Kopytov OS, Bevis RR, Waite DE: Movement of proximal and distal segments after mandibular ramus osteotomies. J Oral Surg 1978;36:263–268.
21. Ive J, McNeill RW, West RA: Mandibular advancement: Skeletal and dental changes during fixation. J Oral Surg 1977;35:881–886.
22. Lake SL, McNeill RW, Little RM, West RA: Surgical mandibular advancement: A cephalometric analysis of treatment response. Am J Orthod 1981;80:376–394.
23. Sandor GKB, Stoelinga PJW, Tideman H, Leenen RJ: The role of intraosseous osteosynthesis wire in sagittal split osteotomies for mandibular advancement. J Oral Maxillofac Surg 1984;42:231–237.
24. Will LA, West RA: Factors influencing the stability of the sagittal

split osteotomy for mandibular advancement. J Oral Maxillofac Surg 1989;47:813–818.
25. Worms FW, Speidel TM, Bevis RR, Waite DE: Posttreatment stability and esthetics of orthognathic surgery. Angle Orthod 1980;50:251–273.
26. Doyle MG: Stability and complications in 50 consecutively treated surgical-orthodontic patients: A retrospective longitudinal analysis from private practice. Int J Adult Orthod Orthogn Surg 1986;1:23–36.
27. LaBlanc JP, Turvey T, Epker BN: Results following simultaneous mobilization of the maxilla and mandible for the correction of dentofacial deformities: Analysis of 100 consecutive patients. Oral Surg Oral Med Oral Pathol 1982;54:607–612.
28. Phillips RM, Bell WH: Atrophy of mandibular condyles after sagittal ramus split osteotomy: Report of case. J Oral Surg 1978;36:45–49.
29. Weinberg S, Craft J: Unilateral atrophy of the mandibular condyle after closed subcondylar osteotomy for correction of mandibular prognathism. J Oral Surg 1980;38:366–368.
30. Poulton DR, Ware WH: Surgical-orthodontic treatment of severe mandibular retrusion. Am J Orthod 1971;59:244–265.
31. Poulton DR, Ware WH: Surgical-orthodontic treatment of severe mandibular retrusion II. Am J Orthod 1973;63:237–255.
32. Finn RA, Throckmorton GS, Bell WH, Legan HL: Biomechanical considerations in the surgical correction of mandibular deficiency. J Oral Surg 1980;38:257–264.
33. Guernsey LH: Stability of treatment results in class II malocclusion corrected by full mandibular advancement surgery. Oral Surg Oral Med Oral Path 1974;37:668–687.
34. Guernsey LH, DeChamplain RW: Sequelae and complications of the intra-oral sagittal osteotomy in the mandibular rami. Oral Surg Oral Med Oral Path 1971;32:176–192.
35. McNeill RW, Hooley JR, Sundberg RI: Skeletal relapse during intermaxillary fixation. J Oral Surg 1973;31:212–227.
36. Steinhauser EW: Advancement of the mandible by sagittal ramus split and suprahyoid myotomy. J Oral Surg 1973; 31:516–521.
37. Ellis E III, Gallo WJ: Relapse following mandibular advancement with dental plus skeletal maxillomandibular fixation. J Oral Maxillofac Surg 1986;44:509–515.
38. Mayo KH, Ellis E III: Stability of the mandible after advancement and use of dental plus skeletal maxillomandibular fixation: An experimental investigation in *Macaca mulatta*. J Oral Maxillofac Surg 1987;45:243–250.
39. Kohn MW: Analysis of relapse after mandibular advancement surgery. J Oral Surg 1978;36:676–684.
40. Arnett GW, Tamborello JA: Condylar movement during intermaxillary fixation sagittal osteotomy. Clinical Congress on Orthognathic Challenges: Predictability, Stability and Complications. AAO/AAOMS Clinical Congress, Scientific Abstract Session, Anaheim, Feb. 1986.
41. Hackney FL, Van Sickels JE, Nummikoski PV: Condylar displacement and temporomandibular joint dysfunction following bilateral sagittal split osteotomy and rigid fixation. J Oral Maxillofac Surg 1989;47:223.
42. Kundert M, Hadjianghelou O: Condylar displacement after sagittal splitting of the mandibular rami. J Maxillofac Surg 1980;8:278–287.
43. Lund E, Sindet-Pedersen S: Postoperative changes after bilateral mandibular osteotomies: A computed tomography study. Oral Surg Oral Med Oral Pathol 1989;67:588–593.
44. Spitzer W, Rettinger G, Sitzmann F: Computerized tomography examination for the detection of positional changes in the temporomandibular joint after ramus osteotomies with screw fixation. J Maxillofac Surg 1984;12:139–142.
45. Timmis DP, Aragon SB, Van Sickels JE: Masticatory dysfunction with rigid and nonrigid osteosynthesis of sagittal split osteotomies. Oral Surg Oral Med Oral Pathol 1986;62:119–123.
46. Tuinizing DB, Swart IGN: Lagerveranderunben des caput mandibulae bei verwendung von zugschrauben nach sagittaler osteotomie des unterkiefers. Dtsch Z Mund Kiefer Gesichtschir 1978;2:94–96.
47. Dawson PE: Optimum TMJ condyle position in clinical practice. Int J Periodontol Restor Dent 1985;3:11–31.
48. Arnett GW, Milam SB, Gottesman L: Progressive mandibular retrusion—idiopathic condylar resorption. Part II: Host adaptive capacity. Am J Ortho Dentofac Orthop in press.
49. Silbermann M, Livne E: Age-related degenerative changes in the mouse mandibular joint. J Anat 1979;129:507–520.
50. Livne E, Weiss A, Silbermann M: Articular chondrocytes lose their proliferative activity with aging yet can be restimulated by PTH-(1–84), PGE1, and dexamethasone. J Bone Miner Res 1989;4:539–548.
51. Forsslund G, Bjurwill B, Orrling S: Bilateral absorption of the capitulum mandibulae in rheumatoid arthritis. Acta Odontol Scand 1961;19:247–257.
52. Goodwill CJ, Steggles BG: Destruction of the temporomandibular joints in rheumatoid arthritis. Ann Rheum Dis 1966;25:133–136.
53. Caplan HI, Benny RA: Total osteolysis of the mandibular condyle in progressive sclerosis (scleroderma). Oral Surg Oral Med Oral Pathol 1978;46:362–366.
54. Lanigan DT, Myall RWT, West RA, McNeill RW: Condylysis in a patient with a mixed vascular disease. Oral Surg Oral Med Oral Pathol 1979;48:198–204.
55. Ogden GR: Complete resorption of the mandibular condyles in rheumatoid arthritis. Br Dent J 1986;160:95–97.
56. Ramon Y, Samra H, Oberman M: Mandibular condylosis and apertognathia as presenting symptoms in progressive systemic sclerosis (scleroderma). Oral Surg Oral Med Oral Pathol 1987;63:269–274.
57. Dick R, Jones DN: Temporomandibular joint condyle changes in patients undergoing chronic haemodialysis. Clin Radiol 1973;24:72–76.
58. Kent JN, Carlton DM, Zide MF: Rheumatoid disease and related arthropathies. Oral Surg Oral Med Oral Pathol 1986;61:423–439.
59. Link JJ, Nickerson JW: Temporomandibular joint internal derangements in an orthognathic surgery population. Int J Adult Orthod Orthogn Surg 1992;7:161–169.
60. Weinburg LA: Role of condylar position in TMJ dysfunction-pain syndrome. J Prosthet Dent 1979;41:636–643.
61. Phillips BA, Okeson J, Paesani D, et al: Effect of sleep position on sleep apnea and parafunctional activity. Chest 1986;90:424–429.
62. Susami T, Kuroda T, Yano Y, Nakamura T: Growth changes and orthodontic treatment in a patient with condylolysis. Am J Orthod Dentofac Orthop 1992;102:295–301.
63. Rabey GP: Bilateral mandibular condylysis—a morphanalytic diagnosis. Br J Oral Surg 1977–78;15:121–134.
64. Kirk WS: Failure of surgical orthodontics due to temporomandibular joint internal derangement and postsurgical condylar resorption. Am J Orthod 1992;101:375–380.
65. Abubaker AO, Arslan W, Sotereanos GC: Estrogen and progesterone receptors in the temporomandibular joint disk of symptomatic and asymptomatic patients. J Oral Maxillofac Surg 1991;49:111.
66. Furstman L, Bernick S, Zipkin I: The effect of hydrocortisone and fluoride upon the rat's mandibular joint. J Oral Therap Pharm 1965;1:515–525.
67. Pellicci PN, Zolla-Pazners S, Rabhan WM, Wilson PD: Osteonecrosis of the femoral head associated with pregnancy: A report of three cases. Clin Orthop Relat Res 1984;185:59–63.
68. Nickerson JW Jr, Boering G: Natural course of osteoarthritis as it relates to internal derangement of the TMJ. Oral Maxillofac Clin North Am 1989;1:27–45.
69. Westesson P-L, Eriksson L, Kurita K: Reliability of negative clinical temporomandibular joint examination: Prevalence of disk displacement in asymptomatic joint. Oral Surg Oral Med Oral Pathol 1989;68:551–554.
70. Westesson P-L: Structural hard-tissue changes in temporomandibular joints with internal derangement. Oral Surg Oral Med Oral Pathol 1985;59:220–224.
71. Eriksson L, Westesson P-L: Clinical and radiological study of patients with anterior disc displacement of the temporomandibular joint. Swed Dent J 1983;7:55–64.
72. de Bont LGM, Stegenga B: Pathology of the temporomandibular joint internal derangement and osteoarthrosis. Int J Oral Maxillofac Surg 1993;22:71–74.
73. Chandra H, Symons MCR: Sulphur radicals formed by cutting α-keratin. Nature 1987;328:833–834.

74. Haskin CL, Athanasiou KA, Klebe R, Cameron IL: A heat-shock-like response with cytoskeletal disruption occurs following hydrostatic pressure in MG-63 osteosarcoma cells. Biochem Cell Biol 1993;71:361–371.
75. Kido MA, Kiyoshima T, Kondo T, et al: Distribution of substance P and calcitonin gene-related peptide-like immunoreactive nerve fibers in rat temporomandibular joint. J Dent Res 1993;72:592–598.
76. Kimball ES: Substance P, cytokines, and arthritis. Ann N Y Acad Sci 1990;594:293–308.
77. Cavagnaro J, Lewis RM: Bidirectional regulatory circuit between the immune and neuroendocrine systems. Year Immunol 1989;4:241–252.
78. Jonakait GM, Schotland S: Conditioned medium from activated splenocytes increases substance P in synthetic ganglia. J Neurosci Res 1990;26:24–30.
79. Jonakait GM, Schotland S, Hart RP: Interleukin-1 specifically increases substance P in injured sympathetic ganglia. Ann N Y Acad Sci 1990;594:222–230.
80. Freidin M, Kessler JA: Cytokine regulation of substance P expression in sympathetic neurons. Proc Natl Acad Sci USA 1991;88:3200–3203.
81. Eskay RL, Eiden LE: Interleukin-1 alpha and tumor necrosis factor-alpha differentially regulate enkephalin, vasoactive intestinal polypeptide, neurotensin, and substance P biosynthesis in chromaffin cells. Endocrinology 1992;130:2252–2258.
82. Schellhas KP, Wilkes CH, Fritts HM, et al: MR of osteochondritis dissecans and avascular necrosis of the mandibular condyle. AJNR 1989;190:3–12.
83. Schellhas KP, Pollei SR, Wilkes CH: Pediatric internal derangements of the temporomandibular joint: Effect on facial development. Am J Orthod Dentofac Orthop 1993;104:51–59.
84. Chuong R, Piper MA: Avascular necrosis of the mandibular condyle—pathogenesis and concepts of management. Oral Surg Oral Med Oral Pathol 1993;75:428–432.
85. Piper MA: Microscopic disk preservation surgery of the temporomandibular joint. Oral Maxillofac Clin North Am 1989;1:279–301.
86. Boyer CC, Williams TW, Stevens FW: Blood supply of the temporomandibular joint. J Dent Res 1964;43:224–228.
87. Bell WE: Temporomandibular Disorders: Classification, Diagnosis, Management, ed 3. Chicago, Year Book Medical, 1990, pp 339–341.
88. Gibbs CH, Mahan PE, Manderlia A, et al: Limits of human bite strength. J Prosth Dent 1986;56:226–229.
89. Bates RE Jr, Gremillion HA, Stewart CM: Degenerative joint disease—part I: Diagnosis and management considerations. Cranio 1993;11:284–290.
90. Mahan PE, Alling CC: Occlusion and occlusal pathofunction. *In* Facial Pain. Philadelphia, Lea & Febiger, 1991, pp 187–193.
91. Gray RJH: Pain dysfunction syndrome and osteoarthritis related to unilateral and bilateral temporomandibular joint symptoms. J Dent 1986;14:156–159.
92. McCord JM: Oxygen-derived radicals: A link between reperfusion injury and inflammation. Fed Proc 1987;46:2402–2406.
93. Nitzan DW: Intraarticular pressure in the functioning human temporomandibular joint and its alteration by uniform elevation of the occlusal plane. J Oral Maxillofac Surg 1994;52:671–679.
94. Gazit D, Ehrlich J, Kohen Y, Bab I: Effect of occlusal (mechanical) stimulus on bone remodeling in rat mandibular condyles. J Oral Pathol 1989;16:345–398.
95. Ehrlich J, Bab I, Jaffe A, Sela J: Calcification patterns of rat condylar cartilage after induced unilateral malocclusion. J Oral Pathol 1982;11:366–373.
96. Ehrlich J, Jaffe A, Shanfeld JL, et al: Immunohistochemical localization and distribution of cyclic neucleotides in the rat mandibular condyle in response to an induced occlusal condyle change. Arch Oral Biol 1980;25:545–549.
97. Mongini F: Condylar remodeling after occlusal therapy. J Prosthet Dent 1980;43:568–577.
98. Peltola JS: Radiologic variations in mandibular condyles of Finnish students, one group orthodontically treated and the other not. Am J Orthod 1993;15:223–227.
99. Walter JM, Gregg JM: Analysis of postsurgical alteration in the trigeminal nerve. J Oral Surg 1979;37:410–414.
100. Martis C: Complications after mandibular sagittal split operation. J Oral Maxillofac Surg 1984;42:101–107.
101. Koblin I, Reil B: Die Sensibiltat der Unterlippe nach Schonnung. Durchtrennung des Nervus Alveolaris Inferior bei Progenieoperationen, Stuttgart. 1974.
101a. Jones DL, Wolford LM: Intraoperative recording of trigeminal evoked potentials during orthognathic surgery. Intern J Adult Orthodon Orthog Surg 5:167–171, 1990.
102. Munger BL, Renehan WE: Degeneration and regeneration of peripheral nerve in the rat trigeminal system. III: Abnormal sensory reinnervation of rat guard hairs following nerve transection and crush. J Comp Neurol 1989;2:169–176.
103. Dellon AL: Wound healing in nerve. Clin Plast Surg 1990;17:545–570.
104. Ducker TB, Kempe, Hayes GJ: The metabolic background for peripheral nerve injury. J Neurosurg 1969;30:270–277.
105. Longo FM, Manthorpe M, Skaper SD, et al: Neuronotrophic activities in fluids accumulated in vivo within silicone nerve regeneration chambers. Brain Res 1983;261:109–115.
106. Gregg JM: Studies of traumatic neuralgias in the maxillofacial region: Surgical pathology and neural mechanisms. J Oral Maxillofac Surg 1990;48:228–237.
107. Scheunemann H, Kuffner HD: Sensory disorders of the trigeminal nerve following trauma, tumor operation and iatrogenic damage. Fortschr Kiefer Gesichtschir 1990;35:138–140.
107a. Campbell J, Meyer R, Davis K, Srinivasa R: Sympathetically maintained pain: A unifying hypothesis. *In* Willis W (ed): Hyperalgesia and allodynia. New York, Raven Press, 1992, pp 41–50.
108. Armer S: Intravenous phentolamine test: Diagnostic and prognostic use in reflex sympathetic dystrophy. Pain 1991;46:17–22.
109. Morris J, Hudson A, Weddell G: A study of degeneration and regeneration in the divided rat sciatic nerve based on electron microscopy I: The traumatic degeneration of myelin in the proximal stump of the divided nerve. A Zellforsch Mikrosk Anat 1972;124:76–102.
110. Zuniga JR, Hegtvedt AK, Pate JD: Future applications in the management of trigeminal nerve injuries. *In* LaBanc J P, Gregg J M, (eds): Trigeminal Nerve Injury: Diagnosis and Management. Philadelphia, W B Saunders, 1992, pp 543–554.

Chapter 18
THE LONG-TERM UNFAVORABLE RESULT IN CLEFT LIP AND PALATE SURGERY

by

John F. Helfrick

Introduction

In September 1995, the American Association of Oral and Maxillofacial Surgeons published the *Parameters of Care for Oral and Maxillofacial Surgery—95.*[1] This publication defines indications for care, therapeutic goals, risk factors, therapeutic standards, and outcome assessment indices for over 90 clinical diagnoses. The section on outcome assessment indices has two components, favorable therapeutic outcomes and known risks and complications associated with therapy. This chapter uses the format of the risks and complications component as an outline for the discussion of complications associated with cleft management. Unfavorable outcomes associated with the following components of cleft care are discussed: primary cleft lip and palate surgery, management of velopharyngeal incompetence, surgical management of alveolar cleft deformities, and correction of secondary maxillofacial deformities.

Controversies in cleft management involve nearly every aspect of surgical care of the patient with cleft lip and/or palate.[2] These controversies exist because of the frequency of unfavorable results that accompany cleft management. Unfortunately, there is a paucity of scientific information on the nature and frequency of complications associated with primary cleft lip and palate surgery.

THE SUBJECTS DISCUSSED IN THIS CHAPTER ARE:

Risk factors for the patient with cleft lip and palate
- Psychosocial and family factors
- Coexisting systemic illness
- Experience of the treatment team
- Patient-related risk factors

- Primary cleft lip and palate repair
  - Therapeutic goals
  - Risks
  - Complications
- Velopharyngeal incompetence (VPI)
  - Therapeutic goals
  - Risks
  - Complications
- Maxillary alveolar cleft deformities
  - Therapeutic goals
  - Risks
  - Complications
- Maxillofacial skeletal deformities requiring management
  - Therapeutic goals
  - Risks
  - Complications

Risk Factors for the Patient with Cleft Lip and Palate

In addition to the scarcity of scientific information relating to complications in these patients, there is even less information relating to risk adjustment. It is well known that patients with cleft deformities may have associated systemic abnormalities that may negatively affect the outcome of care provided by the surgeon. Patients who present with local or systemic abnormalities would most certainly be expected to have a higher incidence of complications than otherwise healthy children. A number of risk factors identified in the *Parameters of Care—95*[1] are inherent to the cleft population and may increase the likelihood of unfavorable outcome.

Psychosocial and Family Factors

From a psychosocial perspective, the patients' and families' poor understanding of the etiology and natural course of the disorder may result in an adverse outcome. Many parents of children with cleft deformities do not understand the complexity of the etiologic factors involved in clefting and blame themselves for the deformity. In addition, they may not have the financial resources or an appreciation for the long course of therapy commonly required in this patient group. These two factors may lead to interpersonal conflicts between the parents and ultimately a breakup of the family unit. Because of the importance of proper sequencing of care over time and the requirements for multiple appointments and procedures, cleft habilitation in the child without supportive parents commonly has an unfavorable outcome.

Coexisting Systemic Illness

Another major risk factor is the presence of a coexisting major systemic disease. If cleft patients are not adequately evaluated by a pediatrician following birth, systemic abnormalities involving the cardiovascular, renal, neurologic, gastrointestinal, or other systems may result in unfavorable outcomes and even death of a patient during or following surgery. Psychiatric disorders can also impact negatively on the outcomes of care. Adolescent cleft patients are particularly vulnerable to depression, and professional counseling is commonly necessary for this group.

Experience of the Treatment Team

It is important for young cleft patients to be treated in a hospital by a surgeon and staff who are familiar with and have had experience in the management of pediatric patients. The anesthetic and perioperative management of these patients is unique and requires the skills of professionals with backgrounds in cleft deformity management. An additional major variable in the surgical management of cleft patients is the surgeon. It is generally assumed that one of the principal reasons for the large number of procedures available to treat cleft patients is that surgeons vary greatly in their abilities and experience. What might work for one surgeon has unfavorable outcomes for others. That is why, in this very complex area of surgery, the Team Standards developed by the American Cleft Palate and Craniofacial Association for assessment of cleft palate teams specify a minimum number of procedures to be performed by the surgeons on a team in order for the team to be approved. A major concern with managed care approach to health care in this country is that cleft patients may not continue to have access to highly qualified and skilled surgeons and the multidisciplinary team approach. Cleft surgery performed by surgeons with limited experience or a lack of current competency certainly results in unfavorable outcomes. This fact has been recognized for many years, and in countries such as Denmark, where the quality of cleft care is respected worldwide, only specific surgeons are allowed by law to manage such disorders. Unfortunately, the concept of surgeon competency equating to favorable therapeutic outcomes is difficult to prove scientifically and is therefore open to challenge by administrators of managed care programs.

Patient-Related Risk Factors

Three risk factors that may result in life-threatening complications are the presence of local or regional infections, the presence of major vascular malformations, and airway abnormalities. These issues are dealt with later in this chapter in the discussion of major complications.

Finally, other factors such as the age of the patient (i.e., too young or too old at the time of surgery), the severity of the cleft deformity (e.g., width, unilateral versus bilateral, complete versus incomplete), the patient's nutritional status, and the patient's inherent potential for keloid or hypertrophic scar formation all play a role in determining the outcomes of care provided. The risk factors mentioned in this section must be considered by the surgeon, and in the quality improvement process, in order to limit unfavorable outcomes and to determine the most appropriate therapeutic approach for each patient.

Primary Cleft Lip and Palate Repair

Therapeutic Goals

The therapeutic goals for cleft lip and cleft palate surgery are listed in Table 18–1.

The primary therapeutic goal in cleft lip surgery is to restore lip form and function. Because the cleft lip deformity is usually accompanied by a significant nasal deformity, however, restoration of nasal form and function is of equal importance (Fig. 18–1). The surgeon must also strive to limit scar formation and growth abnormalities of the maxilla and nose (Fig. 18–2). These sequelae may result from injudicious reflection of mucoperiosteum at the time of surgery or excessive scar formation postoperatively. Inadequate tissue in the upper lip, seen primarily in cases of bilateral cleft lip, can

Table 18–1. Therapeutic Goals of Cleft Lip and Cleft Palate Surgery

Cleft lip surgery	Restore lip function and anatomic features
	Restore nose form and/or function
	Limit growth abnormalities
	Improve maxillary alveolar segment alignment
	Minimize scar formation
	Minimize psychologic impact on patient and family
	Limit period of disability
Cleft palate surgery	Restore palatal form and/or function
	Provide mechanism for normal speech development
	Improve feeding and/or nutritional status
	Improve oral and/or nasal function
	Eliminate need for prosthetic appliance
	Improve social and psychologic development
	Improve eustachian tube and middle ear function
	Limit adverse maxillofacial growth and development
	Limit period of disability

(Data from Parameters of Care for Oral and Maxillofacial Surgery. J Oral Maxillofac Surg 1995; 53 (suppl 5):1.)

also restrict growth; when it is recognized, the surgeon may consider bringing additional tissue into the lip from adjacent anatomic sites. The repair of the lip also positively influences the position of the maxillary alveolar segments if the cleft includes the alveolus and palate. A final major goal of cleft lip repair is to minimize the psychologic impact that this deformity has on the patient and family.

The goal for the repair of the cleft palate is also to restore palatal form and function. An intact palate is necessary for the development of normal speech, and most speech pathologists recommend closure of the palate by 18 months of age. Palate closure also improves feeding and limits nasal regurgitation. Although controversial, one of the therapeutic goals of palate closure is to improve eustachian tube function, thereby preventing the development of otitis media with effusion (OME). Finally, as in cleft lip repair, a major goal of this surgery is limiting the restriction of maxillary growth. The type of procedure selected and the technical skills of the surgeon are both important variables in the limitation of growth abnormalities. Limitation of mucoperiosteal reflection and healing by primary rather than secondary intention are important in preventing excessive scar formation and the resultant restricted growth of the maxilla.

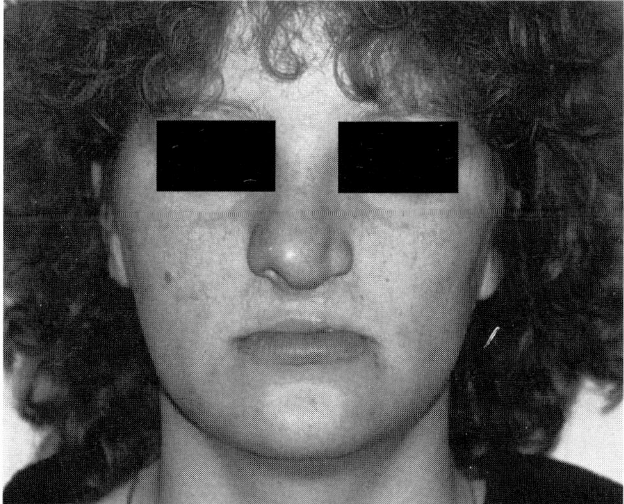

Figure 18–1. This patient has a complication resulting from the primary lip and nose repair—a functional and cosmetic nasal deformity.

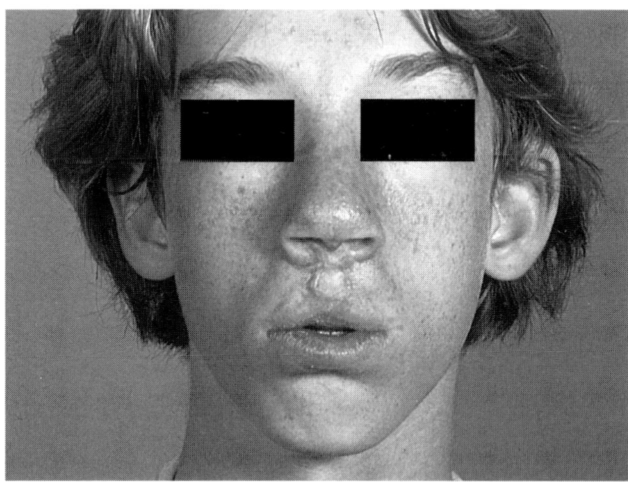

Figure 18–2. Hypertrophic scar formation is not an uncommon complication following bilateral cleft lip repair. Excessive lip scarring can also contribute to limitation of the anteroposterior growth of the maxilla.

These goals for cleft lip and palate surgery must be kept in mind by anyone planning primary reconstructive surgery or assessing postoperative results. Complications and unfavorable results are not uncommon in cleft surgery, and they are most commonly seen when the sequencing of treatment is inappropriate, the wrong procedure is selected, the surgeon is not proficient at performing the repair, or risk factors are present but were not considered in the treatment planning process. Many of these issues are addressed in the parameters of cleft care developed by the American Cleft Palate and Craniofacial Association.[3]

Risks

Following birth, the cleft lip deformity is surgically repaired within the first 6 months, and most centers prefer to perform the primary cheiloplasty at 3 months of age. It is important to understand that this repair also must address the associated nasal deformity. Therefore, unfavorable outcomes relate to both the lip and the nose. In addition, these adverse outcomes must be divided into early and late stages as well as into minor and life-threatening complications.

The palate is generally repaired before the child begins to speak. Although the standard has been by 18 months, many centers in the U.S. close the palate before the child reaches his or her first birthday.

Table 18–2 lists the risks and complications associated with cleft lip and cleft palate repair.

Complications

Because most reports in the literature address complications associated with both the primary lip and palate repairs, these two phases of cleft habilitation are addressed together.

In a retrospective study, British surgeons Lees and Pigott[4] reported a 26.2% incidence of early complications of primary cleft lip and palate surgery. A total of 164 procedures were performed. Isolated cleft lip repair accounted for 16.3% of the total number of complications, whereas simultaneous repairs of the lip and palate (rarely performed in the U.S.) resulted in a total of 34.9% of the total complications. The remaining 48.8% of the unfavorable results occurred in the group undergoing cleft palate repair only.

The majority of the early complications of cleft lip and cleft palate repair in this series occurred within the first 10 days of surgery. The unfavorable outcomes associated with repairs of the lip included one case of wound infection, one case of mucosal dehiscence, and one patient with an elevated temperature who ultimately developed a hypertrophic scar. These researchers did not define the cause of the pyrexia, and its relationship to the hypertrophic scar would be conjecture.

Lees and Pigott[4] also found that the first complication in patients with cleft palate only repairs occurred on the fourth postoperative day. The most common unfavorable result was the development of a palatal fistula, which interestingly was preceded by pyrexia in five of eight cases. In patients in whom the lip and palate were repaired simultaneously, the first complications occurred on the seventh postoperative day and consisted of palatal dehiscence with fistula formation in two cases. Two other patients had palatal fistulas at later dates. In this same group of patients undergoing simultaneous lip and palate closure, three experienced breakdown of the nostril floor; one of these patients developed nostril stenosis, which required secondary surgery for correction.

Table 18–2. Risks and Complications of Cleft Lip and Cleft Palate Surgery

Cleft lip surgery	Wound dehiscence
	Infection
	Hypertrophic and/or keloid scar formation
	Postoperative hemorrhage
	Postsurgical nasal and/or lip deformity—cosmetic and/or functional
	Restricted maxillofacial growth
	Prolonged period of disability
	Adverse effect on patient and family psychologic well-being
Cleft palate surgery	Unacceptable speech development (e.g., hypernasal speech)
	Oronasal fistulas
	Bleeding
	Infection
	Dehiscence
	Restricted maxillofacial growth and development
	Airway compromise
	Chronic otitis media with effusion
	Prolonged period of disability
	Adverse effect on patient and family psychologic well-being

(Data from Parameters of Care for Oral and Maxillofacial Surgery. J Oral Maxillofac Surg 1995; 53 (suppl 5):1.)

These researchers noted complications in their series that were secondary to their procedures but did not involve the lip and palate. Two patients developed acute otitis media following repair of cleft palates. Presumably, these patients had had subclinical infections at the time of surgery. The palate repair, which by definition alters tensor veli palatini muscle and, therefore, eustachian tube function, resulted in an acute otitis media. This complication could have been prevented by the placement of ventilation tubes prior to or during the procedure.

Lees and Pigott[4] also reported the occurrence of conjunctivitis, beginning (or first noted) on the third postoperative day, in four patients. The etiology was unknown, but one must speculate as to whether the conjunctivitis may have represented the clinical presentation of patients with corneal abrasions. This is a complication that is avoidable but can occur following any procedure performed under general anesthesia. Great care must be taken to lubricate and protect the eyes during surgery.

Hemorrhage was reported in three cases immediately following surgery. Two of the patients required transfusions. All three patients were in the group undergoing the cleft palate only repair. There were no cases of reoperation for bleeding, and no cases of secondary hemorrhage.[4]

Of importance and concern in this report was the relative high incidence of major systemic complications. Thirteen patients developed serious intraoperative or postoperative complications related to the respiratory tract. One cheiloplasty patient experienced a respiratory arrest during intubation; fortunately, the patient was resuscitated and the procedure completed. Three patients had "respiratory difficulties" on extubation after cleft palate repair. One of these patients ultimately had breakdown of the palate that required reoperation. Nine other patients developed pneumonia or bronchiolitis postoperatively. Four of the respiratory complications occurred in patients with preexisting cardiorespiratory disease. These problems had been anticipated, and following anesthesia and pediatric consultations, decisions were made to proceed with surgery in all four patients. No cases of life-threatening complications occurred after the sixth postoperative day, and all but one of the most serious complications were apparent by the second postoperative day.

On the basis of this study, Lees and Pigott[4] advocated

a postoperative stay of 3 days following cleft lip repair, because no life-threatening complications occurred after 48 hours in this group, and 5 days following cleft palate repair. They did not recommend earlier discharge in the cleft palate group because of continuing significant morbidity in the cleft palate repair patients up to and including the fifth postoperative day.

Although an uncommon complication of lip repair, excessive lip length can result when large lateral skin flaps are used to lengthen the lip (Fig. 18–3). This excessively long lip can be shortened in a secondary procedure either by raising the entire lip through resection of a segment of tissue at the base of the nose or, in selected cases, by decreasing the amount of the vermilion.

As previously mentioned, nasal reconstruction is an important consideration at the time of primary lip repair. What to do with the nose, however, has been controversial. Randall[5] has recommended that nothing be done to the nose at the time of lip repair. His concern is that early surgery on an infant's nose produces alteration in growth of the nasal cartilage. This concept, however, has been very controversial, because no specific documentation of such growth interference has been published. McCarthy[6] and others believe that unless lifting and reposition of the alar cartilage have been achieved at the time of primary lip repair, any small discrepancy is magnified as the patient grows. McCarthy[6] also stresses the importance of presurgical orthopedic alignment of the bony segments prior to primary repair. Failure to provide a properly aligned bony platform results in displacement of the nasal septum, soft tissues, and alar base, yielding a significant nasal deformity (Fig. 18–4).

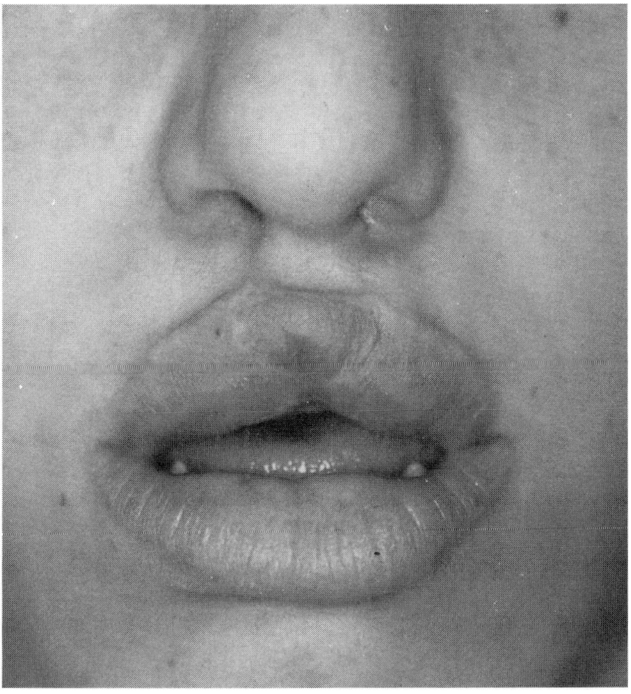

Figure 18–3. Excessive lip length and volume constitute an uncommon but problematic complication of cleft lip reconstruction.

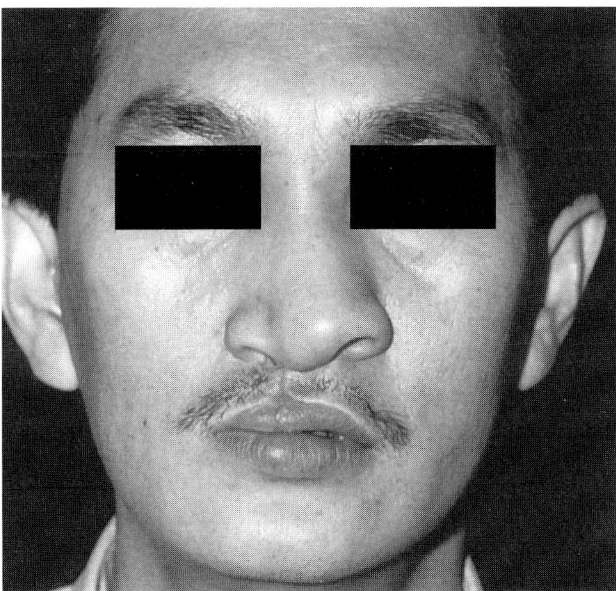

Figure 18–4. This patient exhibits significant displacement of the nasal septum, soft tissues, and alar base secondary to a failure to reconstruct the maxilla.

The nasal deformity associated with bilateral clefts is very complex and difficult to manage. Spira has stated that he's "never repaired a bilateral cleft lip that I've been happy with" (Mel Spira, MD, personal communication, 1990). The principal reason is the magnitude of the nasal deformity associated with bilateral clefts. A wide alar base, depressed nasal tip, and short columella are all components of the unfavorable results seen in bilateral cleft nasal deformities (Fig. 18–5). Sec-

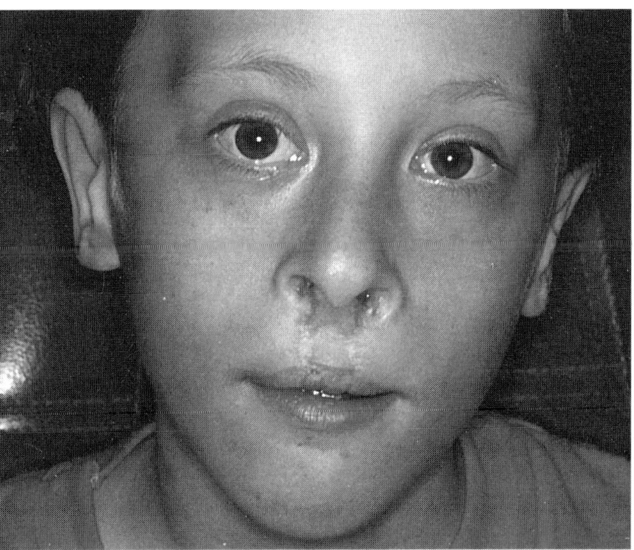

Figure 18–5. This patient has an extremely wide alar base, depressed nasal tip, and short columella—all complications of a bilateral cleft lip repair.

ondary reconstructive surgery is commonly necessary in this group of patients.

Nguyen and Sullivan[2] support the findings of Lees and Pigott[4] and state that the complications following cleft palate repair, in the immediate postoperative period, are bleeding and respiratory distress. They recommend using epinephrine injections at the time of surgery and packing denuded palatal areas with hemostatic agents to control bleeding and limit blood loss. They also note that "respiratory compromise secondary to obstruction from palate lengthening or sedation can be life-threatening."[2]

Lynch and Underwood[7] reported a case of acute upper airway obstruction followed by pulmonary edema in a child undergoing cleft palate repair. The patient, 8 months old, had Pierre-Robin syndrome, and the airway obstruction occurred at the time of extubation following primary palatoplasty. The patient's micrognathia, in combination with a swollen and recently repaired palate, resulted in airway obstruction requiring emergency re-intubation. The obstruction and consequent increase in intrathoracic pressure resulted in pulmonary edema, which was successfully treated with continuous positive airway pressure. Lynch and Underwood recommended that because infants are obligatory nose breathers, a nasopharyngeal airway should be carefully inserted prior to extubation.

Probably the most common complication following palate repair is the development of oronasal fistulas. Nguyen and Sullivan[2] have reported that oronasal fistulas following palate closure are very difficult to manage and are usually secondary to poor tissue quality and excessive wound tension. Other factors may be the type of cleft, type of closure, single-layer repair, the dead space between the mucoperiosteal flap, and postoperative maxillary arch expansion.[8] Because maxillary arch expansion can create or enlarge fistulas, it is best to avoid closure of the fistula until arch expansion is completed. Nguyen and Sullivan[2] noted that the reported incidence of oronasal fistulas ranges from 5% to 29%.

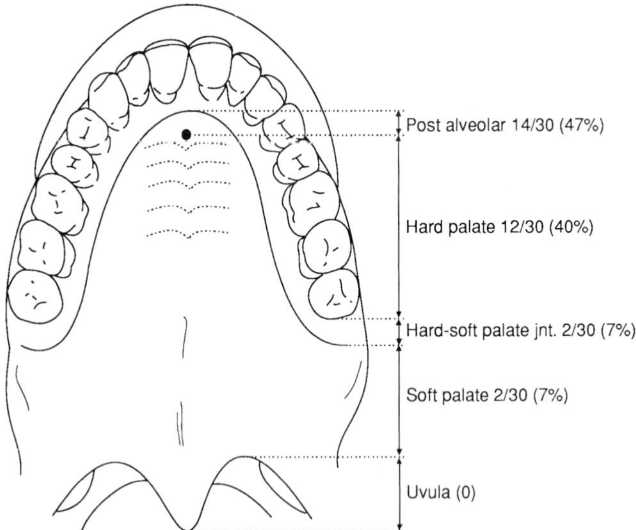

Figure 18–6. The frequency of palatal fistulas is greatest in the anterior hard palate and is lower in the posterior palate, where the blood supply is adequate, the soft tissues are more flexible, and a multiple-layer closure can be achieved.

The fistulas commonly occur in the anterior palate just posterior to the nasal palatine papillae region (Fig. 18–6).[10] This is the region where the palatal mucosa is thin and the blood supply is limited. It is important to close this area passively and to evert the wound edges (Fig. 18–7).

The rate of residual palatal fistulas following primary palatorrhaphy varies in the literature from 0 to 34%.[9–19] Abyholm and colleagues[20] studied 1,108 patients who underwent primary lip and palate repairs from 1954 to 1969. The palatal fistula rate in this series was 18%. The highest incidence of fistulas was noted following the repair of complete clefts (36.1%).

Lindsay[12] reported incidences of fistulas as 16% for unilateral and 23% for bilateral complete clefts, after

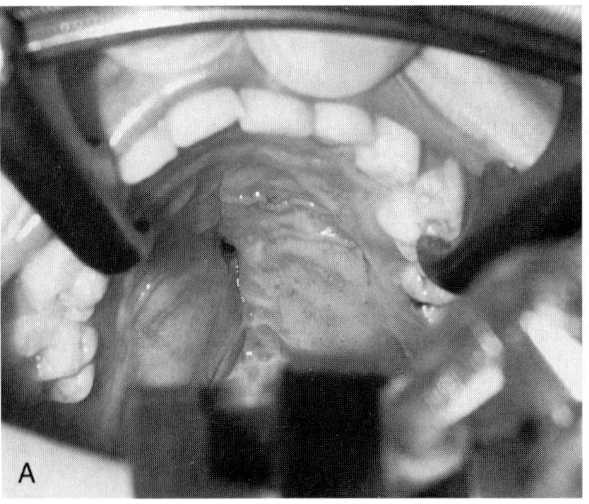

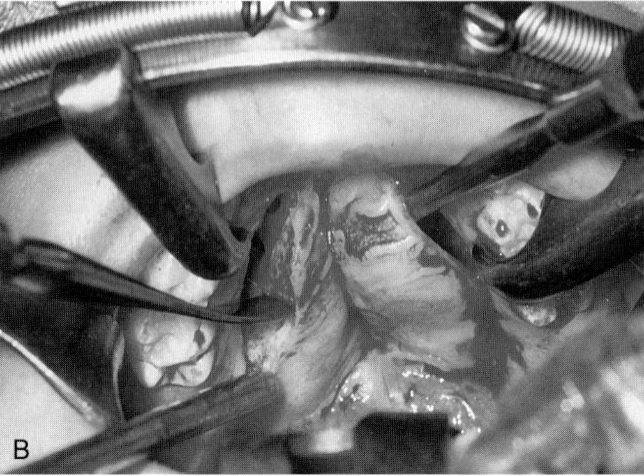

Figure 18–7. *A*, An anterior palatal fistula corresponding to the area of greatest frequency of fistula formation. *B*, An aggressive approach is necessary for the closure of palatal fistulas.

the VonLangenbeck repair in 60 patients. For a push-back palatoplasty, Lindsay[12] found a 10% incidence in unilateral and 21% incidence in bilateral clefts in a group of 45 patients. Amartunga[17] also reported on the prevalence of oronasal fistulas in a series of 346 cases. He reported an incidence of 21% in this series and noted, as did Abyholm and colleagues,[20] that fistulas were found to occur more commonly in bilateral than unilateral cleft repair. Amartunga[17] identified the junction of hard and soft palates as the area of highest incidence (42%).

The repair of the residual fistulas can also be problematic. Amartunga[17] found that fistula closure was successful in only 56% of his series of 73 patients. Abyholm and colleagues[20] reported that in 113 patients requiring fistula repair, closure was achieved in 84.1%.

Rintala[21] reported on the surgical management of 83 palatal fistulas. Closure was achieved in 83% of cases, and complete failure was found in only 4%. This surgeon employed a variety of local flaps, including hinge flaps, rotation flaps, island flaps, and lingual flaps, with or without bone grafting. Rintala[21] encourages surgeons to delay the closure of small fistulas until the alveolar bone graft procedure is performed.

A variety of techniques[10, 19] have been developed and utilized for fistula closure, the most common being local flap mobilization.[8] It is important to remember that fistula recurrence after repair is common and that the repair of even a small fistula requires an aggressive surgical approach with the mobilization of well-vascularized flaps, eversion of wound edges, and closure without tension (see Fig. 18–4).

The most significant complication or unfavorable result of palate closure is velopharyngeal insufficiency. The resonance problem, in the form of hypernasal speech, requires long-term speech therapy and, commonly, secondary reconstructive surgery. These complications are discussed later in the section dealing with velopharyngeal incompetence.

In 1990, Ward and James[8] reported on 410 lip and palate operations performed on 346 patients in the course of 52 operating days. Many of these patients were older, had not been previously treated, or had undergone previous surgery that was unsuccessful. Therefore, the surgeons were treating patients with wide unrepaired clefts of the lip, or palate, or both and with residual deformities complicated by the presence of dense scar tissue and potentially compromised blood supply. In spite of these variables, the incidence of complications was low. In the 220 lip repairs, only two significant complications occurred. In one 4-month-old child with bilateral cleft, an attempt at primary columellar lengthening with forehead flaps resulted in devascularization of the prolabial skin and mucosa. This necrotic tissue was excised on the third postoperative day. The second patient was a 14-year-old girl who had undergone previous failed attempts at repair of a very wide, complete bilateral cleft lip deformity. A repeat attempt at closure was only partially successful because of breakdown of the heavily scarred tissues.

McCarthy[6] noted that wound disruption or excessive scarring is almost always due to excessive wound tension. Associated infection may also be a contributing factor. Prevention of excessive tension on wound edges is important and begins prior to definitive lip repair. Various strap devices have been developed that, when applied, reduce the disparity between the premaxilla and the maxillary segments. The same concept can be applied biologically. The lip adhesion procedure is used in wide cleft to establish lip continuity. The natural forces applied by the intact lip decrease the distance between the prolabium and the greater maxillary segment(s). Regardless of the extent of protrusion of the premaxilla, this important anatomic structure must not be resected. Instead, the previously mentioned techniques should be applied so that the formal lip repair can be completed with minimal amount of wound edge tension. Unfortunately, in spite of excellent technique and minimal skin tension, excessive scarring can still occur secondary to inherent patient factors. The tendency to form hypertrophic scars and keloids can result in an unfavorable outcome in spite of excellent surgery.

A common complication of primary lip repair is the "whistle" deformity, which occurs as the scar retracts vertically or because of inadequate advancement and rotation of the skin flaps (Fig. 18–8). Various lip lengthening procedures performed secondarily, such as V-Y advancements, can correct the deformity and create a normal lip seal.

A complex problem seen in bilateral complete cleft cases, which results from lip and palate closure and a lack of further professional intervention, involves the collapse of the greater segments behind the premaxilla (Fig. 18–9). Palatal or orthodontic retention devices must be utilized postoperatively to prevent greater segment collapse. Although these deformities can be managed, their correction is complex, lengthy, and expensive.

A nasolabial fistula is, by definition, a defect on the

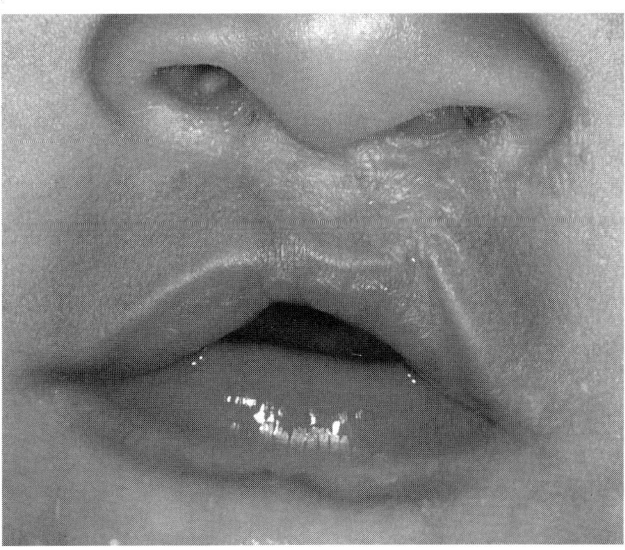

Figure 18–8. Vertical contraction of the lip scar results in a "whistle" deformity.

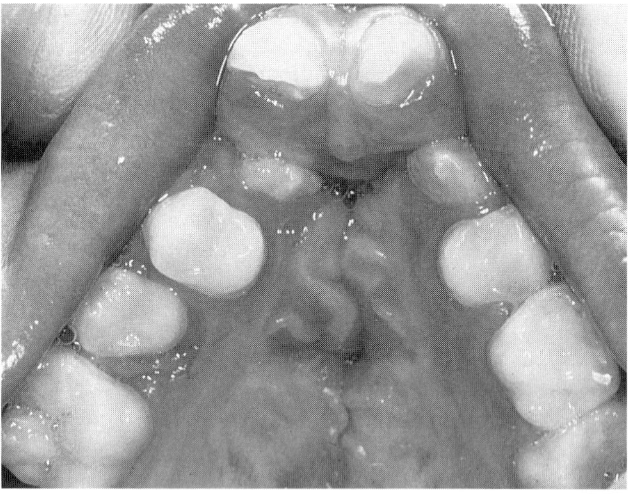

Figure 18–9. Excessive palatal scarring and a lack of professional intervention frequently result in collapse of the greater segments in the patient with bilateral cleft palate.

labial side of the alveolus that often involves the alveolar bone and communicates with the nasal cavity (Fig. 18–10).[22] During primary lip repair, this opening is closed as the floor of the nose is repaired, and a normal labial sulcus is created. In most cases, the primary repair remains intact; however, a nasolabial fistula can occur. It may result from an inadequate closure, excessive tension, infection, or orthodontic arch expansion.

Are nasolabial fistulas a complication? They certainly are if they are present when the cleft patient's habilitation is completed at age 21. A "controlled" fistula, however, that is present following primary lip and palate repair may actually be advantageous during orthodontic expansion and at the time of alveolar bone grafting. Most of these nasolabial fistulas are nonfunctional; however, if the patient regurgitates fluid through the nose or develops a habit of whistling through the defect, they can be considered problematic and may require early closure.

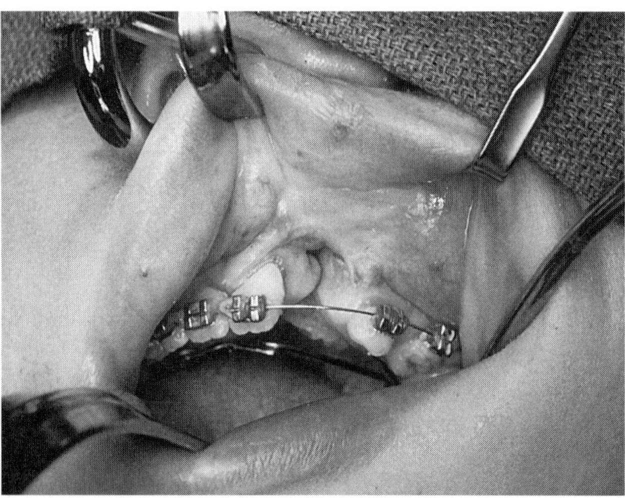

Figure 18–10. Residual nasolabial fistulas are not uncommon following the primary repair of the lip and palate. In the majority of cases, it is preferable to delay closure of the fistula until the arches have been expanded and the alveolar bone graft is performed.

The incidence of residual palatonasal or nasolabial fistulas ranges from 5% to 29% in the world literature. Dufresne[22] stated that in his personal experience, 7% of patients develop fistulas following lip or palate surgery. Secondary surgery successfully corrects 85% of these.

Closure of residual nasolabial fistulas is best deferred until the time of alveolar bone grafting, usually between 9 and 11 years. This approach allows for orthodontic alignment of the maxillary segments prior to fistula closure. In addition, the graft provides a base of bone beneath the repaired fistula that will limit breakdown and recurrence of the oronasal communication. If the oral closure dehisces, the grafted bone functions as a barrier to the nose and allows for healing by secondary intention.

In the series reported by Ward and James,[8] the most common complication in cleft surgery was the development of fistulas following palatal repair. Thirty-eight percent of the Sri Lankan patients in their series developed oronasal fistulas in the region of the alveolus or incisive foramen. This rate compares to an estimated 20% incidence of fistulas in patients treated by the same surgeons in the United Kingdom. They attributed the higher incidence to dissection of scarred and fibrotic nasal and oral tissues secondary to previous failed procedures.

Ward and James[8] also reported excessive hemorrhage after palatal repair in 8 of 189 patients. Except for one 5-year-old girl, these patients were between the ages of 14 and 25 years. All required exploration to control bleeding in the operating room, and one patient, who bled 20 days following surgery, required transfusion.

Bleeding during surgery can usually be controlled by the injection of vasoconstrictors, the application of pressure, and the judicious use of electrocautery. Bleeding must be completely controlled prior to completion of the procedure and transfer of the patient to the postanesthesia recovery unit. If this is not accomplished, the blood pressure elevation that accompanies the emergence from anesthesia will convert oozing to vigorous bleeding, and the patient will have to be returned to the operating room.

Velopharyngeal Incompetence

Therapeutic Goals

One of the most important therapeutic goals of primary palatoplasty is the restoration of the velopharyngeal mechanism and, ultimately, normal speech production. Residual velopharyngeal incompetence is a major unfavorable outcome following cleft palate repair (Fig. 18–11). Speech production depends on the normal development of language, articulation, and resonance. If the velopharyngeal mechanism is inade-

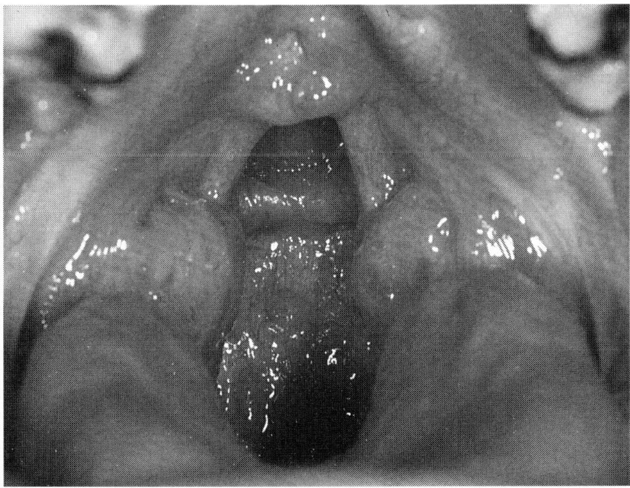

Figure 18–11. A noticeable gap between the velum and the posterior pharyngeal wall is present when the patient says, "Ah." Because of excellent pharyngeal wall motion, this patient would benefit from pharyngeal flap reconstruction.

quate, resonance is altered, and the patient's speech is perceived as being hypernasal.

The major goals in the management of velopharyngeal incompetency (VPI) are shown in Table 18–3.

The pharyngeal flap and various other forms of pharyngoplasty are the procedures most commonly used to correct this structural problem. Pharyngeal wall implants, occasionally in combination with a push-back palatoplasty, are also used if the gap from the residual soft palate to the pharyngeal wall is 4 mm or less as determined by videofluoroscopy. Whether or not to perform tonsillectomy and adenoidectomy prior to reconstructive surgery has been controversial. Clinical judgment must be used in making the final decision; however, unless the tonsils have been totally asymptomatic and have begun to atrophy, it is best to perform a tonsillectomy prior to a pharyngeal flap surgery in order to prevent the airway complications discussed later in this section.

Table 18–3. Management of Velopharyngeal Incompetence: Therapeutic Goals, Risks, and Complications

Therapeutic goals	Provide a mechanism for normal speech production
	Improve social and psychologic well-being
	Avoid compromise of normal respiratory function
	Avoid hyponasality
	Eliminate hypernasality
	Avoid interfering with normal maxillofacial growth and development
	Limit period of disability
Risks and complications	Hyponasal speech
	Persistent hypernasal speech
	Obstructive sleep apnea
	Impaired/delayed healing
	Bleeding
	Infections
	Abnormal maxillofacial growth and development
	Prolonged period of disability
	Adverse effect on patient and family psychologic well-being

(Data from Parameters of Care for Oral and Maxillofacial Surgery. J Oral Maxillofac Surg 1995; 53 (suppl 5):1.)

Risks

The potential risks and complications associated with these surgical procedures are shown in Table 18–3.

Complications

The two most common complications of surgery are residual hypernasality and hyponasality. Critical to avoiding postoperative hypernasality is the preoperative evaluation. Hyponasality, however, is usually secondary to issues related to the surgical procedure or to postoperative nasal or lateral portal obstruction from acute or chronic tonsil or adenoid infections.

McWilliams[23] and colleagues[24] have provided excellent literature reviews on the success of pharyngeal flap surgery. Residual hypernasality following pharyngeal flap surgery is not uncommon and could be anticipated if the patient is older and has developed complex speech compensations, has a neurologic abnormality resulting in little or no lateral wall function, or is mentally impaired and unable or unwilling to cooperate with postoperative speech therapy. The surgeon must remember that the reconstructive surgical procedure is a structural adjunct to the rehabilitation of the patient's speech and that the final determination of the need for surgery is made by and in consultation with a speech pathologist.

Hypernasality may also be secondary to oronasal portals that are too large. Portals may be too large because a flap is too narrow or because placement of a flap to one side has resulted in a wide portal on the opposite side. The flap may be too narrow when elevated or may become narrow through necrosis scar contracture. One technical problem inherent in the creation of the superiorly based flap is that when the vertical incisions are made on the posterior pharyngeal wall, the transverse fibers of the superior constrictor muscle are sectioned. This situation, in combination with the transection of the pharyngeal plexus motor supply to these fibers, frequently results in marked atrophy and narrowing of the flap and enlargement of the portals. One method of avoiding this complication is to raise transverse flaps that are based laterally, as described by Kapetansky.[25]

If the oronasal portals are too large 6 months or more after surgery, the flap can be revised or, more commonly, transected and a new flap raised. Obviously, the new flap will consist of scar tissue resulting from the original procedure; however, residual superior constrictor fibers are present laterally, and the new flaps generally contain adequate muscle tissue to create a new and wider flap.

If the portals are too narrow, the patient presents with some of the following characteristics: hyponasality, snoring, obstructive nasal breathing, and sleep apnea (Fig. 18–12). Although the speech may be quite good, if the patient reports considerable snoring and obstructive nasal breathing, a sleep study should be performed. If hyponasality resulting in sleep apnea is confirmed, the patient should be evaluated closely to determine the etiology. The most common causes are portals that are too small and tonsils or adenoids that have hypertrophied and obstructed the portals. Secondary surgery is definitely necessary in cases of hyponasality or sleep apnea.

The most common initial approach is to surgically enlarge the portals. If the patient is cooperative, this can be accomplished with local anesthesia and progressive enlargement of the portals with electrocautery. Such a procedure has the benefit of having the patient awake and able to speak during it. The procedure may have to be repeated if scarring or portal re-constricture occurs. Another method utilizes the performance of a Z-plasty, which allows for portal enlargement without the potential for scar contracture; however, this is a more extensive procedure that must be performed under general anesthesia.

The third approach is to simply transect the flap. The transection can be done so that a moderate ridge of tissue remains on the posterior pharyngeal wall to provide for some degree of obturation. The procedure may be necessary when (1) there is total or near total nasal obstruction or (2) the more conservative approaches have been unsuccessful. Although some surgeons have advocated injecting the portal areas with steroids during the postoperative period or using stents to enlarge the portals, such approaches are less reliable, and the patient with obstructive sleep apnea is a candidate for more aggressive portal management.

As previously mentioned, adenoidectomy and tonsillectomy prior to pharyngeal flap surgery have been controversial. Because of the potential for airway obstruction, and in order to limit middle ear effusions, most surgeons recommend removal of tonsils and adenoids at least 8 weeks prior to pharyngoplasty.[26–28]

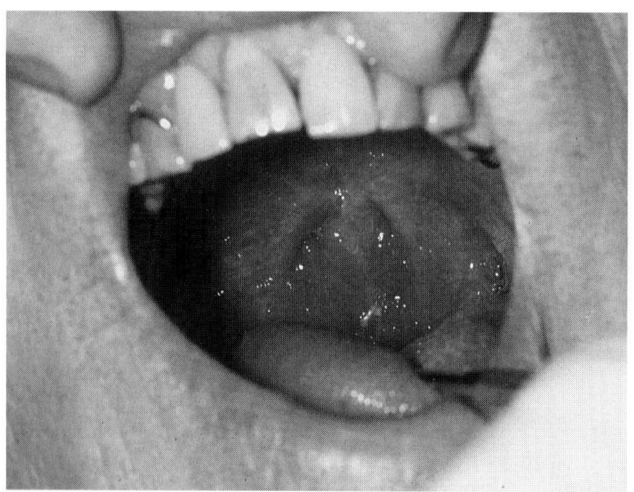

Figure 18–12. Nearly complete obliteration of the nasal portals in this patient resulted in snoring and hyponasality. Management involved surgical enlargement of the portals.

Morris and coworkers[29] have reported on their experience with pharyngeal flap surgery at the University of Iowa. They evaluated 65 patients following superiorly based pharyngeal flap surgery for velopharyngeal function, speech production patterns, and evidence of nasal airway obstruction; 83.1% had normal velopharyngeal function, 66.1% had normal or near-normal speech production, and 89.2% reported that they snored sometimes or often. Nine of the patients had postoperative complications and reoperations. Eight (12.3%) had surgical revision of the flap. Of importance is that seven of the eight were in the older age group of patients (range 11 to 38 years). One patient had revision surgery to reduce oronasal portal size. Six of the remaining seven had portal size increased because of nasal airway obstruction. In one of these, tonsillectomy was performed simultaneously with portal enlargement. Three of the six patients improved, but the other three required flap take-down procedures.

Morris and coworkers[29] further evaluated the patients who reported snoring to determine the severity of the obstruction and whether or not systemic signs of sleep apnea existed. Of the 58 patients who reported snoring, electrocardiogram data from 33 were evaluated for right ventricular hypertrophy indicative of cor pulmonale. Only one patient, in fact, showed such a possibility, but the researchers stated that the evidence for right ventricular hypertrophy in this patient was not conclusive. In spite of these findings clinicians must be aware of the potential for sleep apnea in their patients who have pharyngeal flaps.

Fortunately, complications secondary to hemorrhage and infections are uncommon. Conceivably, if the vertical incisions are made too far laterally or if the internal carotid artery takes an aberrant course, life-threatening hemorrhage could occur. Careful palpation of the incision area prior to surgery should prevent this rare complication.

Infections are also extremely uncommon. The blood supply to this region is excellent, and prophylactic antibiotics, in combination with sterile surgical technique, make infection a rare complication. As previously mentioned, the removal of chronically infected tonsils and adenoids is also advisable prior to pharyngeal flap surgery.

Another uncommon but potential complication is avascular necrosis (Fig. 18–13). It may occur if (1) the base of the flap is too narrow, (2) the flap depth does not extend to the alar-prevertebral fascia, thereby creating a very thin flap, or (3) injudicious cautery is used to control bleeding. In these cases, the flap usually must be revised secondary to residual hypernasality. The effects of pharyngeal flaps on facial growth have been controversial.

Functional skeletal adaptations have been substantiated by studies involving children who have excessive adenoid tissue in the nasopharynx. In these children,

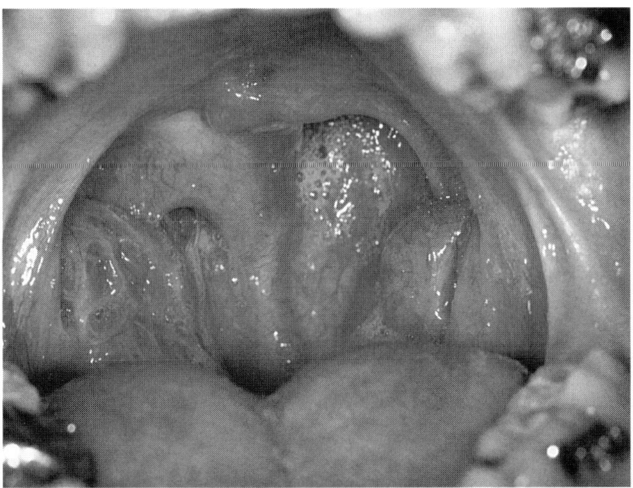

Figure 18–13. Avascular necrosis resulted in the loss of the left side of this superiorly based pharyngeal flap.

there is an increase in anterior facial height, and both the maxilla and mandible are retrusive.[30] The adaptive nature of these characteristics is highlighted by the small but significant improvement in facial form that follows adenoidectomy.[31]

Nasal airway resistance is reported to be high in the cleft lip and cleft palate population, and pharyngeal flaps significantly reduce the nasopharyngeal air space even further.[32] The facial form of the cleft patient has many of the characteristics of the "adenoid facies," and some investigators have reported that the pharyngeal flap and associated increased airway resistance, combined with tongue posturing, might further accentuate these facial skeletal adaptations.[33, 34]

The pharyngeal flap has also been said to restrain the normal forward growth of the maxilla. Semb and Shaw[35] have reviewed the literature and reported on a study, conducted in 257 consecutive patients, that addressed the question of whether or not pharyngeal flap surgery is followed by an altered pattern of skeletal development. They compared matched pairs of patients who did and did not have pharyngoplasties. Group differences failed to confirm that the pharyngoplasty group had intrinsically shorter maxillary length or smaller upper facial height. These researchers pointed out that the differences in the patients were very modest, and they concluded that a superiorly based pharyngeal flap does not appear to significantly alter facial growth in an anteroposterior or vertical dimension.[35] This well-controlled and well-designed study correlates with the findings of Long and McNamara[36] and of Pearl and Kaplan.[37] Although this issue is still controversial, there is currently no evidence that a superiorly based pharyngeal flap alters maxillary growth.

Finally, in spite of successful surgery, failure of the patient to follow through with recommended speech therapy may result in an unfavorable outcome. As previously noted, the flap procedure is merely a surgical adjunct to speech therapy. The lack of an available speech therapist or noncompliance on the part of the patient may result in less than acceptable speech rehabilitation.

Maxillary Alveolar Cleft Deformities

Therapeutic Goals

Most patients with alveolar cleft deformities require bone graft reconstructive surgery. The therapeutic goals for alveolar cleft reconstruction are listed in Table 18–4.

Risks

Reconstruction of the alveolar cleft is a common procedure, and fortunately, surgical complications are unusual. Meeting all the therapeutic goals is not always achievable, however, and unfavorable outcomes are possible. The known risks and complications of alveolar cleft reconstruction are listed in Table 18–4.

The risk factors previously cited in this chapter all

Table 18–4. Alveolar Cleft Reconstruction: Therapeutic Goals, Risks, and Complications

Therapeutic goals	Maxillary alveolar ridge continuity for tooth eruption and the indicated orthodontic correction of malocclusion and crossbites
	Alveolar bone support for adjacent teeth
	Nasal bone support
	Restore alveolar ridge form
	Eliminate oronasal communication(s)
	Improve appearance of the lip
	Improve speech
	Avoid restriction of maxillary growth on the sequelae (e.g., crossbites, midface deficiency)
	Minimize donor site morbidity
	Stable premaxilla in bilateral clefts
	Eliminate need for prosthetic tooth replacement
	Limit period of disability
Risks and complications	Partial or complete loss of bone graft
	Wound dehiscence
	Infection
	Residual oronasal fistulas
	Lack of adequate periodontal bone and/or soft tissue support
	Soft tissue necrosis
	External root resorption
	Failure of teeth in area to erupt spontaneously
	Donor site morbidity
	Collapse of dento-osseous segments
	Loss of vestibular depth
	Inadequate attachment of gingiva to teeth in bone graft area
	Prolonged period of disability
	Adverse effect on patient and family psychologic well-being

(Data from Parameters of Care for Oral and Maxillofacial Surgery. J Oral Maxillofac Surg 1995; 53 (suppl 5):1.)

apply to alveolar cleft grafting. In addition, the severity of the secondary lip or nasal deformities, which frequently relate to the number of previous operations in the area, is a critical determinant of the final outcome of graft reconstruction. The presence of supernumerary teeth in the cleft region, of exposed tooth roots within the cleft, and of infection or lack of health of the adjacent soft tissues, can all be contributors to unfavorable outcomes. As in all facets of cleft management, the timing and coordination of orthodontic intervention and bone graft surgery are critical factors in achieving a desirable outcome.

The age of the patient at the time of grafting has been both controversial and a major recognized risk factor in alveolar cleft grafting. The four principal ages for grafting are prior to 1 year (primary grafting), around 5 or 6 years (early secondary grafting) before the lateral incisor erupts, between 9 and 11 years (secondary grafting) prior to canine eruption, and adulthood (late secondary grafting). The controversies involved in timing relate to which stage results in the most favorable results with minimization of complications and unfavorable outcomes.

Primary bone grafting in conjunction with the primary repair of the palate was popular during the 1950s. Long-term results indicated, however, that grafting before age 2 interfered with maxillary growth and development, and most centers abandoned this approach.[38–40] As a result of a 1982 article published by Rosenstein and Kernahan and others,[41] primary grafting continues to be controversial. These researchers described a surgical technique that they believe does not interfere with maxillary growth and development. Most surgeons and cleft teams, however, still prefer to graft alveolar clefts secondarily.

In 1972, Boyne and Sands[42] published a paper on secondary grafting that outlines the currently accepted rationale for alveolar cleft repair. The rationale is based on the accepted view that maxillary growth in the sagittal and transverse dimensions is completed by 9 to 11 years.[43, 44] Grafting at this age does not interfere with maxillary growth and, in addition to stabilizing the maxillary segments, provides bone support for the erupting cuspid. Because the lateral incisor in the cleft region is commonly missing or is deformed, and because grafting at age 5 or 6 could further impair maxillary growth and development, early secondary grafting is uncommonly performed. Therefore, it is currently believed that the optimal age for alveolar cleft grafting is 9 to 11 years, and the rationale for the timing and management of autologous alveolar bone grafts is well documented.[45–47]

Arch expansion prior to alveolar grafting, once thought to be routine, has also become controversial. Vig and Sindet-Pedersen have made the observation that the quality and quantity of the alveolar bone are better if the majority of arch expansion is completed after graft placement (Katherine Vig, DDS, and Steen Sindet-Pedersen, DDS, personal communication, 1989). The majority of cleft surgeons and orthodontists, however, prefer to correct posterior and anterior crossbites prior to grafting. It is important for arch expansion and surgery to be sequenced properly so that the patient does not have to wear the palatal appliance for a protracted period. Arch expansion can usually be accomplished within 4 to 6 months; therefore, in order to avoid prolonged treatment, a date for surgery should be identified first, and arch expansion should begin 4 to 6 months prior to that date.

Autogenous bone is the most successful grafting material.[35] The most common donor sites are the iliac crest, mandibular symphysis, and cranium. Donor site morbidity must be considered when bone is to be harvested.

If iliac crest is selected, a limited 3-cm incision, placed at least 1 cm posterior and parallel to the anterior crest, avoids injury to the lateral femoral cutaneous nerve and resultant lateral thigh anesthesia. The cartilaginous cap of the iliac crest is exposed without stripping of the muscle attachments, to avoid postoperative gait disturbances. The cartilaginous cap may then be reflected medially, the cancellous bone harvested, and the cap replaced and sutured with wire or nonresorbable sutures. This technique also prevents significant blood loss, peritoneal morbidity, and a cosmetically unacceptable scar.

If the width of the cleft(s) to be grafted is not extensive, and if adequate bone is available, the mandibular symphysis may be selected as a donor site.[48] The surgeon must analyze the donor and recipient sites carefully, as it is possible that adequate symphyseal bone may not be available. In performing this analysis, the surgeon must remember that the cleft is usually wider clinically than it appears radiographically and that the graft, in addition to reconstructing the alveolus, must reconstruct the piriform rim. Bilateral clefts may be of particular concern. The surgeon must also assess the distances between the root apices of the mandibular incisors and the inferior border and between the cuspid roots. Of course, these are the limiting anatomic structures, and damage to adjacent teeth must be avoided at the time of graft harvest. In older patients, the posterior limit is the mental nerve, and injury to this structure, with resultant lip anesthesia, must also be voided. Finally, the harvest technique should preserve the lingual cortical plate, to ensure that bone fills in the defect. Although removing the lingual plate may limit bone healing, it does not result in a cosmetic deformity; however, it may compromise a genioplasty procedure if one is necessary at a later time.

Cranial bone has also been used for alveolar cleft grafting.[43] The parietal eminence is the usual donor site. Once the cranial bone has been exposed, a bur is used to outline the strips to be harvested. Care must be taken to limit the osteotomies to the outer cortex. The edges of the bone cuts are beveled to allow for the placement of the osteotome in a direction that is nearly parallel to the inner cortex, thus avoiding inner table perforation and a dural tear. Care must also be taken to avoid injury to the venous sinuses. Although intracranial bleeding is a rare complication of this procedure, the nondominant side should be selected for harvesting. Because of the cellular density of cranial bone, these grafts vascularize rapidly; however, because of the density of this bone, it is still not clear whether cuspids will erupt as predictably through cranial bone as through cancellous iliac crest grafts.

Complications

Complications associated with alveolar cleft surgery, although uncommon, can occur. Prevention of unfavorable outcomes is critical, and flap design is a major component of this aspect of alveolar cleft reconstruction. The goals are to obtain nasal lining closure, to adequately expose the bony borders of the cleft from the alveolar crest to the piriform rim, and to close on the oral side with well-vascularized tissue that contains attached mucosa at the alveolar crest. Failure to incorporate these factors into flap design may result in exposure of the graft, necrosis and scarring of the soft tissue, obliteration of the vestibule, and a lack of attached mucosa adjacent to the erupting teeth (Fig. 18–14). Hall and Werther[49] reported that the major complication in their series was bone loss as a result of wound breakdown and recurrence of the oronasal fistula. This complication occurred 1% of the time in prepubertal children and 8% in older children and adults. This rate correlates with the reported incidence of bone graft failure in older patients reported by Bergland and associates.[47]

Failure of the canine to erupt through the graft has been an uncommon occurrence. Bergland and associates[47] reported that for the 389 alveolar cleft grafts studied, the canines erupted spontaneously in 292, and 97 required orthodontic positioning.[47] In 90% of their cases, the arch was restored by moving the cuspid into the lateral incisor position, thereby avoiding the need for bridge reconstruction. Bergland and associates[47] also reported that external root resorption was identified in 15 canines in this series. The resorption was noted as early as 9 months and as late as 4 years postoperatively.

El-Deeb and colleagues[50] reported an incidence of 50% for canines that did not erupt through the grafts and required surgical exposure, or orthodontic assistance, or both in order to achieve eruption.[50] Of importance is that these cases involved the use of block rather than cancellous bone grafts.

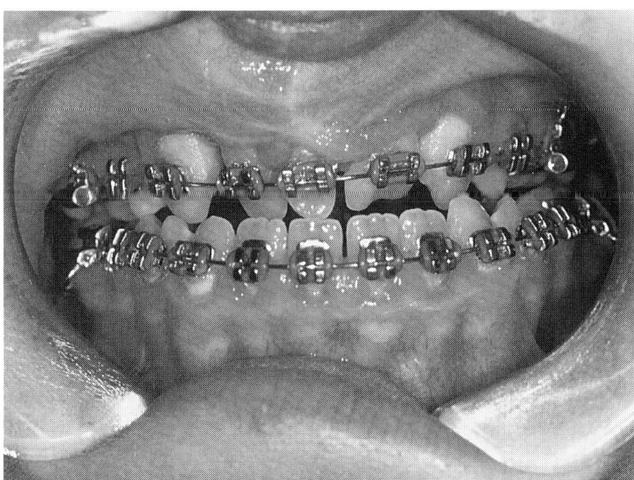

Figure 18–14. The technique for cleft lip repair in this patient resulted in obliteration of the vestibule and absence of attached alveolar mucosa.

Another minor complication is wound dehiscence with or without graft exposure. This can be managed conservatively with saline irrigation and conservative removal of sequestra if they should occur. Finally, care must be taken at the time of flap closure to avoid distortion of the ala of the nose. Advancing a flap from the vestible without proper undermining can pull the ala in the direction of the flap, resulting in a significant nasal deformity.

Other complications and unfavorable outcomes involve the orthodontic and dental restorative phases. Most cleft teams now desire to achieve space closure by movement of the canine into the lateral incisor space, thus avoiding the need for a fixed bridge or a dental implant. If adequate grafted bone is not available in the cleft area, periodontal defects and tooth loss may occur. If an implant is inserted to replace the lateral incisor, it may not integrate and may have to be removed. In addition, the final reconstruction may not be aesthetically acceptable because of ridge form and scarring in the area. Frequently, the central incisor on the side of the cleft is deformed, and the patient has a better aesthetic result if a conventional three-unit bridge is constructed. Finally, an unfavorable result at the time of secondary lip or nose revision may be obtained if the alveolar graft did not contain adequate bulk and did not reconstruct the piriform rim, thereby failing to provide alar base support.

Maxillofacial Skeletal Deformities Requiring Management

Many adolescent and adult cleft patients develop class III skeletal and dental deformities primarily on the basis of maxillary hypoplasia (Fig. 18–15). It is believed that this deformity results from the multiple previous surgical procedures that the patient has undergone. The first procedure, lip closure at age 3 months, may result in significant scarring and a tight lip, particularly in the patient with bilateral clefts. Some of the more aggressive procedures, including some techniques for primary bone grafting, involve extensive reflection of mucoperiosteum, particularly in the area of the premaxillary-vomerine suture. It is believed that this is the principal cause of midface growth problems that follow primary grafting.

The palate surgery and alveolar cleft repair also result in scarring that may interfere with maxillary growth in all three planes of space. For this reason, certain cleft treatment centers, primarily in Europe, prefer to repair only the soft palate prior to speech formation and to defer hard palate closure until the patient is 5 or 6 years old. Finally, these patients may be genetically predisposed to maxillary hypoplasia or mandibular prognathism, which accentuates the skeletal deformity.

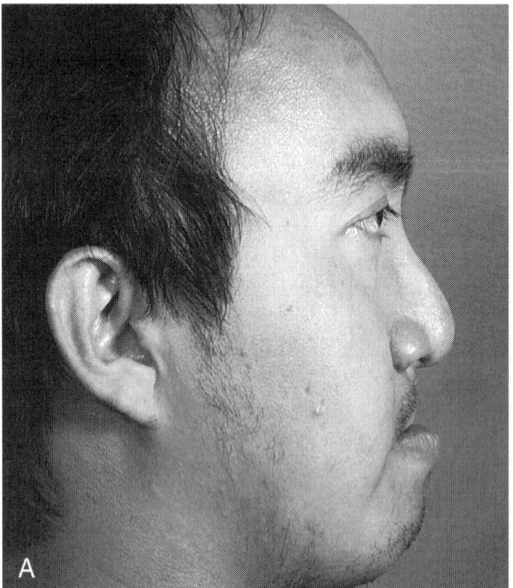

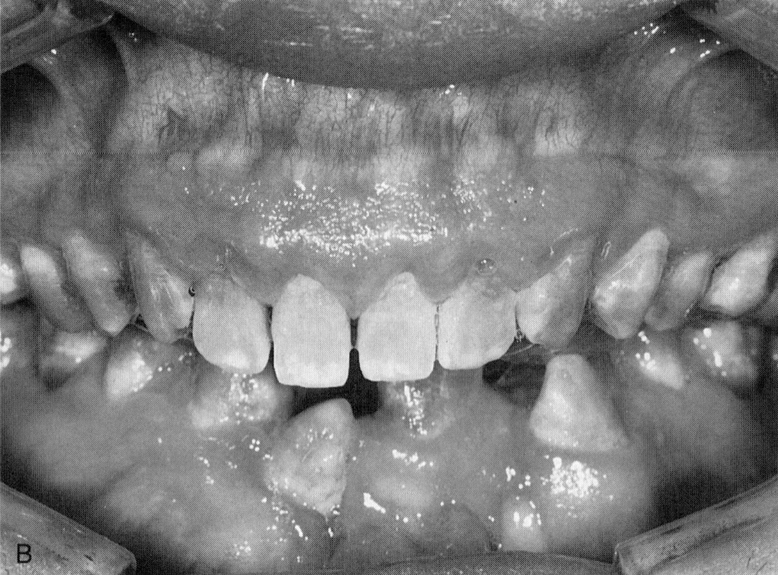

Figure 18–15. *A*, As a result of previous surgeries, this patient developed a significant class III skeletal deformity. *B*, Palatal scarring has resulted in a class III dental deformity with bilateral crossbites.

Therapeutic Goals

The therapeutic goals of surgery to correct maxillofacial skeletal deformities are shown in Table 18–5.

Risks

The risks and complications that have been identified as associated with the correction of maxillofacial skeletal deformities are also listed in Table 18–5.

Complications

Complications in orthognathic surgery were reviewed in Chapter 13. The reader should also refer to that chapter; however, because of the high frequency of complications associated with maxillofacial skeletal surgery in cleft patients, a number of risk factors and unfavorable outcomes must be emphasized here.

It is well recognized that the most significant complication of maxillary advancement surgery in cleft patients is relapse. Hochban and coworkers[51] reported on the long-term results after maxillary advancement surgery in cleft patients. Thirty-one patients were evaluated preoperatively, immediately postoperatively, and 1 year postoperatively by means of clinical and cephalometric examination. Fourteen patients had cleft lip and palate, and 17 did not. These researchers demonstrated a significantly higher tendency to relapse after maxillary advancement in patients with clefts compared with those without. Given a similar amount of maxillary advancement, skeletal relapse was much greater in the cleft group, and Hochban and coworkers[51] recommend surgical overcorrection in cleft patients (Fig. 18–16).

The following factors have been identified as being important contributors to the increased morbidity associated with maxillary advancement surgery in patients with cleft deformities:

- Presence of a pharyngeal flap
- Marginally competent or incompetent velopharynx
- Severely scarred palate
- Unrepaired alveolar cleft or oronasal fistulas
- Nasal septal deformity
- Enlarged nasal turbinates
- Number of previous palatal or maxillary procedures performed
- Severity of anteroposterior discrepancy
- Scarred tight upper lip and vestibular deformity
- Status of the dentition
- Vascular supply to maxilla
- Bilateral versus unilateral cleft
- History of chronic otitis media

Many of these factors are present in each cleft patient requiring maxillary advancement surgery, thereby increasing the potential for unfavorable outcomes.

The presence of a pharyngeal flap limits the amount of maxillary advancement possible (3 to 5 mm) before the flap must be lengthened or sectioned.[52] This factor, in combination with a severely scarred palate, greatly increases the potential for skeletal relapse. As in other maxillary orthognathic surgery, the maxilla must be adequately mobilized and in a passive position at the time of plating in order to limit relapse. Bone grating the osteotomy sites is another important consideration. The surgeon may also want to consider treating the patient reciprocally; that is, advancing the maxilla and setting the mandible back. Doing so limits the amount of maxillary advancement necessary and, therefore, reduces the potential for maxillary relapse. An advancement genioplasty is commonly necessary in these patients in order to avoid the clinical appearance of mandibular hypoplasia. If the flap is to be sectioned,

Table 18–5. Surgical Repair of Maxillofacial Skeletal Deformities: Therapeutic Goals, Risks, and Complications

Therapeutic goals	Improve the musculoskeletal, dento-osseous, and/or soft tissue relationships
	Improve mastication and/or swallowing
	Improve occlusion
	Improve dental and periodontal health
	Improve social and psychologic well-being
	Improve appearance
	Enhance orthodontic result
	Improve quality of speech
	Improve airway
	Close oronasal fistulas
	Stabilize maxillary segments
	Improve associated temporomandibular disorders
	Limit period of disability
Risks and complications	Impaired masticatory function
	Impaired dental occlusion
	Impaired speech
	Impaired social and psychologic well-being
	Deterioration of facial appearance
	Onset or exacerbation of temporomandibular disorders
	Clinical significant neurologic deficit
	Failure of bone to heal (i.e., delayed union or nonunion)
	Unanticipated loss of teeth, bone and/or soft tissue
	Dental pathology requiring treatment
	Infection (acute or chronic)
	Hemorrhage
	Pain
	Restricted mandibular range of motion
	Skeletal relapse
	Impaired growth (e.g., redevelopment of a jaw deformity)
	Onset of parafunctional habits
	Development of hypernasal speech
	Increased incidence of skeletal relapse
	Increased potential for avascular sequelae when maxillary surgery is performed, especially in bilateral cleft with a mobile premaxilla
	Acute otitis media
	Failure to correct, or creation and/or enlargement of, oronasal communications
	Failure of bone grafts
	Failure of maxillary and/or palatoalveolar bone grafts
	Nasal airway obstruction
	Prolonged period of disability
	Adverse effect on patient and family psychologic well-being

(Data from Parameters of Care for Oral and Maxillofacial Surgery. J Oral Maxillofac Surg 1995; 53 (suppl 5):1.)

the patient must be made aware that the flap may have to be replaced secondarily, although this step is rarely necessary.

Another complication of surgery relates to the creation of velopharyngeal incompetence (VPI) as a result of maxillary advancement. Adolescent cleft patients commonly have two basic types of speech abnormalities. The first is VPI, which may be enhanced or created by maxillary advancement, and the other is sibilant distortions that result from abnormal anterior dental relationships. These latter distortions are usually corrected by maxillary advancement surgery and orthodontics. In order to anticipate changes in speech production following LeFort I advancements, a careful preoperative assessment is necessary. Witzel and Vallino[53] and others have noted that the most problematic cleft patient who may develop VPI after maxillary advancement is the one who makes touch contact between the velum and posterior pharyngeal wall during slow, conversational speech. Such a patient, because of this touch contact, occasionally has hypernasality during rapid speech. Multiple-view videofluoroscopy, performed prior to surgery, identifies such patients. It is unlikely that the patient with solid contact will develop VPI postoperatively and, of course, the patient with VPI preoperatively will have it following maxillary advancement. Therefore, the patient of greatest concern is the one with marginal contact during normal conversational speech.

Acute otitis media with effusion (OME), which can occur following maxillary orthognathic surgery, is another complication peculiar to the cleft patient. It usually occurs in patients with a history of OME; therefore, an adequate history is important in anticipating and, it is hoped, avoiding this complication. OME most likely occurs as a result of tensor veli palatini dysfunction and postoperative swelling involving the eustachian tube. If a patient has a recent history of OME, it may be desirable to place ventilation tubes in the tympanic membranes at the time of surgery.

The avascular necrosis problems discussed in Chapter 13 are of great concern in the cleft orthognathic patient. Because of multiple previous procedures and resultant scarring, vascular compromise is a potential problem. In addition, the primary palatorrhaphy procedure may have resulted in an injury to the greater palatine neurovascular bundle, thus compromising palatal blood flow. Finally, in the patient with bilateral clefts, the primary blood supply to the premaxilla comes from the septal and labial soft tissues. Because the septum is detached from the premaxilla during surgery, it is critical to design the vestibular incisions so that the labial soft tissue pedicle is preserved. Failure to maintain this labial soft tissue attachment may result in an avascular premaxillary segment.

Wolford[54] reported on the effects of maxillary orthognathic surgery in the cleft patient on nasal form and function. He noted that this surgery has an adverse effect on the width of the alar base, the tip of the nose, and the nasal airway. He urged extreme caution in performing simultaneous orthognathic surgery and lip or nose revisions and rhinoplasties in these patients. To avoid unfavorable results, he prefers to perform these procedures as a second stage following orthognathic surgery.

Summary

Complications following surgery in cleft patients are not uncommon. Many of these unfavorable outcomes

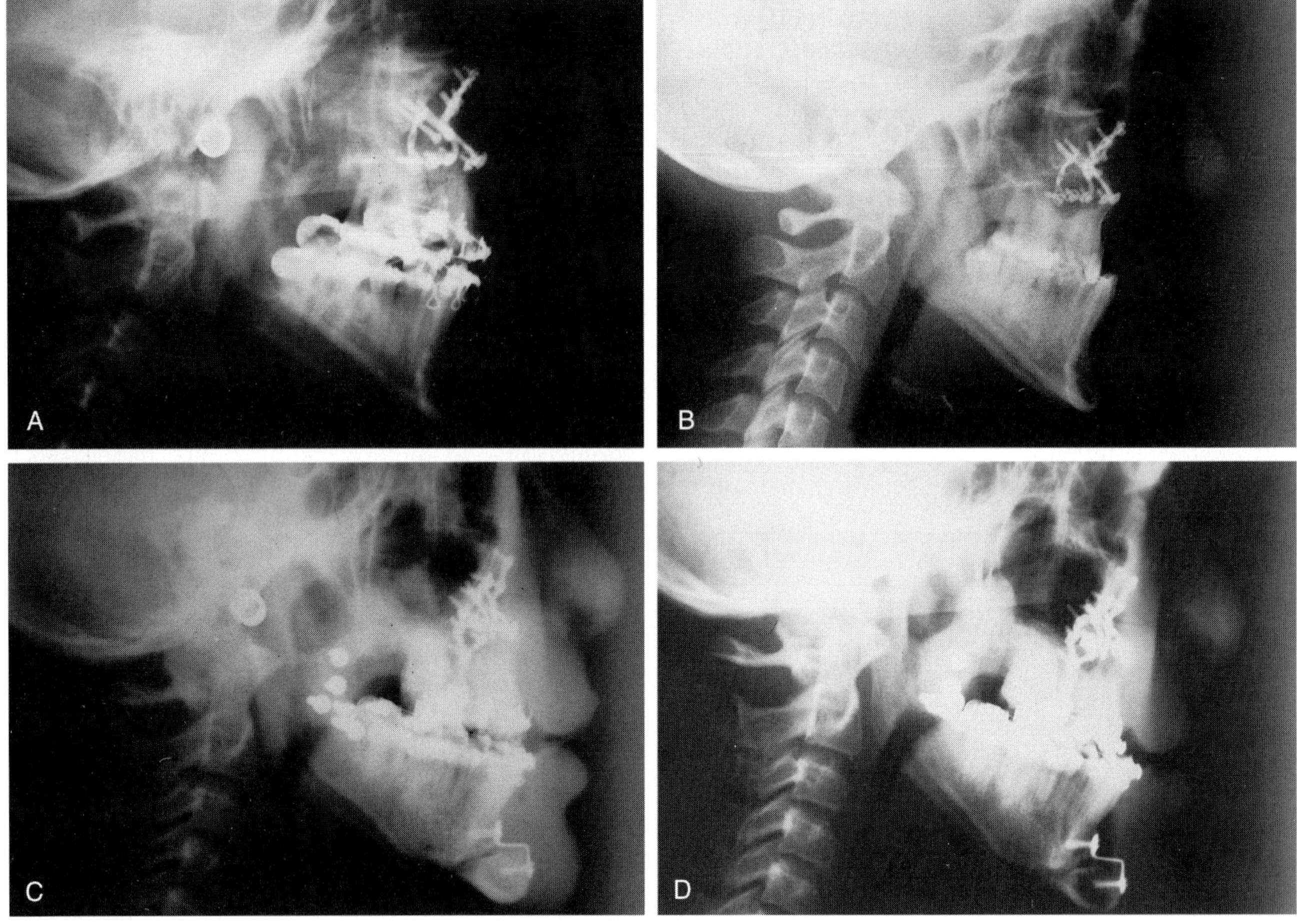

Figure 18–16. *A*, Immediate postoperative cephalometric radiograph disclosing correction of a class III skeletal deformity in a patient with cleft palate. *B*, A cephalometric radiograph of the same patient 1 year postoperatively discloses significant maxillary relapse. *C*, In another patient, a cephalometric radiograph taken 4 months postoperatively discloses relapse of the maxilla. *D*, A cephalometric radiograph taken 1 year postoperatively in the same patient as in *C* discloses significant relapse of the maxilla.

can be anticipated through the performance of a thorough clinical and radiographic examination prior to surgery. It is important for the surgeon to adequately counsel the patient concerning the complexity of the surgical procedures and the potential for complications prior to surgery. It is also imperative that the results of the examination and discussions with the patient are documented in the patient's record. Because of the frequency of complications following cleft surgery, it is advisable to obtain written informed consent describing them, preferably several days prior to surgery.

References

1. Parameters of Care for Oral and Maxillofacial Surgery. J Oral Maxillofac Surg 1995;53(suppl 5):1.
2. Nguyen PN, Sullivan PK: Issues and controversies in the management of cleft palate. Clin Plast Surg 1993;20:671.
3. Parameters for the Evaluation and Treatment of Patients with Cleft Lip/Palate or Other Craniofacial Anomalies. Cleft Palate Craniofac J 1993;30(suppl 1):1.
4. Lees VC, Pigott RW: Early postoperative complications in primary cleft lip and palate surgery—how soon may we discharge patients from hospital? Br J Plast Surg 1992;45:232–234.
5. Randall P: Triangular flap in the repair of unilateral cleft lip. *In* Grabb WC, Rosenstein SW, Bzoch KR (eds): Cleft Lip and Palate: Surgical Dental and Speech Aspects. Boston, Little, Brown, 1971, p 204.
6. McCarthy JG (ed): Plastic Surgery, vol 4. Philadelphia, WB Saunders, 1990, pp 2697–2746.
7. Lynch M, Underwood S: Pulmonary oedema following relief of upper airway obstruction in the Pierre-Robin syndrome: A consequence of early palatal repair? Br J Anaesth 1991;66:391–393.
8. Ward CM, James I: Surgery of 346 patients with unoperated cleft lip and palate in Sri Lanka. Cleft Palate 1990;27:11–15.
9. McClelland RMA, Patterson TJS: The influence of penicillin on the complication rate after repair of clefts of the lip and palate. Br J Plast Surg 1963;16:144.
10. O'Neal R: Oronasal fistulas. *In* Grab WC, Rosenstein FW, Bzoch KR (eds): Cleft Lip and Palate. Boston, Little, Brown, 1971, pp 490–498.
11. Jolleys A, Savage JP: Healing defects in cleft palate surgery: The role of infection. Br J Plast Surg 1963;16:144.
12. Lindsay WK: Von Langenbeck palatoplasty. *In* Grab WC, Rosenstein FW, Bzoch KR (eds): Cleft Lip and Palate. Boston, Little, Brown, 1971, pp 393–403.
13. Musgrave RH, Bremner JC: Complications of cleft palate surgery. Plast Reconstr Surg 1960;26:180.
14. Padgett EC: The repair of cleft palates primarily unsuccessfully operated on. Surg Gynecol Obstet 1936;63:483.
15. Reid DAC: Fistulae in the hard palate following cleft palate surgery. Br J Plast Surg 1986;78:739.
16. Schultz RC: Management and timing of cleft palate fistula repair. Plast Reconstr Surg 1986;78:739.

17. Amartunga NA: Occurrence of oronasal fistulas in operated cleft palate patterns. J Oral Maxillofac Surg 1988;46:834.
18. Posnick JC, Getz SB Jr: Surgical closure of end-stage palatal fistulas using anteriorly based dorsal tongue flaps. J Oral Maxillofac Surg 1987;45:907.
19. Jackson IT: Use of tongue flaps to resurface lip defects and close palatal fistulas in children. Plast Reconstr Surg 1972;49:537.
20. Abyholm FE, Borchgrevink HH, Eskeland G: Palatal fistulae following cleft palate surgery. Scand J Plast Reconstr Surg 1979;13:295.
21. Rintala AE: Surgical closure of palatal fistulae: Follow-up of 84 personally treated cases. Scand J Plast Reconstr Surg 1979;13:295.
22. Dufresne CR: Oronasal and nasolabial fistulas. *In* Bardach J, Morris HL (eds): Multidisciplinary Management of Cleft Lip and Palate. Philadelphia, WB Saunders, 1990, pp 425–436.
23. McWilliams BJ: The long-term speech results of primary and secondary surgical correction of palatal clefts. *In* Bardach J, Morris HL (eds): Multidisciplinary Management of Cleft Lip and Palate. Philadelphia, WB Saunders, 1990, pp 815–819.
24. McWilliams BJ, Morris HL, Shelton RL: Cleft Palate Speech, ed 2. Philadelphia, BC Decker, 1990.
25. Kapetansky D: Transverse pharyngeal flaps: A dynamic repair for velopharyngeal insufficiency. Cleft Palate J 1975;12:44.
26. Gray SD: Airway obstruction and apnea in cleft palate patients. *In* Bardach J, Morris HL (eds): Multidisciplinary Management of Cleft Lip and Palate. Philadelphia, WB Saunders, 1990, pp 418–425.
27. Crockett DM, Bumstead RM: Evaluation and management of nasal airway obstruction in the cleft patient. *In* Bardach J, Morris HL (eds): Multidisciplinary Management of Cleft Lip and Palate. Philadelphia, WB Saunders, 1990, pp 672–680.
28. Warren DW, Hairfield WM: The nasal airway in cleft palate. *In* Bardach J, Morris HL (eds): Multidisciplinary Management of Cleft Lip and Palate. Philadelphia, WB Saunders, 1990, pp 688–692.
29. Morris HL, Bardach J, Jones D, et al: Clinical results of pharyngeal flap surgery: The Iowa experience. Plast Reconstr Surg 1995;96:652–661.
30. Linder-Aronson S: Adenoids—their effect on mode of breathing and nasal airflow and their relationship to characteristics of the facial skeleton and the dentition. Acta Otolaryngol Suppl (Stockh) 1970;265:1.
31. Linder-Aronson S: Effects of adenoidectomy on dentition and nasopharynx. Am J Orthod 1974;65:1.
32. Warren DW, Duany LF, Fischer ND: Nasal pathway resistance in normal and cleft lip and palate subjects. Cleft Palate J 1969;6:134.
33. Harvold EP: The role of function in the etiology and treatment of malocclusion. Am J Orthod 1968;54:883.
34. McKee TL: A cephalometric radiographic study of tongue position in individuals with cleft palate deformity. Angle Orthod 1956;26:99.
35. Semb G, Shaw W: The influence of pharyngeal flap on facial growth. *In* Bardach J, Morris HL (eds): Multidisciplinary Management of Cleft Lip and Palate. Philadelphia, WB Saunders, 1990, pp 415–417.
36. Long RE Jr, McNamara JA Jr: Facial growth following pharyngeal flap surgery: Skeletal assessment on serial lateral cephalometric radiographs. Am J Orthod 1985;87:187.
37. Pearl RM, Kaplan EN: Cephalometric study of facial growth in children after combined pushback and pharyngeal flap operations. Plast Reconstr Surg 1976;57:480.
38. Friede H, Johanson B: A follow-up study of cleft children treated with primary bone grafting. Scand J Plast Reconstr Surg 1974;8:88.
39. Friede H, Johanson B: Adolescent facial morphology of early bone-grafted cleft-lip and palate patients. Scand J Plast Reconstr Surg 1982;16:41.
40. Jolleys A, Robertson NRE: A study of the effects of early bone grafting in complete clefts of the lip and palate—five year study. Br J Plast Surg 1972;25:229.
41. Rosenstein SW, Monroe CW, Kernahan DA, et al: The case for early bone grafting in cleft lip and cleft palate. Plast Reconstr Surg 1982;70:297.
42. Boyne PJ, Sands NR: Secondary bone grafting of residual alveolar and palatal clefts. J Oral Surg 1972;30:87.
43. Turvey TA, Vig K, Moriarty J, et al: Delayed bone grafting in the cleft maxilla and palate: A retrospective multidisciplinary analysis. Am J Orthod 1984;86:244.
44. Bergland O, Semb G, Abyholm FE: Elimination of the residual alveolar cleft by secondary bone grafting and subsequent orthodontic treatment. Cleft Palate J 1986;23:175.
45. Vig KWL, Turvey TA: Orthodontic-surgical interaction in the management of cleft lip and palate. Clin Plast Surg 1985;12:735.
46. Boyne PJ, Sands NR: Combined orthodontic-surgical management of residual palatoalveolar cleft defects. Am J Orthod 1976;70:21.
47. Bergland O, Semb G, Abyholm FE: Elimination of the residual alveolar cleft by secondary bone grafting and subsequent orthodontic treatment. Cleft Palate J 1986;23:175.
48. Sindet-Pedersen S, Enemark H: Reconstruction of alveolar clefts with mandibular or iliac crest bone grafts: A comparative study. J Oral Maxillofac Surg 1990;45:554.
49. Hall HD, Werther JR: Conventional alveolar cleft bone grafting. Oral Maxillofac Surg Clin North Am 1991;3:609–616.
50. El-Deeb ME, Hinirichs JE, Waite DE, et al: Repair of alveolar cleft defects with autogenous bone grafting: Periodontal evaluation. Cleft Palate J 1986;23:126.
51. Hochban W, Gamb C, Austerman KH: Long-term results after maxillary advancement in patients with clefts. Cleft Palate Craniofac J 1993;30:237–243.
52. Eskenazi LB, Schendel SA: An analysis of LeFort I maxillary advancement in cleft lip and palate patients. Plast Reconstr Surg 1992;90:779–786.
53. Witzel MA, Vallino L: Speech problems in patients with dentofacial or craniofacial deformity. *In* Bell WH (ed): Modern Practice in Orthognathic and Reconstructive Surgery, vol 2. Philadelphia, WB Saunders, 1992, pp 1687–1735.
54. Wolford LM: Effects of orthognathic surgery on nasal form and function in the cleft patient. Cleft Palate Craniofac J 1992;29:546–555.

Chapter 19
THE LONG-TERM UNFAVORABLE RESULT IN TEMPOROMANDIBULAR JOINT SURGERY

by

David A. Keith

Introduction

The complications of temporomandibular joint (TMJ) surgery have been discussed in Chapter 7. This chapter comprises a more philosophical discussion based on my experience with the management of patients with a poor outcome. It addresses the issue of when to operate and when to stop operating in the patient who has had multiple temporomandibular joint procedures. Predictors of poor outcome are also discussed. Case histories of patients with unfavorable long-term results after temporomandibular joint surgery are analyzed in an attempt to determine at which point faulty decisions were made.

THE SUBJECTS DISCUSSED IN THIS CHAPTER ARE:

The Most Common Poor Outcomes

The most common poor long-term outcomes are related to pain and mandibular hypomobility. Other unfavorable outcomes are infection, bleeding, poor healing, fifth and seventh nerve deficits, degenerative change, malocclusion, parotid fistula, Frey syndrome, and foreign body reactions to implant materials. A detailed analysis of these more acute complications is given in Chapter 7.

Pain

Relationship Between Pain and Pathology

Pain is a complex neurobiopsychosocial experience that is perceived by different patients differently: No two patients experience pain in the same way. The pain literature is full of examples of positive coping and adaptive strategies, but the difficulty occurs when pain is interpreted as arising from pathology and the pathology can be determined and dealt with by invasive means such as surgery. This progression of thought is common among dentists and oral and maxillofacial surgeons whose training naturally conditions them to such a philosophy. Their clinical role is to determine pathology where it exists. The obverse of that statement, i.e., to state that no demonstrable pathology exists, is somewhat alien to their educational background.

Through either culture or training, the lay public often has a similar view. This philosophy runs into considerable difficulty when one is dealing with conditions that have a psychologic component and for which the etiology is largely functional. Added to this difficulty is the fluctuating and usually self-limiting nature of the conditions, which if given time and appropriate supportive care, will resolve on their own.

Our technology has improved considerably, some may say beyond the bounds of our ability to use it wisely. For example, small joint arthrography was first demonstrated in the temporomandibular joint in the 1940s by Fleming Norgaard.[1] His thesis attracted no great interest until the 1970s, when the technique flourished, largely in the United States.[2–5] A tremendous amount of research effort was directed at perfecting the technique and understanding the internal function of the temporomandibular joint. At the same time, it allowed the dental profession to claim rights over a real problem within the joints. The current climate held that the temporomandibular joint pain–dysfunction syndrome was largely a neuropsychologic condition that, although the symptoms could be modified by dental intervention, was not entirely within the realm of dentistry.

Dentistry's obsession with mechanics no doubt fostered our interest in the origins of clicks, pops, jaw limitation, and pain and gave hope that these symptoms could finally be understood and definitively dealt with now that their cause was apparent. Having a technique to view the inner workings of the joint allowed oral and maxillofacial surgeons and dentists to order arthrography studies in what many viewed as a haphazard fashion. The result of this surge of interest was that now we had definitive evidence of pathology or at least derangement, and if the etiology was now apparent, then surely, we believed, modern techniques could correct it.

Correction of Anatomy and Relief of Pain

Arising from this mass of diagnostic information was a whole new world of dental, prosthetic, orthodontic, and surgical techniques aimed at recapturing the disk. Although studies set out to demonstrate the reduction in pain and increased function of these procedures, it is by no means clear that having the condyle function on the disk is any better than its functioning off the disk. In fact, reliable studies of surgical patients have demonstrated that these recapturing procedures have been largely ineffective in accomplishing that objective, even though the patients' symptoms have improved satisfactorily. Despite the assertion that dental manipulations were conservative, the orthodontic treatment and prosthodontic reconstruction that were subsequently needed were both extensive and expensive and were not particularly conservative at all.

Many of these treatments were based on the assumption that altering the occlusion, or the position of the mandible, or both, and thereby the condyle within the fossa would permit better physiologic function. I know of no credible studies to indicate where the condyle is supposed to be nor any that would indicate where it should be if any changes are deemed necessary. In fact, studies demonstrate the wide variation of normal position of the mandibular condyle in pain-free, functioning individuals.

The failure of these "conservative" treatments invariably led to referrals for surgical repositioning. A whole variety of surgical techniques were developed to recapture the disk, including soft tissue and osseous surgery as well as orthognathic surgery. The results of these procedures indicated a high degree of success irrespective of the particular technique used. Some follow-up studies, however, demonstrated that clinical success and relief of symptoms were not necessarily associated with repositioning of the meniscus. In fact, the results of these procedures may have been a rather rapid remodeling process that might have happened in any case had the patient and surgeon waited.

Arthrography was eventually succeeded by computed tomography (CT scanning), which in retrospect suffered from many artifacts. Magnetic resonance imaging (MRI) currently provides a gold standard for soft tissue imaging within the joint and has provided the ability to define the position and condition of the meniscus with what would appear to be exquisite accuracy. The concurrent development of arthroscopic diagnostic and surgical techniques has correlated these findings with the MRI scans and provides more and more sophisticated information about the condition and function of the joint. Surgical arthroscopic techniques designed either to free up the meniscus or to reposition it have gained in popularity, but again, the long-term results seem to suggest that these techniques do not reliably change the anatomy of the joint despite the fact that most patients improve symptomatically.

With all this information, it became harder and harder not to operate on a temporomandibular joint when there appeared to be so many things that could go wrong and so many different techniques designed to correct the problem. As previously stated, "Just because a procedure can be done does not mean that it should be done."[6] The ability to operate and seemingly to change the internal anatomy and function of the joint led to one of the major disasters in the history of oral and maxillofacial surgery as a specialty.

Having decided to operate on the deranged joint, the surgeon must decide what to do with the damaged meniscus. Should it be repaired and repositioned, with or without osseous surgery, or should it be removed? Once removed, should it be replaced? At the same time that surgeons were getting more involved in surgical approaches to the temporomandibular joint, a family of joint and meniscal replacement materials were manufactured by the Vitek Company in Houston, Texas. Even though the orthopedic literature had condemned the use of polytetrafluoroethylene in joints because of its known ability to fragment and particulate with subsequent development of a foreign body giant cell reaction, this company was allowed to market these implants for the temporomandibular joint.

Although short-term improvements were reported, it rapidly became obvious that what had happened to these implants in other joints was indeed occurring in the temporomandibular joint. Subsequent history has demonstrated the extensive local damage that can occur when these interpositional materials are left in place for several years. The marked destructive changes in the mandibular condyle, articular eminence, posterior aspect of the zygomatic arch, and glenoid fossa have been documented extensively.[7, 8] What is not yet clear is the long-term effects of this condition both locally and systemically. Whereas the orthopedic literature has credible working hypotheses for periarticular breakdown,[9] the majority of studies in our literature are as yet concerned only with the surgical salvage of these joints.

The Complex Physiology of Pain

What is remarkable, but not surprising if the medical literature is reviewed, is that despite these various surgical interventions for the relief of pain, many patients continue to have pain, and indeed, some patients' pain seems to escalate after each surgical intervention.

We need a complete change in philosophy that appears to be anathema to our training. We need to introduce the concept of chronic pain and view it as a diagnosis, not a symptom. Morris,[10] in his book *The Culture of Pain,* summarizes it thus:

> From the time of the ancient hippocratic writings, pain has held a clear and secure status of a symptom. In effect, western medicine has understood pain as a more or less readable inscription that the skilled physician might interpret for its revelations about processes hidden deep within the flesh. Pain on this view is a message composed, sent, and delivered by illness. The medical revolution now underway does not seek to overthrow the ancient—and surely sound—wisdom that interprets pain as a symptom. Rather, alongside this familiar view it introduces a basic change in perspective from which we see that pain is sometimes completely illegible. This more or less unreadable pain no longer resembles a message that passes, by means of a common code or language, in between the physician and the illness. Now the message is the illness.[10]

The literature and professional organizations as well as individuals experienced in the management of these problems are promoting the concept that temporomandibular disorders are chronic pain disorders and need to be managed as such. No longer can we commit ourselves to pain as a sentinel of specific pathology. Rather, we need to identify the highly complex and interrelated psychosocial and behavioral aspects of the patient's presentation and deal with these aspects concurrently with the organic problem.

This viewpoint is unpopular for a whole variety of quite obvious reasons. First, it goes against the grain of our training and education. Second, it moves this group of patients outside the realm of our expertise alone. Third, it relegates temporomandibular disorders to the category of medical rather than dental conditions. This last reason, of course, has philosophical as well as financial implications, but the movement appears to be well under way, and as more and more research of credible quality becomes available, the basis becomes more and more sound.

Interdisciplinary Approach to Pain Management

This philosophy does not, of course, force us as a profession to relinquish our interest in this subject, because we are the professionals who know most about the anatomy, physiology, and function of the masticatory apparatus, but it does suggest that we alone cannot manage many of the patients with these problems. Our primary role is to evaluate patients with masticatory complaints and to determine in a responsible way whether pathology and abnormality exist. Are those abnormalities consistent with and the cause of the patient's complaint, and furthermore, will correction of those abnormalities relieve the patient's symptoms?

It is at this point that we get into some difficulty, because the construct of our training and education has ill prepared us to answer the latter question with any great perception. It is here, however, that a multidisciplinary approach, including input from physical therapists, psychologists, psychiatrists, physiatrists, neurologists, and other health care providers, must play an important role.

The interdisciplinary approach has other advantages. Patients who have psychological problems that contribute to their pain complaints may be entirely relieved of their suffering by behavioral, psychological, or psychiatric treatment and thus become nonpatients. The unrecognized psychogenic nature of many pain complaints is one of the most powerful predictors of poor outcome. If a patient with psychological problems also has organic pathology, then the outcome of surgery can be much enhanced by supportive psychological care.

Case Reports

Case 1

A 45-year-old female had a long history of chronic headaches and bilateral temporomandibular joint clicking and pain. She had undergone orthodontic and restorative treatment with the hope of eliminating the pain. Four years ago, her symptoms worsened, and she was referred to an oral and maxillofacial surgeon. Because she admitted to nocturnal bruxism, a night-time splint was delivered on the same day that an MRI of the right joint was obtained that demonstrated anterior meniscal dislocation without reduction. The following week, an MRI of the left joint revealed similar findings. Owing to continued pain and dysfunction in the left joint, an arthroplasty was performed, and the patient was advised that a right-sided procedure would be necessary. The patient underwent postoperative physical therapy, which was delayed by infection of the surgical site. Two months after surgery, the left side was asymptomatic, but the right temporomandibular joint was painful and the temporal headaches continued. Six months after the first procedure, right temporomandibular joint arthroplasty was performed, and the patient made a good postoperative recovery. She still required Fiorinal, Motrin, and Percocet for pain relief, however.

Two years after the second procedure, the patient was re-evaluated for pain and dysfunction. She was able to open to 35 mm in the midline with left and right lateral excursions of 6 mm. She had an anterior open bite of 2 mm. She had a class I occlusion on the right and a class II occlusion on the left (Figs. 19–1 and 19–2). Tomograms of the temporomandibular joints reveal marked atrophy and loss of the mandibular condyles; the condylar necks were sclerotic with sclerosis of both fossae. In view of the

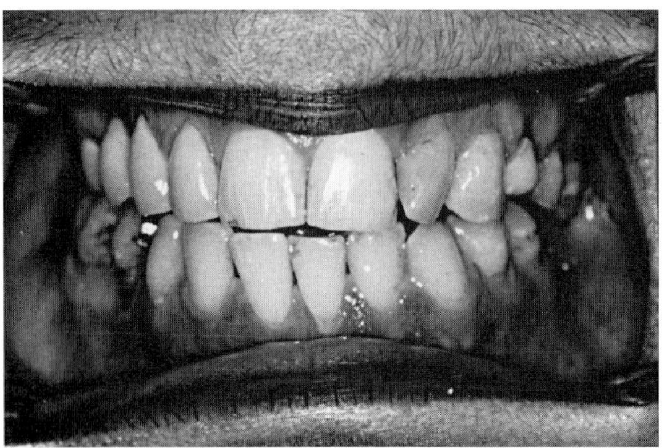

Figure 19–1. *Case 1*: Frontal photographs of occlusion.

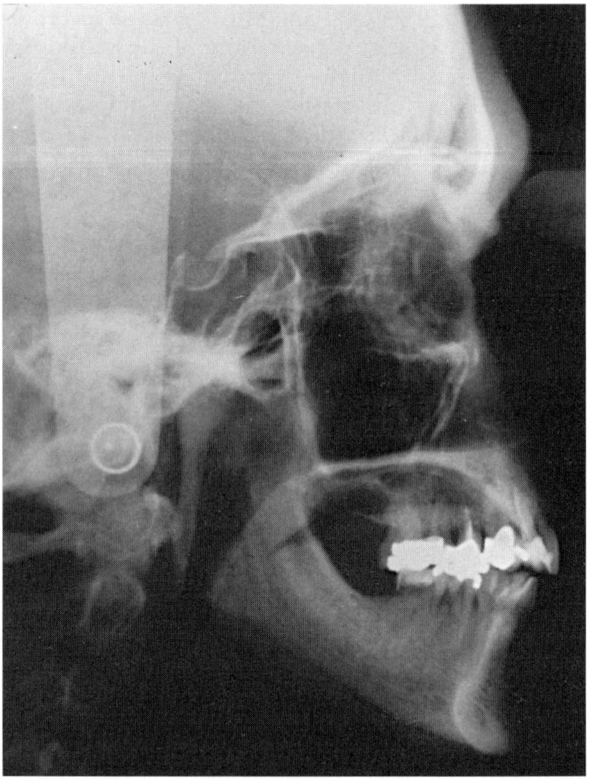

Figure 19–2. *Case 1*: Lateral cephalometric radiograph demonstrating rotation of left mandible with anterior open bite and mandibular retrognathism.

continuing symptoms and malocclusion, it was decided to reconstruct both temporomandibular joints with costochondral junction grafts in association with orthodontic and restorative dental treatment. The patient underwent this procedure and regained a functional range of motion and a stable occlusion. Her joint pain decreased, but the headaches continued.

This case demonstrates the dangers of relating pain to pathology. The patient had a long history of headaches that were diagnosed as tension-type headaches, but because images demonstrated derangements of the temporomandibular joint, it was assumed that operating on the joints would relieve the patient's symptoms. This did not occur, and the surgery produced a significant malocclusion necessitating bilateral joint reconstruction. In hindsight, it was recognized that the patient's joint clicking and derangement were incidental to her chief complaint of headache.

Case 2

The patient has a 16-year history of temporomandibular joint problems that started one morning when she was unable to open her mouth. She consulted her general dentist, who treated her with a soft diet, transcutaneous electrical nerve stimulation (TENS), and splint therapy. She subsequently saw a chiropractor. Her chief complaints were pain in the temporomandibular joints and ears, headaches, muscle spasms, and neck, back, and shoulder pain. She was treated by a neurologist with diazepam and by a gastroenterologist for irritable bowel syndrome. She underwent a further course of TENS, biofeedback, physical therapy, speech therapy, relaxation techniques, and splints.

Eight years later, the patient had a fall, and her symptoms worsened. Temporomandibular joint films were taken (Fig. 19–3). She was referred to a temporomandibular joint specialist, and further splint therapy was undertaken. She was finally referred to an oral and maxillofacial surgeon who recommended surgery on the right temporomandibular joint. A second opinion suggested that the patient not undergo surgery because of the chronicity and multifactorial basis of her pain problem. She decided, however, to go ahead with a right condylectomy (Fig. 19–4).

On reevaluation 1 year after the surgery, the patient still had the same spectrum of headaches and facial pain and in addition had a bite change with deviation to the right side on opening. The bite was visibly premature on the right. The surgeon recommended a similar procedure on the left joint; however, the patient again sought a second opinion, which recommended aggressive medical management of the pain and dental treatment to attempt to equilibrate the occlusion. The patient's symptoms did not resolve with this approach, so it was decided to reconstruct the right temporomandibular joint by way of an extraoral sliding osteotomy to restore the anatomy (Fig. 19–5). No assurance that the headache problems would resolve was given.

This patient has myofascial pain dysfunction and tension-type headaches. Surgical treatment created an iatrogenic malocclusion, and a recommendation to perform similar surgery on the contralateral side would no doubt result in a retrognathic mandible and a need for subsequent mandibular advancement. The decision was made to correct the result of the previous operation to restore the patient's native occlusion. The pain problem was not expected to change, and chronic pain management strategies were put in place to handle it.

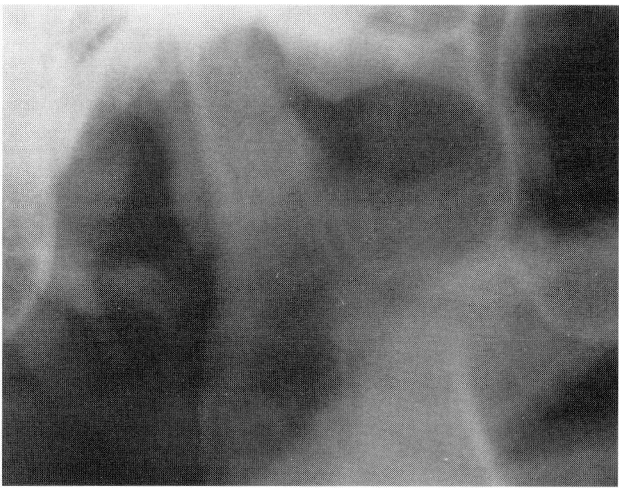

Figure 19–4. *Case 2*: Right temporomandibular joint after surgery.

Mandibular Hypomobility

Normal Range of Motion

Decreased mandibular mobility is the other common complaint and reason for surgical intervention; however, it is invariably secondary to pain as the patient's chief complaint. Previously published reports,[11–13] as well as personal observation (Cho Y-M, Keith DA:

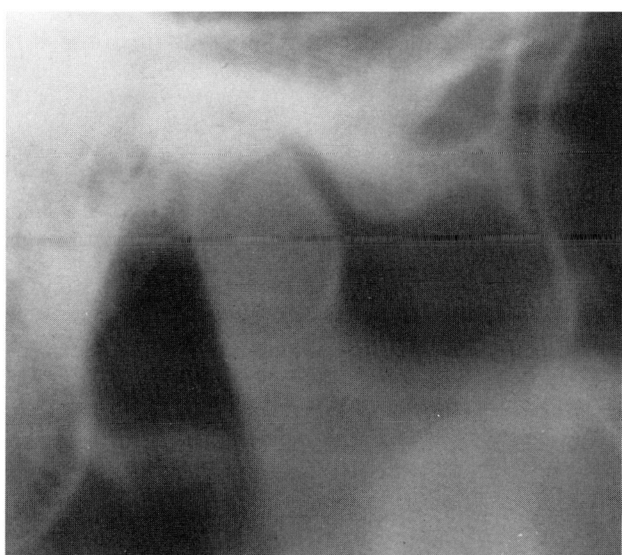

Figure 19–3. *Case 2*: Normal right temporomandibular joint anatomy prior to surgery.

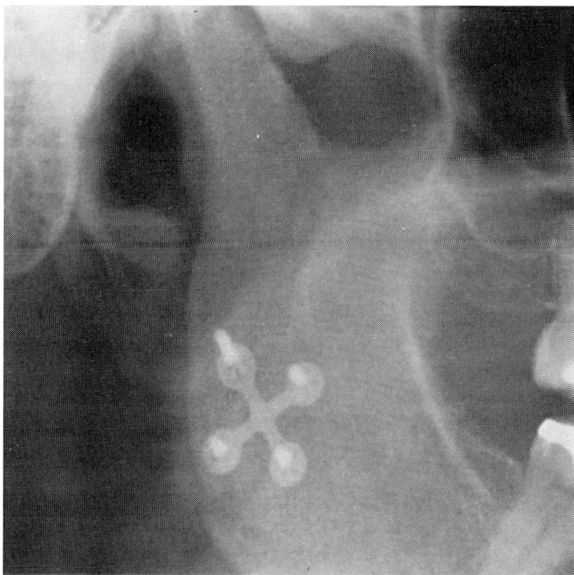

Figure 19–5. *Case 2*: Right temporomandibular joint after sliding osteotomy to correct occlusion.

Mandibular mobility in temporomandibular dysfunctions, unpublished, 1993), demonstrate, based on combined mean analysis, that the mean interincisal opening is 50.7 ± 6.4 mm for the total population (with a range of 31.5 to 69.9 mm). For males, the figure is 53.1 ± 7.3 mm (with a range of 31.2 to 75.0 mm) and for females 48.5 ± 5.6 mm (with a range of 31.7 to 65.3 mm). As these figures demonstrate, there is a wide range of normal mandibular motion, and although dentists may complain about treating patients on the low end of the normal scale, such patients have no complaints themselves.

Relationship of Range of Motion to Mastication, Speech, and Various Joint Conditions

The primary functions of the masticatory system are speech, deglutition, and mastication. Little information is available regarding the range of motion necessary to perform these activities.

Gibbs and colleagues[14] have studied chewing patterns and jaw movement during mastication and have determined that masticatory movements occur within one half or less of maximal interincisal opening. The maximum amount of vertical movement from occlusal contact was plotted to be 21.6 mm. Prehensile (grasping) movements are not considered essential to mastication, because food may be portioned in smaller sizes prior to initiation of masticatory movements.

All speech sounds are made by controlled expulsion of air from the lungs. Vertical jaw positions during common speech sounds have been reported. Sounds made by rapid transition from one vowel to another (diphthongs) require 5 to 10 mm of interincisal space. Nasal consonants require 2 to 4 mm, and sibilant sounds are produced with only 1 to 1.5 mm of incisal separation.[15]

Patients with bony ankylosis have no mandibular motion at all. Those with fibrous ankylosis may be limited to 10 to 20 mm of opening. Patients presenting with other diagnoses have mandibular motion as shown in Table 19–1.

Patients with acute close lock may have a maximum interincisal opening of 20 to 25 mm, which although inconvenient appears to be compatible with most oral functions. For patients with internal derangement, one of the driving forces for surgical intervention is to increase that range of motion, and most surgeons would aim for 35 mm or so, after rehabilitation. In the ankylosis patient who has undergone multiple operations, maintaining an interincisal opening of 20 mm would probably be considered a success.

Table 19–1. Amount of Mandibular Motion Associated with Various TMJ Disorders

TMJ Disorder	Opening (mm)
Capsulitis	45.7 ± 4.0
Capsulitis and myofascial pain dysfunction	43.0 ± 6.5
Myofascial pain alone	42.6 ± 7.0
Degenerative joint disease	40.3 ± 6.9
Internal derangement	
With reduction	45.8 ± 5.2
Without reduction	30.5 ± 5.6

(From Cho Y-M, Keith DA: Mandibular mobility in temporomandibular dysfunction. Unpublished observations, 1993.)

Table 19–2. Chronologic Summary for Patient in Case 3

Year	Event(s), Treatment(s), Result(s)
1974	Hit in face with baseball bat
	Splint therapy, physical therapy, ultrasound, etc
1981	Arthrogram
July	Right temporomandibular joint arthroplasty
October	Left temporomandibular joint condylectomy
1982	
January	Right temporomandibular joint condylectomy
	Trigger point injections
	Outpatient pain management program
1984	
May	Bilateral reconstruction of temporomandibular joints with costochondral junctions
	Bilateral coronoidectomies and muscle stripping
	Physical therapy
December	Bilateral coronoidectomies and muscle stripping
1985	
June	Inpatient pain program
	Grafts removed; bilateral total joints placed
	Postoperatively, left joint dislocated; relocated manually
1986	
October	Muscle stripping and release of ankylosis
1988	
January	Release of scar tissue
1989	
January	Release of scar tissue
November	Condylar implants removed
1991	
January	Glenoid fossa implants removed
July	Coronal flap; bilateral zygomatic osteotomies; bilateral costochondral grafts and temporalis muscle flaps
1994	
October	Coronal flaps; release of scar tissue
	Bilateral costochondral grafts and temporalis muscle flaps
	Chronic pain evaluation
1995	
March	Manipulation under anesthesia
September	Manipulation under anesthesia

Case Report

Case 3

A 34-year-old woman has had pain for over 20 years, beginning with the onset of local aching in the left temporomandibular joint and then involving the right temporomandibular joint. A chronologic summary of her history is shown in Table 19–2.

Evaluation for Inpatient Pain Program, August 1985

This 34-year-old female has had facial pain since 1974. She has had multiple surgical procedures of both temporomandibular joints, including replacement of mandibular condyles and glenoid fossae with prosthetic joints. She has had trials of nerve blocks and outpatient therapy with no resolution of her pain problem. There were several signs of reactive depression, including insomnia, weight loss, and feelings of hopelessness and helplessness. Her life has been revolving around the pain. She has been unable to return to work because of the pain. She is totally inactive at this point and complaining of anxiety attacks and fainting spells. Because the pain is unresponsive to conventional outpatient approaches and is associated with marked life disruption, this patient is appropriate for admission to an inpatient pain program with milieu as an important component. The extent of pain and disability is such that the goal of changing her pain behavior syndrome probably could not be accomplished in a lesser setting. She seems motivated and agreeable to this approach.

Chronic Pain Evaluation, December 1994

The patient has had jaw and head pain for about 20 years but has noted increased frequency and intensity and a new location of this pain since her last operation about 2 months ago. She describes this pain as being bilateral now, whereas before it was only on the left side of her face, extending from the periauricular region down to the angle of the jaw. Now it is also in the right periauricular region down to the angle of the right side of the jaw.

The pain is continuous, shooting, stabbing, sharp, cramping, hot, burning, throbbing, and aching in nature, with acute interspersed paroxysms of pain. The patient relates that when her pain flares up, her face will become erythematous, and she notes some blanching and swelling of the periauricular regions.

The patient is currently not employed and is receiving disability compensation. The pain increases with cold temperatures, fatigue, stress, alcohol, and noise, and she is unable to chew solid foods. Her pain also increases with talking. She is on a soft-solid diet. It is quite probable that she will require further procedures for the continuing problem of ankylosis of her temporomandibular joints.

The patient's medications consist of Percocet, 1 tablet by mouth every 6 hours, which helps to take the edge off her pain somewhat. Today, the patient states her pain level is at 7/10 on a scale of 1/10 to 10/10, but at times it can rise to 10/10 with no apparent provocation. The Percocet brings the level down to about 5/10. Her only other medications are Premarin and Provera. The patient is reluctant to take long-term medications for any reason. She recently tried indomethacin, 3 times a day for 6 weeks, but did not find it helpful.

The patient notes that she is unable to sleep on her back. She has to sleep in a lateral decubitus position with many changes from one side to the other throughout the night because of the pain.

The other therapies she has tried include trigger-point injections in the early 1980s, which served only to aggravate her pain, causing muscle spasm and severe headache. She participated in the Inpatient Pain Program in 1985, in which she learned physical therapy, relaxation, biofeedback, psychotherapy and ice massage techniques, which did not help whatsoever. Heat helps her to relax but does not really decrease the pain.

The patient's previous medical history is significant for hiatal hernia with gastroesophageal reflux, which does not require any therapy currently. She has had three spontaneous vaginal deliveries and a subsequent tubal ligation. She had a "small cerebrovascular accident," which resulted in a left footdrop, around 3 years ago after one of her operations; the footdrop resolved spontaneously after 3 months. Past surgical history includes arthroscopy of the right knee, cholecystectomy, and tubal ligation. The patient has allergies to codeine, which gives her chest pain. Fentanyl patch was tried recently and gave her skin irritations, and morphine causes respiratory depression.

Physical examination showed the patient to be a moderately obese, pleasant female in no acute distress. On examination of her head and neck, she had a slightly ruddy complexion. There was minimal mouth opening, about 15 mm, which was limited by pain. She had decreased lateral range of motion of the neck secondary to pain and mild decrease in extension and flexion of the neck. She had no audible click at the temporomandibular joint, although it was very tender to palpation bilaterally from the periauricular area, both anterior and posterior to the ears bilaterally, down to the angle of the jaw. She had bilateral neck scars that were nontender to light touch and scars from her scalp to the posterior auricular area. Cranial nerves II through XII were intact, although she tended to squint her left eye a little more than the other. The extraocular motions were intact, and pupils were equal, round, and reactive to light and accommodation testing. The rest of the physical examination was benign. There were no areas of hypesthesia or hyperesthesia on the face and no areas of allodynia or hyperpathia. In fact, the only finding was severe tenderness on palpation of the previously described areas. In addition, there were some vascular and autonomic changes, which consisted of the erythematous complexion; however, temperature was symmetric bilaterally, and there was no blanching on palpation of the face.

The patient's anatomic diagnosis appears to be neuropathic pain from multiple surgical interventions. She does exhibit some pain behavior, in terms of guarding the facial muscles and trying not to open her mouth too much or to touch the area too much. This has had an effect on many of her activities, in the sense that she is no longer able to read with enjoyment as she did in the past secondary to resurgence of pain, and as mentioned, it has limited her eating and her interacting and talking in a social manner.

Pain Diagnostic Tests

Stellate Ganglion Blocks × 3: No change.
IV Lidocaine: 8/10–5/10.

Pain Medications

Twenty-three different medications have been tried for pain relief, including narcotics, nonsteroidal anti-inflammatory drugs, muscle relaxants, calcium channel blockers, tricyclic antidepressants, anticonvulsants, and monoamine oxidase inhibitors. Side effects included allergies, gastrointestinal upset, confusion, hypotension, urinary retention, and sedation.

This patient represents a typical patient with intractable pain and severe mandibular hypomobility who has undergone multiple operations. The problem spans two decades and was apparently precipitated by a blow to the jaw. The symptoms were treated noninvasively for the first several years. Why she was referred for surgery is unknown, other than that her symptoms persisted. It is important to recognize that surgery is not the last resort for these patients, and certainly this patient would by definition be a chronic pain patient; therefore, surgery would perhaps not be indicated. The fact that an abnormality was seen on an arthrogram does not alter the argument in any way. Once a decision was made for surgery, future procedures were rapidly necessary. The iatrogenic contracture, scarring, and heterotopic bone formation that developed as a result of the numerous interventions have left her with severe mandibular hypomobility requiring repeated brisement forcé procedures and an anterior open bite. The pain crescendoed after each intervention and is now largely uncontrolled by even heavy narcotic use. The family and social impacts of this problem have been severe. After the first operation, the patient's family suffered severe financial hardship. As a result of subsequent procedures, her medical insurance was terminated. As a result of her inability to work, she is now on disability.

Predictors of Poor Outcome

To develop outcome predictors, investigators have attempted to determine what differences, if any, exist between patients who have been treated successfully and those treated unsuccessfully for temporomandibular disorders.[16, 17] Comparison of these groups has found that both have more emotional problems than the control population. The unsuccessful TMD treatment outcome group had emotional distress to a greater degree, however, than those who had a successful outcome. The level of anger, agitation, and depression was greater in the unsuccessful treatment group.

The longer patients suffer from pain of one sort or another, the more difficult it seems to treat them.[18] Psychologic factors seem to be involved. The pain has altered these patients' lives to such an extent that they have difficulty living without it. Although a patient's response to the pain may have been appropriate originally, it has been maintained because of reinforcement by family, friends, and doctors.[19] The patient receives attention and sympathy because of the pain and may also be able to avoid some undesirable activity. In fact, the patient's entire life may revolve around the pain.[20] This maintenance of the pain to gain some advantage from the environment is referred to as *secondary gain*.[21]

Another factor that makes therapy for these patients difficult is their past experience with the medical community. It may be said that the greater the extent of previous therapy, the more difficult the patient will be to treat. Many of these patients have had a great deal of medical and surgical treatment for their conditions, and, because the attempts have failed, they may distrust further attempts.

In a study of over 400 patients with chronic craniofacial pain who were attending an interdisciplinary facial pain group, several predictors of poor outcome for pain management were identified. In this group, predictors of bad outcome were previous history of depression, somatoform pain disorder, neurogenic pain, and narcotic abuse.[22]

Treatment failures were associated with (1) incorrect diagnosis, (2) incorrect or inadequately delivered treatment, and (3) unrecognized factors.

Incorrect Diagnosis

It goes without saying that a correct diagnosis is essential before a decision to perform an operation is made. In the area of craniofacial pain, a whole host of conditions may mimic masticatory system pain and dysfunction. Space does not permit a full discussion of these conditions nor a full consideration of how to arrive at a correct diagnosis. Suffice it to say that any surgeon who suggests an operation to a patient should be conversant with the other potential diagnoses and convinced that the current diagnosis is the source of the patient's chief complaint. A careful history and physical evaluation are mandatory and will help to ensure that the correct diagnosis has been made. Practitioners should also be aware that temporomandibular disorders, as other craniofacial pain disorders, have a natural history of their own and that the clinical condition can deteriorate or ameliorate as a function of time. An open mind should be kept as to the patient's status at the time of diagnosis and the possible sequelae of different treatments.

As an example, internal derangement may be a stable condition, with the patient complaining of clicking and intermittent locking of the jaw over a period of years. Some patients may eventually have no locking; others, however, may progress to a closed lock, and beyond that to degenerative change. Patients with a closed lock may regain a normal functional range without pain by simple adaptation of their tissues. At this point, it is difficult to predict the outcome of palliative treatment or simply longitudinal observation, but both approaches should be given adequate opportunity to relieve the patient's symptoms prior to a decision for surgery, if at all possible.

Incorrect or Inadequately Delivered Treatment

Treatment may also fail because the diagnosis is correct but the treatment has been delivered incorrectly or inadequately. In the majority of cases, practitioners treating this problem are skillful in their own treatment modalities, so incorrectly delivered therapy is rarely a problem. Inadequate treatment is a major problem, however.

It is very important to recognize the multifactorial nature of temporomandibular joint problems. There is no single cause and therefore no single treatment that will be universally successful. The symptoms reported by each patient include a variety of structural, functional, and psychologic components. The objective is to identify these components and to address each of them appropriately, recognizing that their relative importance may change over time. Dentists and oral and maxillofacial surgeons commonly feel uncomfortable in addressing psychologic problems and often reinforce a patient's belief in pathology or derangement as etiologic factors, to the exclusion of dealing with the emotional issues. This situation can be very damaging in the long run, because neglecting the emotional input invariably has a detrimental effect on outcome.

Unrecognized Factors

The category of unrecognized factors is where the most errors lie. Failure to respond to initial treatment in an appropriate way may indicate that significant etiologic factors have been overlooked. For example, an internal derangement has been unrecognized and the patient has been treated only for myofascial pain. Masticatory muscle pain may be part of a regional myofascial pain problem involving the upper body muscles. This condition, however, can be a precursor of a global muscle pain problem, such as fibromyalgia. The practitioner may not ask for and the patient may not offer information that there is pain in other parts of the body. Under these circumstances, it is unrealistic to expect that dealing with the masticatory system will have any long-term beneficial effect on the systemic problem.

The more difficult case is that of a patient who for a time has pain confined to the masticatory system and receives what would appear to be appropriate treatment for that condition. The pain then begins to involve other parts of the body. Later, and with hindsight, it is recognized that the patient was in the early stages of developing fibromyalgia. One hopes that the initial treatment did not produce any long-term harm. How such a situation can be predicted is unknown at this time.

Psychologic factors are, in my experience, the most common unrecognized problems that contribute to poor outcome in treating craniofacial pain or temporomandibular disorders. The patient usually has depression, anxiety, somatoform pain disorder, or psychosis. The comorbidity rate of Diagnostic and Statistical Manual of Mental Disorders III psychiatric diagnosis with facial pain was 65% in my study.[22] The fact of the matter is that patients who come to dentists or oral and maxillofacial surgeons are reluctant to discuss their emotional lives, and most practitioners are reluctant to ask the right questions. Both may suffer from the illusion that emotional state has nothing to do with physical symptoms. A good answer is to have every patient fill in a psychologic profile, which would identify those with significant psychopathology. Its presence does not eliminate them as patients for treatment but does suggest that their other needs should be addressed concurrently. Failure to adequately evaluate the patient's psychologic profiles will undoubtedly lead to many cases of poor outcome.

Case Reports

Case 4

A 45-year-old female presented with complaints of pain in her left temporomandibular joint and limitation of jaw motion. Conservative therapy had failed to resolve the symptoms. Imaging studies of the left temporomandibular joint demonstrated a large osteophyte from the mandibular condyle which traversed the joint space (Fig. 19–6). A diagnosis of degenerative joint disease of the left temporomandibular joint and possible perforation of the meniscus was made, and the patient was taken to surgery. The operative findings confirmed the presence of an osteophyte that had perforated the meniscus and was causing degenerative changes in the glenoid fossa. An arthroplasty was performed, and the condyle smoothed. The meniscus was repaired. The patient was discharged on the second postoperative day.

She was readmitted one week later because of increasing pain, decreasing mandibular mobility, and dehydration. During the next few days in the hospi-

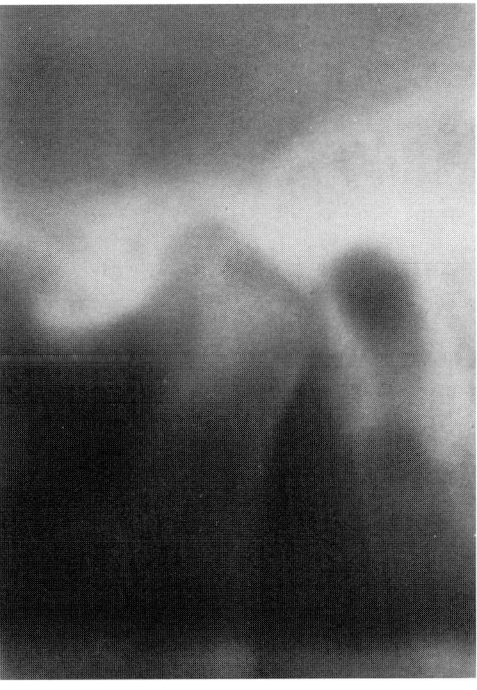

Figure 19–6. *Case 4*: Osteophyte demonstrated on left mandibular condyle.

tal, the patient lay in bed curled up in a fetal position, unresponsive to the administrations of the medical staff. A psychiatrist was consulted, who diagnosed depression and started treating the patient with tricyclic antidepressant medications. The depression was long-standing and had previously been denied by the patient and her family. It had started two decades earlier, when the patient had given birth to a stillborn child while her husband was away in the armed forces. Her husband, now a long-distance truck driver, was frequently absent from the house. With treatment over the course of the next several weeks, the patient recovered a functional range of mandibular motion with no significant pain complaints. She has been maintained on a low dose of tricyclic antidepressant for the past 10 years.

This patient had two diagnoses, temporomandibular joint arthritis severe enough to account for the presenting symptoms and a covert depression that prevented her from making an appropriate recovery. It is hard to say whether the two diagnoses were related or whether indeed a more thorough psychologic history preoperatively would have uncovered the depression. In any case, the key to the patient's full recovery lay in dealing with both diagnoses.

Case 5

A 26-year-old female had complained of left facial pain and jaw clicking for 2 years, which she related to a bicycle accident in which she broke her left collar bone and struck her face. Splint therapy had not relieved the symptoms, and a CT scan of the left temporomandibular joint demonstrated a displaced meniscus, which was repaired surgically.

Four months later, the patient complained of similar symptoms in the right temporomandibular joint. A CT scan of that joint demonstrated a displaced meniscus without reduction, and the patient was scheduled for surgery. The procedure was deferred 1 month because of a prolonged bleeding time subsequent to aspirin use. Postoperatively, the patient continued to do poorly and stated that the bilateral facial pain was getting worse, requiring an occasional Percocet. She could open to 2.0 cm without pain and to 2.8 cm with discomfort, and she was back to using a splint 24 hours a day. The pain interfered with her lifestyle: She became inactive and spent a lot of time sleeping, though on occasion the pain kept her from sleep. Her concentration deteriorated, and she found it impossible to work. She was limited to soft foods because of the pain. She also complained of pain on swallowing and pain in her neck and back.

Evaluation revealed evidence of diffuse muscle tension and depression (Fig. 19–7). A tricyclic antidepressant was prescribed (doxepin, 25 mg h.s., increasing to 100 mg h.s.), which gradually reduced her symptoms over a period of 3 months. Nine months later, the patient described herself as "100% better and very happy." The right side was symptom-free, and she experienced only occasional discomfort on the left. She had regained a normal range of mandibular opening, including lateral excursions and protrusion. Her appetite, concentration, and sleep were restored to normal, and she wore a splint at night only.

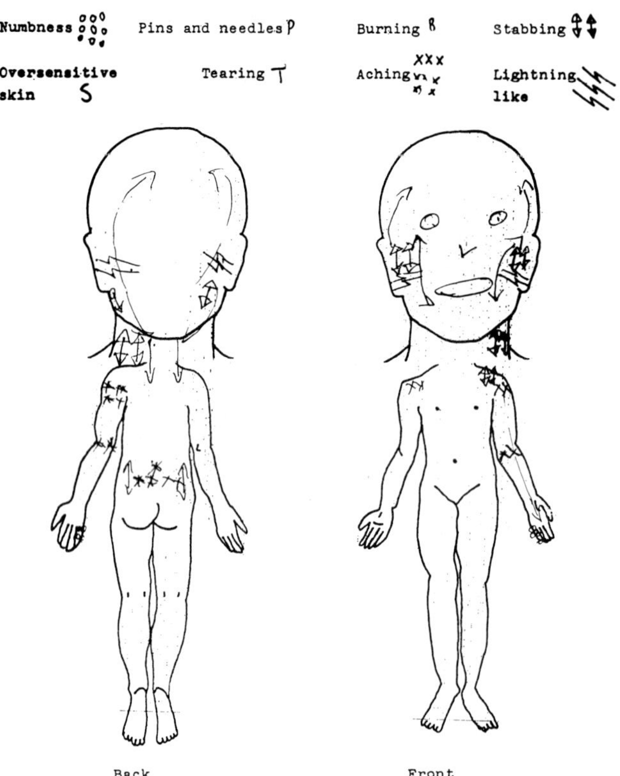

Figure 19–7. *Case 5*: Pain drawing indicating diffuse distribution of pain associated with patient's depression.

This patient had the usual progression of events leading to left joint surgery. A recurrence of symptoms on the right side led more rapidly to a surgical decision without appropriate investigation of other factors. In retrospect, it was apparent that this patient had recurring bouts of depression and came from a dysfunctional family. Subsequently, several of her siblings were treated for the same condition. The patient's somatic focus during her time of depression was on her temporomandibular joints, driving her pattern of treatment and referrals. A more adequate family, social, and psychologic history may have raised a red flag; whether it would have prevented the first or second operation is unknown.

Conclusions

The argument has been made both ways: One philosophy is that other than for clearly defined pathologic conditions (e.g., condylar hyperplasia, tumors, infections, and certain arthritic conditions), surgery has no place in managing temporomandibular disorders. The opposing philosophy puts surgery on a par with other modalities in dealing with conditions such as derangement. In our current state of knowledge, this dilemma cannot adequately be resolved. Clearly, the results of surgery in carefully selected patients indicate the efficacy of this approach. The devastating results of hastily prescribed invasive treatment in poorly defined clinical situations, however, lead the cautious practitioner to step back and reconsider.

The two most important lessons would seem to be these: Most patients can function very adequately with a range of motion exceeding 30 mm. Surgery designed to give them a greater range of motion is likely to be met with partial success at best. In general, patients (except in the extreme) do not complain of mobility problems. The medical literature on surgery solely for the relief of pain is dismal, especially in a field where behavioral and psychologic problems are at least part of the problem. We need to be exceptionally cautious in offering our patients pain relief unless we are quite certain that the pathology that we see is indeed the major source of their complaints. Although surgery can be beneficial, it can also have disastrous results.

On a more optimistic note, it should be recognized that because pain is a multifactorial experience, many different modalities can help relieve it. Behavioral, psychologic, and physical therapy interventions, although outside the scope of dental practice, can indeed be extremely beneficial and sometimes pivotal in alleviating pain symptoms.

References

1. Norgaard F: Temporomandibular arthrography [thesis]. Copenhagen, Munksgaard 1947.
2. Toller PA: Opaque arthrography of the temporomandibular joint. Int J Oral Surg 1974;3:17.
3. Wilkes C: Arthrography of the temporomandibular joint in patients with TMJ pain dysfunction syndrome. Minn Med 1978;61:645.
4. Farrar WB, McCarty WL: Inferior joint space arthrography and characteristics of condylar paths in internal derangements of the TMJ. J Prosthet Dent 1979;41:548.
5. Katzberg RW, Dolwick MF, Helms CA, et al: Arthrotomography of the temporomandibular joint. Am J Roentgenol 1980;134:995.
6. Keith DA: Surgery of the Temporomandibular Joint. Edinburgh, Blackwell Scientific, 1988, p xv.
7. Ryan DE: Alloplastic implants in the temporomandibular joint. Oral Maxillofac Surg Clin North Am 1:427–441, 1989.
8. Yih WY, Merrill RG: Pathology of alloplastic inter-positional implants in the temporomandibular joint. Oral Maxillofac Surg Clin North Am 1989;1:415–426.
9. Wang J-T, Goldring SR: The role of particulate orthopaedic implant materials in peri-implant osteolysis: Mechanisms of granuloma formation and particle-induced osteolysis. *In* BF Morris (ed): Biological Material and Mechanical Considerations of Joint Replacement. New York, Raven Press, 1993, pp 119–126.
10. Morris DB: The Culture of Pain. Berkeley, University of California Press, 1991.
11. Agerberg G: Longitudinal variation of maximal mandibular mobility: An intraindividual study. J Prosthet Dent 1987;58:370–373.
12. Sheppard J, Sheppard S: Maximal incisal opening—a diagnostic index? J Dent Med 1965;20:13–15.
13. Mezitis M, Rallis G, Zachariades N: The normal range of mouth opening. J Oral Maxillofac Surg 1989;47:1028–1029.
14. Gibbs CH, Mahan PE, Lundeen HC, et al: Occlusal forces during chewing: Influences of biting strength and food consistency. J Prosthet Dent 1981;46:561–567.
15. Hickey JC, Zarb GA, Bolender CL: Boucher's Prosthodontic Treatment for Edentulous Patients, ed 9. St Louis, CV Mosby, 1985.
16. Millstein-Prentky S, Olson RE: Predictability of treatment outcome in patients with myofascial pain—dysfunction syndrome. J Dent Res 1979;58:1341–1345.
17. Schwartz RA, Greene CS, Laskin DM: Personality characteristics of patients with myofascial pain dysfunction (MPD) syndrome unresponsive to correctional therapy. J Dent Res 1979;58:1435–1439.
18. Hackett TP, Bouckoms A: The pain patient: Evaluation and treatment. *In* Hackett TP, Cassem NH: Massachusetts General Hospital Handbook of General Hospital Psychiatry. Littleton, MA, PSG Publishing, 1987, pp 42–68.
19. Gerschman JA: The determinants of chronic orofacial pain. Clin J Pain 1987;3:45–53.
20. Burton RC: The problem of facial pain. J Am Dent Assoc 1969;79:154–160.
21. Burdette BH, Gale EN: Pain as a learned response. J Am Dent Assoc 1988;116:881–885.
22. Keith DA: Differential Diagnosis of Facial Pain and Headache. Oral Maxillofac Surg Clin North Am 1989;1:7–11.

Chapter 20
THE LONG-TERM UNFAVORABLE RESULT IN MIDFACE TRAUMA

by

Michael F. Zide, DMD

Introduction

In this chapter four common long-term periorbital complications of midface trauma are discussed. Characteristically, these complications may occur despite adequate reduction of the facial bones during treatment of the acute injury. Each complication is discussed in relation to the surgical anatomy and with suggestions for its prevention and management. The complications are illustrated by case presentations.

The Subjects Discussed in This Chapter Are:

- Assessment for reconstruction
- Displaced medial canthus
  Applied local anatomy
  Prevention and management
- Hollowed temporal region
  Applied local anatomy
  Prevention and management
- Enophthalmos
  Applied local anatomy
  Prevention and management
- Ectropion
  Applied local anatomy
  Prevention and management

Long-term complications in facial trauma patients may be related to healing or may result from treatment during any period after the traumatic episode. Severity of the injury, method of repair, and adequacy of the healing process may all play a role in the unfavorable result. The truly agonizing complications are those that occur even after the surgeon has treated the initial injuries adequately and has noted that the bones were anatomically positioned in the postoperative radiograph. These complications are extruding plates, nasal cartilage deformities, adherent scars, and periorbital deformities.

Even experienced surgeons have an occasional patient with unfavorable residual posttraumatic deformities, the most obvious occurring after severe midface injuries. These complications have been reviewed extensively.[1] In this chapter, I focus on specific periorbital deformities that may coexist while the bones are in proper position.

Assessment for Reconstruction

The definition of a successful outcome may be variable and unclear. The goal of "restoration to exact preinjury anatomy" may not be realistically possible in the setting of complex facial trauma. Under these circumstances, the patient and surgeon must be willing to accept "symmetry and appearance close to normal" as an end result. The benefit of additional surgery may not warrant the risk. In order to evaluate the reconstructive process, it is helpful to consider the following five aspects of the patient's care:

- Mechanism of injury.
- Review of initial hospitalization examinations and operative notes.
- Reconstructive maneuvers that have already been carried out.
- Review of acute, postoperative, and current radiographs and computed tomographic (CT) scans.
- Consultant input.

The surgeon and patient must then reevaluate goals in light of the patient's desires and expectations and of what is realistically possible to achieve by additional operations. Although it is often convenient to place blame, the best results can be obtained only through convergence of ideas toward correction of what the patient views as wrong.

Displaced Medial Canthus

Applied Local Anatomy

The signs and symptoms of an acutely displaced medial canthus may be masked by swelling in the early postinjury period. The muscle-free zone of the nose is composed of very thin skin that can swell to huge proportions in the presence of injury. As the swelling resolves, the deformity becomes all too clear.

The configuration of the medial canthus may be rounded. This, in effect, shortens the horizontal measurement of the palpebral fissure. Although some patients have a widened intercanthal distance through ethnic inheritance, their premorbid photographs may be a beneficial guide to individual situations. Additionally, the lid may be lax, and excessive scleral show may be present. This canthal displacement laterally may produce epicanthal folds that were not originally present.

The underlying bone injuries may complicate the soft tissue problem. As the frontal process of the maxilla and the nasal bones are forced into the interorbital space, the medial wall of the orbit is outfractured into the comminuting ethmoid air cells. Uncorrected, these problems produce either a hollow appearance medially or a fullness at the frontal process. Clinically, these anatomic deformities become even more evident if the nose is crushed or depressed into a pug shape, because the normally distinct topographic boundaries of the medial maxillary area become confluent or malpositioned in relation to one another.

The symptoms of the anatomic aberrations may be particularly disconcerting. Visual disturbances, tearing problems, and nasal obstruction may functionally all be part of what may appear to be only a displaced canthal tendon.

Acute fracture displacement of the medial canthus or its bony insertion requires aggressive early reduction. The goal should be overcorrection with a visibly reduced intercanthal measurement on the operating table. It is almost impossible to overcorrect traumatic telecanthism. Unfortunately, the locally intricate anatomy may make a perfect outcome difficult to obtain.

The medial canthal tendon is a tripartite arrangement consisting of strong anterior horizontal and verti-

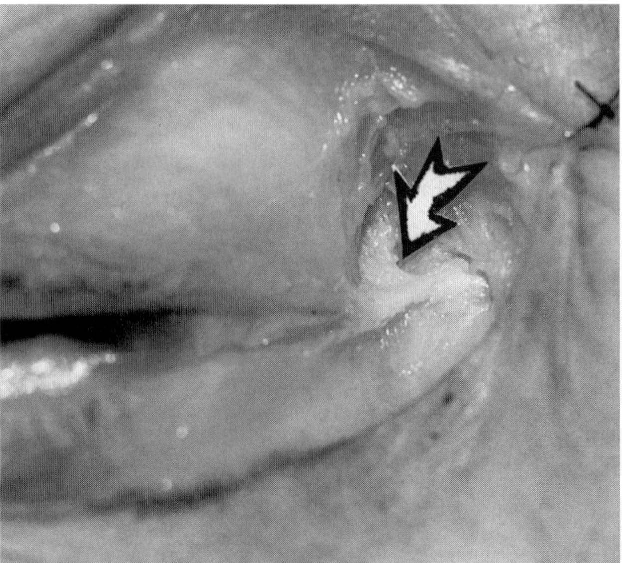

Figure 20–1. The canthal tendon must be controlled at the anterior lacrimal crest or close to the medial corner of the eye. A 7-mm to 10-mm incision made 2 mm medial to the corner of the palpebral fissure (canthus) provides direct access to the tendon. Capture of the tendon further medially and placement of the tendon into a bony hole more posteriorly than the anterior lacrimal crest will, in effect, move the canthus laterally.

cal components and a deeper, less tenuous horizontal component.[2] The anterior horizontal tendon inserts onto the anterior lacrimal crest and beyond onto the nasal bones. Any suture method to replace the tendon should pierce the tendon just at the anterior lacrimal crest, because more medial placement in effect worsens telecanthism (Fig. 20–1). If only the anterior components are dissected off the bone, the posterior component supplies significant residual support.[3, 4] Unfortunately, in naso-orbital fractures, the posterior support may be in a separate segment from the anterior components. Additionally, for fracture treatment, the horizontal anterior component may be the only controllable utilizable component of the three.

The second anatomic concern is the central fragment of bone itself. The central fragment of bone abuts the lateral nose, inferior orbital rim, medial orbital ethmoidal wall, nasomaxillary puriform buttress, and frontal process of the maxilla at the internal angular process of the frontal bone. The medial canthal tendon attaches to this fragment, which may itself be fractured.

Anatomic reduction and stabilization require wide exposure via subciliary, transoral, and coronal incisions. Small fragments may have to be united as a matrix prior to plate stabilization. The comminution in the area may inadvertently allow the surgeon to displace or rotate the internal components of the fracture laterally. As a result, the nasal root is widened as well as any attached anatomic structures, especially the medial canthal tendons.

Case 1

A 30-year-old male patient was in a motor vehicle accident and sustained severe nasoethmoidal fractures. The policeman at the scene retrieved part of the patient's cartilaginous nasal septum from the dashboard of the car and brought it to the hospital. The septum was replaced at surgery, and the bones were reduced anatomically. Late surgical result reveals good bony contour but unfavorable shape of the canthal tendon area (Fig. 20–2).

Prevention and Management

Methods of treating telecanthus resulting from naso-orbital fractures are well described.[5] Transnasal wiring, plate fixation holding canthal segments in place,[6] primary bone grafting, canthopexy, and external bolsters have all been suggested for acute fracture therapy.

Late correction of telecanthus may involve repair of soft tissues or bone or a combination of the two. If telecanthus is associated with epicanthus, the repair may correct both problems. Mild telecanthism requires correction of the canthus alone by plication to a fixed object, e.g., screw, plate, bone piton. Most posttraumatic cases, however, also involve transnasal wiring to the stable contralateral bone.

Osteotomy of the frontal process of the maxilla with or without the nasal bones may be an integral part of late correction. These procedures are complex because of the proximity of the canthal attachment and the nasolacrimal apparatus. Additionally, internal bone consolidation in the ethmoid or nasal area may restrict movements, and access for easy removal of bone may be limited. For these reasons, onlay nasal bone grafting is a significantly more practical choice in surgical cor-

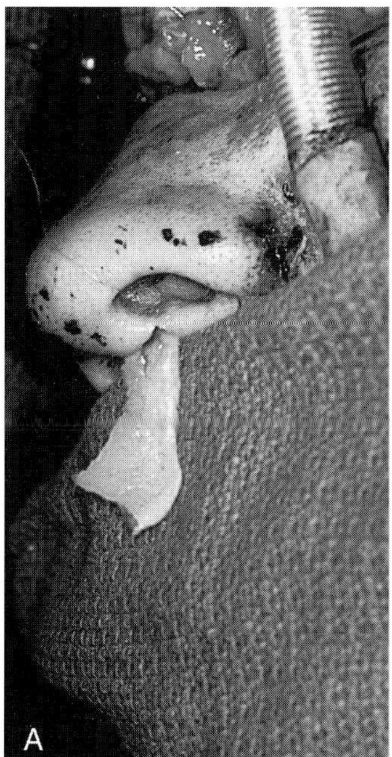

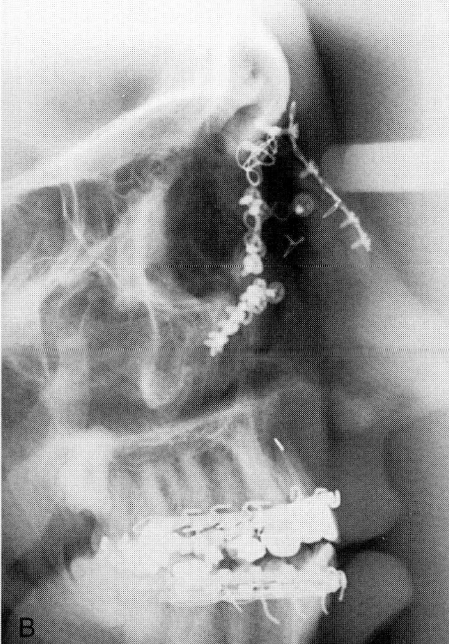

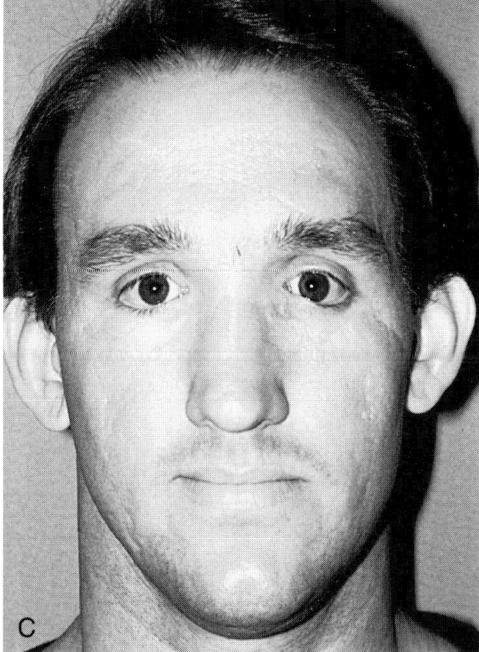

Figure 20–2. *A*, Initial patient presentation with cartilaginous septal avulsion prior to replacement with pull-in suture. *B*, Postoperative radiograph, with good projection noted in lateral view. *C*, Clinical view reveals unfavorable anatomic contour with small palpebral fissures horizontally and slight left ectropion.

rection of the late medial canthal deformity. It provides an immediate positive improvement in appearance.

Late deformities secondary to medial canthal and naso-orbital ethmoid injuries remain difficult problems to treat. Patients need to be advised of probable revisions. One contributing factor in this situation is that the injury is uncommon and yet demands a high level of experience. Some observations that may be helpful for the surgeon are as follows:

1. Early aggressive surgery produces better results than late reconstruction.
2. Measurements of intercanthal distance never lessen after the patient is off the operating table. Wire, not nylon or resorbable suture, should be used to control the area surgically.
3. Correct orientation of the central fragment and its attached canthus produces the best result. Transnasal wiring and plate stabilization appear to be effective. External lead plates or bolsters have no effect on the canthal tendon position.
4. Primary orbital and nasal bone grafting has low morbidity and is indicated to preserve bone height and to mask irregularities.
5. Late reconstruction is rarely perfect. Soft tissue procedures and osteotomies are helpful. The final result may depend on masking bone grafts to blunt the deformity by increasing the height of the nasal bony radix.

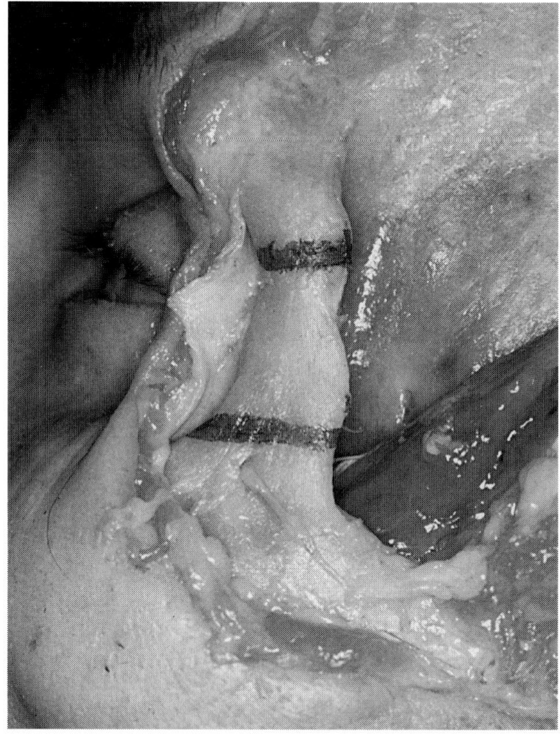

Figure 20–3. The hollow area is just behind the lateral orbital wall, reflected temporal muscle on cadaveric specimen.

Hollowed Temporal Region

Applied Local Anatomy

The hollowed temporal defect noted after facial fracture reduction is usually an hourglass-shaped defect. There are typically no associated symptoms unless the facial nerve has been injured. With injury to the temporal branch of the seventh cranial nerve, forehead-eyebrow and eyelid movements are diminished or absent.

This deformity may be masked by a hairstyle that covers the area. The patient commonly presents, however, with a pronounced lateral orbital rim or arch depression behind the affected orbit. This is noticed as an asymmetry in comparison with the unaffected side. The complication may also occur in association with the use of a coronal flap. The surgical events that result in a hollowed temporal area are (1) reflection of the temporalis muscle from behind the lateral orbital rim, (2) cauterization of temporal fat during reflection of the flap, (3) failure to resuspend or reelevate tissues over the arch after flap surgery, (4) adherence of periosteal scar around the zygomatic arch after coronal flap elevation, and (5) multiple coronal flaps causing atrophy of fat.

Anatomically, the defect is behind the orbital rim and above the zygomatic arch (Fig. 20–3). Dissection in this area places the temporal branches of the facial nerve at risk,[8] at least superficially. After the facial nerve emerges from the upper pole of the parotid, it passes anterosuperiorly over the arch to reach the muscles. The nerve is vulnerable superficially to a point 1 to 1.5 cm above the lateral margin of the orbital rim. The nerve enters the frontalis muscle from its deep surface, above where the vertical lateral fibers of the frontalis muscle meet the circumferential fibers of the orbicularis oculi. Before the nerve enters the frontalis muscle, it travels in the deep superficial musculo-aponeurotic system layer adherent to the temporal fascia. Assessment for reconstruction must factor in protection of the facial nerve.

Case 2

The patient had a severe zygomatic complex fracture and was left with a facial nerve palsy as well as a hollowed temporal area (Fig. 20–4*A*). The area was reconstructed with methyl methacrylate. Her eyebrow was suspended. The defect was filled adequately, but the result is marred by lack of elevation of the eyebrow and persistent depression in the temporal region (Fig. 20–4*B* to *D*).

Prevention and Management

Treatment of the hollowed temporal region should be planned to include the defect in the skin as well as the deep tissues. For example, the deformity associated with a detached temporalis muscle may be maskable with resuspension of the muscle to bony holes placed along the lateral orbital rim and internal graft.[7] Temporalis muscle itself is relatively easy to rotate but difficult to elevate. Isolated soft tissue defects may respond to rotation of a fat-fascia flap from behind the hairline,[9] free flap, or soft tissue–dermal fat graft. A pronounced zygomatic arch may respond to osteoplasty or fascial overlay. A reduction of the height of the temporalis

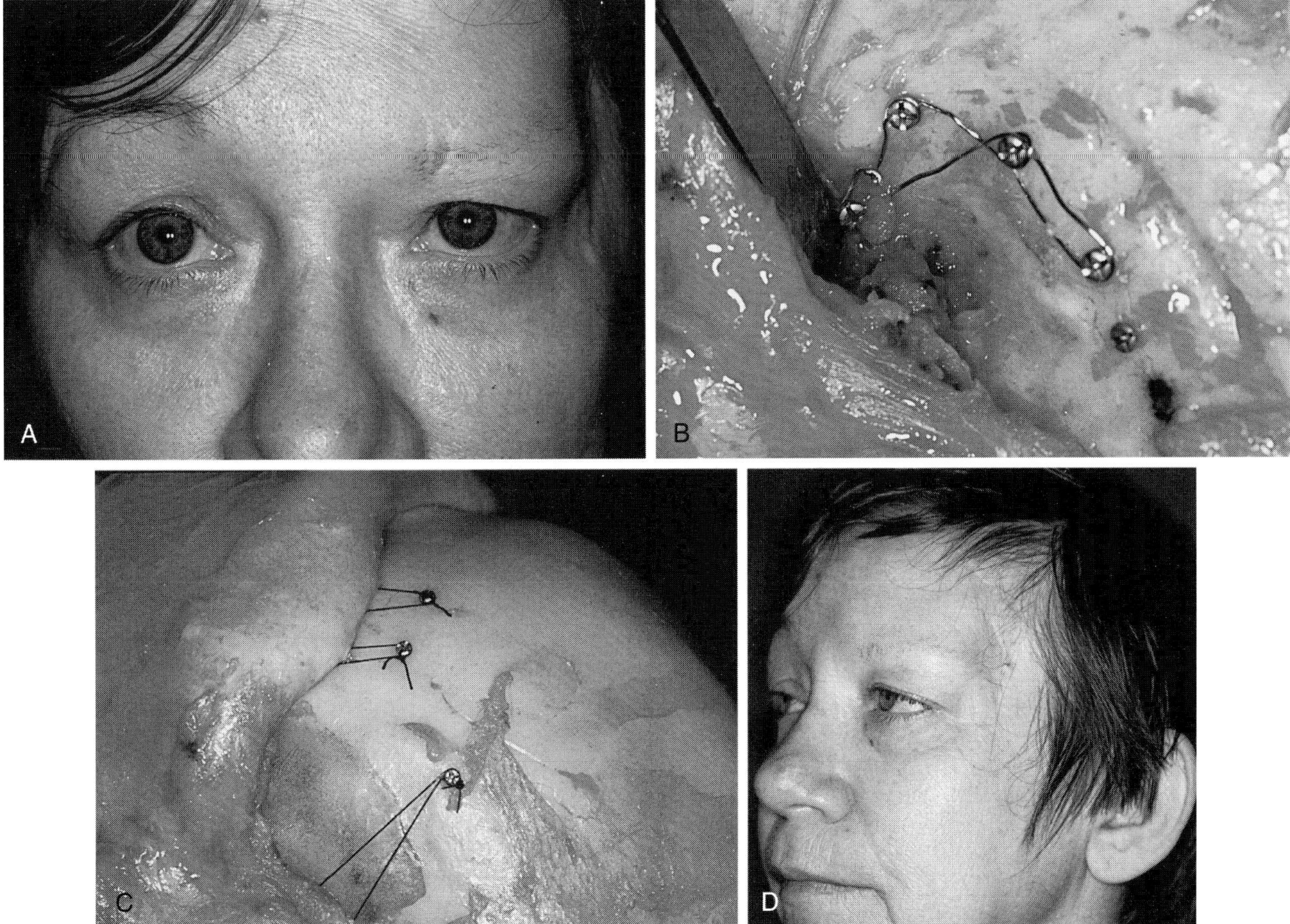

Figure 20–4. *A,* Hollowed left temporal area and facial nerve palsy. *B,* Temporal substructure of wires and screws. *C,* Nylon-screw suspension of the eyebrow and cheek flap in addition to methyl methacrylate reconstruction of hollowed defects. *D,* Filled temporal area is acceptable but eyebrows are asymmetric.

muscle may be masked by alloplastic or autogenous onlay. This last defect merits comment.

Tissue augmentation currently has two conceptual options, alloplastic or autogenous tissues. Alloplastic options include granular materials (e.g., hydroxylapatite) and solid materials (e.g., Medpor, methyl methacrylate).[10] Autogenous materials include muscle, fat, and fascia.

The attractions of alloplastic material are obvious. There is no need to consider a donor site. Alloplastic material, unlike autogenous or allogeneic bone and cartilage, has no potential for unpredictable resorption. The options are not limited by the amount of autogenous material available. The considerations for use of an alloplast are (1) type of tissue defect (soft tissue as opposed to bone), (2) soft tissue coverage, and (3) preexisting problems such as limiting anatomy, (e.g., sinus) and prior radiation therapy.

Polymers and ceramics have been valuable to craniofacial reconstruction. Polymer chemistry has produced multiple implantable products whose biologic behavior, strength, and elasticity vary. Usually, the body walls off or encapsulates these implants, although some allow for porous ingrowth. The two most popular polymers are porous polyethylene (Medpor) and methyl methacrylate.

High-density polyethylene (Medpor) appears almost inert[11] when implanted, and its direct placement on or within bone may encourage bony ingrowth. Prefabricated blocks and easily carvable sheets and blocks make this implant attractive.[12] Infection has been rare compared with its "ingrowth" predecessor, Proplast.

Methyl methacrylate is most commonly used as a cold-cured polymerizing implant shaped in vivo. The material is strong and biocompatible, and it becomes encapsulated. The material may be anchored to the skull with mesh, screws, wires, or bur holes. Exothermic reactions should be prevented by cold irrigation as the material cures, but problems associated with the exothermic reaction appear minuscule. Final contouring with a bur has produced excellent results in small and large areas; however, late, bacterially seeded infections have occurred decades after implantation.[12]

Ceramic materials, specifically hydroxylapatite (HA), are made from sintering[13] crystals together with high heat[13] or through a chemical transfer process with a coralline matrix.[14] These calcium phosphate ceramics are inert, are highly compatible,[15] and do not resorb. A capsule does not form around the implanted HA. Block-shaped coralline HA can act as a scaffold for new bone formation and is, therefore, osteoconductive. When bony ingrowth does occur, the brittle, fragile nature of the material improves, because load-bearing properties are shared with infiltrating bone.

Granular HA does not, however, achieve great bony growth. Its mobile nature induces a soft tissue matrix that remains mobile or moldable for a few weeks. When it is placed subperiosteally on bone, both plaster and collagen matrices have aided in stability. Unfortunately, when HA is placed in soft tissue or under a thin skin cover, balling and settling have been problematic.[4]

The most important suggestion to counteract the hourglass defect involves prevention through avoidance of reflection of muscle behind the orbit and resuspension of the flap after coronal flap surgery. All reconstructive efforts should be aimed at masking the deformity where it lies.

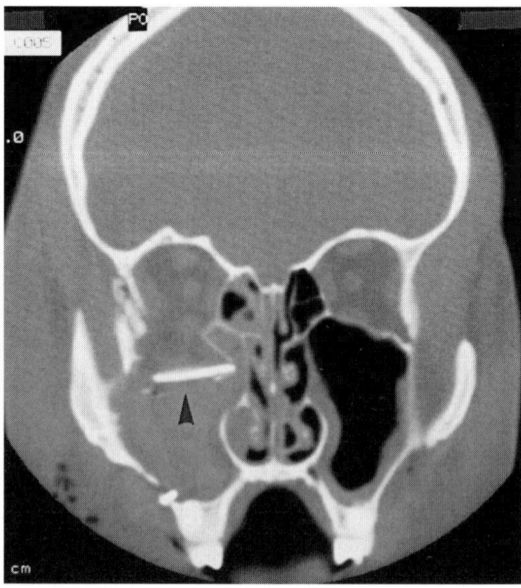

Figure 20–5. CT scan of bone graft improperly placed. The volume of the reconstructed orbit is too large. This patient should be brought back to the operating room.

Enophthalmos

Applied Local Anatomy

Enophthalmos is not an isolated anatomic entity. Associated abnormalities are superior sulcus depression, palpebral fissure diminution, and vertical globe or orbital displacement. Double vision may also be present.

Posttraumatic enophthalmos is primarily the result of volumetric orbital expansion[16] with, perhaps, some contribution by fat atrophy[17] and scar contraction. Correlation of CT scanning and clinical findings reveals that fractures involving more than 25% of the orbital floor often lead to significant enophthalmos.[18] Although CT scans of the two sides may not be exactly comparable, volume expansion, in addition to bony fracture displacement, should always be considered.[19, 20] Direct sagittal and transverse CT scans are useful in evaluating globe position in the presence of orbital injury.

Surgeons often do not consider orbital volumetric changes and the possibility that they may lead to enophthalmos (except when globe injury, such as commotio retinae, has caused a delay in operation for several weeks). The surgeon retrieves herniated tissue from the sinus and repairs the orbital floor with bone or an implant. The size of the implant is often selected arbitrarily, larger for more severe injuries. Why, then, does enophthalmos sometimes occur? We now suspect several causes. Perhaps the implant or graft that was placed did not satisfactorily restore normal preoperative anatomy (Fig. 20–5).

Postoperative CT scan is critical for evaluation of orbital grafts and implants. The shape and position of the implant can be judged, and the orbital volume can be compared with the contralateral side. The medial orbital wall, for example, is not wholly concave, and bulges into the orbit. This shape may be hard to mimic with a graft or implant. The type of floor or wall replacement may limit the shape and long-term stability of the new orbital cavity. For example, cranial bone grafts are difficult to contour and may have to be bent or cut to adapt to curves. Bone grafts placed "on top" of plates may resorb.

The surgeon's fear of complete exploration of the orbit or swelling may result in inadequate exposure of the entire circumference of the defect. Confined space and proximity to the globe, optic nerve, and structures of the superior orbital fissure restrict access. Failure to recognize or restore an outbuckled orbital floor may have a poor result. All these factors are of concern in the prevention of enophthalmos.

Case 3

A 40-year-old woman suffered nasal and zygomatic fractures in a motor vehicle accident (Fig. 20–6*A*). Late zygomatic osteotomy and nasal surgery corrected the position of the zygoma and nose to a great extent. The enophthalmos is still present, however, as evidenced by the superior sulcus depression (Fig. 20–6*B*).

Prevention and Management

An orbital floor fracture anterior to a plane from the anterior lacrimal bone to the anterior lateral orbital rim does not produce enophthalmos. In other fractures, prevention of enophthalmos can be accomplished only by restoring the orbital anatomy behind the equator of the globe. Hence, the medial blowout, the posterior blowout, and the lateral displacement of the wall of the zygoma all produce enophthalmos. Orbital rim osteotomy has been suggested as one adjunctive surgical exposure method[21] when the zygoma itself does not need to be repositioned. Failure to reestablish orbital shape and volume anatomically may result in a progressively worsening enophthalmic deformity.[5]

Surgeons have implanted autogenous and alloplastic

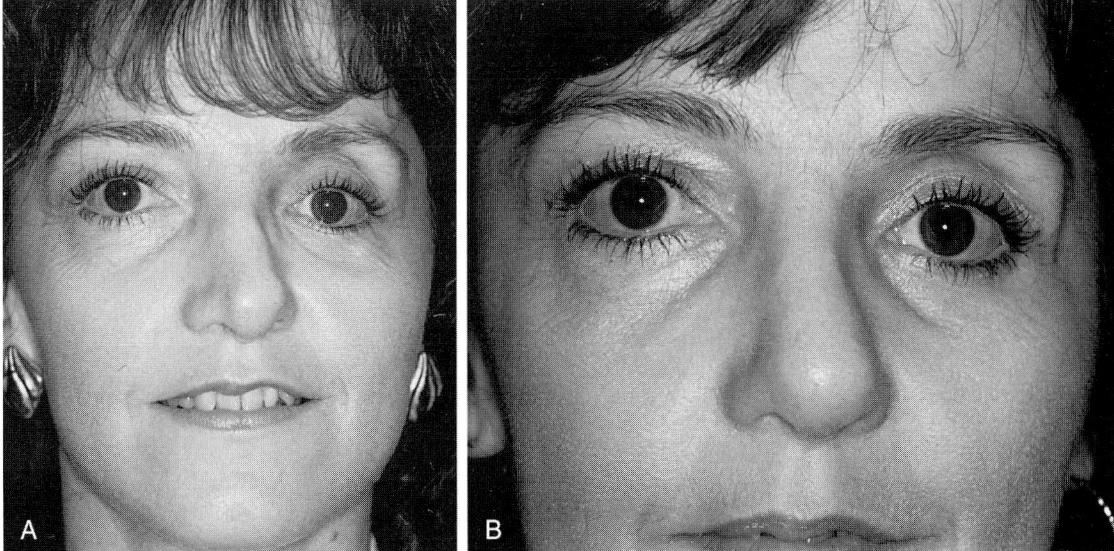

Figure 20–6. *A,* Preoperative nasal and zygomatic deformity. The nasal fracture pushed the nose to the left. The cheekbone fracture was unrepaired initially. The entire globe is down and the cheeks are flat on the left. *C,* After late correction with zygomatic-nasal osteotomies and Medpor grafts, the patient still has enophthalmos and sulcus depression albeit with improvement.

materials all around the internal orbit to reconstruct volumetric orbital defects and resolve late enophthalmos. With the use of either autogenous or alloplastic material, late enophthalmos may or may not totally be eliminated. It appears that even though fat atrophy and tissue fibrosis are not the primary causes of enophthalmos, they may contribute to the inability to correct the problem easily.

Late augmentation of the orbital floor alone is rarely successful in correcting enophthalmos. That is to say, late surgical placement of autogenous or alloplastic materials to recreate the bony anatomy of a floor fracture tends to leave the globe short of the desired projection. Preoperative judgment of the magnitude of the problem is helpful but may not be predictive of the result. The Hertel and Luedde exophthalmometers are often useless in the presence of associated bony injuries to the lateral orbital rim. Likewise, judgment in the operating room that the globe is projected adequately, or is overcorrected or undercorrected may be erroneous. Patients have had to be re-treated. This poses the question as to whether or not severe, long-standing enophthalmos can be treated in a single operation. Further scarring or fibrosis can occur as swelling resolves. Careful assessment of publications of the best cases by experts reveals significant improvement but undercorrection of the deformity. Mustarde[22] has stated that there may be cases in which total correction is impossible.

The complexity of the initial injury may also cloud late results. The globe is seen in relationship to the adjacent adnexal structures. The globe position may be anatomically excellent, but cheek or lid position might make it appear unaesthetic. Additionally, superior sulcus depression is significantly improved when vertical position of the globe is good. Unfortunately, full superior sulcus correction has been noted as impossible unless accompanying enophthalmos is fully addressed. Fortunately, many patients who wear glasses are happy with orbital symmetry in spite of the lid sulcus depression.

The surgical approach for correction of late enophthalmos should be varied, depending on the anatomy of the defect. Easier exposure can be accomplished with rim orbitotomy, although this maneuver has not proved necessary in most cases. My technique involves choosing any infraorbital incision that allows access to the floor and the lateral and medial orbit. Care should be taken with the medial wall exploration, lest dissection poke through into the ethmoid air cells. Large pieces of smoothed Medpor are placed along the entire lateral wall and behind the equator along the floor and medial wall. I stop adding volume filler when vertical forced duction is tightly limited.

The greatest risk of the operation is catastrophic vision loss. Although retinal artery occlusion is possible, the complication of direct implant pressure causing choroidal or retinal folds is more likely. Visual acuity should be checked immediately in the recovery room and then every 2 hours for the next 6 hours. The fundus should be evaluated by an ophthalmologist in high-risk cases. Tonometry has not been a routine procedure in my experience unless there appears to be proptosis or pain.

Ectropion

Applied Local Anatomy

Ectropion or scleral show may manifest as a minor aesthetic problem or as a major functional problem with eversion of the lower eyelid. Ectropion may be congenital or may occur after blepharoplasty or trauma.

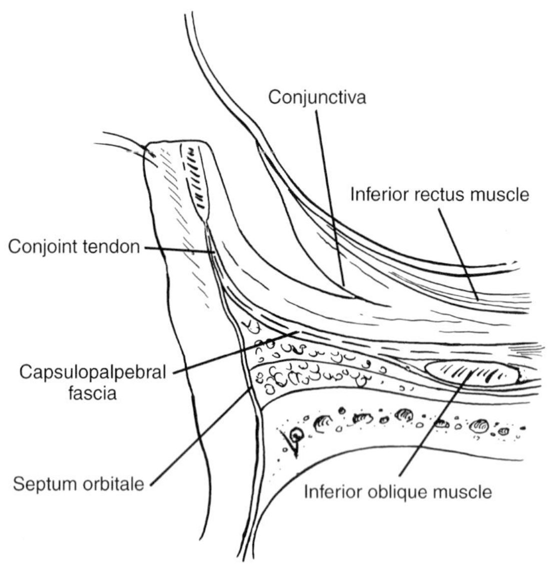

Figure 20–7. Anatomy of lower eyelid showing relation of septum and capsulopalpebral fascia.

The surgeon should have an understanding of the anatomic structures that maintain lower eyelid position; they are as follows:

- Canthal ligaments and tarsus supporting superiorly.
- Orbicularis muscle supporting the lid (pretarsal).
- Forces of skin, septum orbitale, and capsulopalpebral fascia (extending from the rectus muscle to the tarsus) (Fig. 20–7).

Anatomically, lower lid support is a delicate balance among these structures. The elastic capsulopalpebral fascia and nonelastic septum orbitale are at greatest risk for injury with orbital trauma. The capsulopalpebral fascia, known as the lower lid retractor system, inserts onto the lower border of the tarsus and the conjunctival fornix. The capsulopalpebral fascia is the anterior projection of the inferior rectus muscle sheath. It thickens to become the Lockwood suspensory ligament, an inelastic structure that attaches to both retinacula. (A retinaculum is any structure that retains an organ or tissue in place, such as the canthal tendons.) The function of the capsulopalpebral fascia is to lower the eyelid in unison with the globe during downward gaze.

Ectropion is the most common complication associated with cosmetic approaches to and traumatic repair through the lower eyelid.[23] Some authors report a 28% incidence of scleral show with the skin-muscle subciliary approach (Fig. 20–8), compared with a 3% rate for a transconjunctival approach. Others suggest that this ectropion is transient unless a skin-only subciliary flap is used.

It is evident that no anatomic approach guarantees against ectropion or eyelid retraction. Entropion, in fact, is possible with the transconjunctival approach. The preseptal transconjunctival approach, however, seems to offer a significantly lower incidence of lid problems, whether used alone or combined with lateral canthotomy.[25] In this technique, the incision is made just below the tarsus on the internal surface of the lower eyelid. From here, the conjoint tendon of the lower eyelid retractors is cut, and the approach goes atop the septum orbitale just like the subciliary skin-muscle flap. Surgeons who use this approach report no difference in complications whether the transconjunctival approach proceeded preseptally or retroseptally[26] and whether the conjunctiva is sutured after surgery.

Case 4

A 20-year-old male was in a motor vehicle accident (Fig. 20–9*A*). His right periorbital fractures through a subciliary incision resulted in significant ectropion (Fig. 20–9*B*). A lateral canthotomy approach was used to correct the ectropion as well as the enophthalmos. Postoperatively, scleral show and upper lid deformity (slight levator dehiscence) remain (Fig. 20–9*C*).

Prevention and Management

Ectropion resolves spontaneously or with massage in the vast majority of cases. Many reconstructive pro-

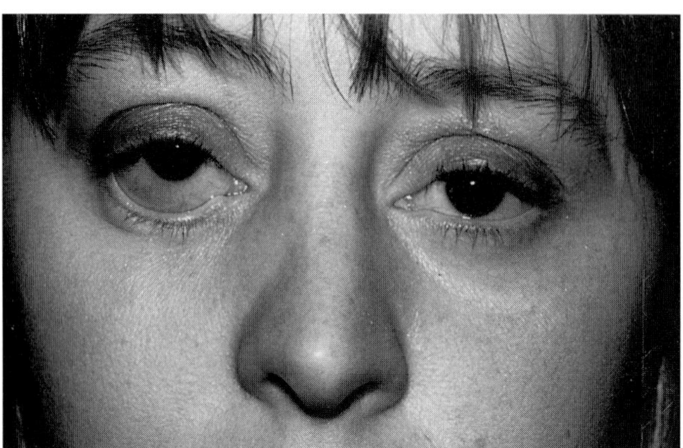

Figure 20–8. Severe unrepaired ectropion noted 3 years after surgery. Subciliary incision.

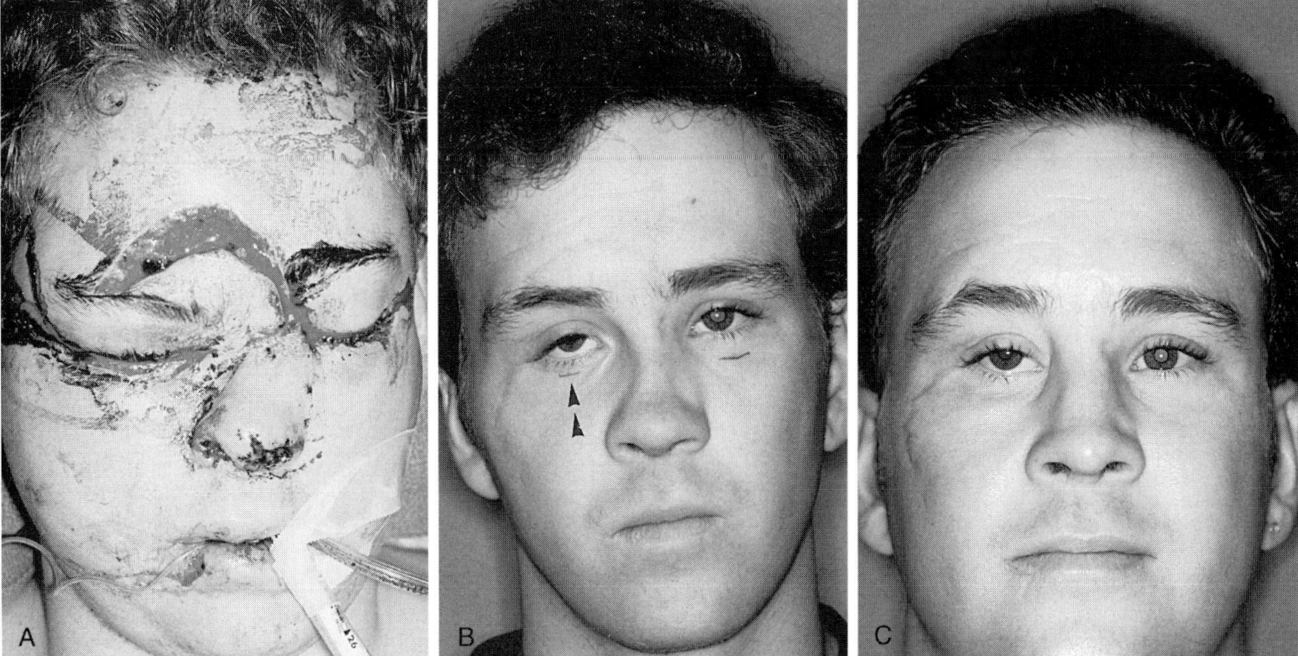

Figure 20–9. *A,* Severe trauma after motor vehicle accident, with nasoorbital and soft tissue injuries. *B,* Early ectropion, before transconjunctival insertion of hydroxylapatite blocks and lateral canthopexy. Short horizontal marks show position of infraorbital rims; the globes are level. *C,* Late result after enophthalmos treatment, scar revision, and nasal surgery.

cedures have been described to correct persistent ectropion. They include tarsal strip procedure, lateral canthal sling, full-thickness skin grafting, and scleral interpositional grafting.[27] Perhaps the most effective technique, in patients with deep scar contracture refractory to simple elevation, is the use of a nasal septal cartilage graft.[28] The cartilage is placed on the septum orbitale to elevate the lid and to support it intrinsically.

Recommendations have been made to reduce the incidence of ectropion with the subciliary approach. They include but are not limited to the following:

1. Preservation of a 1-cm strip of pretarsal orbicularis muscle during the dissection.
2. Avoidance of deep lateral dissection.
3. Not suturing the septum down or reducing its height vertically by any method.
4. Not suturing periosteum after primary fracture surgery.
5. Fastidious hemostasis.
6. Periosteal suspension of lateral tissues.[29]
7. Use of a Frost suture or intermarginal tarsorrhaphy.[26]
8. Taping the eyelid postoperatively.
9. Prevention of edema and hematoma.
10. Early massage of eyelids (beginning at 10 days to 3 weeks postoperatively) for 10 seconds, 10 times a day.[27, 30]

Others have suggested modifications when lid laxity is present, such as wedge resection tarsectomy in older patients and lateral canthopexy. Alternatively, one might avoid the subciliary approach altogether and use a transconjunctival approach.[24]

There is no experienced surgeon who has not noted ectropion after an infraorbital incision. Although many ways of counteracting ectropion have been suggested, none is foolproof. Rare ectropion has been noted even with the transconjunctival approach. Obviously, although ectropion may be limited in occurrence, other complications unique to the internal route do exist, including globe injury, chemosis, canthal malposition, and eyelid retraction.[7]

Appling and colleagues[24] suggest that the transconjunctival approach be considered for the following patients:

- Children.
- Older patients with existing lid laxity.
- Patients who form hypertrophic scars.
- Patients undergoing reoperation.
- Patients with eyelid or cheek lacerations, to avoid going through a scar or creating adhesions between the skin and deep tissues.

Contraindications to the transconjunctival approach are (1) operation on the functioning eye in a monocular patient, (2) acute or chronic conjunctival disease, (3) dry eye syndrome, (4) anophthalmic socket, and (5) history of previous scleral buckle procedure for retinal detachment, depending on the risk of exposing the alloplast next to the globe to contamination.

The best approach appears to be a selective one. The ease of the subciliary approach and the routinely excellent results suggest that the technique should continue to be used in the adult population, but the recommendations noted should not be taken lightly. Controversy as to what exactly is the cause of ectropion will continue. I personally know surgeons who claim excellent results with utilization of their favored techniques, such as placing a small piece of rubber band as a drain to avoid hematoma for 1 day.

References

1. Eisele DW: Complications in Head and Neck Surgery. St Louis, CV Mosby, 1993, p 534.
2. Rodriguez RL, Zide BM: Reconstruction of the medial canthus. Oculoplastic Surgery 1988;15:255.
3. Zide BM, Jelks GW: Surgical Anatomy of the Orbit. New York, Raven Press, 1985, p 45.
4. Zide BM, McCarthy JE: The medial canthus revisited: An anatomical basics for canthopexy. Ann Plast Surg 1983;11:1.
5. Mathog RH, Bauer W: Post traumatic pseudohypertelorism (telecanthus). Arch Otolaryngol 1979;105:81.
6. Markowitz BL, Manson PN, Sargent L, et al: Management of the medial canthal tendon in nasoethmoid orbital fractures: The importance of the central fragment in classification and treatment. Plast Reconstr Surg 1987;5:843.
7. Westfall CT, Shore JW, Nusery WR, et al: Operative complications of the transconjunctival inferior fornix approach. Ophthalmology 1991;98:1525.
8. Perino G, Zide MF, Kinnebrew M: Late treatment of malunited malar fractures. J Oral Maxillofac Surg 1984;42:20.
9. Block M, Zide MF, Kent JN: Proplast augmentation for post-traumatic zygoma fractures. Oral Surg Oral Med Oral Pathol 1984;57:123.
10. Ruben LR: Polyethylene as a bone and cartilage substitute: A 32 year retrospective. *In* Biomaterials in Reconstructive Surgery. St Louis, CV Mosby, 1983, p 474.
11. Iliff NT: The ophthalmic implications of the correction of late enophthalmos following severe midfacial trauma. Trans Am Ophthalmol Society 1991;84:477.
12. Leipziger LS, Dufresne CR: Autogenous and allogenic materials. *In* Dufresne CR, et al (eds): Complex Craniofacial Problems. New York, Churchill Livingstone, 1992, p 489.
13. Kent J, Quinn J, Zide M: Alveolar ridge augmentation using nonresorbable hydroxylapatite with and without autogenous cancellous bone. J Oral Maxillofac Surg 1983;41:629.
14. Holmes RE: Alloplastic implants. *In* McCarthy JG (ed): Plastic Surgery, vol 1. Philadelphia, WB Saunders, 1990, pp 698–731.
15. Jarcho M: Calcium phosphate ceramics as hard tissue prosthetics. Clin Orthop 1981;157:259.
16. Pearl RM: Surgical management of volumetric changes in the bony orbit. Ann Plast Surg 1987;19:349.
17. Manson PN, Clifford CM, Su CT, et al: Mechanisms of global support and post-traumatic enophthalmos. I: The anatomy of the ligament sling and its relation to intramuscular cone orbital fat. Plast Reconstr Surg 1985;77:193.
18. Bite U, Jackson IT, Forbes GS, et al: Orbital volume measurements in enophthalmos using three-dimensional CT imaging. Plast Reconstr Surg 1985;75:507.
19. Manson PN, Grivas A, Rosenbaum A, et al: Studies on enophthalmos. II: The measurement of orbital injuries and their treatment by quantitative computed tomography. Plast Reconstr Surg 1985;77:203.
20. Manson PN, Iliff NT: Post traumatic enophthalmos. Curr Ther Plast Reconstr Surg 1989, p 123.
21. Antonyshyn O, Gruss JS, Gallbraith DJ, et al: Complex orbital fractures: A critical analysis of immediate bone graft reconstruction. Ann Plast Surg 1989;22:230.
22. Mustarde JC: Repair and Reconstruction in the Orbital Region: A Practical Guide, ed 2. Edinburgh, Churchill Livingstone, 1980.
23. Heckler FR, Songcharoen S, Sultani FA: Subciliary incision and skin muscle eyelid flap for orbital fractures. Ann Plast Surg 1983;10:309.
24. Appling WD, Patrinely JR, Salger TA: Transconjunctival approach vs subciliary skin-muscle flap approach for orbital fracture repair. Arch Otolaryngol 1993;119:1000.
25. Goldberg RA, Lessner AM, Shore N, et al: The transconjunctival approach to the orbital floor and orbital fat: A prospective study. Ophthal Plast Reconstr Surg 1990:6:241.
26. Ellis E, Zide MF: Surgical Approaches to the Facial Skeleton. Baltimore, Williams & Wilkins, 1995, p 9.
27. Carraway JH, Mellow CG: The prevention of and treatment of ectropion following blepharoplasty. Plast Reconstr Surg 1990;85:971.
28. Carraway JH, OLoughlin KC: The use of nasal septal cartilage grafts in lower eyelid reconstruction for ectropion. Techniques in Plast Surg 1994;1:127.
29. Phillips JH, Gruss JS, Wells MD, Chollet A: Periosteal suspension of the lower eyelid and cheek following subciliary exposure of facial fractures. Plast Reconstr Surg 1991;87:145.
30. Waite PD, Carr DD: The transconjunctival approach for treating orbital trauma. J Oral Maxillofac Surg 1991;49:499.

Chapter 21
LONG-TERM COMPLICATIONS OF OSSEOINTEGRATED IMPLANTS

by

Richard A. Smith

Introduction

Compared with complications of many surgical procedures performed by oral and maxillofacial surgeons, complications related to the surgical implantation of osseointegrated implants are usually relatively minor. Some complications may be severe, but many may be considered only inconveniences, correctable nuisances, or prolongation or modifications of the treatment plan. Some of the complications may require minor or major surgical interventions or antibiotic therapy. As the utilization of dental implants increases in both conventional and expanded applications, so do the reports on the number, variety, and severity of the surgical complications.

Despite the minor nature of most such complications, the surgeon should not trivialize their significance to the patient. Many patients consider implantation a major decision because of the extent of disability, fear of the unknown, the knowledge of potential complications from the informed consent process, and potential monetary loss. Because some patients plan major social events or work-related activities around completion of the oral reconstruction, complications and delays can be quite demoralizing and disappointing, leading to loss of confidence in the clinician. Occasionally, a patient cannot accept these "setbacks," interprets them as negligence and malpractice, and files legal claims against the treating surgeon.

The complications of osseointegrated implant therapy related to the perioperative period are well known and have been described in the literature. They range from minor events to life-threatening hemorrhages and air emboli. This chapter attempts to categorize and review only the long-term complications related to osseointegrated implants. One must be cognizant that the long-term experience in North America with osseointegrated implant systems is only about 10 years; and the international experience is closer to 30 years. Thus, some of the long-term complications may not be readily apparent to surgeons with the shorter experience. Because many patients receiving osseointegrated implants are geriatric patients, the medical risks of surgery and anesthesia to this population must also be taken into consideration.

THE SUBJECTS DISCUSSED IN THIS CHAPTER ARE:

- Patient selection
- Psychological factors
- Medical factors
- Bone quantity and quality
- Dentate status and type of reconstruction
- Anatomic factors
- Imaging errors
- Bony concavities
- Implant displacement or migration
- Mandibular fractures in patients with endosseous implants
- Surgical technique
- Peri-implant reactions
- Biomaterials
- Systemic effects of titanium implants
- Biomechanical complications
- Special clinical situations
- Ancillary surgical procedures

Complication avoidance and favorable outcome should be the goals of the surgeon. Complications can be minimized by proper patient selection, appropriate consultation particularly with the restorative dentist, proper treatment planning, meticulous attention to detail in the surgical procedure, proper implant maintenance and loading, and adequate short-and long-term follow-up.

Shortcomings in the preoperative planning and performance of the procedure may not have immediate complications, but they may manifest later and lead to long-term complications. Some of the implant failures occur before or at the abutment connection procedure, but others appear at variable times after loading. Later failure may be due to occlusal or biomechanical factors, but problems encountered during the surgical phase may have predisposed the case to delayed complications or failure. For example, an implant that was placed in bone of marginal quality or was not precisely fitted to the recipient site may demonstrate biomechanical failure once loaded.

The American Association of Oral and Maxillofacial Surgeons (AAOMS)[1] has enumerated the known risks and complications of dental maxillofacial implants (Table 21–1). Numerous articles have also classified and reported specific implant-related complications.[2–11] Complications that appear beyond the intraoperative and immediate postoperative periods are considered long-term complications and are discussed in this chapter; they include problems that occur in the immediate perioperative period and produce long-term complications and affect clinical outcome (e.g., nerve injury). Postoperative swelling, pain, and hematomas should not be considered complications, but rather, expected sequelae.

Table 21–1. Known Risks and Complications Associated with Dental and Maxillofacial Implant Therapy

- Unstable implant
- Loss of implant
- Excessive vertical and horizontal bone loss
- Presence of signs and symptoms such as pain, infection, neuropathies, and paresthesia
- Infection (acute or chronic)
- Mandibular fracture
- Injury to adjacent teeth
- Loss of bone graft or augmentation material, resulting in implant failure
- Nasal or sinus fistulas
- Implant not restorable
- Implant or component fracture
- Improper implant positioning, causing prosthetic compromise
- Hemorrhage
- Hyperplastic soft tissue response
- Presence of an outcome indicator(s) listed in the preamble section of the AAOMS *Parameters of Care*[1] on generic clinical indicators for oral maxillofacial surgery in inpatient or outpatient facilities

Data from American Association of Oral and Maxillofacial Surgeons: Parameters of Care for Oral and Maxillofacial Surgery. Rosemont, Illinois, AAOMS, 1995.

Because the most significant complication in implant reconstruction is premature implant failure,[6] the patient must be properly asked for informed consent after being apprised of potential adverse outcomes. The AAOMS implant informed consent form can be modified to suit the needs of the individual practitioner. The clinician must also discuss with the patient the alternatives, risks, and complications of the proposed procedure, and not rely solely on the written consent form. The surgeon should indicate specific risk factors and potential risks and complications as they apply to the given individual patient, rather than quoting the national and international reported statistics from various centers that may not be applicable to a given patient every time. The clinician should exercise caution when interpreting data regarding success rates of dental implants. Life-table analysis with proper study design and implementation is the statistical method of choice to assess the survival of osseointegrated implants. Invalid statistical analysis gives a distortion of success rates that can be misleading to the patient.

Patient Selection

Certain complications can be related to poor patient selection rather than to a surgical mishap. The surgeon must recognize that all totally or partially edentulous patients are not candidates for dental implants and must not be compelled by pressures from patients or referring practitioners to perform procedures that are contraindicated or have a very poor prognosis or high complication rate. Additionally, the surgeon requires specific criteria for the evaluation and selection of candidates for restoration with tissue-integrated prostheses. In 1986, Laney[12] described three categories of edentulous patient that clearly indicate the possible use of implant supported dentures; they are as follows:

- The patient with previous conventional complete denture experience who has considerable residual ridge resorption.
- The individual who psychologically has not been able to accept a removable prosthesis or whose exaggerated gag reflex precluded the possibility of tolerating a conventional prosthesis.
- The patient with acquired or congenital defects that severely compromise the physical conditions necessary for the retention and stability of a non–tooth-supported prosthetic restoration.

Since Laney's report, the applications for dental implants have been expanded. The current indications for osseointegrated implants, as delineated by the AAOMS,[1] are shown in Table 21–2. The surgeon should be cognizant of the factors affecting risk when applying these expanded indications for care (Table 21–3) and should inform every patient of these risk factors as they apply to that patient.

Psychological Factors

Blomberg[13] identified specific psychological contraindications to implant therapy. They included psychotic

Table 21–2. Indications for Dental and Maxillofacial Implant Therapy

- Clinical or imaging evidence of hard or soft tissue deformity in the maxillofacial region, including tooth loss
- Masticatory dysfunction
- Aesthetic deficiency and/or compromise
- Speech impairment
- Behavioral and/or psychological impairment
- Neurologic dysfunction
  - — Pain: nerve compression, soft tissue irritation
  - — Parafunctional habits (e.g., bruxism, clenching)
- Inadequate orthodontic anchorage
- Allergy to materials used in conventional prosthetic reconstruction

Data from American Association of Oral and Maxillofacial Surgeons: Parameters of Care for Oral and Maxillofacial Surgery. Rosemont, Illinois, AAOMS, 1995.

syndromes such as schizophrenia or paranoia, severe character disorders, and neurotic syndromes (i.e., hysteroid and borderline personality, dysmorphophobia), extreme or unrealistic expectations about the cosmetic results, syndromes of cerebral lesions, and presenile dementia. In a patient who appears suspicious and distrustful, any surgical complication may aggravate a latent paranoid psychopathology. The surgeon should be aware of the details of any current troubling life situation (e.g., divorce, loss of a job), because with a patient who is acting under duress, cooperation and prosthesis acceptance are likely to be less than optimal.[12] Some patients may distort the nature of the surgical procedure and exaggerate the painful and traumatic episodes, and others may underestimate the invasiveness of the procedure and expect it to be painless with virtually no postoperative recovery necessary. "Many patients with stormy histories of unsatisfactory experience find the denture prosthesis or its maker suitable repositories for claims of dissatisfaction actually based in their own personality disorders."[14] Some patients with alcohol or other drug-related problems or with underlying emotional disorders may be poor candidates for implant surgery.

Table 21–3. Factors That Increase Risk and the Potential for Known Complications

- Inadequate patient and family understanding of the etiology and natural course of the condition or disorder, therapeutic goals, and proposed treatment
- Presence of coexisting major systemic disease identified during the patient assessment (e.g., disease that increases a patient's ASA classification to II, III, or IV)
- Inadequate preoperative clinical preparation (i.e., history and physical evaluation, indicated laboratory and other diagnostic studies)
- Presence of systemic conditions that may interfere with the normal healing process and subsequent tissue homeostasis (e.g., diabetes mellitus, bleeding disorder, steroid therapy, immunosuppression, malnutrition)
- Inadequate prosthetic treatment planning
- Inadequate review of the factors that are known to influence the creation of osseointegration
  - — Implant material
  - — Implant geometry (macrostructure)
  - — Implant surface (microstructure)
  - — Status of recipient bone (inadequate bone quality and volume)
- Improper selection of surgical technique
- Improper performance of surgery
- Unfavorable prosthetic design and loading conditions
- Presence of bone and/or soft tissue pathology
- Severity of deformity
- Trauma to mandibular nerve and adjacent teeth
- Parafunctional habits
- Inadequate oral hygiene
- History of radiation therapy
- Presence of behavioral, psychological, or psychiatric disorders
- Habits (e.g., tobacco, alcohol, drug abuse) that may affect surgery, healing, or response to therapy
- Extent of patient's and/or family's cooperation and/or compliance

Data from American Association of Oral and Maxillofacial Surgeons: Parameters of Care for Oral and Maxillofacial Surgery. Rosemont, Illinois, AAOMS, 1995.

The informed consent process must take place to prepare patients for possible complications and failure. The process may also help identify patients who would be unable to tolerate any adverse effects of the proposed treatment. I have observed patients who, after having implant failures, claim they were emotionally immobilized or could not return to work or school or get on with their life until the problem was fixed. Some patients cannot accept inconveniences and delays in treatment or the financial loss related to treatment. The surgeon should avoid giving justification to a patient's belief that he or she would never have undergone the procedure if he or she "had known."[15] Thus, written communication with the patient is essential in delineating the possibility of implant failure and complications as well as what happens in case of failure—repeat-procedures, replacement parts, and other costs. If there is a complication, sympathetic questioning and listening as well as willingness to help ameliorate the situation are often appreciated by the patient.

The complication rate related to patient dissatisfaction declines if the surgeon makes the effort to recognize psychological disorders and is selective about the patients in whom procedures are performed.

Medical Factors

The only paucity of information in the dental implant literature documenting implant complications is that related to medical factors. Coexisting major systemic disease (i.e., disease that increases a patient's American Society of Anesthesiologists [ASA] classification to II, III, or IV) or an uncontrolled systemic condition that may interfere with the normal healing process and subsequent homeostasis (e.g., diabetes mellitus, bleeding dyscrasia, steroid therapy, immunosuppression, malnutrition) are medical factors that may be expected to affect risk for the prospective dental and maxillofacial implant patient (see Table 21–3).

Smith and colleagues[16] studied 104 consecutive patients treated with 313 Nobelpharma implants (Nobelpharma AB, Gothenburg, Sweden) to determine the medical risks associated with dental implants. Implant failure rate and perioperative morbidity did not appear to increase in patients with compromised medical status. Age, sex, and concurrent use of hypoglycemic agents, supplemental female hormones, or steroids also did not correlate with increased implant failure or perioperative morbidity. Implant procedures using a variety of pain or anxiety control agents failed to reveal any increase in anesthesia-related complications. Linkow[17] regarded health status as one of the factors influencing long-term implant success. He defined good health as the absence of predisposition to poor wound healing. Uncontrolled diabetes mellitus, alcohol or other drug abuse, and blood dyscrasias were conditions that he regarded as compromising the healing processes of soft tissue and bone. The association between the failure of dental implants and cigarette smoking[18] and the relationship of cigarette smoking with impaired intraoral wound healing[19] have been identified.

Cigarette smoking has a direct effect on exposed tissues as well as acute and chronic effects that decrease tissue perfusion and oxygen delivery. Bain and Moy[18] studied the association between failure of dental implants and cigarette smoking and reviewed the outcome of 2,194 Braånemark implants placed in 540 patients over 6 years. The overall failure rate was 5.92%; however, when patients were subdivided into smokers and nonsmokers, it was found that a significantly greater percentage of failures occurred in smokers (11.28%) than in nonsmokers (4.76%) ($P < .001$). These differences were significant for all areas except the posterior mandible. When fixture length was considered, it was found that in the maxilla, failure rates of shorter implants in smokers were extremely high and in several cases exceeded 25%. Recognizing the absence of any research-based data, Bain and Moy[18] suggested that the patient cease smoking at least 1 week prior to the surgery to permit reversal of the higher levels of platelet adhesion and blood viscosity seen with smoking as well as the shorter-term effects associated with nicotine. The patient should continue to avoid tobacco for at least 2 months after implant placement, to enable the early stages of osseointegration to occur.

The potential adverse effects of glucocorticoids on bone and soft tissue are generally well understood, but their effect on osseointegration of dental implants is less well known. Steiner and Ramp[20] recognized this medical risk factor but concluded that endosseous implants should not be absolutely contraindicated in the glucocorticoid-dependent patient. They did, however, postulate an increased risk of potential failure.

Patients commonly inquire whether osteoporosis is a risk factor in osseointegration of dental implants. The orthopedic literature indicates that osteoporotic fractures heal readily. The prevalence of osteoporosis increases among the elderly and after menopause, but in a study by Dao and associates,[21] implant failure rate was not correlated with age and sex. These researchers believed that implant reconstruction should not be denied to a patient because of a diagnosis of osteoporosis and that treatment planning for any dental implant therapy should be based on a local assessment of the potential surgical site.

Bone Quantity and Quality

Most surgeons concur that complications increase when bone volume and bone quality are compromised. *Bone quality* involves density and vascularity. Jaffin and Berman[22] found that the quality of the bone appeared to be the single greatest determinant of fixture loss. Bone of type I, II, or III usually offered adequate strength. Type IV bone, however, has a thin cortex and poor medullary strength with low trabecular density. In this study, 90% of 1,054 implants were placed in type I, II, or III bone, and only 3% of these fixtures were lost. Of the 10% of fixtures placed in type IV bone, 35% failed.

Van Steenberghe and associates[23] delineated the complications and failures related to a prospective multicenter study of 558 fixtures placed in edentulous jaws. Of the total 558 implants placed, 19 failed and were removed during the healing period or the stage II abutment connection operation. Nevertheless, 10% of the patients in this study suffered from one or more fixture losses. Most failures occurred in groups with less favorable bone quality. Patients who had been partially edentulous for a longer period could be identified in the group with decreased bone quality and were at higher risk for nonintegration. The shortest fixtures in the maxilla (7 mm) had an associated failure rate of 10.7%.

My clinical experience confirms the finding of others that the incidence of implant failure is higher when quality and quantity of bone are compromised (Fig. 21–1). The clinician is obliged to use shorter implants, resulting in a smaller surface area for osseointegration, less initial stability of the implant, and predisposition to micromovement. When the clinical condition of decreased quantity and quality of bone is identified, the clinician should consider ancillary treatment, such as bone grafting or guided bone regeneration, to allow for more ideal implant reconstruction that is engineered to have a more favorable long-term outcome.

Dentate Status and Type of Reconstruction

Fixed Detachable Prostheses in the Totally Edentulous Jaw

Problems and complications may be related to the dentate status of the patient and the type of prosthetic reconstruction utilized. The standards to which all situations are compared are the long-term follow-up studies of osseointegrated implants in the treatment of the totally edentulous jaw using the Brånemark system. In their study, Adell and colleagues[24] reported on the long-term outcome of prostheses and implants in 759 totally edentulous jaws of 700 patients. A total of 4,636 standard implants were placed and followed for a maximum of 24 years. A life-table approach was applied for statistical analysis. More than 95% of maxillas had continued prosthesis stability at 5 and 10 years, and at least 92% at 15 years. The figure for mandibles was

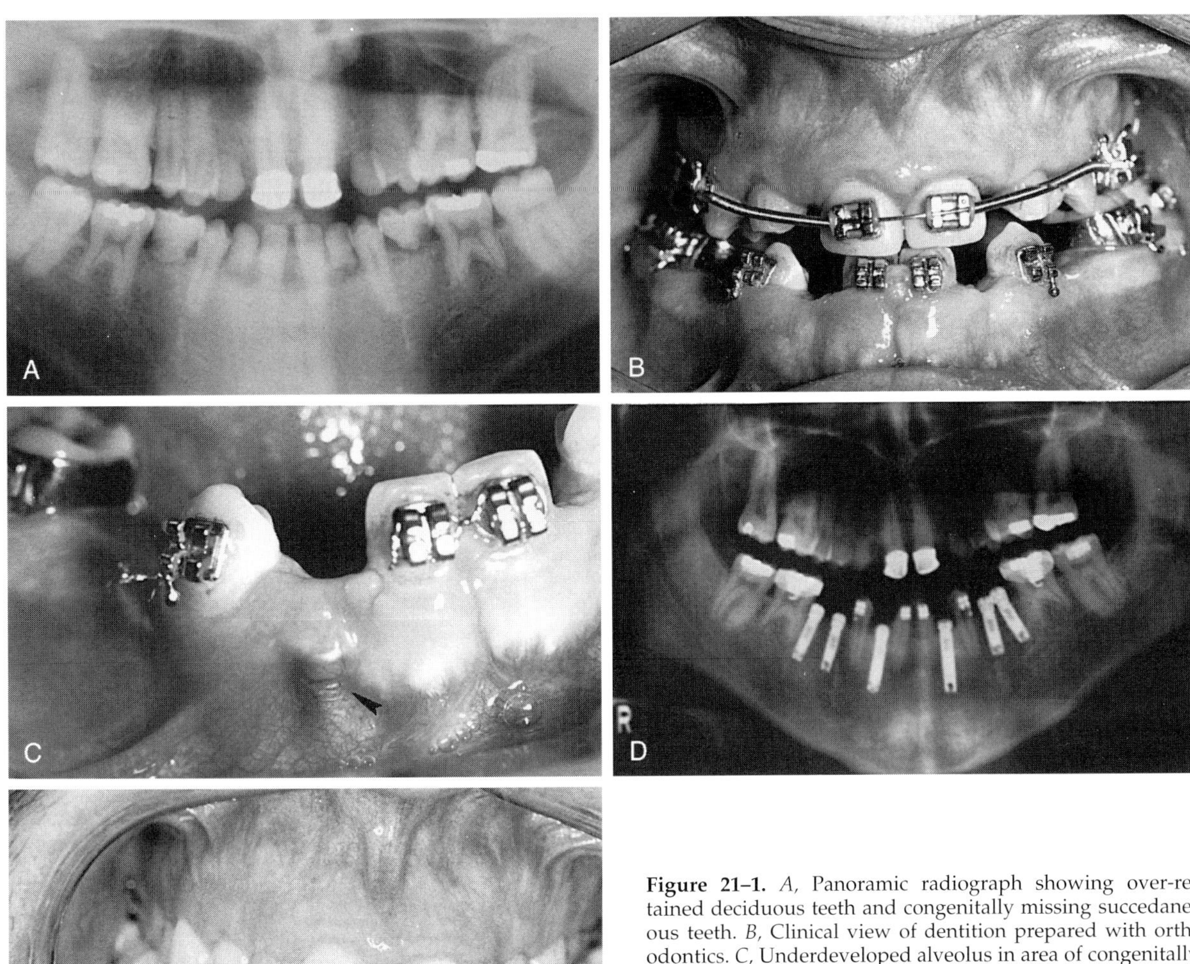

Figure 21–1. *A,* Panoramic radiograph showing over-retained deciduous teeth and congenitally missing succedaneous teeth. *B,* Clinical view of dentition prepared with orthodontics. *C,* Underdeveloped alveolus in area of congenitally missing tooth, demonstrating implant visible through mucosa overlying a labial fenestration. No additional treatment required. *D,* Panoramic radiograph is showing implants in place. *E,* Final mandibular restorations.

99% at all intervals. Individual fixture survival was less than prosthesis survival, with higher success rates in the mandible than in the maxilla. A multicenter American and Swedish report[25] on osseointegrated oral implants reported a 5-year success rate similar to that of the Adell study.

Problems and complications encountered in reconstruction of the edentulous jaw with fixed detachable prostheses (Fig. 21–2) are shown in Table 21–4. Methods of minimizing such complications are listed in Table 21–5. It appears that success rates in patients who are partially edentulous, who need single-tooth replacement, or who are completely edentulous and require overdentures are similar to the success rate in the totally edentulous patient treated with fixed detachable prostheses, but the longest follow-up is only about 5 years. Conditions specific to reconstruction of the posterior jaw, however, suggest a reduced success rate and higher incidence of complications (Table 21–6), but there are measures the clinician may take to reduce the risks (Table 21–7).

Fixed Partial Prostheses

Jemt and Lekholm[26] reported on 67 partially edentulous patients treated with freestanding, implant-supported prostheses and followed for 5 years. A total of 70 jaws were provided with 94 prostheses supported by 259 implants. Seven implants were found to be loose and were removed, with no effect on prosthesis stability. The survival rates were 97.2% and 100% for implants and prostheses, respectively. On average, 0.8 mm of marginal bone was lost around implants in the maxilla, compared with 0.6 mm in mandible. Fatigue fractures of resin veneer material and loosening of gold alloy screws were the major clinical problems. Nevins and Langer[27] reported a retrospective study of 1,203 Nobelpharma (Nobelpharma AB, Gothenburg, Swe-

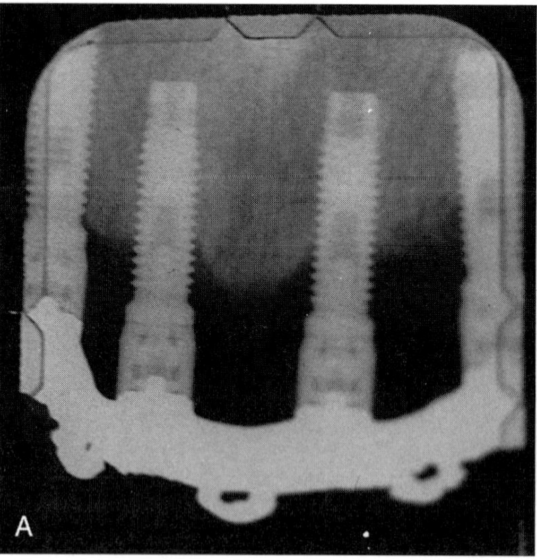

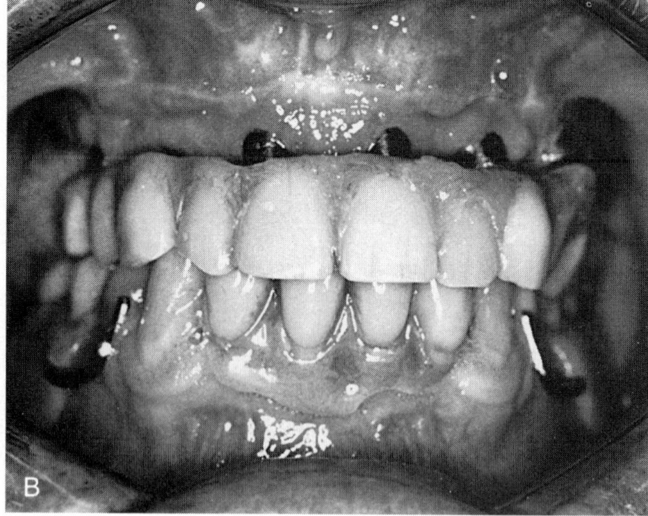

Figure 21–2. *A,* Radiograph illustrating generalized crestal bone loss occurring over 7 years in otherwise successful fixed detachable maxillary reconstruction opposing a natural dentition in a patient with bruxism. *B,* Clinical view of maxillary reconstruction.

den) implants. Of the 551 implants placed in the mandible, 25 failed, for an implant success rate of 95.5%. Of the 247 mandibular prostheses fabricated for 200 mandibles, 8 failed, for a prosthesis stability rate exceeding 97%. Of the 652 implants placed in the maxilla, 31 failed, for a success rate of 95.2%. Of the 250 maxillary prostheses fabricated for 193 maxillas, 2 failed, for a success rate exceeding 99%. Only one mandibular implant and no maxillary implants were lost prior to stage II surgery. The mandibular failures comprised 10 unloaded and 15 loaded implants, whereas the maxillary failures consisted of 21 unloaded and 10 loaded implants.

Table 21–4. Problems and Complications Associated with Reconstruction of the Edentulous Jaws with Fixed Detachable Prostheses

- Mucosal perforations
- Gingival hyperplasias
- Fistulas
- Paresthesias/dysesthesias
- Mandibular fractures
- Maxillary sinus and nasal fossae perforations
- Perforations of the inferior border of the mandible
- Malalignment/malposition of implants
- Infections
- Osteomyelitis
- Chronic pain
- Hygiene access problems
- Speech and salivary spray problems, mostly related to maxillary prostheses
- Fractured gold and abutment screws, prostheses, or implants
- Aesthetic problems
- Instability problems with a complete denture in the opposing arch
- Possible accelerations of bone loss in the opposing edentulous arch with a complete denture (combination syndrome)
- Inadequate intermaxillary space
- Abnormal ridge relationships (developmental or acquired through resorptive patterns) requiring unfavorable cantilevers for aesthetic and occlusal requirements.

Jemt and colleagues[28] reported on failures and complications in 127 consecutively placed, fixed partial prostheses. Problems during the first year of function were related to loose gold screws and aesthetic complaints, complications that the researchers described as easily resolved. Van Steenberghe and associates[23] concluded that after 1 year, success rates in the partially edentulous jaw equal to or better than those obtained in edentulous jaws may be expected. Failures (implant loss) were primarily attributable to unfavorable bone quality and smaller fixture size. Pylant and colleagues,[29] in a retrospective study, also achieved a high level of success in reconstruction of the partially edentulous jaw using osseointegrated implants.

Single-Tooth Replacement

The long-term experience with the single-tooth implant is not extensive, and only a limited number of studies have been reported. Preliminary reports and clinical experience document success rates of at least 97% 1 to 3 years after loading.[30–32] Single-tooth replacement is performed most commonly in the maxillary incisor region because of congenitally missing teeth, teeth lost to trauma, failed endodontic therapy, cracked teeth, caries, or periodontal disease. In the short term, biologic, functional and aesthetic results range from good to excellent, although failures and complications do occur (Table 21–8). There are methods to reduce the incidence of these problems (Table 21–9). The predominant complications are loose screws, loss of interdental papilla, fistulas (Fig. 21–3), and an aesthetic compromise. They usually are managed by employing proper torque control devices for screw joint stability, by limiting incisions in the interdental papilla, and by appro-

Table 21–5. Methods of Reducing the Incidence of Problems and Complications in Reconstruction of the Edentulous Jaw with Fixed Detachable Prostheses

- Use surgical stents to indicate the correct position of the incisal edges for proper implant placement
- A buccal-lingual ridge diameter of at least 5 mm should be present for placement of a standard 3.75-mm–diameter implant; if such a diameter not present, consider graft or guided bone regeneration
- Allow longer healing periods if bone quantity and quality are compromised
- Perform alveolar ridge reduction, if possible, when there is inadequate intermaxillary space
- Remove all sources of infection prior to placing the implants
- Initial implant stability is essential and can usually be achieved by placing the implant in vascularized, osteogenic bone
- Avoid wound dehiscenses by limiting prosthesis usage immediately postoperatively and then periodically relining the relieved prosthesis; exposed implants may cause crestal bone loss in cases of compromised hygiene
- Avoid micromovement of implant through transmucosal loading by proper relief and relining of the prosthesis
- For adequate load distribution to the bone and implant, place the implant along a curve or in any arrangement other than a straight line
- The interimplant distance should not be less than one implant diameter for adequate interimplant bone support and hygiene access
- If a dehiscence or fenestration occurs at time of implant placement, place a graft and/or perform guided bone regeneration
- Achieve enhanced implant stability and ability to withstand load with bicortical fixation in mandibular cases
- Remove all soft tissue around bone preparation during stage I surgery, to prevent migration into the preparation and to produce fibrous encapsulation of the implant
- Contour the ridge, avoid sharp or thin areas, and create a plateau for adequate buccal-lingual width to accommodate the implant
- Do not perforate the inferior border of the mandible, because bacteria may be introduced into this area, creating a submental infection
- When uncovering implants, attempt to bisect the keratinized crestal tissues and transpose if necessary to provide keratinized tissue circumferetially around the abutments
- Preoperative antimicrobial prophylaxis, rinsing with chlorhexidine, and brushing of teeth in dentate cases reduce the incidence of postoperative infections
- Minimize cantilevers
- If the bone tissue in the preparation does not bleed spontaneously, probe the area to stimulate bleeding
- Keep saliva out of the preparation, irrigate and let bony site fill with blood, and then place the implant to create a favorable environment to achieve osseointegration
- Place the implant at ridge crest or below to prevent tissue dehiscence and transmucosal loading

priate treatment planning, obtaining of proper implant trajectory, and reconstruction of tissue-deficient areas, respectively. Many of the failures are due to bony deficiencies, which compromise the precise ideal placement of the implant, create dehiscenses or fenestrations during implant placement, produce inadequate initial implant stability, create aesthetic problems with the prosthesis, or allow for future bone loss when thresholds are reached after loading (Fig. 21–4). The surgeon should reconstruct these bony deficiencies with bone grafts or guided bone regenerative techniques. If the deficiency is significant, the ridge should be reconstructed, and implant placement delayed 3 to 6 months.

Table 21–6. Conditions Specific to the Posterior Jaw with Potential to Increase the Failure or Complication Rate After Reconstruction

- Smaller volumes of available bone
- Shorter implant lengths generally used
- Decreased available space to place additional implants
- Inability to obtain bicortical fixation
- Unfavorable biomechanical situation when fewer implants are placed, increasing the bending forces on individual implants
- Presence of natural teeth that may create problems in designing a harmonious prosthesis
- Less favorable bone quality
- Limits imposed by mandibular canal and maxillary sinus
- Increase in occlusal forces with closer placement of teeth to the temporomandibular joint
- Greater likelihood that implants are placed in linear rather than curvilinear arrangement, resulting in an unfavorable load distribution
- Periodontal pathogens, which may infect implant sites
- More difficult technically owing to access and visualization problems
- Risk of microscopic movement of implants during healing period due to more substantive diet of the dentate patient

Table 21–7. Methods of Reducing the Incidence of Complications in Treatment of the Posterior Jaw

- Through appropriate imaging, determine length of implant contiguous to maxillary sinus or mandibular canal
- Obtain proper screw joint stability with appropriate amount of screw torque
- Achieve adequate engineering by using as many implants as appropriate
- Use grafting or guided bone regeneration in cases of bone deficits
- Make implants as long as possible without violating vital structures
- Use wide-diameter implants when conditions allow
- Design freestanding bridges rather than combining bridges with natural teeth
- Place implants in a nonlinear arrangement
- Consider the use of self-tapping screws when screw-type implants are inserted
- Avoid distal inclination of implants to facilitate prosthetic reconstruction
- Utilize surgical stent after reviewing setup with restorative dentist
- Place the implant in the area of tooth to be replaced rather than the interproximal region
- Appreciate the opposing occlusion to avoid buccal or lingual cantilevers
- Obtain proper trajectory emergence profile of implant
- Place implant and coverscrew flush with or just below crestal bone
- Space implants to allow for adequate interproximal tissue health and access for hygiene
- To place two 3.75-mm implants, confirm presence of 17 mm of mesial-distal space; for three implants, space should be 24 mm

Table 21–8. Complications Associated with Single-Tooth Replacement

- Loose restorations related to loose or fractured abutment screws, due to inadequate tightening of screws
- Aesthetic compromise, usually due to tissue deficiencies, poor alignment or trajectory of implant, or poor prosthetics
- Loss of interdental papilla, resulting in interproximal spaces, due to tissue deficiencies and incisions and reflection of the tissues
- Supragingival visibility of portions of the implant or abutment, due to crestal bone loss or gingival recession
- Disproportionate size of restoration compared with adjacent teeth, due to tissue deficiencies
- Crestal bone loss, due to inadequate available crestal bone, dehiscences at the time of surgical placement, or exceeding of the load threshold
- Fistula formation, due to loose restoration, inadequate hygiene, or cement entrapment
- Peri-implantitis, due to poor hygiene or excessively thick soft tissue interface
- Fenestrations or dehiscenes of facial bone, due to labial plate collapse after tooth extraction, to resorption after implant placement, or to anatomic labial concavities
- Peri-implant abscess
- Damage to the periodontium or root of the adjacent tooth

If a fenestration or dehiscense occurs at the time of implant placement, the defect should be grafted using one of many available techniques.

Overdentures Supported by Osseointegrated Implants

Clinical experience and data from published articles indicate that high success rates are achievable with overdentures supported by osseointegrated implants, but complications and problems do occur.[33–38] In one study of overdentures supported by osseointegrated implants in edentulous mandibles over a 2.5-year period, there was a 97.7% success rate in 44 patients.[33] In a second mandibular study, 25 overdentures were supported by 68 implants with a success rate of 92.65% over 5 years.[34]

Maxillary overdentures were consecutively inserted in 92 severely resorbed maxillas and followed for 1 year.[35] The dentures were supported by a total of 430

Table 21–9. Methods of Reducing the Incidence of Complications Associated with the Single-Tooth Replacement

- Exercise caution in the patient with bruxism, short upper lip and high dynamic smile line, vertical or horizontal alveolar ridge resorption, or deep overbite
- Avoid injury to the periodontal ligament of the adjacent tooth
- Be prepared to place a narrow-diameter implant in thin ridges and to understand their reduced strength
- Consider that the morphology of the alveolar ridge may not correspond to the optimal trajectory of the fixture and that the implant may need to be placed more vertically
- Place the fixture palatal to the incisal edge of the tooth to be restored, to optimize screw access hole and the trajectory
- Use the longest implant that is anatomically allowable; the shortest implant should be about 10 mm
- Be prepared to use long burs or burs with extensions and long fixture mounts, so the handpiece head does not interfere with the teeth
- Use correct tightening torque for proper screw-joint stability
- Use nonrotating abutments
- Use surgical stents for optimal implant position, alignment, and trajectory
- Avoid repetitive incision and reflection of the interdental papilla, to preserve papilla
- Do not sacrifice gingival tissues at the abutment connection procedure unless there is excess tissue
- The shoulder of the abutment should be positioned about 2 mm subgingivally
- Wait about 6 weeks before having an impression taken after stage II surgery, because the gingiva tends to recede
- A minimum of 5 mm of vertical interarch distance is needed to stack the prosthetic components
- Use self-tapping fixtures
- Consider the use of a wide-diameter implant when allowable, or fabricate a transitional crown by taking an impression at stage I surgery to allow for a wider emergence profile of implant; the latter allows for gingival healing that is more elliptic and natural than with round, conventional abutments
- Do not expose implant to heavy occlusal forces
- The width and height of the remaining alveolus will determine the ultimate position of the implant and subsequent emergency profile of the definitive restoration. Therefore, consider bone grafting or a guided bone regeneration procedure before implant placement
- Collapse of the facial or buccal plate is a common sequela of tooth extraction. Insertion of an implant following initial socket healing but prior to buccal plate collapse will help maintain the bone and allow optimal labial lingual placement of the fixture, avoiding the need for a ridge lap restoration
- When extracting a tooth in anticipation of later implant placement, curette the socket well, and if there is a deficiency, use a graft or guided bone regeneration. If there is a loss of the buccal plate, consider placing a barrier membrane to prevent prolapse of the labial gingival tissues and a resultant deficient ridge
- Evaluate smile line and dynamic lip activity to ascertain whether cervical area will be clinically evident
- Place implant apical to the cementoenamel junction of the adjacent tooth to allow for the subgingival veneering material to be placed that gives an aesthetic and naturally emerging appearance. This is particularly important when there is facial plate collapse, which requires the implant to be placed more palatally and results in a ridge-lapped restoration. The restorative dentist can then design a more favorable cervical-labial contour in the restoration
- Do not place the implant in interproximal region, because it is impossible to create an aesthetic restoration in this position
- Inform patient preoperatively that grafting may be necessary, a donor site may be required, and implant placement may have to be delayed
- Avoid prematurely loading the implant transmucosally with the transitional prosthesis

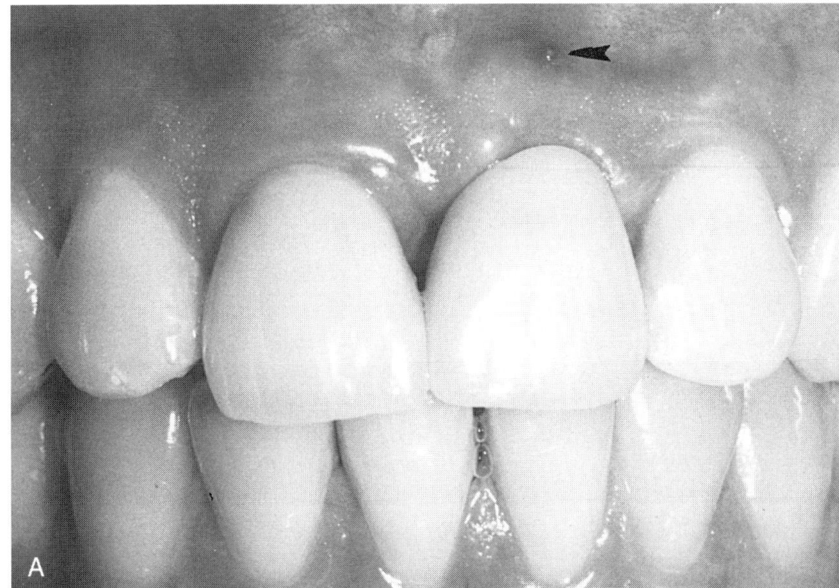

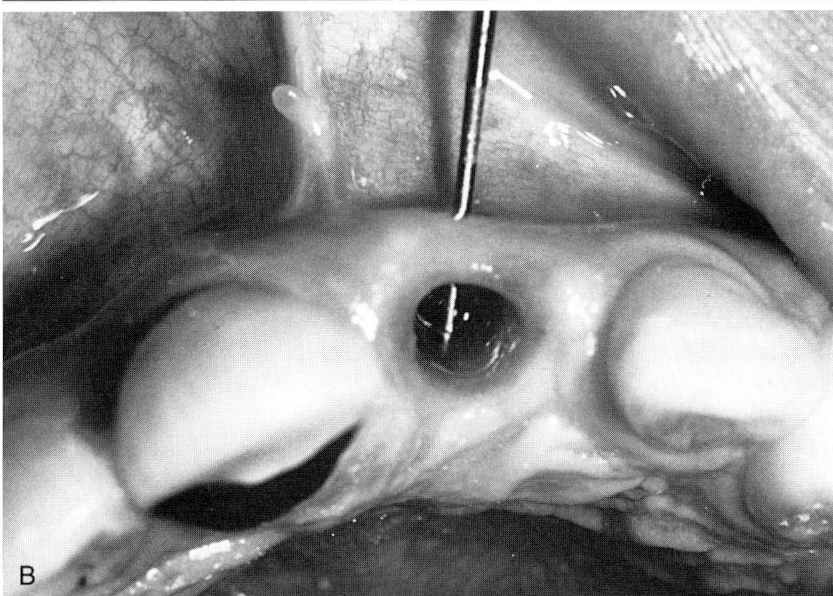

Figure 21–3. *A*, Single tooth implant with soft tissue fistula. *B*, Abutment removed, osseointegrated implant placed deep in the alveolus; probe in fistula.

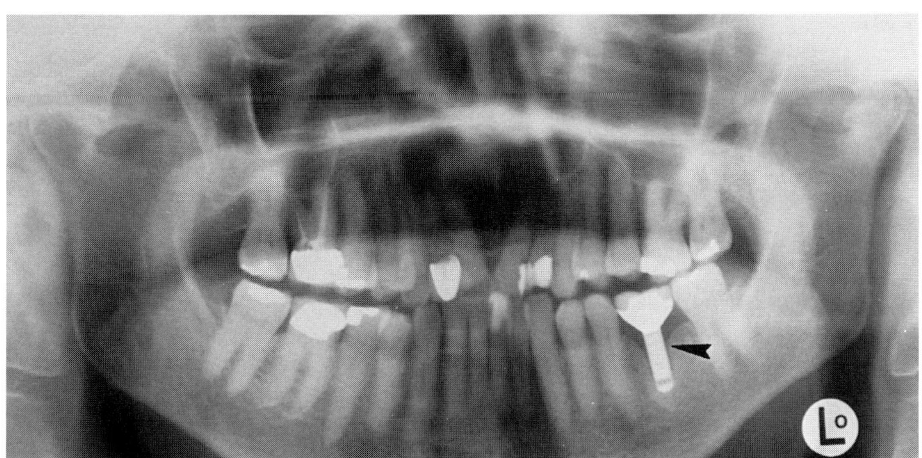

Figure 21–4. Panoramic radiograph showing progressive bone loss in stable implant.

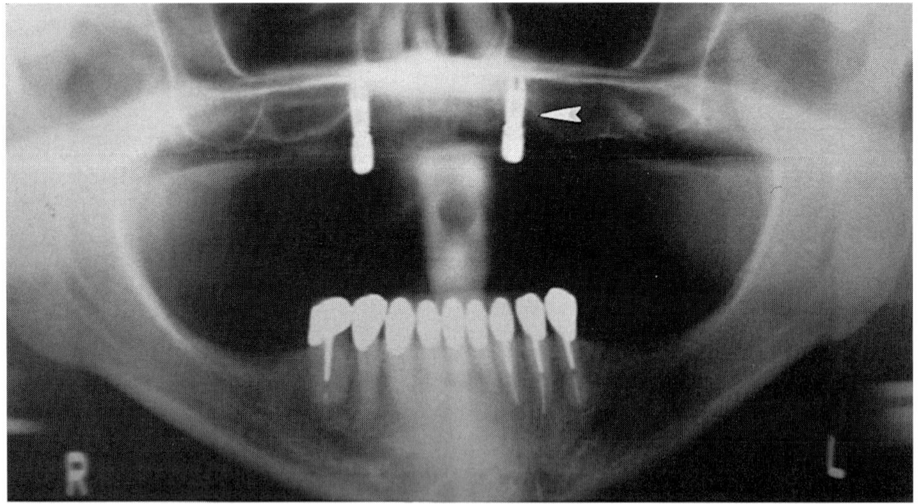

Figure 21–5. Panoramic radiograph of crestal bone loss (coning) in unsplinted but stable maxillary implants opposing a natural dentition.

implants. Of these, 69 (16%) became loose and were removed during the follow-up period. In another maxillary overdenture study, only 2 of 19 patients lost an implant.[36]

A multicenter prospective study of overdentures supported by implants in the maxilla and mandible comprised 133 patients provided with 117 maxillary implants and 393 mandibular implants.[37] The preliminary results indicated a success rate in the mandible comparable to that achieved with fixed prostheses. Results of overdenture treatment in the maxilla, however, appeared to be less favorable than those of fixed prostheses. Another multicenter study of osseointegrated implants supporting overdentures in the maxilla had a fixture survival of 99% in the mandible, but in the maxilla, 58 of 191 were lost.[38]

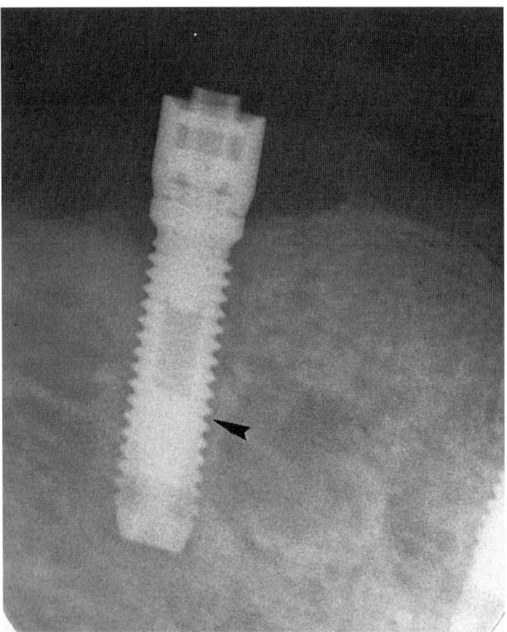

Figure 21–6. Failing implant, progressive bone loss at 6 months after clip bar overdenture construction.

These studies appear to indicate that overdentures supported by implants are a biologically sound and predictable alternative for restoration of the edentulous jaw. Most failures occur at stage II surgery or shortly after loading (Figs. 21–5 and 21–6). Higher failure rates can be anticipated in patients with inferior bone quality and in maxillary cases, particularly when implants less than 10 mm are placed. Numerous problems and complications are possible (Table 21–10), but the most frequently encountered and reported are peri-implant inflammation and hyperplasia, abutment screw loosening, gold screw fracture, and clip loosening. Methods of minimizing problems and complications in this type of reconstruction are listed in Table 21–11. Inflammatory hyperplasia can be minimized by placing the abutment approximately 2 mm above the gingiva and by relining and placing a transitional denture to compress the gingival tissues. Home care instructions, meticulous oral hygiene, and massage of the tissues are helpful. Palatal grafting to eliminate movable, nonkeratin-

Table 21–10. Complications and Problems Associated with Overdentures Supported by Osseointegrated Implants

- Abutment and gold screw loosening and fracture
- Acrylic-resin fracture, particularly in cases with inadequate intermaxillary space
- Clip loosening and fracture
- Peri-implant inflammation and hyperplasia
- Mandibular fracture
- Paresthesia or dysesthesia
- Fixture fracture
- Marginal bone loss
- Palatally placed implants in atrophic maxillae, resulting in bulky prosthesis on palatal side
- Lingual placement of implants in the mandible, which may interfere with Wharton's ducts or require a bulge in the prosthesis that invades the tongue space
- Decubitus ulcer
- Creation of instability in the opposing, complete denture
- Rotational movement identified by patient
- Collection of food under the posterior denture flanges

Table 21–11. Methods of Reducing the Incidence of Complications Associated with Overdentures Supported by Osseointegrated Implants

- Place the implants so that they fit under the denture base to avoid unfavorable cantilevers
- Identify the severely retroinclined anterior mandible to avoid disorientation and placement of malaligned implants
- Position both fixtures at the anterior residual ridge crest as its largest dimension (usually the canine region), and make sure the straight line connection between the two sites is as closely parallel as possible to the terminal mandibular hinge axis
- Consider placing a third fixture in the mandibular midline when there is concern about the success of one of the two implants
- Use soft liners, because converted metal-base removable partial dentures may damage implant components
- Trim or reduce excessive tissue thickness around abutment
- Place implants so that bar will lie over the residual crest; this may vary when a U- or V-shaped ridge is present
- Ascertain a passive fit of the bar
- Ensure good horizontal stability of overdentures to decrease bone resorption
- Place implants far enough apart to allow two clips to be used in the denture, because the prosthesis will be more retentive
- Evaluate intermaxillary available space in the patient recently rendered edentulous and consider alveolar ridge reduction
- Confirm abutment seating radiographically and use a torque driver to tighten screws
- Use abutment caps as protectors of the internal threads of the abutments during the transitional phase of the prosthetic reconstruction
- Splint implants together for greater strength and stability
- Design bar shape and contour to allow rotation and avoid torquing forces

ized tissue is occasionally required, as is excision of the hyperplastic tissue. The use of torquing devices generally eliminates the loosening of components. The most common patient complaints and dissatisfactions with overdentures are related to movement of the prosthesis during function and trapping of food under the flanges. The use of additional implants gives further support, better retention, improved function, and enhanced satisfaction.

Anatomic Factors

The objective of reconstructive implant surgery is to utilize the available bone, modify it if necessary, and produce minimal insult to the regional anatomy. Careful clinical examination, digital palpation, and appropriate imaging enable the clinician to appreciate deficiencies, contour defects, morphologic variances, concavities, and contiguous vital structures.

Injury to Blood Vessels

Although the oral and maxillofacial region is well vascularized, two blood vessels appear to be most susceptible to injury during endosseous implant surgery, the sublingual and inferior alveolar arteries. Two reports of life-threatening hemorrhage from injury to the sublingual artery indicate the potential damage to this vessel when the lingual cortical plate is perforated during preparation of an implant site in the anterior mandible.[39, 40] Staying within a subperiosteal plane, preventing laceration of the soft tissue, and appreciating the angle and trajectory of the drills minimize this potential complication. Injury to the inferior alveolar artery can result in brisk bleeding. Because this vessel is intrabony, hemostasis with pressure packing is usually easily achievable; however, this treatment may result in additional injury to the inferior alveolar nerve.

Injury to Sensory Nerves

Nerve injuries have been reported following placement of implants.[41, 42] The nerves likely to be injured are the inferior alveolar, mental, lingual, and infraorbital. When such injuries are inflicted during the surgical procedure, their potential long-term effects take the form of paresthesias, anesthesias, and dysesthesias (Figs. 21–7 to 21–9). Nerve injuries caused by the dissection, drills, or the implant may result in neurapraxia, axonotomesis, or neurotmesis. Lip and chin numbness are the most common areas of sensory impairment. The incidence of altered sensation is unclear and variable, and most cases are transient paresthesias that resolve. If a nerve injury is identified intraoperatively, radiographic verification of the implant must be made in order to ascertain that the implant has not violated the mandibular canal. If it has, the implant should be immediately "backed out" either through reversal of the implant with the drill or through the use of a reverse mallet in the case of a press-fit cylindric implant. Protocols for management of peripheral nerve injuries have been established and should be followed (see also Chapter 6).[43] Injuries to the mandibular canal can usually be prevented through proper assessment of the available bone above the canal.

The anterior loop of the mental nerve is vulnerable to injury during soft tissue dissection, drilling, or implant insertion. The most distal implants should be no closer than 4 to 5 mm from the anterior aspect of the foramen. The mental foramen can be explored and identified intraoperatively, but it is not necessary to dissect out the nerve, a procedure more likely to produce injury. The mental nerve is vulnerable in cases of severe mandibular atrophy, in which the nerve is lying on the superior aspect of the ridge-crest. A palpating finger often helps identify the nerve's presence. One way to determine the location of the mental nerve relative to the clinical ridge and implant site is to use a radiographic stent. An anatomic relationship that can help localize the mental nerve position is that the supraorbital and infraorbital foramina, the pupil, and the mental foramen are aligned in a vertical plane. The infraorbital nerve is more likely to be injured during an augmentation procedure for an atrophic maxilla or during a maxillary sinus lift procedure.

Imaging Errors

Sonick and coworkers[44] performed a cadaver study comparing the accuracy of periapical radiography, pan-

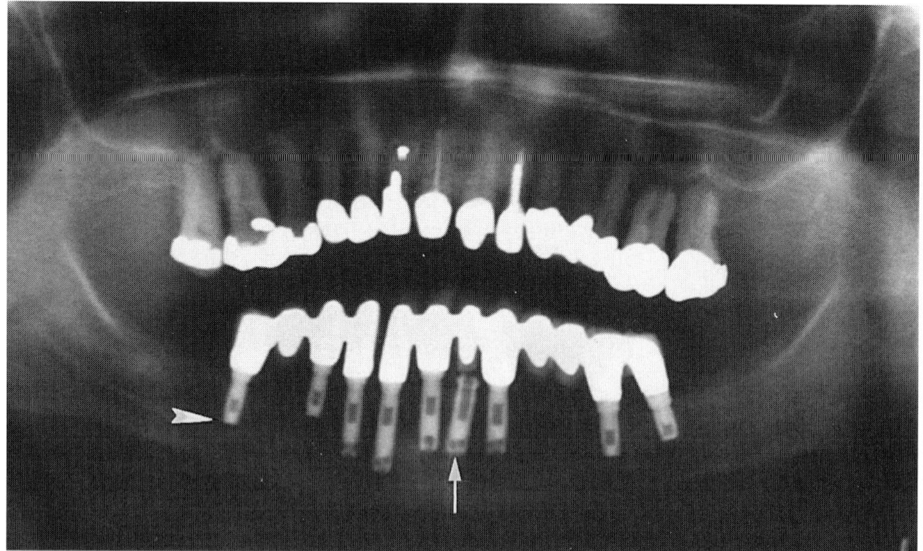

Figure 21–7. Patient presented with persistent painful dysesthesia in lower right lip subsequent to implant violation of the mandibular canal *(arrow)*. A "sleeping" implant is also present in the anterior mandible *(arrow)*.

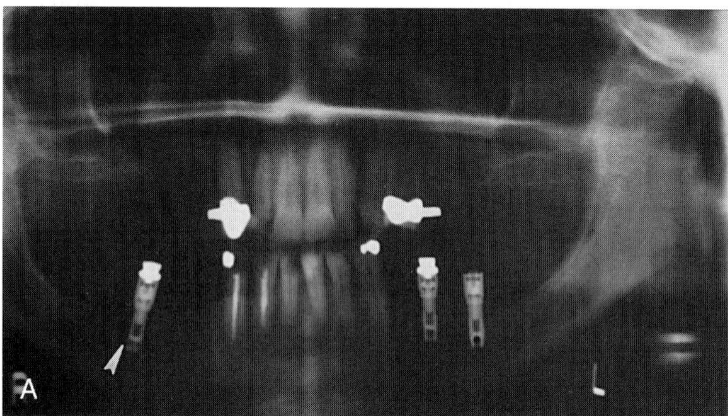

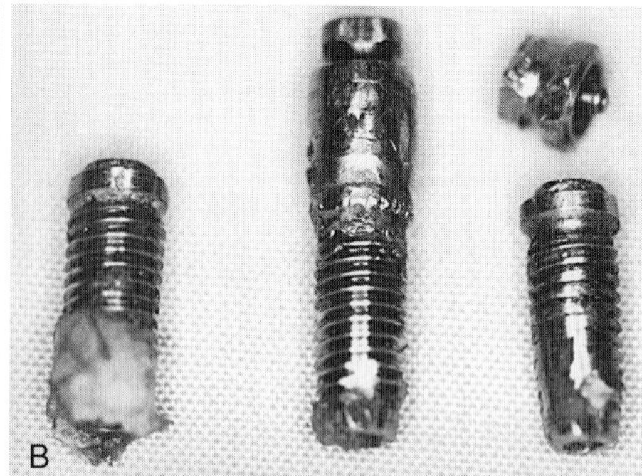

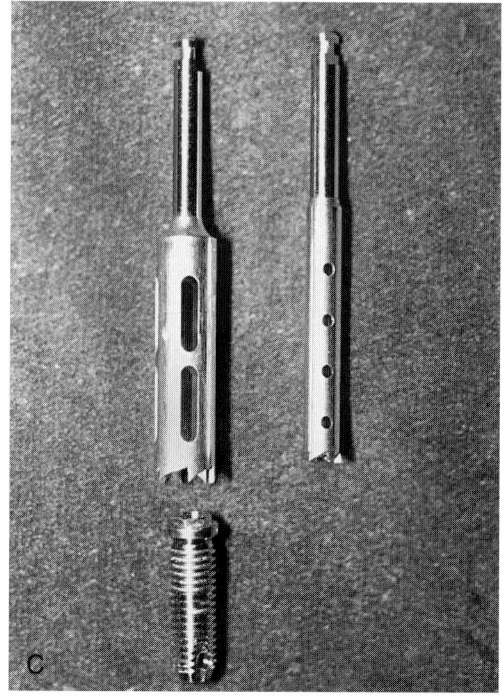

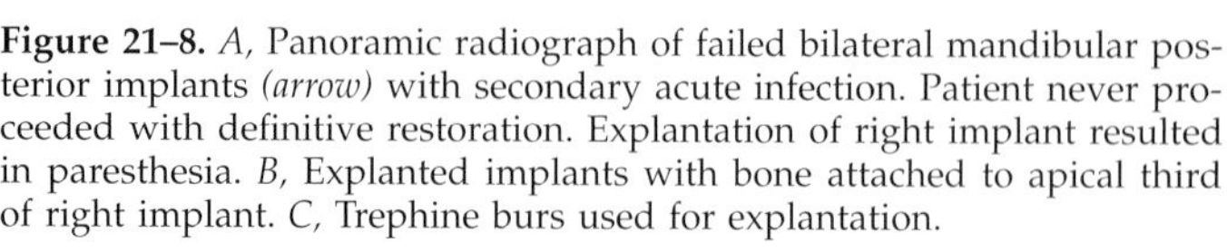

Figure 21–8. *A*, Panoramic radiograph of failed bilateral mandibular posterior implants *(arrow)* with secondary acute infection. Patient never proceeded with definitive restoration. Explantation of right implant resulted in paresthesia. *B*, Explanted implants with bone attached to apical third of right implant. *C*, Trephine burs used for explantation.

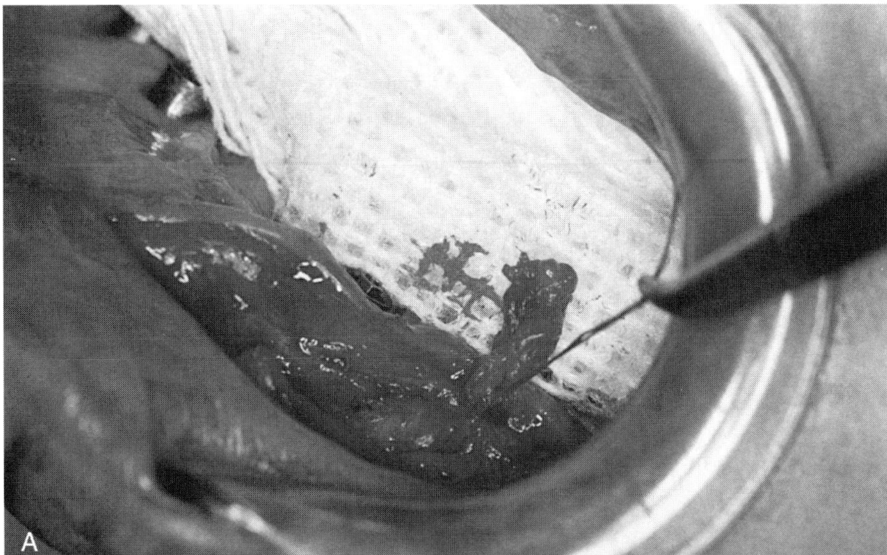

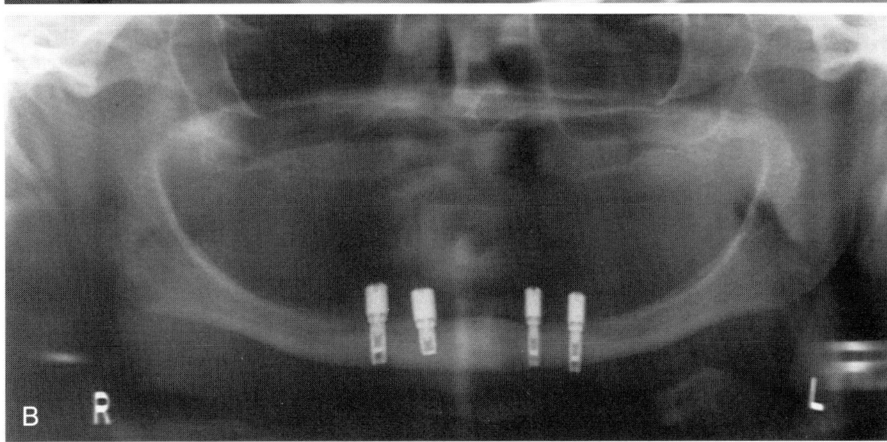

Figure 21–9. *A,* Neuroma at site of bone graft augmentations and implant placement. Alteration in sensation did not occur until fabrication of the prosthesis. *B,* Radiograph of implants in augmented mandible.

oramic radiography, and computerized tomographic (CT) scanning in locating the mandibular canal. The average amounts of distortion for the periapical radiographs, panoramic radiographs, and CT scans were 1.9 mm (14%), 3.0 mm (23.5%), and 0.2 mm (1.8%), respectively. Cross-sectional CT scanning for implant site assessment is an excellent alternative to characterize the alveolar crest and visualize anatomic structures in a buccolingual dimension while providing an accurate estimation of available vertical space from the ridge-crest.[45] Radiation absorbed from dental implant radiography should be a consideration.

In a comparison study of linear tomography, computerized tomography, and panoramic and intraoral techniques, lithium fluoride thermoluminescent dosimeters were placed at selected anatomic sites within and on a humanoid x-ray phantom.[46] CT examination delivered the greatest dose, whereas linear tomography had generally the lowest dose. Panoramic and intraoral doses were similar to that of linear tomography.

There is considerable variability in the utilization of imaging techniques. Most surgeons agree that a panoramic radiograph would be required in most cases, but others argue the need for additional linear tomography or CT scanning for more accurate assessment. In the average case, a panographic radiograph and periapical radiographs of dentate areas are adequate, provided that the clinician understands the pitfalls of panoramic radiology in implant surgery—i.e., the amount of alveolar bone seen on the radiograph may vary from the amount of alveolar bone actually present.[47] When the mandibular canal along its S-shaped course lies in a more lingual position, as it does at its origin at the mandibular foramen, its image is seen in a more superior location. When the canal lies in a more buccal position, as it does inferior to the first molar tooth and in the region of the mental foramen, the image is cast relatively less superiorly. When the image of the mandibular canal is less distinct, the canal may be situated more deeply in this region.

The resorption pattern in the buccal and lingual surfaces of the alveolar ridge after dental extraction is not uniform. In panographic imaging, if the alveolar bone is situated farther lingually, the image of the bony height gives the appearance of having more bone than actually exists. The panoramic radiograph also does not represent the third dimension, and the buccolingual width and the inclination of the alveolar ridge cannot be assessed. Because of horizontal foreshortening, it is essential not to attempt to make accurate linear measurements on the radiograph, particularly in the mental foramen area. The variability of focus-to-film distances results in a greater magnification in particular regions, contributing to the unreliability of the panoramic radiograph to accurately determine available height.

Use of a radiographic splint may be beneficial to determine whether the alveolar ridge is correctly placed in the focal trough. Metal balls placed in an acrylic splint appear round if the patient is properly positioned, and oval if not. The magnification can be measured as well as the distance from the distal part of the ball to the mental foramen. Despite these pitfalls, limitations, and inaccuracies of panographic radiography, this imaging technique is commonly suitable for treatment planning, as long as the surgeon understands these shortcomings, takes into consideration at least a 25% enlargement factor, and adds 1 to 2 mm as a margin of error in calculating the amount of available bone.

Bony Concavities

Unanticipated bony concavities in implant surgery can result in implant failure through the creation of identified or unidentified fenestrations or dehiscences. If mucoperiosteal flaps are not adequately reflected or the concavities are not detected on clinical examination, violations of the alveolus may go unidentified, leading to failure of osseointegration. When these perforations are identified, they can be grafted, allowing for an improved prognosis. Two anatomic areas exist that preclude this situation: concavities in the labial maxillary incisor or canine region (Fig. 21–10) and in the lingual mandibular molar region (see Figs. 21–6 and 21–7).

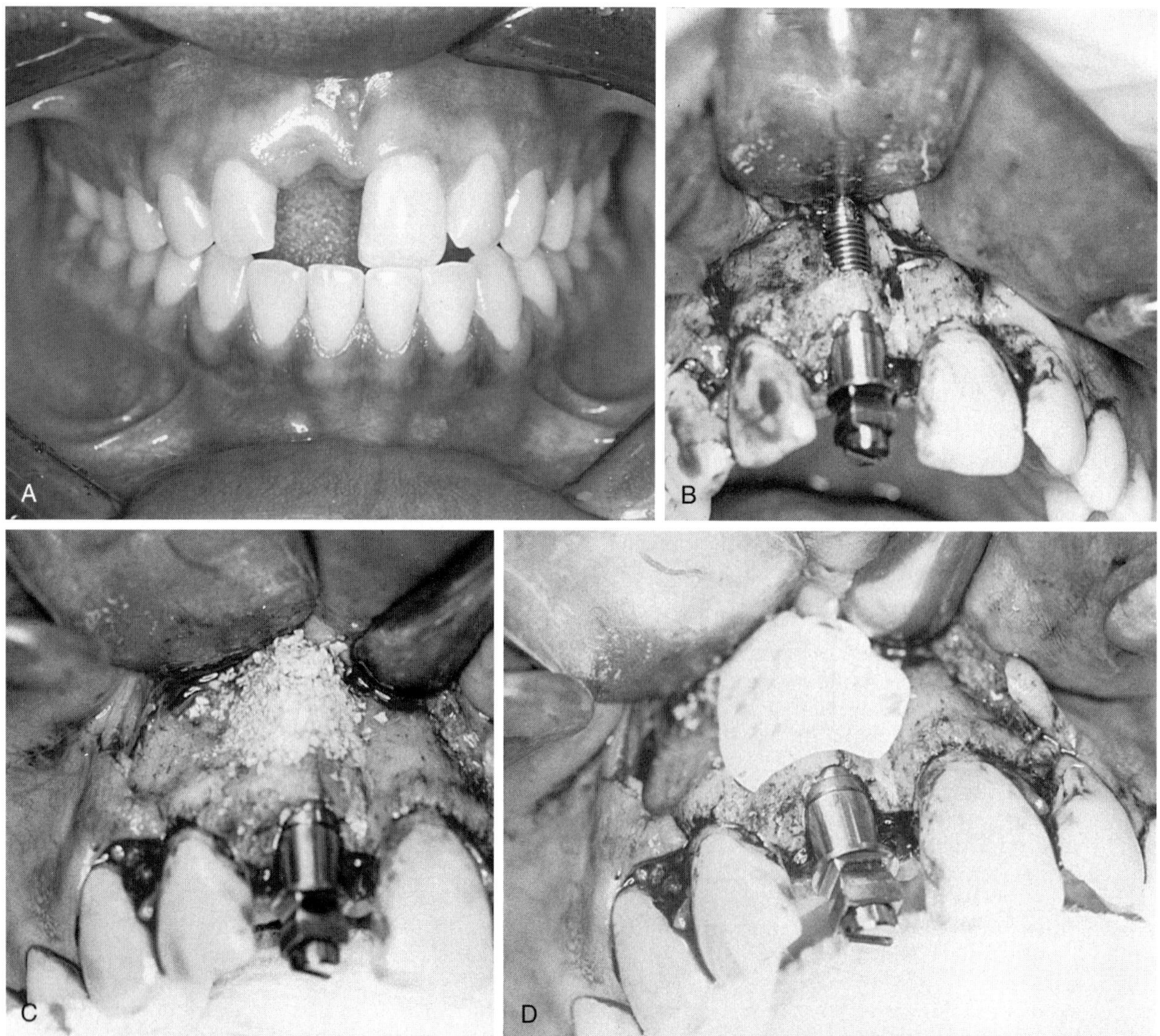

Figure 21–10. *A,* Preoperative view of edentulous area with labial concavity. *B,* Implant with large dehiscence increased by attempt to achieve proper trajectory in the presence of a severe labial concavity. *C,* Composite autogenous graft and xenograft. *D,* Barrier membrane in place.

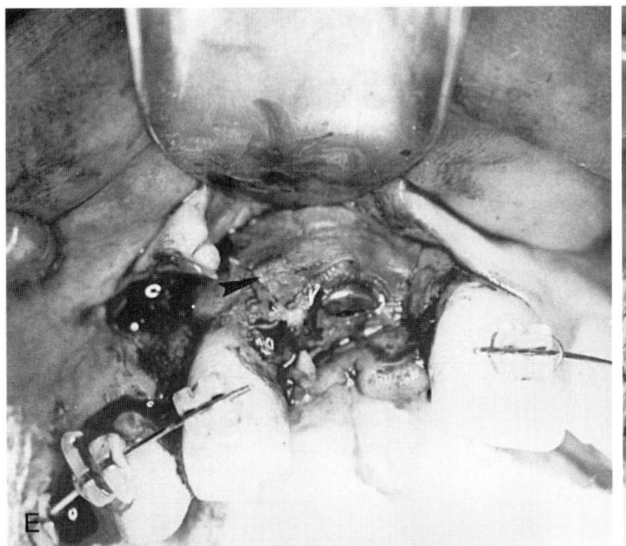

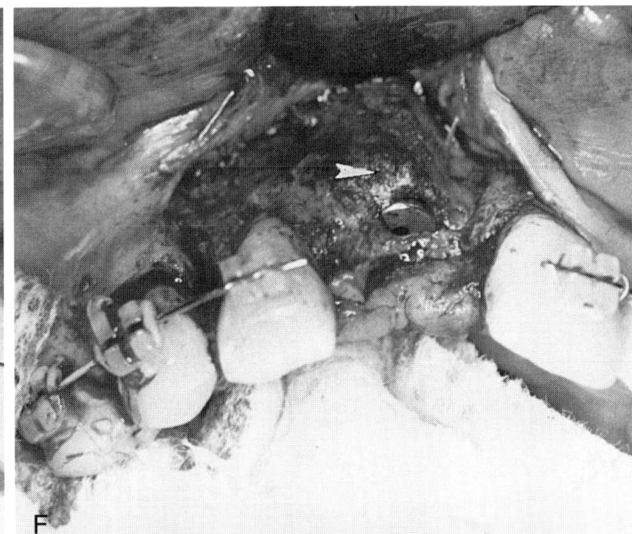

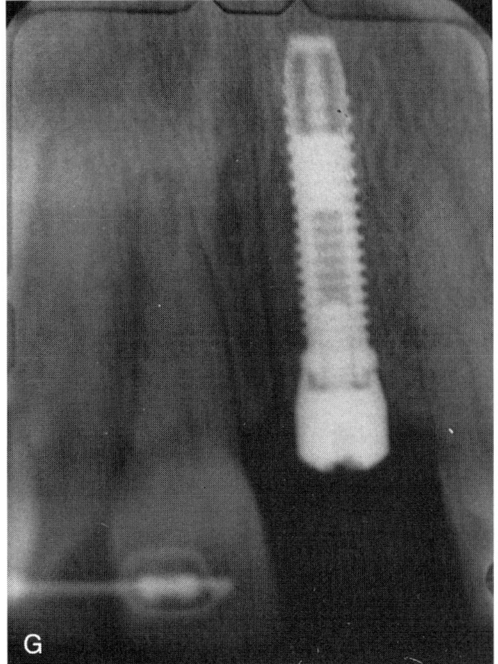

Figure 21–10. *Continued E,* Implant at abutment connection procedure 6 months postoperatively, showing healed composite autogenous graft and xenograft with membrane in place. *F,* Membrane removed to show new bone formation. *G,* Radiograph of implant 6 months after procedure.

When placing implants in the anterior maxilla in the aesthetic zone, the surgeon must be cognizant of the importance of proper trajectory and emergence profile and must utilize a surgical stent to assist in implant placement. In the attempt to satisfy the prosthetic and aesthetic requirements, the perimeter of the alveolus may be perforated. A clinical decision whether to graft first, manage a perforation with a graft material, or accept a compromised implant position must be made. If its position is severely compromised, the implant should not be placed.

Resorptive processes in certain anatomic situations in the posterior mandible can deceive the surgeon, and a concavity on the lingual aspect of the mandible must be appreciated. This must always be assessed as part of the clinical evaluation. Perforation into the submandibular fossa may occur (Fig. 21–11) causing the implant to be in part extraosseous, with resultant failure to osseointegrate. Damage to the salivary glands, by violation of these structures during the preparation phase, can lead to mucus retention phenomenon.

Implant Displacement or Migration

During or subsequent to implant placement or abutment connection procedures, implants or instruments used during the procedure can be displaced into aberrant locations. Implants can be displaced into the maxillary sinus during stage I surgery or, if the implant is not osseointegrated, at stage II surgery (Fig. 21–12) Entry of the implant into the nasal fossae, mandibular medullary space, submandibular fossae, submental space, or mandibular canal[48] can occur, requiring additional surgery to retrieve the foreign body. An implant

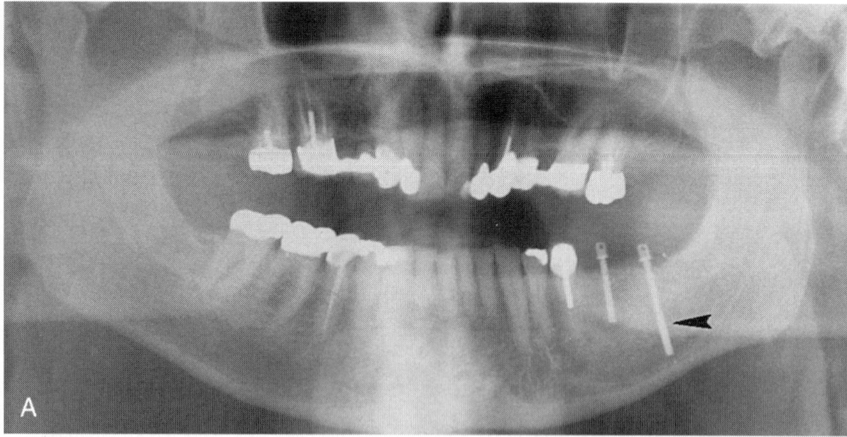

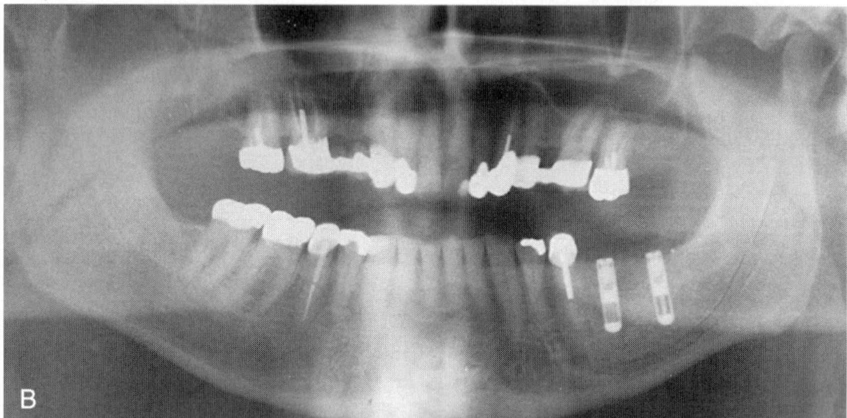

Figure 21–11. *A,* Panoramic radiograph of 22-mm depth gauge probe placed in 15-mm preparation *(arrow)* that appeared to be in the mandibular canal. Probe had entered a perforation in the lingual plate and entered the submandibular space. *B,* Panoramic radiograph of 4.0-mm × 15-mm cylindrical implants in place. There were no neurosensory deficits.

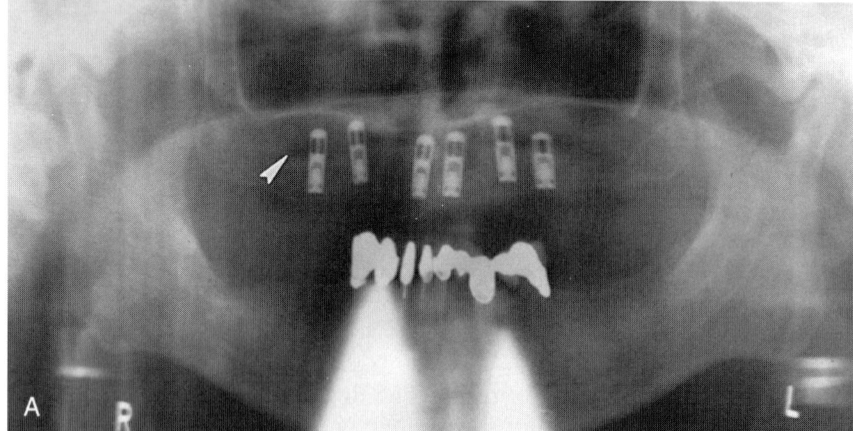

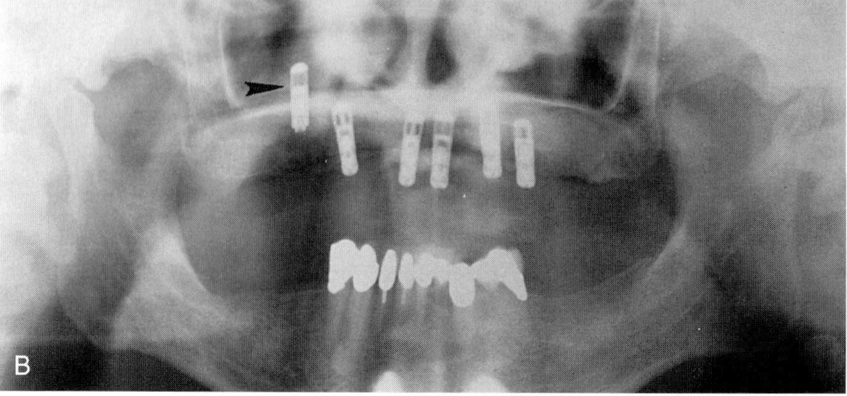

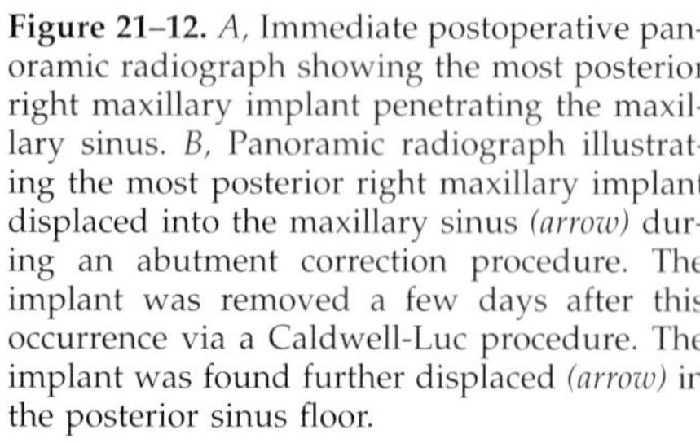

Figure 21–12. *A,* Immediate postoperative panoramic radiograph showing the most posterior right maxillary implant penetrating the maxillary sinus. *B,* Panoramic radiograph illustrating the most posterior right maxillary implant displaced into the maxillary sinus *(arrow)* during an abutment correction procedure. The implant was removed a few days after this occurrence via a Caldwell-Luc procedure. The implant was found further displaced *(arrow)* in the posterior sinus floor.

is capable of migrating into ectopic positions and, when contiguous to the nasal fossa, can be expelled spontaneously (Fig. 21–13C). Small instruments, components, or implants can be swallowed or aspirated. Swallowed instruments or implant components are usually passed but can lead to obstruction or perforation, requiring endoscopic or even open surgical procedures. A life-threatening complication involving intraoperative aspiration of an implant screwdriver has been reported (Fig. 21–14).[49] The patient did not cough or show any other signs of respiratory distress. The instrument was removed by rigid bronchoscopy. This event was followed by a chain of further complications, including pneumothorax treated with thoracocentesis and placement of a water-sealed chest tube. Late laryngeal obstruction required tracheostomy, and a pleural effusion required drainage.

Patients who have undergone ablative tumor resec-

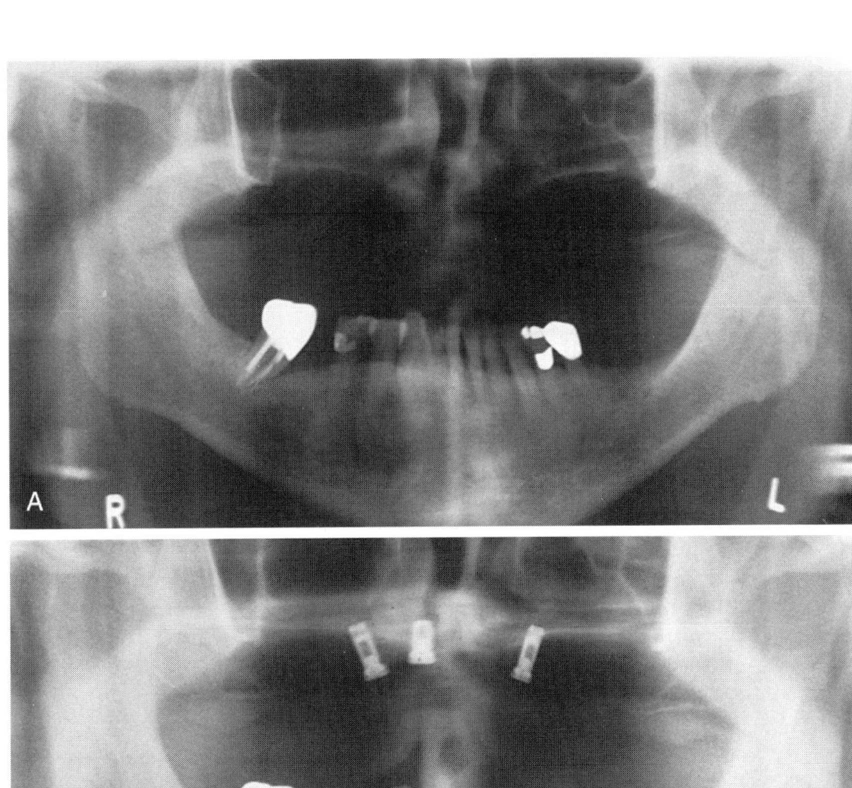

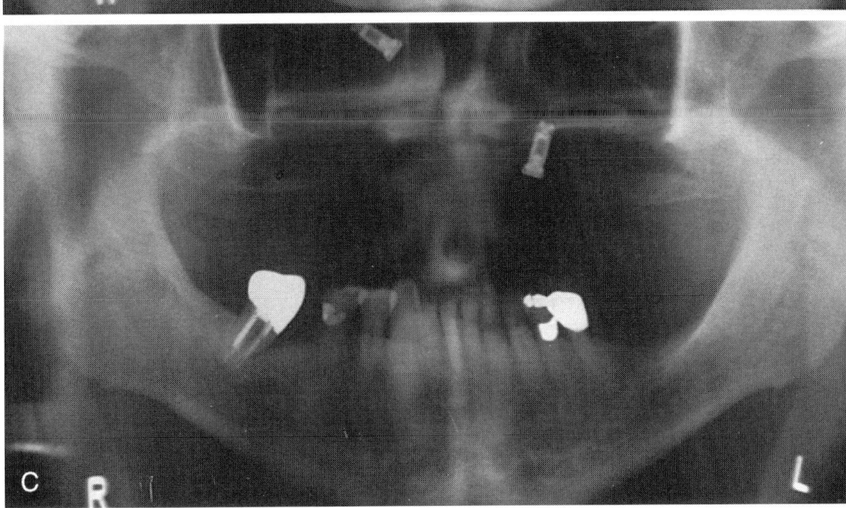

Figure 21–13. *A*, Preoperative panoramic radiograph of atrophic edentulous maxilla. *B*, Panoramic radiograph showing three endosseous implants in autogenous maxillary graft. *C*, Panoramic radiograph illustrating displacement of one implant into the maxillary sinus. The other missing implant was expelled spontaneously through the nose after the patient sneezed.

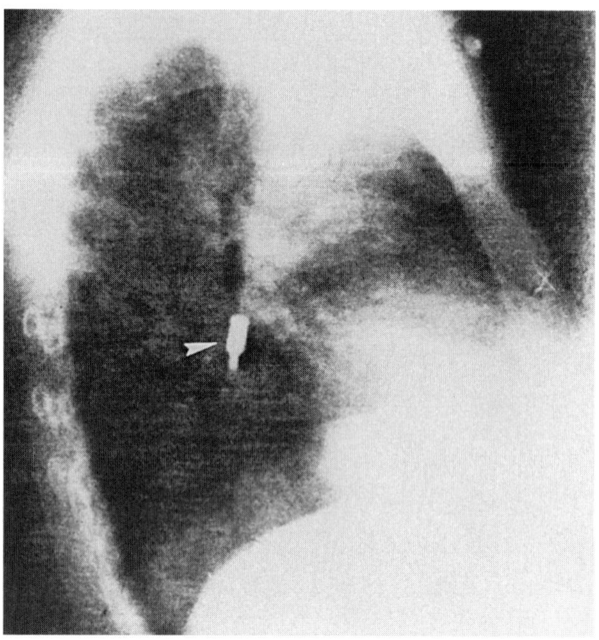

Figure 21–14. Lateral chest radiograph with aspirated screwdriver in right main-stem bronchus.

tions or radiation in the oral and maxillofacial region may be at higher risk for displacement and aspiration of foreign bodies because of limited access in such cases. To help prevent this occurrence, use pharyngeal screens and handpiece-held screwdrivers, and if the patient is unable to be cooperative, use a general anesthetic with endotracheal intubation, throat packs, and pharyngeal screens.

Mandibular Fractures in Patients with Endosseous Implants

Mandibular fractures through endosseous implants (Fig. 21–15) have been reported, and several etiologies have been expounded, as follows:[50, 51]

- Osteoporotic (decreased bone mass) changes affecting the atrophic mandible
- Deficient mineralization, which may occur subsequent to bone grafting
- Stress concentration at the implant site during implant placement
- The tensile forces that occur within the mandible during function

Binger[52] reported on osteomyelitis and pathologic fracture after implant placement in the edentulous jaw.

Avoidance of this complication in the atrophic mandible can be achieved by limiting the number of implants placed, providing adequate interimplant distance(s), and avoiding overtightening of screw implants and use of excessive forces in seating cylindric implants. There should be at least 6 mm of vertical height and width of mandible available; otherwise, bone grafting is indicated. A transversely placed 7-mm implant can be placed in a 6-mm mandible but can result in an unfavorable inclination (Fig. 21–16).

Surgical Technique

Long-term iatrogenic complications can be the result of errors committed during one of the surgical phases of endosseous implant reconstruction. As with other surgical procedures, there is a learning curve for each surgeon. As applications of implants expand with more complex procedures, a new learning curve is established, and just as a surgeon's failures and complications were on the decline, they begin to rise once again. The complications encountered may not be so trivial with more invasive procedures.

Mucoperiosteal Flap Design and Implant Site Preparation

Paying meticulous attention to detail and following established surgical protocols are essential. Failures related to the reflection of mucoperiosteal flaps are possible when there is excessive vertical flap reflection, which

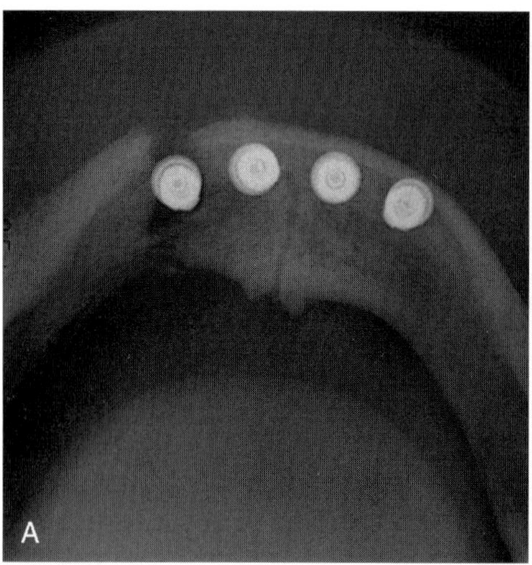

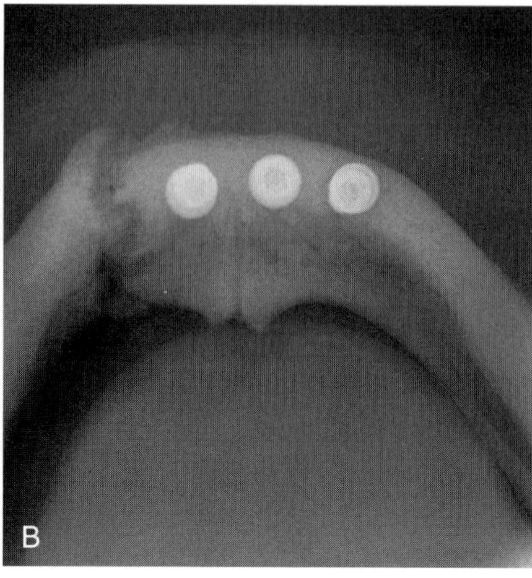

Figure 21–15. *A*, Radiograph of fractured mandible secondary to implant placement. *B*, Radiograph showing fractured mandible after implant removal.

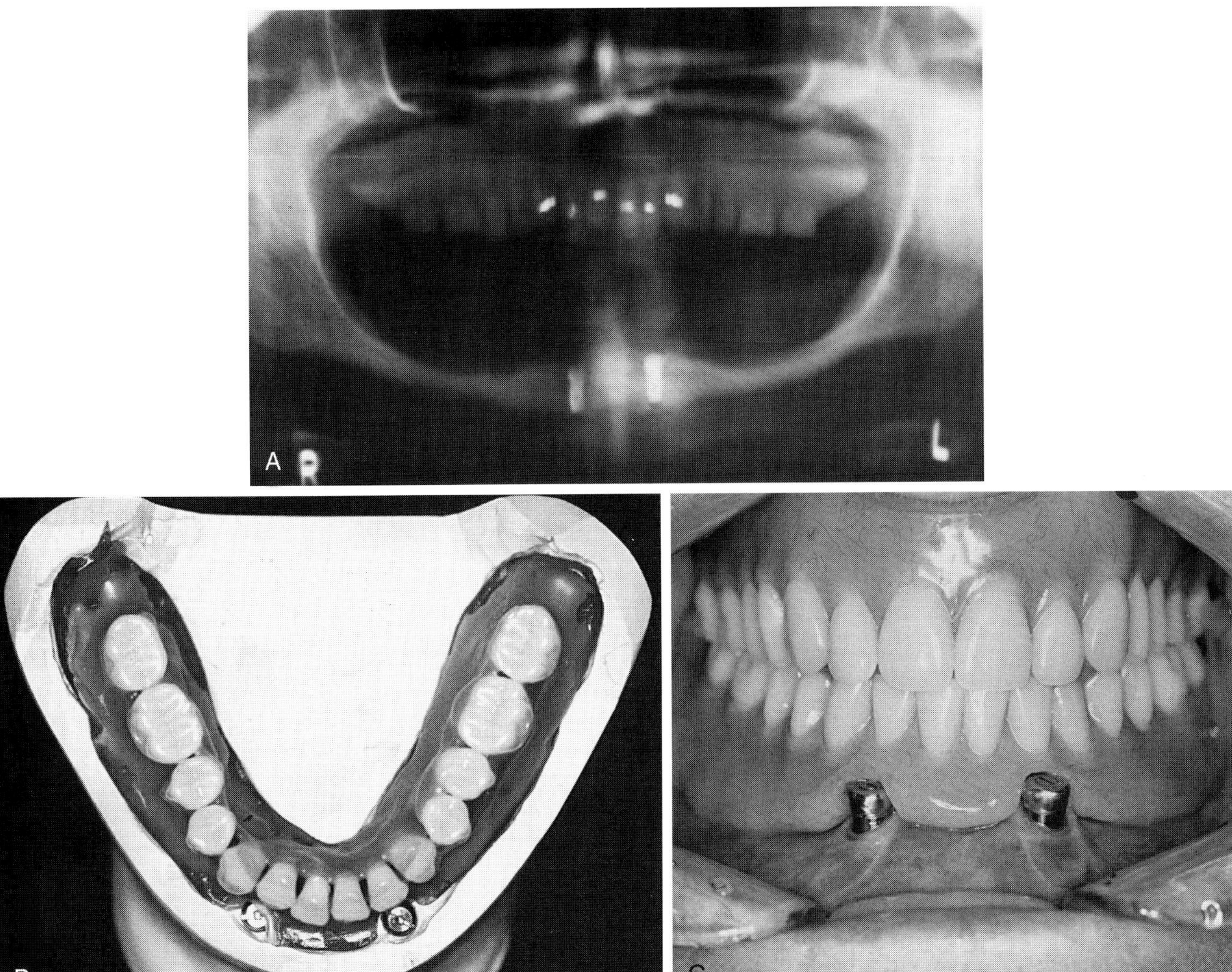

Figure 21–16. *A,* Panoramic radiograph illustrating 7-mm screw implants placed in atrophic mandible. *B,* Model of wax-up showing labially placed implants. *C,* Clinical view of implants with cantilevered bar resulting from labial inclination of the implants.

can compromise the blood supply to the atrophic mandible and implant recipient site as well as cause chin ptosis. Care must be taken not to traumatize the flaps, to work in a subperiosteal plane, and to close the flap primarily without tension. Flap dehiscences not only delay healing but may jeopardize complete healing, and some long-term crestal bone loss may persist. If a flap dehiscence occurs, it is not necessary to mobilize a flap to reclose it, as wound breakdown may recur. Wound débridement and home care can be used to manage this type of complication.

Failure to achieve concentricity of the bony preparation produces an imprecise, oval or elliptic preparation, which produces gaps at the bony interface and compromises implant stability. Generating high temperatures during the drilling procedure can cause hyperthermically induced osteonecrosis at the bone-implant interface, resulting in failure of osseointegration. Using specially designed implant drilling equipment, slow, intermittent drilling with proper cooling irrigants, and new sharp débrided burs reduce the chance of producing osteonecrosis, which results in fibrous encapsulation and eventual implant loss. During drilling, the bur is moved up and down in the preparation, so that saline solution may reach down into the prepared site to cool the bone and flush away surgical debris. A bone tap can destroy its own threads if it continues to turn once the bottom of the preparation is reached. Also, excessive forces during implant placement and excessive countersinking can lead to crestal bone loss, cratering and saucerization, or failure of osseointegration. Excessive countersinking can cause progressive bone loss or "coning," particularly if occlusal forces beyond the threshold of the bone-implant interface are achieved. When screw-shaped implants are placed using fixture mounts in a deep bony preparation, the fixture mount may bind in the bone, making removal from the fixture mount difficult and damaging the implant hex during the process, leading to future difficulty in abutment connection. If the hex distortion is minimal, burnishing with an instrument corrects the problem. If the hex is severely damaged, a round rather than hexed abutment must be used, but the nonrotating feature of the abutment is eliminated.

Small perforations created in the bone preparation away from the ridge-crest are generally well tolerated. For larger fenestrations or dehiscences, however, grafting procedures should use autogenous, allogeneic, alloplastic, or composite grafts with or without barrier membranes. Leaving larger fenestrated areas of implants in direct contact with the overlying mucoperiosteal flap generally does not result in bone growth over the exposure and may lead to eventual failure. Improper placing of cover-screws, once the implant has been placed, can lead to potential problems. The cover-screw should be turned slowly without force; otherwise, there may be cross-threading and inability to seat the cover-screw, preventing future use of the internal threads of the implant to accommodate an abutment. Fracture of the stem of the cover-screw within the implant body and stripping of the screwdriver hex or slot are other potential complications. If the cover-screw hex or slot is stripped, carefully deepening a slot in the screw with a high-speed bur makes retrieval possible. If the threads were stripped in the internal portion of the implant, a temporary abutment may be rotated clockwise and counterclockwise in the implant body until the threads are retapped. Some implant systems include retapping tools. Improper seating of the cover-screw leads to bone growth around the implant, requiring its removal and predisposing it to injury. When cover-screws are properly seated and there is bone growth over them, the use of bone mills easily and precisely removes the bone without injuring the implant.

Instrumentation and Equipment

Titanium and stainless steel instruments should be kept separated to avoid contact. Contamination of the implant with other metals may cause breakdown of the titanium oxide layer essential for osseointegration.

Only drilling equipment that does not use air-and-water spray should be used in implant surgery. Three patients treated by the same surgeon suffered fatal cardiac arrest during surgery as a result of air emboli.[53] Two of the patients who died had received general anesthesia, and the third had received intravenous sedation; the three patients were treated by three different anesthetists. All three patients had sudden cardiac arrest developing profound cynanosis and electromechanical dissociation, underwent prolonged resuscitative efforts, and showed marked hypoxemia and hypercapnea. Two other patients had signs of injection of air but survived, one suffering cardiac collapse and the other sustaining massive subcutaneous emphysema. The air emboli were produced by inadvertent injection of a mixture of air and water, passing through the hollow dental drill, directly into the mandible to the facial and pterygoid plexus veins and then to the superior vena cava and right atrium.

Disorientation of the Surgeon

Loss of orientation by the operating surgeon can result in improperly aligned implants, creating aesthetic compromise, difficult prosthetic construction (Fig. 21–17), or useless implants. A useless implant must be either explanted or "put to sleep" by removing the transmucosal component, burying it in the bone, and closing the soft tissue over it. Angled and bendable abutments are poor substitutes, because they may by unaesthetic and may lead to mechanically unfavorable loading in the long term.[54] The surgeon's disorientation may produce injury to the adjacent tooth root and periodontum (Fig. 21–18). Planning the procedure on articulated study casts with a setup of the proposed occlusion, using surgical templates, having other members of the operating team assist in the orientation and angulation of the implant, and continual reference to the opposing arch and point of emergence through the mucosa reduce the incidence of complications related to loss of orientation. Preventing surgeon disorientation can avoid prosthetic compromise due to unfavorable cantilevers, ridge laps, and biomechanical compromise.

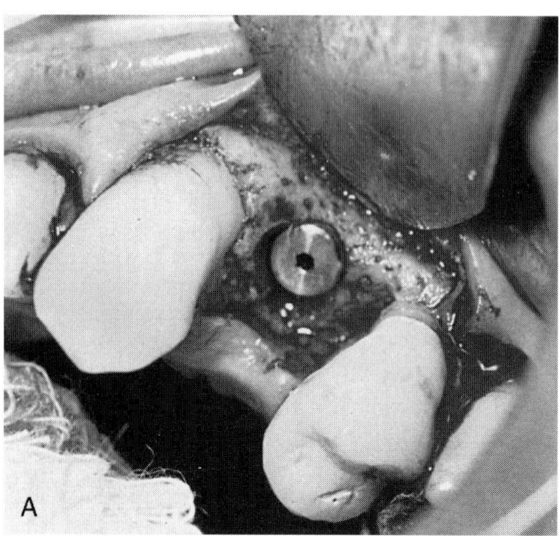

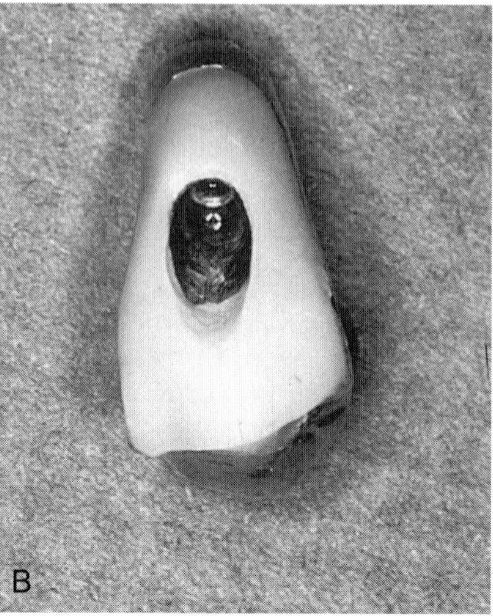

Figure 21–17. *A,* Single-tooth implant placed with buccal inclination. *B,* Crown with screw access hole through labial surface creating unaesthetic situation.

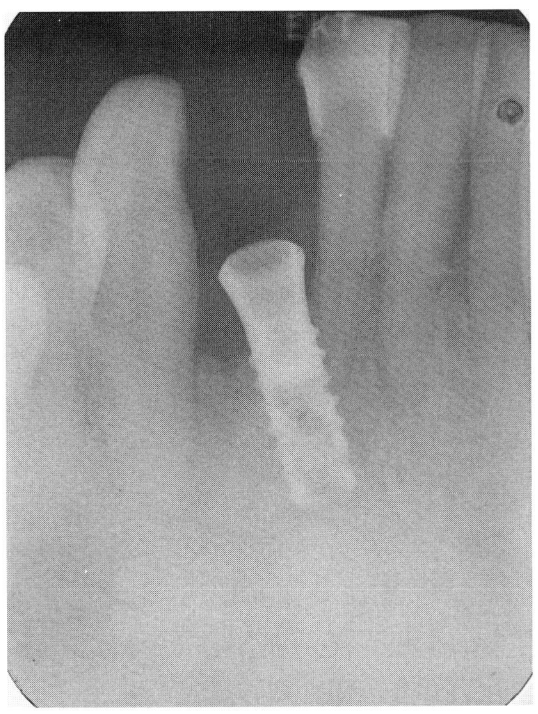

Figure 21–18. Injury to adjacent tooth root during implant preparation.

Handedness of the Surgeon

The handedness of the operator can influence the angulation of the implant. During placement of implants in the anterior mandible, with the surgeon positioned behind the patient, there is a tendency to slope the implants in one direction off the vertical plane (Fig. 21–19). In the edentulous situation, there is no reference point for orientation. A surgical stent, frequently constructed by duplication of the patient's denture, can be very helpful. During placement of implants in the posterior mandible, with the mouth wide open, there is a tendency to place the implants with a posterior slope, creating an unfavorable path of insertion for components and screwdrivers and creating nonaxial occlusal forces (Fig. 21–20). Implant placement adjacent to natural teeth may be difficult because of hindrance by the teeth that may cause deflections in the angle of the bone preparation or insufficient intermaxillary room for the handpiece. Use of drill extenders or long shafted burs may address this problem.

Contamination of the Implant and Implant Site

Implant surface contamination can be caused by touching the surface with nontitanium instruments, surgical gloves, surgical cotton products, suction tips, surgical flaps, and patient's tongue and saliva. This contamination must be avoided by proper retraction and suction, flap reflection, and appropriate implant preparation. The implant may also become contaminated when placed in an implant site with residual dental pathology that was not managed prior to the implant procedure. All soft tissue surrounding the prepared bony site should be removed, because it can proliferate and invaginate into the preparation, causing fibrous encapsulation and eventual failure.

Abutment Connection Errors

Problems and complications can result from errors committed at the abutment connection stage. Faulty seating of the abutment (Fig. 21–21) allows soft tissue ingrowth, producing an inflammatory response and possibly requiring a secondary procedure if not promptly identified and corrected. A postoperative radiograph must be taken to confirm proper abutment seating. If an error in seating goes unidentified, the abutment will most certainly become loose, can create stresses within the abutment screw and implant, and may even cause component fracture. Selecting an abutment with inadequate height can result in tissue creep over the top of the abutment, leading to hyperplasias that require excision (Figs. 21–22 and 21–23). Poor oral

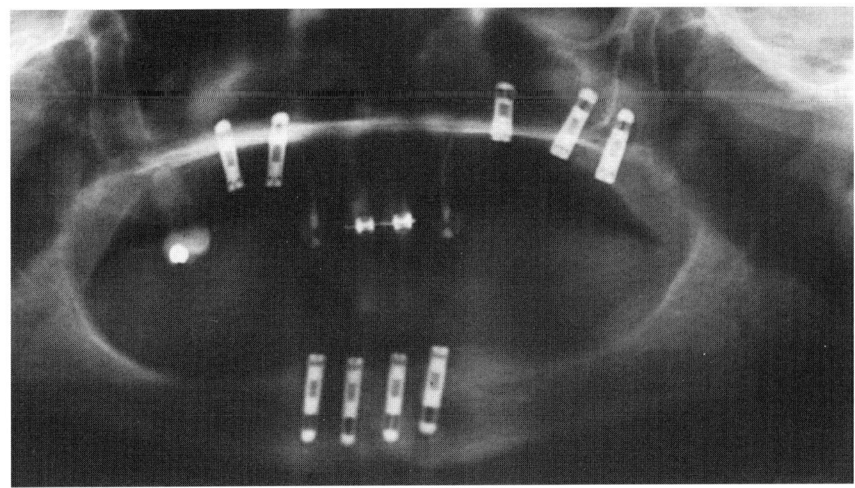

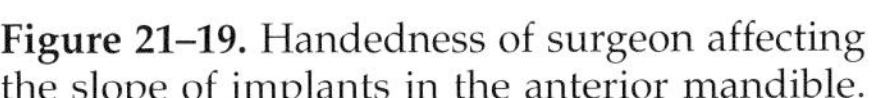

Figure 21–19. Handedness of surgeon affecting the slope of implants in the anterior mandible.

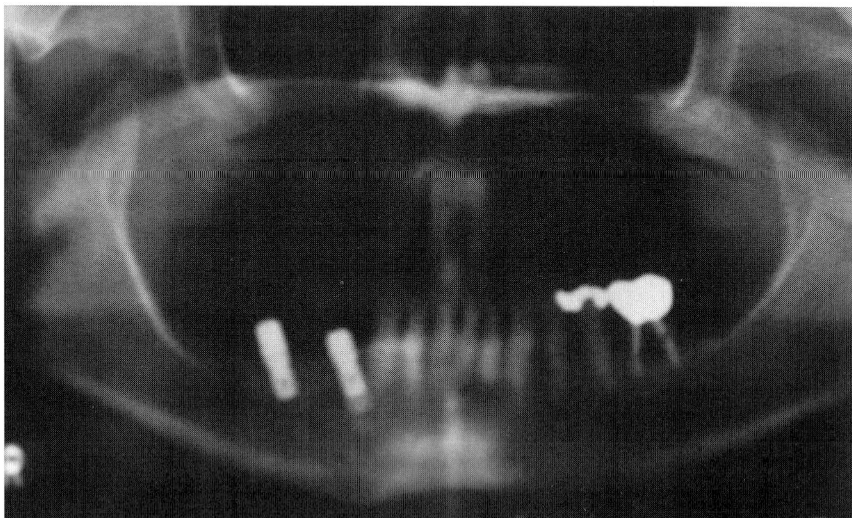

Figure 21–20. Radiograph illustrating tendency for distal inclination of implants with mouth in wide-open position, making component attachment very difficult.

hygiene and movable, nonkeratinized tissue aggravates this situation. The abutment should project 1 to 2 mm above the level of the soft tissue. If there is a question as to the type of abutment to be incorporated into the final restoration, a temporary abutment should be used. It is essential to anticipate the type of abutment and to determine whether the surgeon or restorative dentist will provide it, to prevent disputes and unanticipated costs. A complete inventory of components is necessary for the abutment connection procedure as for other aspects of the treatment.

To prevent loosening of and potential damage to the components, proper tightening with a torque wrench that meets manufacturer specifications should be used. When a prosthesis is to be worn over abutments, they must be adequately relieved and relined with a soft-tissue liner. This will help adapt the peri-implant tissue. Modified metal-based, removable partial dentures can be damaging to the underlying abutments. When abutments are removed to make changes, the procedure should be done expeditiously; otherwise, the soft tissue may rapidly contract and cover the implant.

Peri-implant Reactions

A report by Block and Kent[55] identified factors associated with soft tissue and hard tissue compromise of endosseous implants. Their prospective analysis determined factors associated with implant removal as well as with implant morbidity resulting in nonscheduled visits. The most important factors in implant success were surgery without compromise in technique, placement of implants into sound bone, avoiding thin bone or implant dehiscence at the time of implant placement, avoiding premature implant exposure during the healing period, establishing a balanced restoration, and ensuring appropriate follow-up hygiene care. Perforations of the maxillary sinus occurred with 45% of those implants placed into the posterior maxilla without sinus grafting. No adverse sequelae were noted.

Articles have been published specifically focusing on the peri-implant, periodontal, and marginal soft tissue reactions to osseointegrated titanium implants.[56–58] Failures and complications are likely if a perimucosal soft tissue seal to the implant surface is not achieved.[59] If

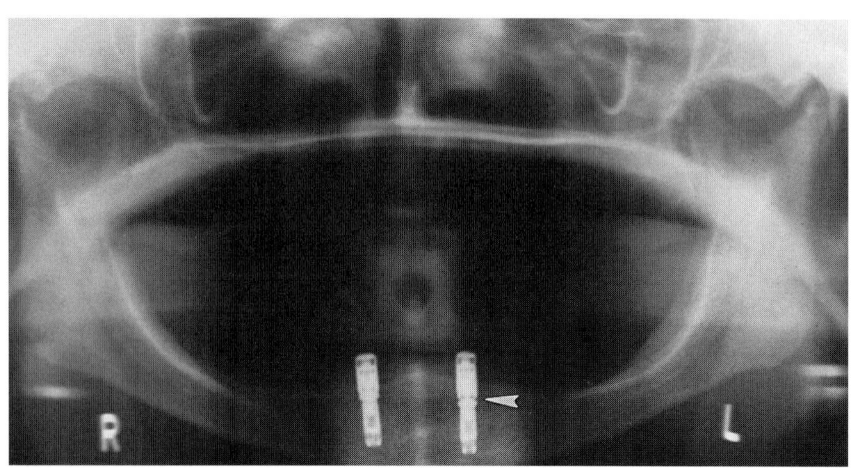

Figure 21–21. Immediate post–stage II surgery radiograph demonstrating unseated left mandible abutment. Failure to seat abutment must be immediately identified and corrected at stage II operation.

such a seal is not achieved or maintained, there may be apical migration of the epithelium into the interface of the implant and bone, resulting in possible complete or partial soft tissue encapsulation of the implant. If the seal is not achieved or deteriorates, a periodontal type pocket develops, predisposing the implant to a periodontal-type disease.

Conflicting data exist regarding the necessity of having attached gingiva surrounding the implants. Long-term findings from the Brånemark Clinic indicate that the lack of attached keratinized tissue had little or no bearing on the success of the bone response around the fixture,[60] but Kirsh and Menteg[61] emphasize the importance of keratinized gingiva around coated implants. It is their conception that keratinized tissue is more resistant to peri-implantitis and its sequela, progressive bone loss. Oral hygiene is facilitated and aesthetics are enhanced when attached keratinized tissue is present. When there is mobile unattached tissue, however, inflammatory changes and clinical symptoms often become evident, particularly in areas of muscle attachments.

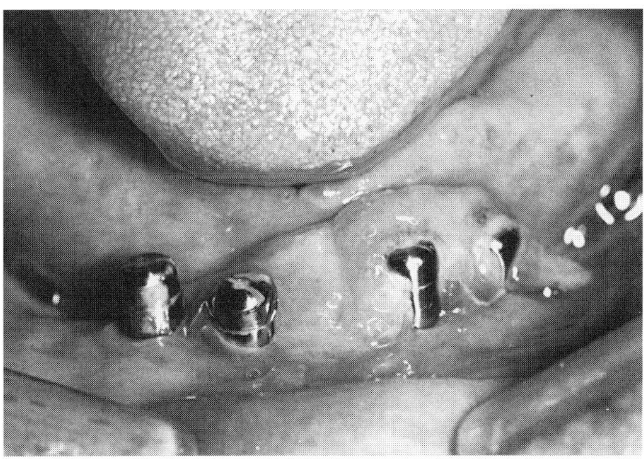

Figure 21–23. Edentulous jaw with inflamed gingiva around abutments 3 weeks after abutment correction procedure. Hyperplasia was managed by excision of the hyperplastic tissue, removal and sterilization of the abutments, and antibiotic therapy.

The bacteriology related to peri-implantitis and its correlation with adult periodontitis have been described.[62] There appear to be more subgingival spirochetes associated with failing endosseous implants owing to increased pocket formation. The failing implants also had more gram-negative anaerobic rods, mainly *Bacteroides* and *Fusobacterium* species that were not frequently found in nonpathologic sites. Clinical and DNA probe analysis were used to evaluate 36 failing implant sites in 13 patients.[63] There was evidence of greater mobility and a high incidence of peri-implant radiolucencies in radiographs in the failing implants. The DNA probe analysis revealed moderate levels of *Actinobacillus actinomycetemcomitans, Bacteroides intermedius,* and *Bacteroides gingivalis,* microorganisms associated with adult periodontitis. It has been shown that the surface of natural teeth, smooth titanium, and plasma-sprayed titanium, and hydroxyapatite support the maturation of microbial plaque. In this environment, a critical mass of microorganisms could result in an inflammatory response and peri-implant disease.[64] This phenomenon must be taken into consideration for possible potential metastatic infection problems related to endoprosthesis replacing joints and cardiovascular structures.[65] Although there are no data available regarding infected joint replacements or endocarditis, consultation with the patient's physician should be obtained to discuss the risk-benefit of implant reconstruction.

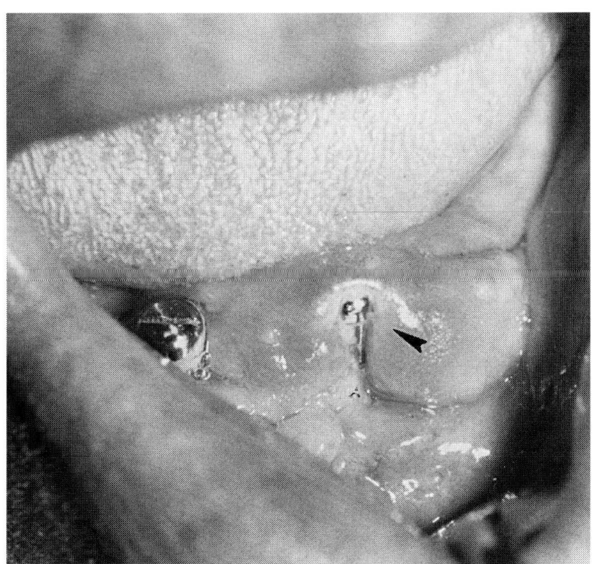

Figure 21–22. Edema and inflammation 2 weeks after abutment correction procedure managed by irrigation, improved home care, and antibiotics.

Special consideration must be given to the patient with rapidly progressive periodontitis when osseointegrated implant placement treatment is planned. The postoperative sequelae reported in such a patient revealed peri-implantitis as well as bone and implant loss.[66] A chemotactic defect in the patient's neutrophils was identified. It was recommended that patients with aggressive forms of periodontal disease should be subjected to appropriate mechanical and antimicrobial therapy to produce a healthy oral flora prior to implant insertion.

Peri-implantitis may produce a failing implant, which is characterized by bone loss, pocketing, bleeding on probing, purulence, and indications that the bone loss patterns are progressive. The failed implant has mobility, a dull sound on percussion, and a peri-implant radiolucency on radiographs.[59] There are treatment options for salvaging the ailing and failing implant, but the only treatment for the failed implant (with mobility) is explantation (Figs. 21–24 to 21–26).

The failing implant has an endotoxin-contaminated surface and as long as endotoxin is present, there can be no biologic repair.[59] In a study by Zablotsky and associates,[67] various chemotherapeutic agents were evaluated for their ability to remove radioisotope-labeled lipopolysaccharide endotoxin from hydroxyapa-

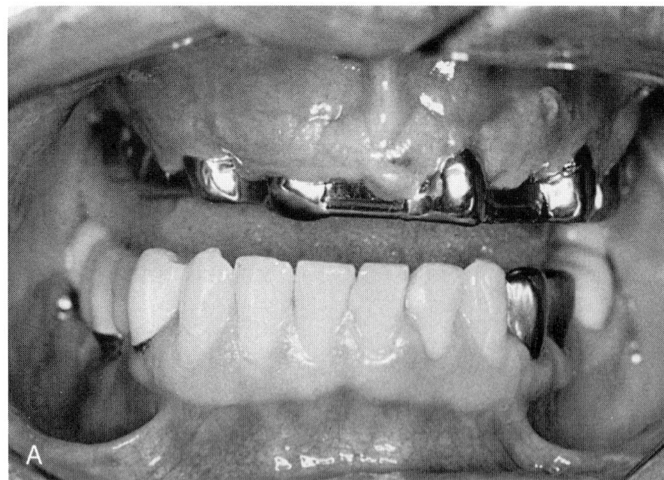

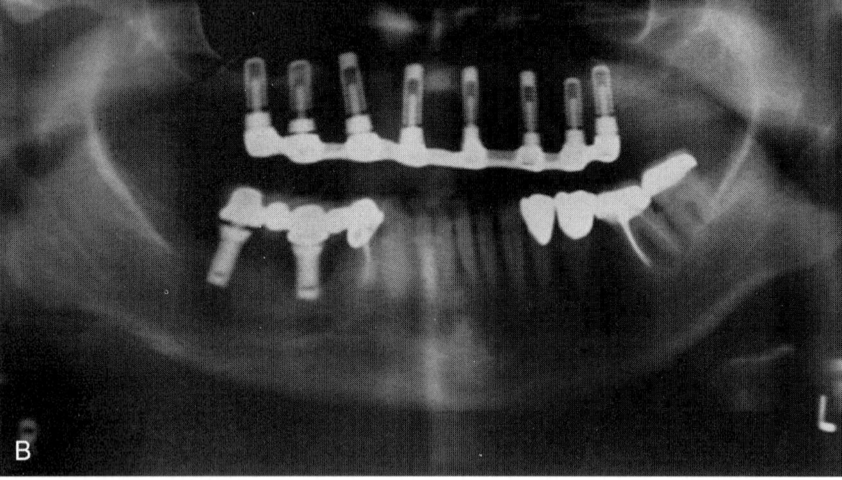

Figure 21–24. *A*, Gingival hyperplasia under prosthesis substructure. *B*, Panoramic radiograph of failing maxillary fixed reconstruction opposing a natural dentition.

tite surfaces.[67] From these studies, it was determined that the most effective treatment for removing endotoxin from the hydroxyapatite-coated surface is citric acid applied to the surface for 30 to 60 seconds. If application times of 2 to 3 minutes are used, there appears to be a weakening of the hydroxyapatite substrate. Further findings demonstrated that tetracycline is relatively ineffective in detoxification of a hydroxyapatite-coated substance but effective on a metallic surface. Meffert and colleagues[59] developed a protocol to repair the failing implant, as follows:

- If an active infection is present, the tissue should be reflected and the defect degranulated with hand instrumentation. When the implant is coated with hydroxyapatite, it is considered contaminated and should be removed, exposing the metallic substrate. The surface is detoxified with tetracycline paste (250 mg mixed with saline) and applied to the implant surface for 2 to 3 minutes with a cotton pledget or camel's hair brush and left on the surface. The defect is then grafted with either nonresorbable hydroxyapatite or freeze-dried bone.
- In the absence of active infection, and if the hydroxyapatite shows no evidence of pitting, cracking, resorption, or change of color, the surface may be detoxified with citric acid, pH 1 (40%), for 30 to 60 seconds with a camel's hair brush. The area is then irrigated and grafted.
- If the surface of the implant is clean and has been detoxified, biologic healing may take place with the use of demineralized freeze-dried bone. If, however, the surface is not clean and detoxified because of tortuous osseous defects not amenable to instrumentation, an alloplast such as hydroxyapatite should be used. A barrier membrane may be used if there is a need to retain the grafting material.

Although techniques have been described to repair the failing implant, there is no long-term data to substantiate its efficacy. There is a tendency for both patient and doctor to retain a failing implant beyond a reasonable time because of the effort and cost invested by both parties. Delaying the decision to remove a nonsalvageable implant only leads to further deterioration of the implant site and extends the time to resolution of the problem.

Biomaterials

Titanium or titanium-aluminum-vanadium alloys are the most commonly used metallic biomaterials in den-

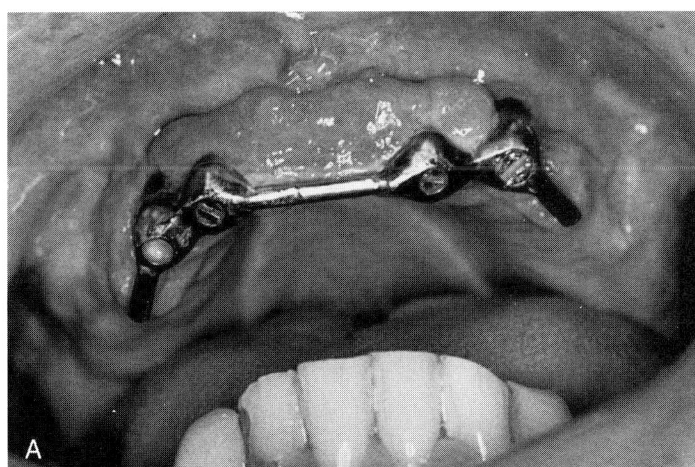

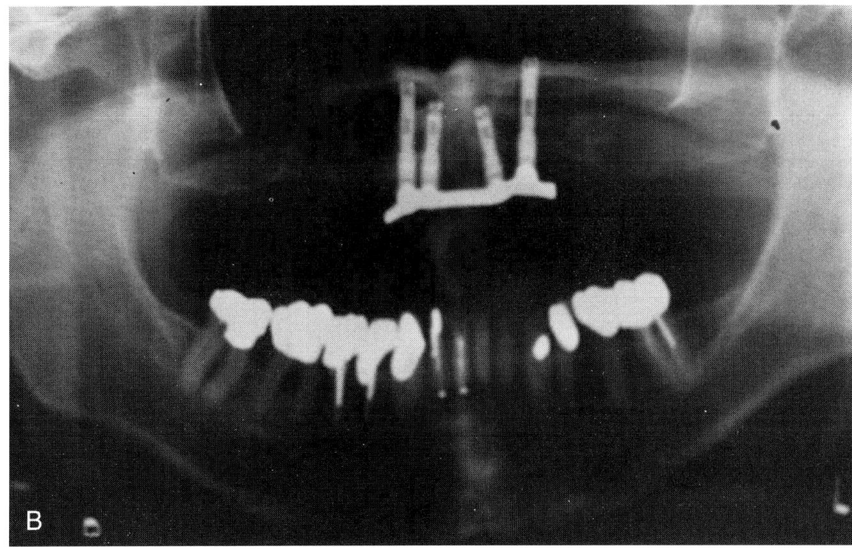

Figure 21–25. *A,* Gingival hyperplasia under prosthesis substructure. *B,* Panoramic radiograph of failing maxillary removable reconstruction opposing a natural dentition.

tal implantology. Commercially pure titanium oxidizes when it contacts air or tissue fluids, thereby minimizing corrosion. Titanium has a low density, which gives it a high strength-to-weight ratio, and it can be alloyed with aluminum and vanadium. Aluminum increases the strength and decreases the weight of the material, and vanadium acts as an aluminum scavenger, to prevent corrosion.[59] Use of other metals has not been demonstrated to yield the predictability of long-term osseointegration. It has been shown that noncoated, coated, and plasma-sprayed implants can achieve osseointegration of different degrees and rates.[68]

Although long-term complications occur in endosseous implants in all types of surfaces, four patterns of peri-implantitis with hydroxyapatite-coated implants have emerged.[69] Type I peri-implantitis involves rapid and complete loss of osseointegration and an approximately 0.25-mm peri-implant radiolucuency on radiography. Type II shows rapid bone loss after functional loading to a point of stability, the percentage and radius of bone loss are variable, and the gingival tissues appear clinically healthy. Type III peri-implantitis produces progressive bone loss with minimal signs of early inflammation. Mobility of the implant cannot be detected until advanced bone loss has occurred, and there is a typical 0.5-mm-wide radiolucent defect. Type IV exhibits progressive bone loss with obvious signs of clinical inflammation and symptoms. The percentage of bone loss is variable but more severe than with the other types. The bone loss ranges in radius from 3 to 7 mm and is associated with infection. Mobility is not present until the bone loss is advanced, but edema, suppuration, and bleeding on probing are seen. Kirsch and Mentag[61] reported that all hydroxyapatite coatings resorb as a function of the amount of amorphous material in the coating. This amorphous material is created when the hydroxyapatite changes as it is plasma sprayed onto the implant body. These researchers also reported that hydroxyapatite-coated implants approximately parallel the success rates of titanium plasma spray–coated implants for the first 7 years, but at the seventh year, there is a dramatic increase in the number of hydroxyapatite-coated implant failures.

The clinician must be cautioned about the routine use of hydroxyapatite-coated implants, because they are subject to soluble dissolution and cellular degradation, and this biodegradability factor has long-term retention implications (Fig. 21–27). When a new tech-

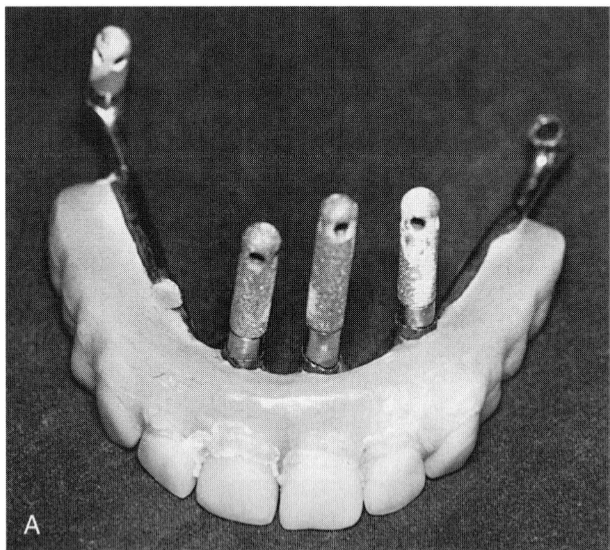

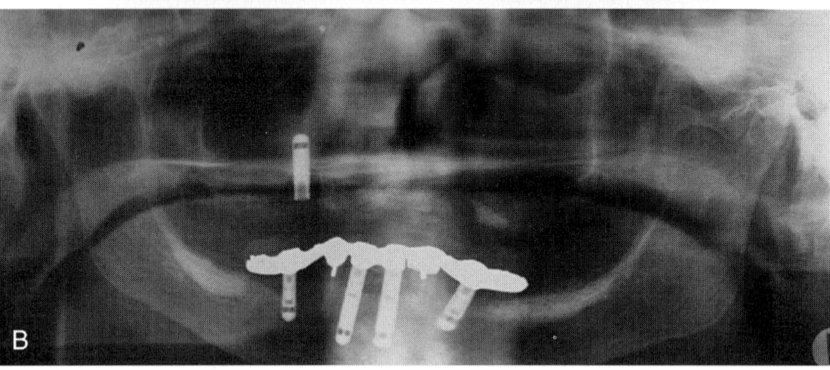

Figure 21–26. *A,* Spontaneously exfoliated implants and prosthesis while still attached. *B,* Panoramic radiograph of failed exfoliated implants and prosthesis with one remaining implant.

nology emerges in the surgical arena, it is imperative that the clinician study the literature, including long-term clinical and animal research as well as the experience in other specialties and countries. Of interest is a report in the orthopedic literature, by Bloebaum and Dupont,[70] on the clinical and histologic findings in a case in which the hydroxyapatite coating separated in a press-fit total hip arthroplasty. Semiquantitative histologic analysis showed grade 3+ mononuclear histiocytes and giant cells present in a retrieved capsule and the periprosthetic tissues. Back-scattered electron and correlated elemental analysis confirmed that the hydroxyapatite coating had migrated to the articulating surface of the polyethylene insert, causing third-body wear. Bloebaum and Dupont[70] recommended that the surgeon use caution in the routine use of hydroxyapatite-coated implants if osteolysis associated with hydroxyapatite separation and migration is to be avoided.

Systemic Effects of Titanium Implants

Assessment of the Safety and Efficacy of Dental Implants

The safety and efficacy of dental implants are determined by animal and laboratory testing followed by human clinical trials. Standardized tests for determination of the toxicity and general biocompatibility responses of dental implants have been developed by the American Dental Association, the American National Standards Institute, and the Fédération Dentaire Internationale.[71] The local and systemic toxicity, carcinogenicity, and animal tissue responses are evaluated.

Human Ingestion of Titanium

A considerable amount of titanium is ingested daily by humans in their diet.[72] Approximately 40% of the total amount ingested, or about 300 μg per day, is metabolized. This is about 10,000 times the amount that the oxidation of a titanium implant can "deliver."

Degradation Products of Titanium Implants and Their Biologic Interactions with Host Tissue

Quantitative metal analysis was used to study the deposition of titanium in distant organ sites resulting from the presence (52 to 76 months) of porous root titanium alloy (Ti-6Al-4V) dental implants in the mandibles of three adult rhesus monkeys.[73] Light microscopy and atomic absorption spectrophotometry allowed for correlation of histopathologic observations with the concentration of titanium in the tissues after

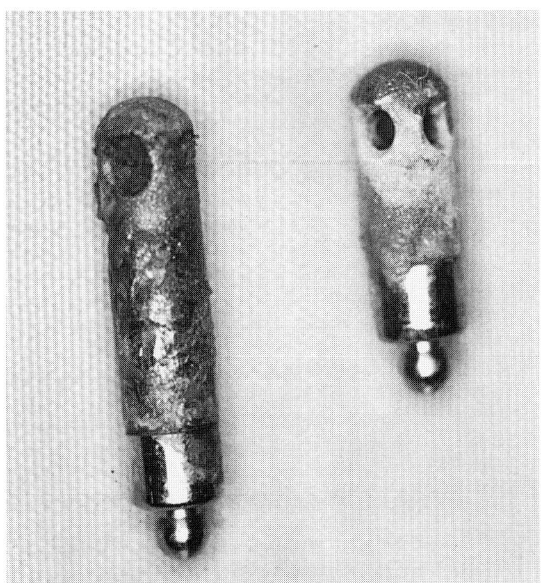

Figure 21–27. Infected explanted maxillary hydroxyapatite-coated cylindric implants with evidence of delaminated surface.

implantation. Tissue specimens of liver, lung, spleen, kidney, cardiac muscle, skeletal muscle, and regional lymph nodes of the neck were harvested for histopathologic examination using light microscopy. The results of this study demonstrated the presence of detectable titanium only in lung tissue. The researchers believed, however, that owing to the small number of animals sampled, it could not be known whether the approximately 10-fold increase in deposition in the lungs of the experimental monkeys was due to the long-term presence of the porous dental implants. It also was not determined whether the small concentration of titanium present in the lung tissue elicited subcellular biochemical effects. There was no histopathologic evidence of any tissue alterations that were a direct result of titanium deposition.

Although titanium and its alloys demonstrate good corrosion resistance, Bruneel and Helsen[74] were able to detect titanium compounds in tissues adjacent to unalloyed titanium implants. These investigators believed that there is low if any toxicity of titanium to the human body but were more concerned about the effects of aluminum and vanadium in the alloy implants. Metal ions can be toxic, sensitizing, and oncogenic. If metallic ionic components are released from an implant surface, portions remain free in the tissue, and some bind to serum albumin and erythrocytes, which are transported to and eventually accumulate in organ sites or are excreted. Release of titanium from implants is believed to occur at a very slow rate. The presence of a titanium implant can be considered irrelevant to the total titanium "load" to the body, and systemic reactions (allergy) and deposition in the organs do not appear to occur.[72] The biologic half-life of titanium (320 days) is too short for this element to accumulate in the body.

Schliephake and associates[75] carried out a study in Gottingen minipigs to study metal release from titanium fixtures during placement in the mandible.[75] They showed that the use of titanium screw taps or the placement of self-tapping fixtures may produce abrasion of particles from the surface, because of the low wear resistance of the material. Immediately after implant placement, the abraded particles were deposited at the implant-bone interface. Deposition of particles at the site of implantation, cellular uptake, and subsequent lysosomal degradation of particles and transportation to lymph nodes and distant parenchyma of organs were observed to occur. Five months after implant placement, particles were no longer observed on the bone surface adjacent to the implants. The titanium concentration was highest in the lungs and much lower in the kidneys and liver. According to these researchers, the biologic relevance of these release effects may be considered uncritical, because titanium is known to be nontoxic and well tolerated.

Malignant Neoplasms Associated with Implants

The carcinogenic potential of unalloyed titanium and Ti-6Al-4V implants was investigated in the bones of albino inbred (Sprague-Dawley) rats.[76] The development of malignant tumors at or away from the implant recipient site was determined. The preliminary results of this study suggested that animals with metal implants may be at greater risk for the development of malignancy, particularly sarcomas and lymphoreticular neoplasms. Sunderman[77] reviewed case reports of malignant tumors at sites of metal orthopedic implants in humans and domestic animals. He concluded that the actual incidence of sarcomas in association with metal implants cannot be reliably estimated and that the apparent associations may be coincidental. Smith and colleagues[78] and Friedman and Vernon[79] reported on malignancies occurring in dental implant patients but suggested no cause and effect.

Despite the fact that titanium may be a potential carcinogen, the American Dental Association Council on Dental Materials, Instruments, and Equipment recommends the use of endosseous implants in selected cases in which the of risks and benefits are carefully evaluated and discussed with the patient. The long-term toxic, oncologic-mutagenic, and hypersensitivity effects of dental implants require further investigation.

Biomechanical Complications

Prosthodontic Design

Biomechanical complications of osseointegrated implants must be given consideration, because unfavorable force distribution may result in long-term failures. The force distributions in multiple tooth–supported and implant-supported prostheses is completely different.[80] The biomechanics of combined implant and natural tooth–borne prostheses, rigid and nonrigid connections, cantilevers, lateral forces versus axial forces, surface area of osseointegrated surfaces, occlusal loads,

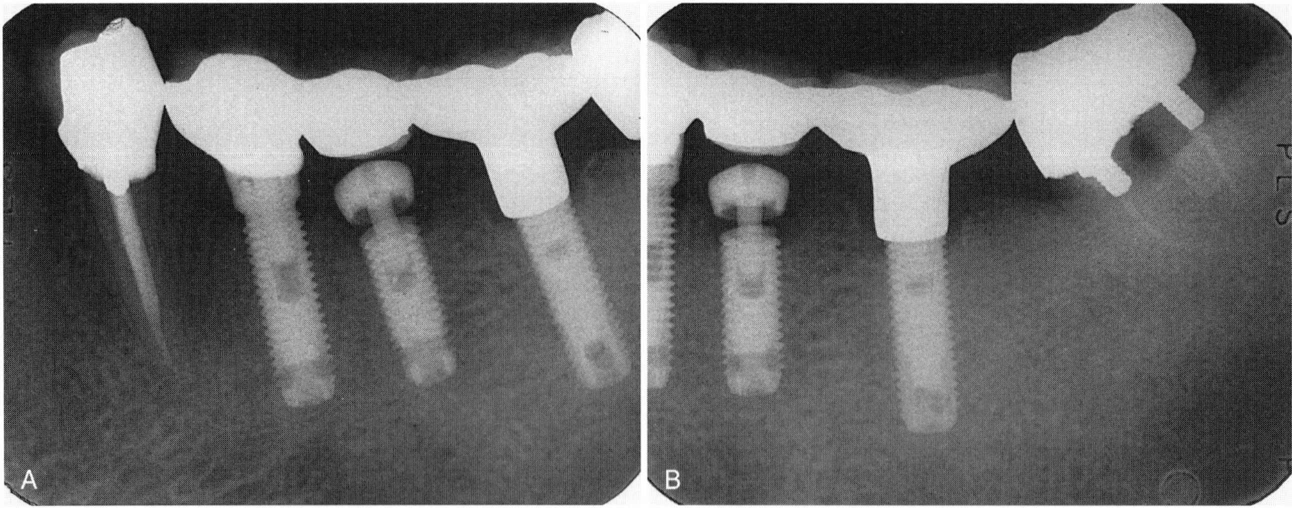

Figure 21–28. *A,* Periapical radiograph demonstrating fracture of heads of two endosseous screw implants. One implant was buried with cover screw. *B,* The most posterior implant was also fractured and received a "custom" abutment.

parafunctional habits, and length of edentulous spans must be considered in the design of a prosthesis using an endosseous implant. Biomechanical failure may lead to prosthesis loosening, component fracture, or bone loss and eventual implant loss (Figs. 21–28 to 21–31). From a force distribution standpoint, implant-supported prostheses are best designed to be freestanding. When natural tooth–supported and implant-supported prostheses are combined, however, the attachment between the two should relieve stress to prevent overload of the implant and retaining screws.[80] Occlusal loads should be axial in direction, eliminating lateral forces. Cantilevers should be minimized, the number of implants maximized, and harmful parafunctional habits managed. Understanding lever arm principles and adjusting the occlusion and cusp geometry can reduce the number of biomechanical failures.

Natural tooth intrusion can occur when internal nonrigid connectors are used in combining implants and natural teeth (Fig. 21–32). The natural tooth is observed to intrude apically, so that the male portion of the attachment extends above the originally designed occlusal level.

System and Component Failure

When the force threshold for bone is surpassed, bone resorption occurs; when the threshold for the implant is surpassed, component fracture occurs. If the fracture occurs in the implant, the options range from placing a headless screw in the fractured implant body, leaving the implant buried in the bone, attempting a custom abutment, or trephining out the fractured implant and replacing it. The design and occlusion of the prosthesis should be reassessed, parafunctional habits addressed, and night guards considered. A small occlusal table without lateral interferences is beneficial. The use of more and wider implants and possibly stronger alloy implants may prevent this complication. The patient should be informed that if the abutment comes loose,

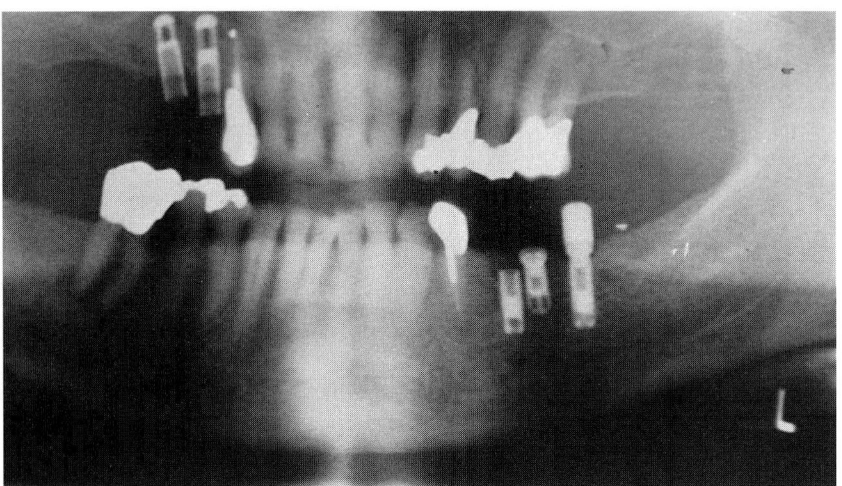

Figure 21–29. Panoramic radiograph illustrating fractured implant managed by inserting a headless screw, putting the implant "to sleep," and inserting a third implant.

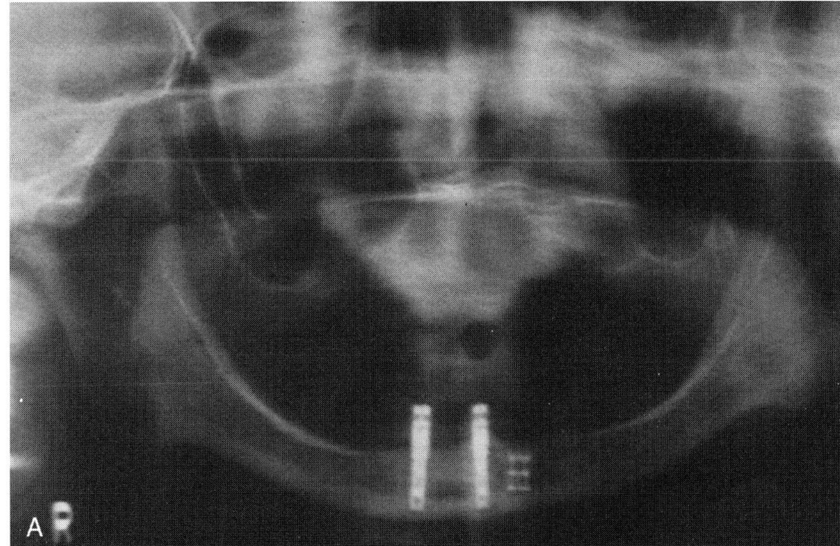

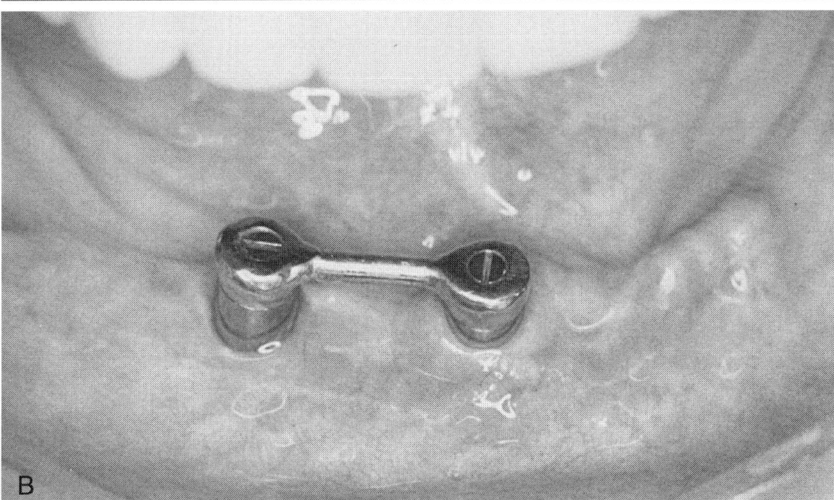

Figure 21–30. *A*, Panoramic radiograph of failed basket-type implant reconstruction with one fractured burred implant. Two screw-type implants were placed subsequently. *B*, Clinical view of clip bar and secondary reconstruction.

immediate retightening is essential to avoid metal fatigue fractures. Fractures may occur in the implant when there has been some crestal bone loss because the superior flange of the implant no longer assists in force distribution (see Figs. 21–16 to 21–18). The importance of passive fit of the prosthesis and use of competent laboratory technicians cannot be overemphasized.

The surgeon is most often requested to remove fractured abutment screws (Fig. 21–33). This procedure is usually simple because the abutment screw fractured is preceded by abutment screw loosening. The use of one or two rigid endodontic explorers allows the fractured abutment screw to be "backed out." Prosthodontic treatment planning concepts that help avoid complications have been summarized by Beumer and colleagues,[81] and the prosthodontic results and longitudinal clinical effectiveness of osseointegrated implants have been reported.[82] The surgeon must understand the prosthodontic concepts as they relate directly to the surgical aspects and ultimate outcome. The surgeon must also collaborate with restorative dentists who are trained in the discipline of implant prosthodontics to avoid preventable iatrogenic problems.

Special Clinical Situations

Implants in the Growing Child

It has been recognized that placement of implants in the growing child requires special considerations.[83–86] Osseointegrated implants lack the compensatory growth mechanism of the natural dentition. Remodeling associated with skeletal growth in the site of implantation could cause the implant to become either unsupported by bone or submerged like an ankylotic tooth.[87] The submergence of the implant in the growing child is the result of an inability of the implant to erupt as needed for vertical growth of the alveolar process. Vertical dentoalveolar development, in the area of implant placement, can be retarded. In the growing child with a strong rotational pattern of growth, implants placed in the posterior mandible may tend to become deeply embedded below the occlusal plane.

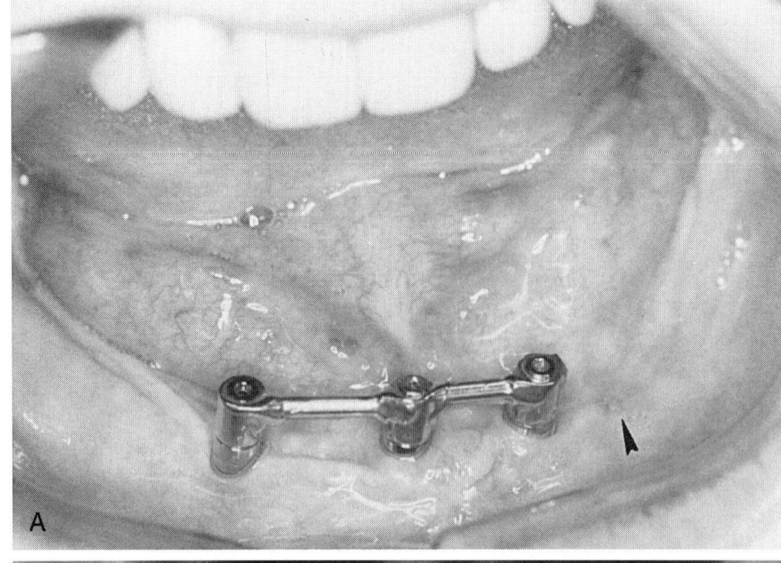

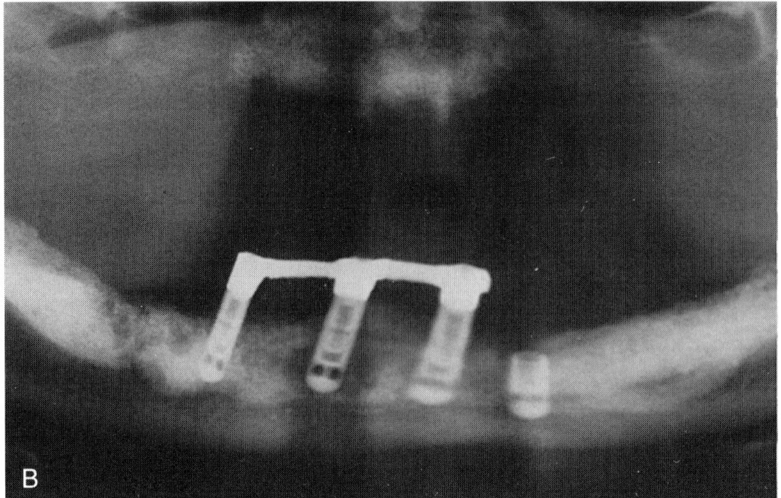

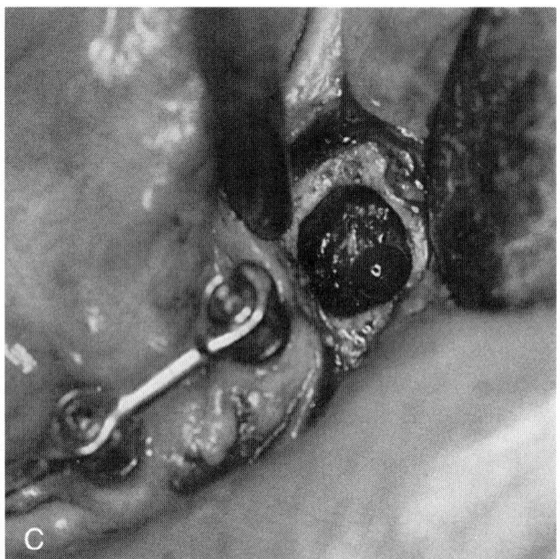

Figure 21–31. *A,* Buried implant with fistula *(arrow)* formation. *B,* Radiograph of infected buried implant. *C,* Intraoperative view of removed buried implant.

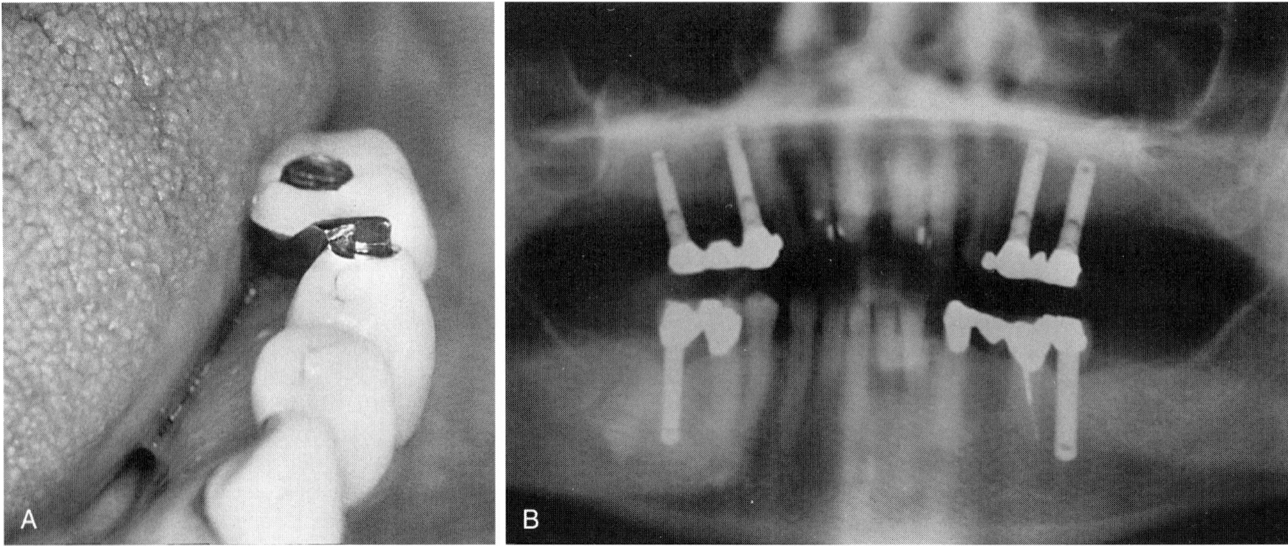

Figure 21–32. *A,* Clinical view showing intrusion of natural tooth attached to the posterior implant via a nonrigid connector. *B,* Panoramic radiograph illustrating well-osseointegrated implants.

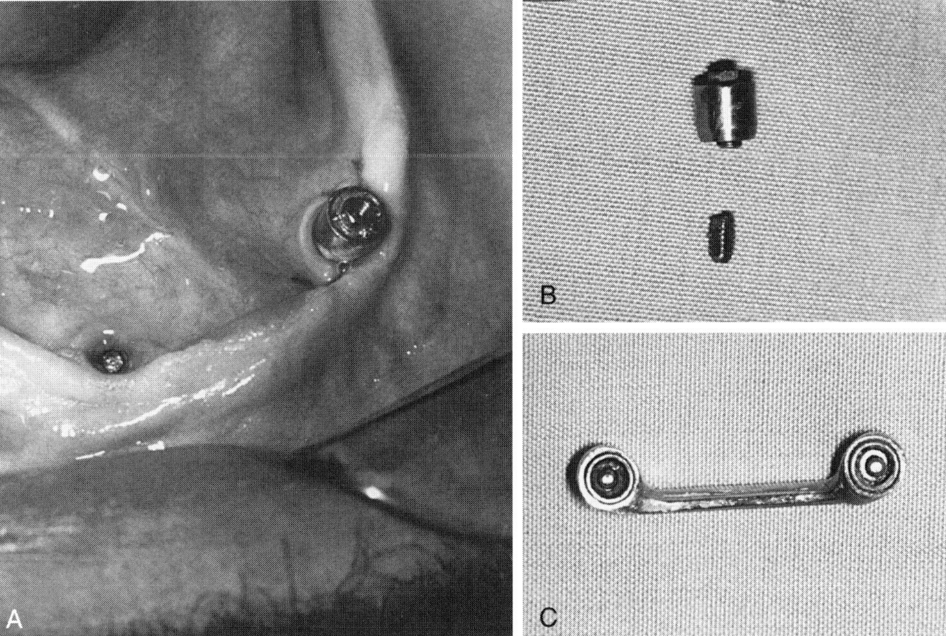

Figure 21–33. *A*, Clinical view of fractured abutment supporting a clip-bar overdenture. *B*, Fractured abutment screw removed with endodontic explorer. *C*, Poorly designed rectangular bar that created torquing forces and did not permit prosthesis rotation.

Because the symphyseal suture begins to close soon after birth, implant placement in this region is not likely to injure a growth center, and a prosthesis placed across the mandibular midline should not limit transverse growth. Prostheses do need to be monitored and altered as growth continues, however. Also, longer abutments may be required as the implant becomes more submerged. Submerged implants in the mandible could alter normal tooth relationships, affecting occlusal force distribution, total jaw growth patterns, and long-term occlusal relationships.

Prostheses that cross the midpalatal suture and are attached to implants may potentially restrict transverse growth of the maxilla. When implants are placed in the aesthetic zone (anterior maxilla) in the growing child, cosmetic compromise results as the discrepancy between the incisal edges becomes apparent. Ideally, growth should cease before implants are placed in the jaw. Therefore, implant placement should be delayed until age 15 for girls and age 18 for boys. This practice is not always feasible, however. Smith and colleagues[84] reported on placement of a single endosseous mandibular midline implant in a 5-year old patient with hereditary hypohidrotic ectodermal dysplasia. There were no aesthetic considerations in this patient with partial anodontia, because an overdenture was planned. As of 1996, 7 years after implant placement, the implant is still osseointegrated and functionally useful. Abutment change and refabrication of the prosthesis were required as growth occurred. Distinction must be made between the adult patient and growing patient because of the effect of osseointegrated implants on the growth and development of the dental and craniofacial growth patterns, in order to avoid potential long-term complications.

Implants in Irradiated Tissues

Several studies have suggested that placement of implants into irradiated bone may be possible. Jacobsson inserted 35 endosseous implants in nine patients aged 4 to 72 years.[88] There was a great range among these studies in the quality of radiation, absorbed dose, fractionation schedule, time since radiation, and site of implantation. Follow-up time ranged from 15 to 44 months. Six of the 35 implants had to be removed because of lack of osseointegration, but no osteoradionecrosis occurred. Albrektsson and colleagues[89] published data from a combined Swedish and international follow-up study of 54 implants in radiated mandibles and 26 in radiated maxillas. Only three fixtures were lost from the maxillary group 1 to 5 years after implantation.

The ideal time delay between irradiation therapy and implant placement is unclear from the literature. The use of hyperbaric oxygen therapy (HBO) and certain reconstructive techniques, however, makes early reconstruction more feasible. Granstrom[87] proposed a protocol for HBO when implants are planned in irradiated bone, involving 20 HBO sessions prior to implant placement, which is followed as soon as possible by another 10 HBO sessions, using 2 to 2.4 atm absolute pressure.

It is also unknown whether implants in situ present an unacceptable risk when radiation is planned. Hatjigiorgis and associates[90] suggested that a dose enhancement as great as 10% might occur at the tissue interface with hydroxyapatite implants. Whether the increase in radiation dose to the bone due to backscatter radiation from the implant increases the incidence of osteoradionecrosis is not known. If radiation is required in a patient with endosseous implants, explantation may not be necessary. The prosthesis, abutments, and frameworks should be removed prior to irradiation, but the implants may be left in situ.

When a patient who presents for implant placement has undergone therapeutic doses of radiation therapy for a head and neck malignancy, certain factors deserve assessment. The patient's prognosis for survival should be reasonable, and the acute post-radiation stomatitis should have resolved. The patient's oral hygiene must be good, and all dental disease eliminated. Smoking and alcohol consumption should have ceased. There should be no signs of osteoradionecrosis or bony changes at the site of implantation. The oral tissues in the region of implant insertion should not have severe radiation-induced changes. A good prognostic sign is uneventful healing of sites of postradiotherapy tooth extractions. If there is significant concern about the potential for healing, a small flap can be drilled in the planned implant recipient site. If the bone bleeds freely, there is a reasonable chance for healing, and the implant procedure can proceed. Although the experience is not vast, there is some suggestion that the prognosis for osseointegration in the irradiated patient is worse the longer the delay after radiation therapy. Each case must be assessed individually, and the alternatives and risks must be frankly discussed with the patient, in order to reduce the incidence of complications.

Implants in Extraoral Sites

Large defects of the maxillofacial complex often are not amenable to reconstructive surgical procedures and must rely on prosthetic rehabilitation. Osseointegrated implants allow for additional retention, comfort, and security for patients with these large defects. Reports indicate, however, that problems are encountered and that certain groups of patients are more prone to complications than others. A 6-year follow-up report on 30 patients treated with 92 craniofacial implants indicated an overall success rate of 73.3% but that the rate varied according to implant location and radiation status.[91] Of these implants, 86 were uncovered, 8 were subsequently buried because of soft tissue problems, and 15 failed to achieve or maintain osseointegration. The most reliable site was the temporal bone (92.5%), followed by the nasal floor (72.2%) and the orbit (65.0%). There was a significant reduction in success for the irradiated group (58.3% for the orbital reconstructions). A report from 13 U.S. centers and Sweden had similar findings in 95 patients treated with 319 craniofacial osseointegrated implants.[92] Of interest is that in the irradiated patients, implants were lost at the same rate in the less and greater than 1 year (i.e., from the time implants were placed to loss of the implant) groups.

In both the nonradiated and radiated patients, the number of total implants lost early (< 1 year after placement) and lost late (> 1 year after placement) was similar, with only a slightly worse outcome in the radiated group. The region of greatest risk was the orbit.

The bone-anchored hearing aid is an alternative to the conventional bone-conduction hearing aid, without the disadvantages of pressure pain or skin irritation and with direct sound transmission to the skull.[93] The clinical results of 68 percutaneous implants placed in the mastoid process in 65 patients, with a follow-up of 8 to 45 months, revealed that 97% of the implants were anchored in bone. In 86% of the implants, no potentially dangerous skin reactions occurred. Skin reactions were related to poor skin condition around the implant, thick skin, and movement of the skin. Others have reported that complications with extraoral osseointegrated implants are mostly minor and primarily inflammatory.[94] Lack of sufficient trimming of the subcutaneous tissue was one of the factors considered to contribute to the inflammatory response.

The microflora surrounding percutaneous titanium implants in two groups of patients were studied: one with local irritation and one without irritation.[95] Staphylococci were the most commonly isolated species. Nevertheless, Enterobacteria, group B streptococci, and *Pseudomonas,* bacteria not considered part of the normal skin flora, were also isolated from implants both with and without local tissue irritation.

Implants in Fresh Extraction Sites

In order to reduce potential alveolar ridge resorption after extraction, decrease the number of surgical procedures and anesthetics, and reduce treatment time and possible costs, the concept of immediate placement of osseointegrated implants in fresh extraction sites evolved. Several publications have been reported on the long-term results. One hundred ninety immediate implantations—93 primary immediate implantations and 97 secondary immediate implantations (performed at 6 to 8 weeks after extraction)—were performed and followed for an average of 12.4 months.[96] A life-table approach applied for statistical analysis showed no difference between primary and secondary implants. Peri-implant pocket depth, the gingival index, the hygienic index, and the amount of bone resorption were examined. The group of primary immediate implants showed a tendency toward deeper pocket formation and an increased frequency of membrane dehiscences that may be due to the poor quality of the soft tissue cover. The advantage of secondary immediate implantation is to allow soft tissue regeneration for better primary closure. When a flap is reflected to obtain primary closure, the mucogingival relationship is altered, creating a possible aesthetic compromise. In 114 of the implantations, it was unnecessary to use membrane techniques, because the implants fit well into the recipient sites. The group with primary immediate implants showed a markedly higher frequency of dehiscence development than the group with secondary immediate implantations.

Another paper reported on predictably successful results in 61 patients followed for up to 6 years.[97] All 301 implants that were uncovered at stage II surgery were osseointegrated and prosthetically loaded. Two implants were lost in the same patient, presumably because of infection. Block and Kent[98] describe their 4-year experience with placement of hydroxyapatite-coated implants into extraction sites immediately after tooth extraction. Small defects evident after implant placement were treated with dense, nonresorbable hydroxyapatite. Larger defects were treated with demineralized bone. All implants had integrated at the time of exposure. Forty-two implants were placed in the maxilla and 20 in the mandible. Two implants were lost within 6 months of function. The immediate implant appears to be a biologically sound procedure with predictable results,[99, 100] but long term experience is limited.

When an implant is placed in a fresh extraction site, there is a tendency to use an un-ideal trajectory (Fig. 21–34). The bony preparation may have to extend outside the perimeter of the fresh extraction site to obtain the proper angulation.

Ancillary Surgical Procedures

In order to manage more complex and compromised cases with endosseous osseointegrated implant reconstruction, a series of ancillary procedures have been developed to create a more favorable and hospitable environment in which the implants are inserted. These procedures are guided bone regeneration, bone grafting, maxillary antroplasty (sinus lift), and mandibular

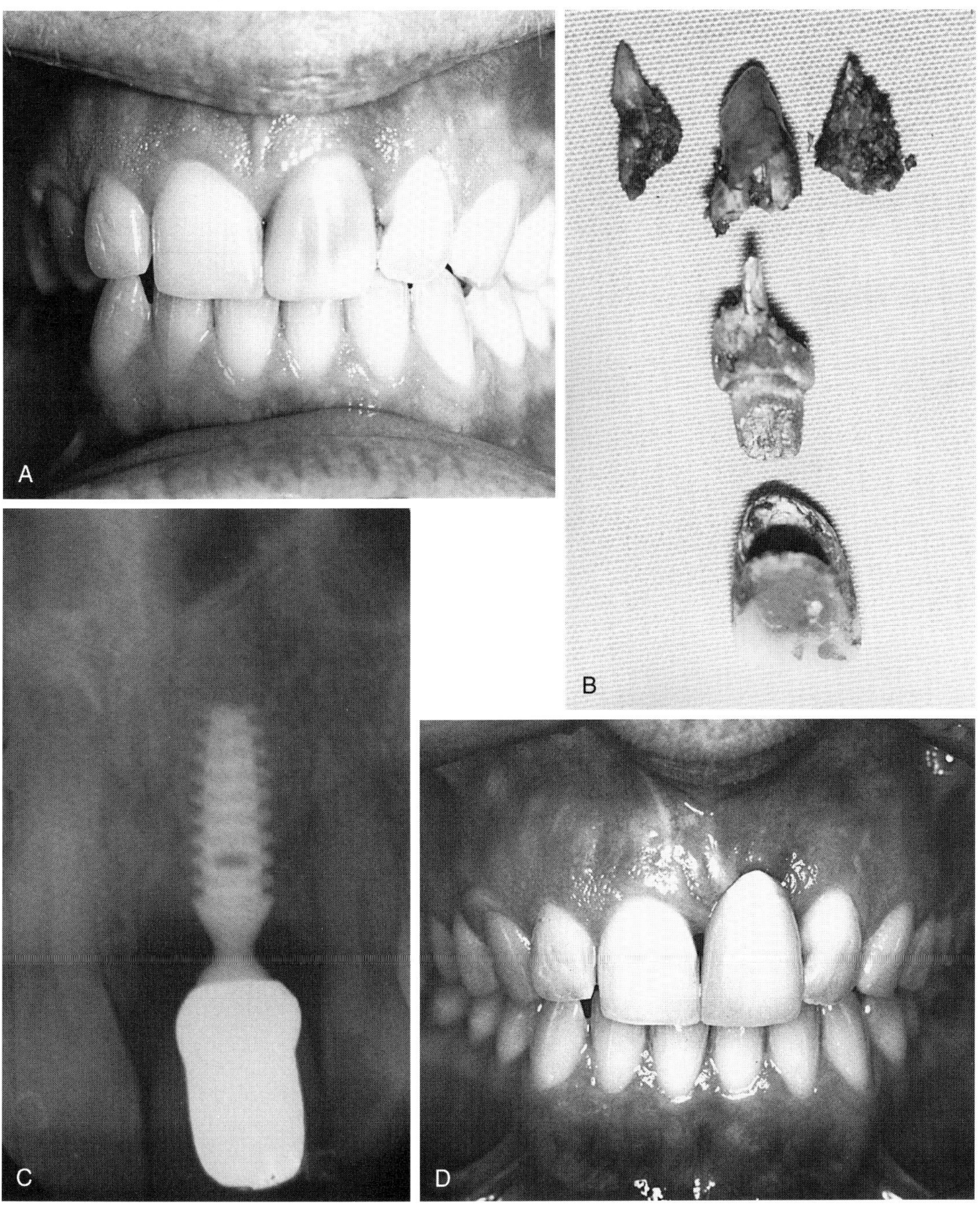

Figure 21–34. *A,* Fractured, discolored, devitalized maxillary left central incisor requiring extraction. *B,* Fragments of extracted tooth. *C,* "Finned" implant placed in fresh extraction site using autogenous and demineralized freeze-dried bone and barrier membrane technique. *D,* Lingual placement of implant due to defect in labial plate requiring ridge lap restoration with discrepancy in the occlusal-gingival length of the restoration and the adjacent tooth.

nerve lateralization. These procedures in themselves present specific problems and complications inherent to the given regional anatomy and the particular procedure performed.

Guided Bone Regeneration

When insufficient bone is available or morphology is inadequate, guided bone regenerative procedures can alter, in a more favorable manner, the bony recipient site. This procedure can be performed simultaneously with implant placement or as a staged procedure. The term *guided bone regeneration* is more appropriate than *guided tissue generation,* because it is bony tissue that is indicative of a successful outcome. Guided tissue regeneration, producing fibrous connective tissue, can result but is an unfavorable and undesired outcome.

Rominger and Triplett[101] used 63 expanded polytetrafluoroethylene membranes in 40 patients receiving implants. Their prospective clinical study examined the use of guided tissue regeneration for the bony augmentation of alveolar bone around, or in preparation for, titanium endosseous implants. Postoperative infections were identified in nine membranes (14%), and dehiscence with exposure of the membrane to the oral cavity occurred in nine membranes (14%). Forty-five of the augmentations (71%) healed uneventfully, and all membranes were removed at an average of 4.5 months. Sixty-one of the augmentations (96.8%) were considered successful, as determined by the clinical success of the implants and the presence of bone in a previous osseous defect. The two unsuccessful cases (3.2%) were complicated by infection. Although the early complication rate appeared to be relatively high, the long-term success of the augmentation was apparently unaffected. In this study, freeze-dried demineralized bone allografts were placed in the spaces created by the membranes. Other materials, including autogenous bone, fleece collagen, xenograft material, and resorbable hydroxyapatite, have also been used.

Attempts should be made to keep the barrier in place and buried until the next surgical procedure. If the membrane becomes exposed, an attempt should be made to keep it in place for at least 6 weeks. The patient can irrigate the membrane and use chlorhexidine swabs for home management. If suppuration occurs, the membrane should be removed immediately. The clinician must be aware that nonresorbable membranes may become adherent to the tissue and fragmentation may occur, predisposing to portions of the membrane being left in situ. The wound must be examined carefully to ensure complete removal. If there is any pressure from overlying transitional prostheses, premature membrane exposure, fibrous healing, and bone resorption may result (Fig. 21–35).

Ridge Augmentation with Bone Grafts

Alveolar ridge defects may be caused by trauma, loss of teeth, alveolar clefts, ablative tumor surgery, and other congenital and developmental abnormalities. Quite often, an insufficient volume of bone is available, beyond the biological capabilities of guided tissue regenerative techniques. There are generally two major categories of clinical situations, (1) the severely atrophic, usually edentulous maxilla or mandible requiring major bone grafting and patient hospitalization and (2) the local ridge defect in the usually partially edentulous maxilla or mandible requiring a smaller volume of bone graft material. Each category has complications related and proportional to the extent of the defect to be augmented as well as to the donor site. Severe mandibular atrophy may require onlay bone grafts in combination with endosseous implants. Keller and Tolman[102] placed autogenous onlay iliac bone graft and titanium cylindrically threaded implants simultaneously in seven patients with advanced bone resorption. All seven patients experienced uncomplicated healing and continuous, uninterrupted prosthesis use without soft tissue or mechanical complications for 1 to 4 years. The long-term implant stability in these patients is unknown, but the early results appear optimistic. All 32 composite graft implants were uncovered and placed in function with a loss of only 2 implants. One to 2 mm of crestal bone loss was observed after the first year of loading.

An extraoral approach to the simultaneous placement of osseointegrated implants and iliac crest bone grafting to the mandible also has been reported to have a successful outcome. Lew and associates[103] performed the procedure in 10 patients, and the longest follow-up was 3 years. They achieved a 93% success rate. Bone resorption at the implant sites was considered negligible (less than 1 mm). The three implants that failed were the most distal ones placed. Long-standing mental nerve dysfunction was noted in 3 patients. Six patients subsequently required palatal or split-thickness skin grafts to create better quality peri-implant soft tissue.

A 2-year longitudinal study was conducted on the simultaneous placement of implants and bone grafting for the severely resorbed maxilla using a horseshoe-shaped iliac bone graft.[104] The average percentage of surviving fixtures in the study was 77.4%. Three patients lost all fixtures. Most implant losses were in the more distal regions. Adell and colleagues[105] reported on reconstruction of the severely resorbed edentulous maxilla using osseointegrated fixtures in immediate autogenous iliac bone grafts. The results in the first 23 consecutive patients they treated, with a mean observation time of 4.2 years (range 1 to 10), were reported. A total of 124 implants were originally placed into the grafts but required supplementation with an additional 16 implants placed in seven jaws. Throughout their observation period, 17 of the patients had continuously stable prostheses. The remaining five had overdentures, and one patient had resorted to a conventional complete denture. Four years after delivery, 12 of 16 patients had continuously stable prostheses. From the date of fixture placement, approximately 75% of the original fixtures were clinically and radiographically osseointegrated. The mean marginal bone loss after the first year of prosthesis function was 1.49 mm. The

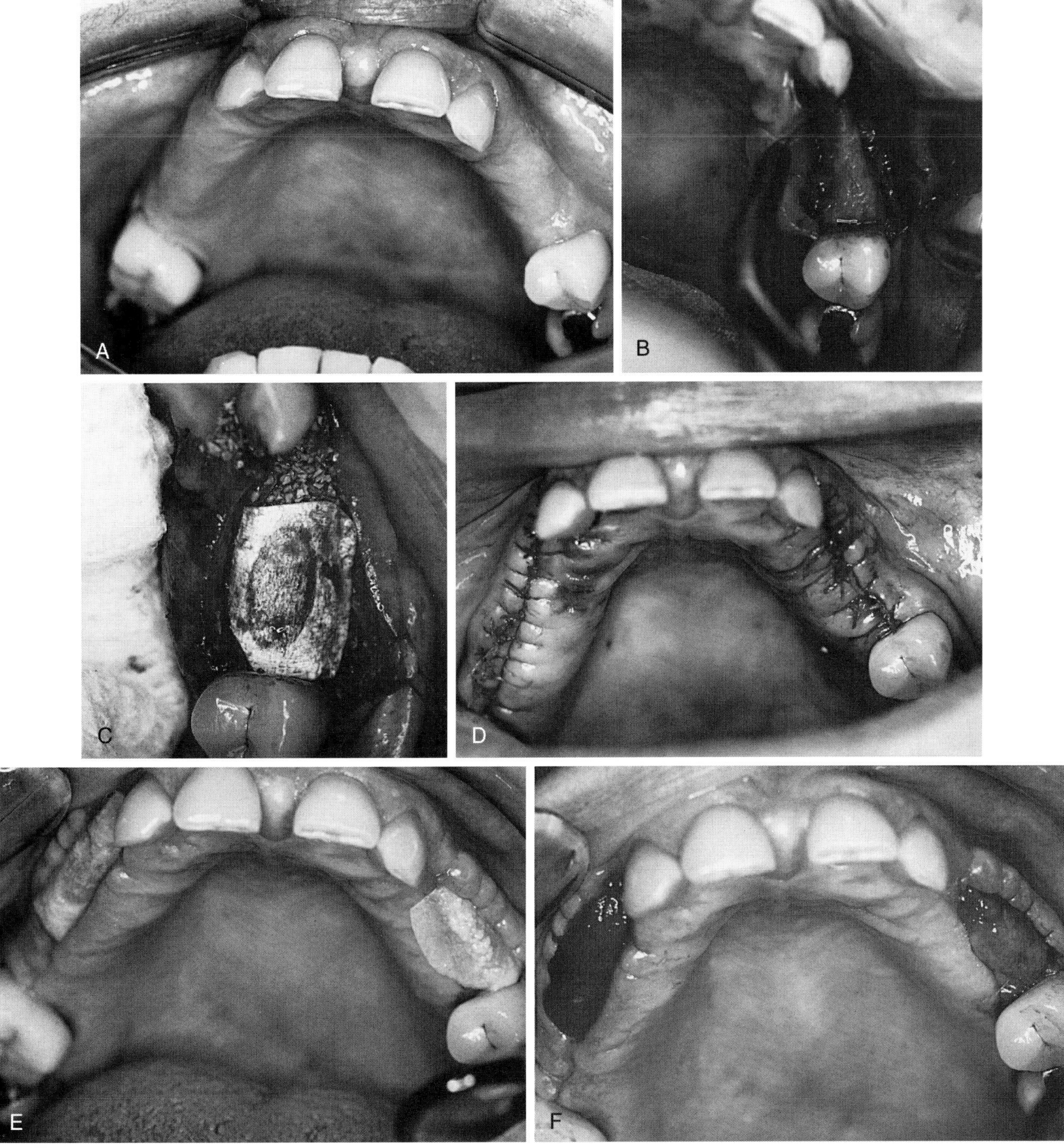

Figure 21–35. *A,* Preoperative view of narrow edentulous maxillary ridges. *B,* Flaps reflected, exposing underlying thin bony ridge, the magnitude of which was not readily detectable during clinical evaluation. *C,* Composite autogenous graft and xenograft with nonresorbable barrier membrane. *D,* Primary closure after grafting. *E,* Bilateral exfoliation of membranes 6 weeks after placement. *F,* Removal of membranes to leave well-granulated bases.

annual marginal bone loss thereafter was about 0.1 mm.

Jensen and associates[106] described reconstruction of the severely resorbed maxilla with bone grafting followed by implant placement at a second operation. They described five cases with a median follow-up time of 16 months (range 10 to 29 months). A total of 51 implants were installed. Nine of the 36 implants placed in grafted bone and 7 of the 15 implants placed in nongrafted bone were lost. These researchers believe that the load-bearing capacity of cancellous bone is less than that of cortical bone and was probably the most important factor in the prognosis. It has been suggested that in view of the observed rapid resorption of endochondral iliac crest onlay bone grafts, the number of failed implants can be significantly reduced if intramembranous mandibular symphyseal bone is used for placing titanium implants.[107]

Jensen and Sindet-Pedersen[108] reported the results of local augmentations of alveolar ridge defects in 16 partially edentulous patients using bone grafts harvested from the iliac crest. The mean period of functional loading was 27 months (range 2 to 80). Two implants were lost during initial healing because of wound dehiscences. Two implants were left buried, so that 51 out of 55 implants were in function at the time of follow-up. Twenty-five implants had been placed at the time of bone grafting, and 30 implants were in place after an average of 3.2 months. The pocket depth values ranged from 1 to 6 mm, with a mean of 3.3 mm. Marginal bone loss averaged 0.6 mm before functional loading.

There have also been reports of the successful use of calvarial bone grafts and implants,[109] of demineralized freeze-dried bone allografts around implants,[110] and of fresh-frozen allogeneic bone for maxillary and mandibular reconstruction.[111] The most significant complication of calvarial bone grafts is related to the donor site. The most significant potential complication of fresh-frozen allogeneic bone is the possibility of disease transmission. Although there is some variation in the reported values, it is apparent that the failure and complication rate is higher when bone grafts are placed in conjunction with endosseous implants and that the maxilla has a higher failure rate. There is evidence, however, that the grafted bone does not significantly resorb when implants are successfully osseointegrated and loaded compared with bone grafts placed without implants.

When there are local bone defects to be reconstructed, usually in the partially edentulous patient, the use of corticocancellous onlay bone grafts harvested from the mandibular symphysis appears to have predictable success with low morbidity and can be accomplished in the office setting. The grafts are contoured and fixed with miniscrews after they and the residual ridge have been perforated to improve vascularity. Primary, tension-free closure is essential, as is avoidance of pressure from transitional prostheses.

Maxillary Antroplasty (Sinus Lift)

There are limiting factors to reconstruction of the edentulous posterior maxilla. Often, available bone is insufficient to place implants of satisfactory dimension, the quality of the cancellous bone is compromised, and

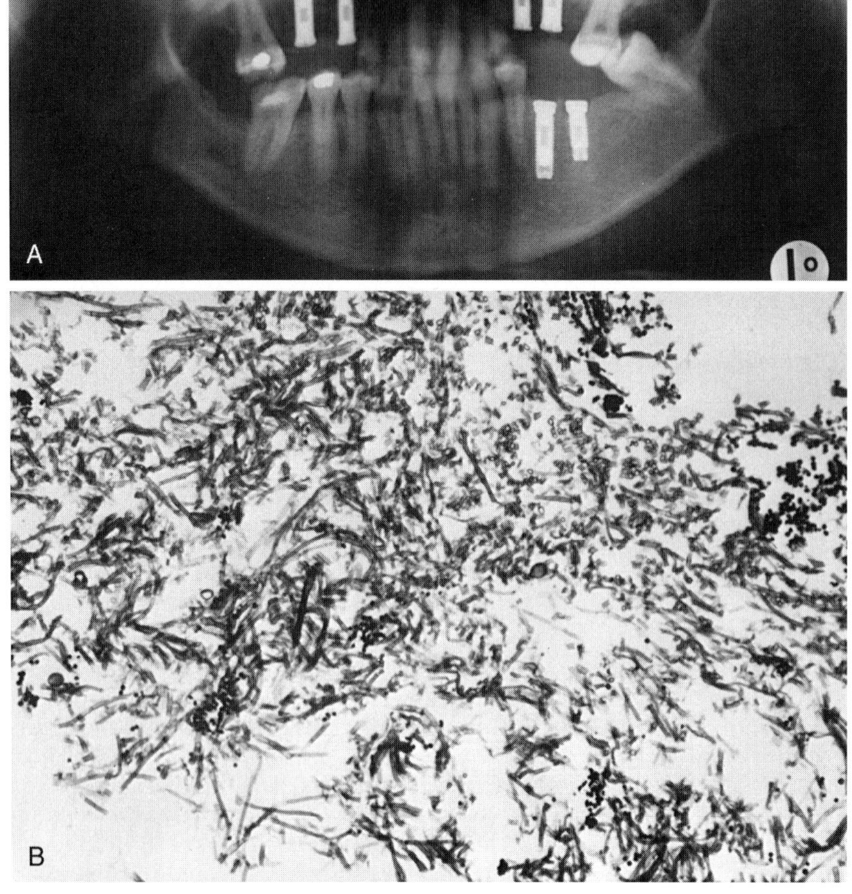

Figure 21–36. *A,* Implants placed simultaneously in the posterior maxilla with autogenous bone grafts. *B,* Postoperative aspergillosis infection requiring multiple operative procedures that resulted in explantation of the right maxillary implants and chronic right infraorbital pain. (Magnification × 100; silver stain)

the maxillary sinus presents anatomic limitations. In order to overcome these shortcomings in this anatomic area, the maxillary antroplasty (sinus augmentation, sinus lift, sinus graft) procedure was developed. As with other ancillary procedures, problems and complications have been encountered. They include infection of the graft requiring removal, wound dehiscences, sinus membrane perforations, maxillary sinusitis, poor quality or insufficient quantity of bone formed, failure of osseointegration, malposition of the implant, fungal infections, chronic pain, displacement and migration of the implant, and biomechanical failure, particularly when there is an opposing natural dentition (Figs. 21–36 and 21–37). Failure rates may increase in the smoker, so cessation of smoking should be strongly encouraged, particularly in the perioperative period.

Different grafting materials have been used to augment the maxillary sinus. Most clinicians would agree, however, that the use of autogenous bone alone or as a composite graft yields the most predictable successful results. The sinus should not be overpacked with bone that may block the ostium. The graft should be compacted to eliminate any voids. If the host residual ridge is adequate (approximately 5 mm) to stabilize the implant, a simultaneous graft–implant placement procedure can be done. Otherwise, it would be prudent to delay the implant procedure 4 to 6 months. Patients are started on systemic antibiotics and are instructed not to blow their noses or perform any Valsalva maneuvers. Sequential loading should be considered with a transitional prosthesis, particularly for the patient with parafunctional habits.

Jensen and colleagues[112] performed 128 sinus lift and 34 nasal lift procedures in a cohort of 98 patients. There were 45 cases (35%) of sinus membrane perforation. In 18 of 65 (28%) sinus lift procedures in partially edentulous patients, and 4 of 63 (6%) sinus lift procedures in totally edentulous patients, significant intraoperative bleeding was encountered. The investigators attribute the higher bleeding potential in the partially edentulous cases to be related to the greater vascularity in dentulous jaws. Intraoperative hemorrhage may lead to hematomas, infection, and, possibly, long-term or eventual failures. Two patients developed postoperative sinus infections.

Perforation of the nasal mucosa occurred in 5 of 34 nasal lift procedures.[112] Minor postoperative bleeding was controlled by conventional anterior nasal packs. Complications, including sinusitis and nasal obstruction, were not reported. Two of the patients required hospitalization for 24 hours after surgery. The implant survival in this study was 88.2%. The high success rate was attributed to the use of intramembranous versus endochondral bone, the short storage time used for the graft material, and the limited use of onlay grafts.

Inferior Alveolar Nerve Repositioning (Transposition, Lateralization)

In situations in which less than 10 mm of bone is available above the mandibular canal, shorter implants, which have a higher failure rate, must be used to reconstruct the edentulous posterior mandible. Success rates improve when larger surface areas of implants are osseointegrated and when initial bicortical stabilization is achieved. In order to accomplish bicortical stability, the inferior alveolar nerve must be repositioned laterally to allow implant placement (Fig. 21–38). This procedure should be limited to very special situations and carried out by surgeons experienced in nerve exposure and repair procedures.[113]

Various publications have reported on the outcomes of inferior alveolar nerve repositioning. In 100 patients with edentulism of the posterior mandible, 250 endosseous screw implants were placed after transposition of the inferior alveolar nerve.[114] Implant survival was 95.2% at 6 months, 94.2% at 12 months, and 93.6% at 18 months postoperatively. During the 12-month period

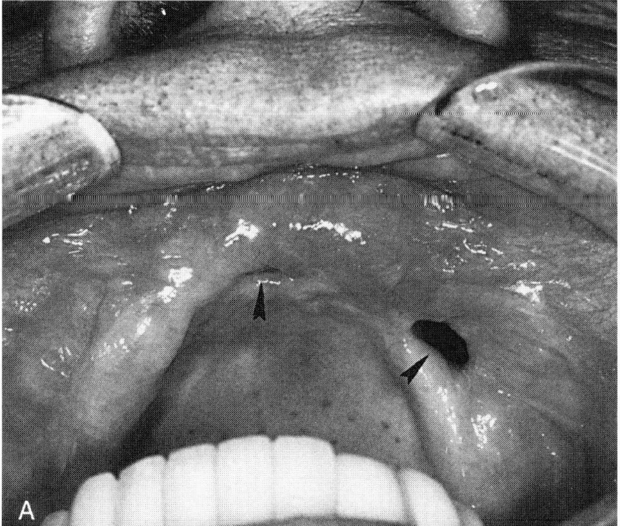

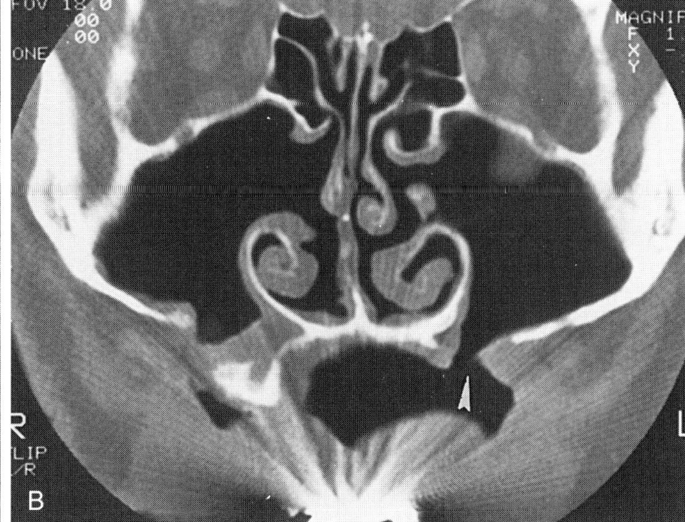

Figure 21–37. *A,* Oral-antral and oronasal fistulas after bone graft, sinus lift, and implant failures. *B,* CT scan showing oral-antral fistula.

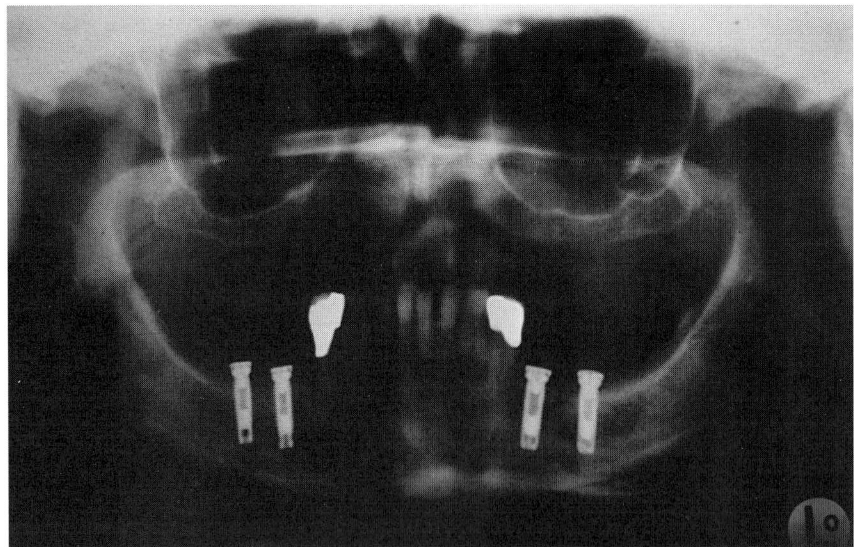

Figure 21–38. Bilateral inferior alveolar nerve repositioning resulted in transient bilateral paresthesias without achieving bicortical fixation.

following abutment connection, the mean marginal bone loss was 0.3 mm (range 0.1 to 5.1 mm). One week after implant placement, 21% of the patients had normal neurosensory function, 32% had diminished function, and 47% had no function. Six months postoperatively, however, 77% of patients had normal function, 21% had diminished function, and 2% had no function. At 18 months postoperatively, 94% had normal sensation, 4% had diminished sensation, and 1% had no sensation. Postoperative infections developed in 7 of the study patients, 2 of whom had symptoms resembling osteomyelitis with severe pain of long duration, and 1 had rapid marginal bone loss. Thick buccal cortices and thin neurovascular bundles created inherent technical difficulties.

Others have reported on their results, technical aspects, and potential complications of this nerve repositioning procedure.[115–117] Complications include the risk of producing neural lesions, paresthesias, anesthesias, painful dysesthesias, and hyperesthesias. Accidental laceration or transection of the nerve is also a potential complication. When adequate intermaxillary space is available in the posterior regions, bone grafting augmentation procedures should be considered first, because the potential neurosensory deficits created do not appear to be as common, prolonged, or profound.

References

1. Parameters of Care for Oral and Maxillofacial Surgery. Rosemont, Illinois, American Association of Oral and Maxillofacial Surgeons, 1995.
2. Worthington P, Bolender CL, Taylor TD. The Swedish system of osseointegrated implants: Problems and complications encountered during a 4-year trial period. Int J Oral Maxillofac Implants 1987;2:77.
3. Smith RA: New developments and advances in dental implantology. Curr Opin Dent 1992;2:42.
4. Sones AD: Complications with osseointegrated implants. J Prosthet Dent 1989;62:581.
5. Beirne O: Problems and complications in implant surgery. Oral Maxillofac Surg Clin North Am 1991;3:993.
6. Shulman LB, Shepherd NJ: Complications of dental implants. Oral Maxillofac Surg Clin North Amer 1990;2:499.
7. Maeglin B: Difficulties and Complications of Oral Implantology Basics: ITI Hollow Cylinder Systems. *In* Schroeder A, Sutter F, Krekeler G (eds): Implantology. New York, Thieme Medical Publishers, 1991, p 331.
8. Smith RA, Kaban LB: The use of dental implants in oral and maxillofacial reconstruction. Adv Plast Reconstr Surg 1994;10:231.
9. Zarb GA, Schmitt A: The longitudinal clinical effectiveness of osseointegrated dental implants. Part I: Surgical results. J Prosthet Dent 1990;63:451.
10. Zarb GA, Schmitt A: The longitudinal clinical effectiveness of osseointegrated dental implants: The Toronto Study. Part II: The prosthetic results. J Prosthet Dent 1990;64:53.
11. Zarb GA, Schmitt A: The longitudinal clinical effectiveness of osseointegrated dental implants: the Toronto study. Part III: Problems and complications encountered. J Prosthet Dent 1990;64:185.
12. Laney WR: Selecting edentulous patients for tissue-integrated prostheses. Int J Oral Maxillofac Implants 1986;1:129.
13. Blomberg S: Psychological response. In Brånemark PI, Zarb GA, Albrectson T (eds). Tissue-Integrated Prostheses. Chicago, Quintessence Publishing, 1985, p 165.
14. Pilling LF: Psychiatric aspects of diagnosis and treatment. *In* Laney WR, Gibilisco JA (eds): Diagnosis and Treatment in Prosthodontics. Philadelphia, Lea & Febiger, 1983, p 129.
15. Harris D: Osseointegrated implants: I would never had had it done had I known. Br Dent J 1993;9:261.
16. Smith RA, Berger R, Dodson TB: Risk factors associated with dental implants in healthy and medically compromised patients. Int J Oral Maxillofac Implants 1992;7:367.
17. Linkow LL: Factors influencing long-term implant success. J Prosthet Dent 1990;63:64.
18. Bain CA, Moy PK: The association between the failure of dental implants and cigarette smoking. Int J Oral Maxillofac Implants 1993;8:609.
19. Jones JK, Triplett RG: The relationship of cigarette smoking to impaired intraoral wound healing: A review of evidence and implications for patient care. J Oral Maxillofac Surg 1992;50:237; discussion, p 239.
20. Steiner M, Ramp WK: Endosseous dental implants and the glucocorticoid-dependent patient. J Oral Implantol 1990;16:211.
21. Dao TT, Anderson JD, Zarb GA: Is osteoporosis a risk factor for osseointegration of dental implants? Int J Oral Maxillofac Implants 1993;8:137.
22. Jaffin RA, Berman CL: The excessive loss of Brånemark fixtures in type IV bone: A 5-year study. J Periodont 1991;62:2.
23. van Steenberghe D, Lekholm U, Bolender C, et al: Applicability

of osseointegrated oral implants in the rehabilitation of partial edentulism: A prospective multicenter study on 558 fixtures. Int J Oral Maxillofac Implants 1990;5:272.
24. Adell R, Eriksson B, Lekholm U, et al: Long-term follow-up study of osseointegrated implants in the treatment of totally edentulous jaws. Int J Oral Maxillofac Implants 1990;5:347.
25. Albrektsson T: A multicenter report on osseointegrated oral implants. J Prosthet Dent 1988;60:75.
26. Jemt T, Lekholm U: Oral implant treatment in posterior partially edentulous jaws: A 5-year follow-up report. Int J Oral Maxillofac Implants 1993;8:635.
27. Nevins M, Langer B: The successful application of osseointegrated implants to the posterior jaw: A long-term retrospective study. Int J Oral Maxillofac Implants 1993;8:428.
28. Jemt T, Linden B, Lekholm U: Failures and complications in 127 consecutively placed fixed partial prostheses supported by Braånemark implants: From prosthetic treatment to first annual checkup. Int J Oral Maxillofac Implants 1992;7:40.
29. Pylant T, Triplett RG, Key MC, et al: A retrospective evaluation of endosseous titanium implants in the partially edentulous patient. Int J Oral Maxillofac Implants 1992;7:195.
30. Ekfeldt A, Carlsson GE, Borjesson G: Clinical evaluation of single-tooth restorations supported by osseointegrated implants: A retrospective study. Int J Oral Maxillofac Implants 1994;9:179.
31. Jemt T, Laney WR, Harris D, et al: Osseointegrated implants for single tooth replacement: A 1-year report from a multicenter prospective study. Int J Oral Maxillofac Implants 1991;6:29.
32. Laney WR, Jemt T, Harris D, et al: Osseointegrated implants for single-tooth replacement: Progress report from a multicenter prospective study after 3 years. Int J Oral Maxillofac Implants 1994;9:49.
33. Naert I, De Clercq M, Theuniers G, et al: Overdentures supported by osseointegrated fixtures for the edentulous mandible: A 2.5-year report. Int J Oral Maxillofac Implants 1988;3:191.
34. Hemmings KW, Schmitt A, Zarb GA: Complications and maintenance requirements for fixed prostheses and overdentures in the edentulous mandible: A 5-year report. Int J Oral Maxillofac Implants 1994;9:191.
35. Jemt T, Book K, Linden B, et al: Failures and complications in 92 consecutively inserted overdentures supported by Braånemark implants in severely resorbed edentulous maxillae: A study from prosthetic treatment to first annual check-up. Int J Oral Maxillofac Implants 1992;7:162.
36. Palmqvist S, Sondell K, Swartz B: Implant-supported maxillary overdentures: Outcome in planned and emergency cases. Int J Oral Maxillofac Implants 1994;9:184.
37. Johns RB, Jemt T, Heath MR, et al: A multicenter study of overdentures supported by Braånemark implants. Int J Oral Maxillofac Implants 1992;7:513.
38. Engquist B, Bergendal T, Kallus T, et al: A retrospective multicenter evaluation of osseointegrated implants supporting overdentures. Int J Oral Maxillofac Implants 1988;3:129.
39. Mason ME, Triplett RG, Alfonso WF: Life-threatening hemorrhage from placement of a dental implant. J Oral Maxillofac Surg 1990;48:204.
40. ten Bruggenkate CM, Krekeler G, Kraaijenhagen HA, et al: Hemorrhage of the floor of the mouth resulting from lingual perforation during implant placement: A clinical report. Int J Oral Maxillofac Implants 1993;8:329.
41. Berberi A, Le Breton G, Mani J, et al: Lingual paresthesia following surgical placement of implants: Report of a case. Int J Oral Maxillofac Implants 1993;8:580.
42. Ellies LG, Hawker PB: The prevalence of altered sensation associated with implant surgery. Int J Oral Maxillofac Implants 1993;8:674.
43. Pogrel MA, Kaban LB: Injuries to the inferior alveolar and lingual nerves. J Calif Dent Assoc 1993;21:50.
44. Sonick M, Abraham J, Faiella RA: A comparison of the accuracy of periapical panoramic and computerized tomographic radiographs in locating the mandibular canal. Int J Oral Maxillofac Implants 1994;9:455.
45. Kassebaum DK, Nummikoski PV, Triplett RG, et al: Cross-sectional radiography for implant site assessment. Oral Surg Oral Med Oral Pathol 1990;70:674.
46. Clark DE, Danforth RA, Barnes RW, et al: Radiation absorbed from dental implant radiography: A comparison of linear tomography, CT scan, and panoramic and intra-oral techniques. J Oral Implantol 1990;16:156.
47. Serman NJ: Pitfalls of panoramic radiology in implant surgery. Ann Dent 1989;48:13.
48. Theisen FC, Shultz RE, Elledge DA: Displacement of a root form implant into the mandibular canal. Oral Surg Oral Med Oral Pathol 1990;70:24.
49. Bergermann M, Donald PJ, à Wengen DF: Screwdriver aspiration: A complication of dental implant placement. Int J Oral Maxillofac Surg 1992;21:339.
50. Mason ME, Triplett RG, Van Sickels JE, et al: Mandibular fractures through endosseous cylinder implants: Report of cases and review. J Oral Maxillofac Surg 1990;48:311.
51. Tolman DE, Keller EE: Management of mandibular fractures in patients with endosseous implants. Int J Oral Maxillofac Implants 1991;6:427.
52. Binger T: Osteomyelitis and pathological fracture after implant placement in the edentulous jaw. Z Zahnärztl Implantol 1989;5:12.
53. Davies JM, Campbell LA: Fatal air embolism during dental implant surgery: A report of three cases [see "Comments"]. Can J Anaesth 1990;37:112.
54. Krogh PHJ, Collins TA: Complications of osseointegrated implants. Oral Maxillofac Surg Clin North Am 1994;6:837.
55. Block MS, Kent JN: Factors associated with soft- and hard-tissue compromise of endosseous implants. J Oral Maxillofac Surg 1990;48:1153.
56. Lekholm U, Adell R, Lindhe J, et al: Marginal tissue reactions at osseointegrated titanium fixtures. (II) A cross-sectional retrospective study. Int J Oral Maxillofac Surg 1986;15:53.
57. Quirynen M, Naert I, van Steenberghe D, et al: A study of 589 consecutive implants supporting complete fixed prostheses. Part I: Periodontal aspects. J Prosthet Dent 1992;68:655.
58. Weyant RJ: Characteristics associated with the loss and peri-implant tissue health of endosseous dental implants. Int J Oral Maxillofac Implants 1994;9:95.
59. Meffert RM, Langer B, Fritz ME: Dental implants: A review. J Periodontol 1992;63:859.
60. Strub JR, Gaberthuel TW, Grunder U: The role of attached gingiva in the health of peri-implant tissue in dogs. I: Clinical findings. Int J Periodont Restor Dent 1991;11:317.
61. Kirsch A, Mentag PJ: The IMZ endosseous two phase implant system: A complete oral rehabilitation treatment concept. J Oral Implantol 1986;12:576.
62. Mombelli A, van Oosten MA, Schurch EJ, et al: The microbiota associated with successful or failing osseointegrated titanium implants. Oral Microbiol Immunol 1987;2:145.
63. Becker W, Becker BE, Newman MG, et al: Clinical and microbiologic findings that may contribute to dental implant failure. Int J Oral Maxillofac Implants 1990;5:31.
64. Gatewood RR, Cobb CM, Killoy WJ: Microbial colonization on natural tooth structure compared with smooth and plasma-sprayed dental implant surfaces. Clin Oral Implants Res 1993;4:53.
65. Haanaes HR: Implants and infections with special reference to oral bacteria. J Clin Periodontol 1990;17:516.
66. Malmstrom HS, Fritz ME, Timmis DP, et al: Osseo-integrated implant treatment of a patient with rapidly progressive periodontitis: A case report. J Periodontol 1990;61:300.
67. Zablotsky MH, Meffert R, Mills O: The macroscopic, microscopic, spectrometric effects of various chemotherapeutic agents on the plasma sprayed HA-coated implant surface. Clin Oral Implants Res 1992;3:189.
68. Albrektsson T, Sennerby L: State of the art in oral implants. J Clin Periodontol 1991;18:474.
69. Henry P, Johnson B, Kirsch A: Solutions for specific soft tissue situations. Int J Oral Maxillofac Implants 1994;9:30.
70. Bloebaum RD, Dupont JA: Osteolysis from a press-fit hydroxyapatite-coated implant: A case study. J Arthroplasty 1993;8:195.
71. Natiella JR: The meaning of biocompatibility. Oral Maxillofac Surg Clin North Am 1991;3:755.
72. Steinman S: Oral Implantology Basics: ITI Hollow Cylinder Systems. *In* Schroeder A, Sutter F, Krekeler G (eds): Implantology. New York, Thieme Medical Publishers, 1991, p 37.

73. Keller JC, Young FA, Hansel B: Systemic effects of porous Ti dental implants. Dent Mater 1985;1:41.
74. Bruneel N, Helsen JA: In vitro simulation of biocompatibility of Ti-Al-V. J Biomed Mater Res 1988;22:203.
75. Schliephake H, Reiss G, Urban R, et al: Metal release from titanium fixtures during placement in the mandible: An experimental study. Int J Oral Maxillofac Implants 1993;8:502.
76. Memoli VA, Woodman JL, Urban RM: Malignant neoplasms associated with orthopaedic implant materials. Trans Orthop Res Soc 1982;7:164.
77. Sunderman FW: Carcinogenicity of metal alloys in orthopedic prostheses: Clinical and experimental studies. Fundam Appl Toxicol 1989;13:205.
78. Smith RA, Silverman SJ, Auclert O: Recognition of malignancy and dysplasia in the dental implant patient. J Oral Implantol 1989;15:255.
79. Friedman KE, Vernon SE: Squamous cell carcinoma developing in conjunction with a mandibular staple bone plate. J Oral Maxillofac Surg 1983;41:265.
80. Weinberg LA, Kruger B: Biomechanical considerations when combining tooth-supported and implant-supported prostheses. Oral Surg Oral Med Oral Pathol 1994;78:22.
81. Beumer J III, Hamada MO, Lewis S: A prosthodontic overview. Int J Prosthodont 1993;6:126.
82. Naert I, Quirynen M, van Steenberghe D, et al: A six-year prosthodontic study of 509 consecutively inserted implants for the treatment of partial edentulism. J Prosthet Dent 1992;67:236.
83. Cronin RJ, Oesterle LJ, Ranly DM: Mandibular implants and the growing patient. Int J Oral Maxillofac Implants 1994;9:55.
84. Smith RA, Kearns G, Bosch C: Placement of an endosseous implant in a growing child with ectodermal dysplasia. Oral Surg Oral Med Oral Pathol 1993;75:669.
85. Oesterle LJ, Cronin RJ, Ranly DM: Maxillary implants and the growing patient. Int J Oral Maxillofac Implants 1993;8:377.
86. Perrott DH, Sharma AB, Vargervik K: Endosseous implants for pediatric patients. Oral Maxillofac Surg Clin North Am 1994;6:79.
87. Granstrom G: The use of hyperbaric oxygen to prevent implant loss in the irradiated patient. *In* Worthington P, Brånemark PI (eds): Advanced Osseointegration Surgery. Chicago, Quintessence Publishing, 1989, p 336.
88. Jacobsson M, Tjellstrom A, Thomsen P, et al: Integration of titanium implants in irradiated bone: Histologic and clinical study. Ann Otol Rhinol Laryngol 1988;97:337.
89. Albrektsson T, Dahl E, Enbom L, et al: Osseointegrated oral implants: A Swedish multicenter study of 8139 consecutively inserted Nobelpharma implants. J Periodontol 1988;59:287.
90. Hatjigiorgis CG, Shiu AS, Fleming TJ, et al: Influence of calcium phosphate hydroxylapatite on dose distribution in electron beam radiation therapy. Int J Oral Maxillofac Implants 1987;2:65.
91. Roumanas E, Nishimura R, Beumer J: Craniofacial defects and osseointegrated implants: Six-year follow-up report on the success rates of craniofacial implants at UCLA. Int J Oral Maxillofac Implants 1994;9:579.
92. Parel SM, Tjellstrom A: The United States and Swedish experience with osseointegration and facial prostheses. Int J Oral Maxillofac Implants 1991;6:75.
93. Mylanus EAM, Cremers CWRJ, Snik AFM: Clinical results of percutaneous implants in the temporal bone. Arch Otolaryngol Head Neck Surg 1994;120:81.
94. Tolman DE, Desjardins RP: Extraoral application of osseointegrated implants. J Oral Maxillofac Surg 1991;49:33.
95. Holgers KM, Paulsson M, Tjellstrom A: Selected microbial findings in association with percutaneous titanium implants. Int J Oral Maxillofac Implants 1991;9:565.
96. Mensdorff-Pouilly N, Haas R, Mailath G: The immediate implant: A retrospective study comparing the different types of immediate implantation. Int J Oral Maxillofac Implants 1994;9:571.
97. Tolman DE, Keller EE: Endosseous implant placement immediately following dental extraction and alveoloplasty: Preliminary report with 6-year follow-up. Int J Oral Maxillofac Implants 1991;6:24.
98. Block MS, Kent JN: Placement of endosseous implants into tooth extraction sites. J Oral Maxillofac Surg 1991;49:1269.
99. Krump JL, Barnett BG: The immediate implant: A treatment alternative. Int J Oral Maxillofac Implants 1991;6:19.
100. Barzilay I: Immediate implants: Their current status. Int J Prosthodont 1993;6:169.
101. Rominger JW, Triplett RG: The use of guided tissue regeneration to improve implant osseointegration. J Oral Maxillofac Surg 1994;52:106.
102. Keller EE, Tolman DE: Mandibular ridge augmentation with simultaneous onlay iliac bone graft and endosseous implants: A preliminary report. Int J Oral Maxillofac Implants 1992;7:176.
103. Lew D, Hinkle RM, Unhold GP, et al: Reconstruction of the severely atrophic edentulous mandible by means of autogenous bone grafts and simultaneous placement of osseointegrated implants. J Oral Maxillofac Surg 1991;49:228.
104. Nystrom E, Kahnberg KE, Gunne J: Bone grafts and Brånemark implants in the treatment of the severely resorbed maxilla: A 2-year longitudinal study. Int J Oral Maxillofac Implants 1993;8:45.
105. Adell R, Lekholm U, Grondahl K, et al: Reconstruction of severely resorbed edentulous maxillae using osseointegrated fixtures in immediate autogenous bone grafts. Int J Oral Maxillofac Implants1990;5:233.
106. Jensen J, Simonsen EK, Sindet-Pedersen S: Reconstruction of the severely resorbed maxilla with bone grafting and osseointegrated implants: A preliminary report. J Oral Maxillofac Surg 1990;48:27.
107. Schliephake H, Neukam FW, Scheller H: Local ridge augmentation using bone grafts and osseointegrated implants in the rehabilitation of partial edentulism: Preliminary results. Int J Oral Maxillofac Implants 1994;9:557.
108. Jensen J, Sindet-Pedersen S: Autogenous mandibular bone grafts and osseointegrated implants for reconstruction of the severely atrophied maxilla: A preliminary report. J Oral Maxillofac Surg 1991;49:1277.
109. Donovan MG, Dickerson NC, Hanson LJ, et al: Maxillary and mandibular reconstruction using calvarial bone grafts and Braånemark implants: A preliminary report. J Oral Maxillofac Surg 1994;52:588.
110. Landsberg CJ, Grosskopf A, Weinreb M: Clinical and biologic observations of demineralized freeze-dried bone allografts in augmentation procedures around dental implants. Int J Oral Maxillofac Implants 1994;9:586.
111. Perrott DH, Smith RA, Kaban LB: The use of fresh frozen allogeneic bone for maxillary and mandibular reconstruction. Int J Oral Maxillofac Surg 1992;21:260.
112. Jensen J, Sindet-Pedersen S, Oliver AJ: Varying treatment strategies for reconstruction of maxillary atrophy with implants: Results in 98 patients. J Oral Maxillofac Surg 1994;52:210.
113. Krogh PHJ, Worthington P, Davis H: Does the risk of complication make transpositioning the inferior alveolar nerve in conjunction with implant placement a "last resort" surgical procedure? Int J Oral Maxillofac Implants 1994;9:249.
114. Rosenquist B: Implant placement in combination with nerve transpositioning: Experience with the first 100 cases. Int J Oral Maxillofac Implants 1994;9:522.
115. Jensen J, Reiche-Fischel O, Sindet-Pedersen S: Nerve transposition and implant placement in the atrophic posterior mandibular alveolar ridge. J Oral Maxillofac Surg 1994;52:662.
116. Haers PE, Sailer HF: Neurosensory function after the lateralization of the inferior alveolar nerve and simultaneous insertion of implants. Oral Maxillofac Surg Clin North Am 1994; 6:707.
117. Ruskin JD: Surgical approaches to repositioning of the inferior alveolar nerve for placement of osseointegrated implants. Oral Maxillofac Surg Clin North Am 1994;2:9.

Chapter 22
LONG-TERM COMPLICATIONS AFTER VASCULARIZED BONE GRAFTS

by

Martin B. Hirigoyen
Daniel Buchbinder

Introduction

As microsurgery enters its fourth decade, the level of reconstructive sophistication that is achievable using free tissue transfer continues to evolve. In particular, advances in flap design have transformed the possibilities for reconstruction of bony defects of the head and neck. Whereas the restoration of mandibular continuity using nonvascularized bone and alloplasts was once the only achievable goal, a range of functional modalities can now be included in the reconstruction as vascularized tissues.

The Subjects Discussed in This Chapter Are:

- Microvascular complications
- Success rates
- Causes of failure
  Preoperative factors
  Operative factors

The prime concern in reconstruction of mandibular defects has gone beyond restoring structural support and cosmesis and has become the restitution of oromandibular function.[1] Although nonmicrovascular methods retain their use in specific cases, single-stage primary reconstruction using free bone transfer is the only technique that offers optimal restoration of form and function with success rates approximating 96%.[2] Vascularized bone avoids the threat of infection and resorption associated with allografts, as well as the danger of infection and extrusion associated with alloplastic materials, and is unrivaled in its ability to overcome the problem of non-union in wound beds compromised by prior irradiation and salivary fistulas.[3–6] In addition, at the time of reconstruction, endosseous implants can be implanted directly into the bone and retentive dentures placed in a second procedure, greatly improving mastication.[7, 8]

Many of the problems encountered during staged reconstruction, such as atrophy and scarring of the soft tissue envelope, are avoided by a single procedure,[6, 9] which provides the utmost[1] and most cost-effective[10] opportunity to restore anatomy and function to the oral cavity. For example, the use of an interpositional nerve graft to reestablish continuity to the inferior alveolar nerve is associated with a high level of return of lower lip sensation and oral competence.[11, 12] In a similar fashion, the creation of composite osteomyocutaneous flaps has made possible the accurate restoration of sulcular anatomy, and modification of soft tissue flap design to incorporate vascularized nerve grafts has allowed the restoration of functional sensation to the oral lining. Most importantly, it has been demonstrated in large series that an optimal return to premorbid quality of life can be achieved most readily, in terms of the excellent aesthetic[13] and functional[6, 12, 14, 15] results, by reconstruction using vascularized bone grafts.

In spite of the versatility and superior results obtained using free tissue transfer, however, they are not without morbidity. The specter of a failed free flap weighs heavily upon both patient and surgeon, and other complications that may occur at either the donor or recipient site of a tissue transfer make it a frequently exacting procedure. It behooves the surgeon to understand the etiology of potential complications associated with vascularized bone grafts, so as to minimize the risk of their occurrence.

MICROVASCULAR COMPLICATIONS

Transfer of vascularized bone has so far been the single greatest advance in oromandibular reconstruction. As a consequence of continuously improving success rates, advances in flap design, and overall expanding enthusiasm for microsurgery, an ever-increasing number of bone flaps are being used in head and neck reconstruction. The small failure rate still poses a menace, because a failed flap incurs substantial morbidity to the patient[16] and because the associated waste of surgical resources has become an increasingly sensitive issue.[10] This section discusses the microvascular complications that may occur during vascularized bone transfer, and some recommended measures to avoid them.

SUCCESS RATES

A greater understanding of the pathophysiology of ischemia-reperfusion injury,[17] improved methods of flap monitoring,[18] and better selection of donor flap and of recipient vessels[19] have all contributed to making free tissue transfer a more reliable operation. The success rates for microvascular transfers have steadily risen over the past two decades and in expert hands can be expected to reach 98.8%, with a reexploration rate of 3.7%.[19] Despite the impressive statistics quoted in these individual series, multicenter surveys of free flap success rates that poll statistics from surgeons at all points on the learning curve of microsurgery report lower figures.[20, 21]

Series that report results of vascularized bone transfers are smaller but indicate that anastomotic patency results can be obtained with the composite flaps used in head and neck reconstruction similar to those with other free flaps.[2] Sullivan and colleagues[22] report a single thrombotic failure in 17 cases using the free scapula osteocutaneous flap (6%); the failure occurred when infection supervened in a postirradiated bed.[22] David and associates[3] report an 8.6% failure rate in 35 cases of mandibular reconstruction using the iliac crest flap. Also using iliac crest, Riediger[8] reported no complete losses in reconstructing 41 defects of the mandible and maxilla, although several partial losses occurred. In an analysis of 36 cases of second metatarsal and iliac crest osteocutaneous transfers, Duncan and coworkers[5] experienced three failures (0.8%), two of which were attributable to occlusion of the venous pedicle. Boyd and colleagues[6] compared 60 cases using vascularized iliac crest (three flap losses, one flap salvaged) with 13 cases of radial osteocutaneous flaps (one flap salvaged); in a summary review of 140 vascularized bone grafts, Boyd and Mulholland[23] found their flap failure rate to be 5.7%. Similarly, Urken and associates[11] reported a 6% failure rate with 71 cases of oromandibular reconstruction using microvascular composite free flaps.

Although these data indicate that success rates for vascularized bone match those for reconstruction of the extremities, the figures that compare heterogeneous types of flaps should be interpreted with caution. The complexity of reconstruction imposed by individual defects may greatly influence the conditions for microvascular surgery, as may the presence of salivary fistulas, infection, or a previously irradiated bed.[24]

Retrospective reviews clearly indicate that operative experience is the single most important factor related to improved success rates.[21, 24–27] In an in-depth analysis of why free flaps fail, Khouri[19] observed that anastomotic technique is often not to blame and that the majority of microvascular disasters occur because of some technical error in overall craftsmanship that eventually leads to circulatory impairment within the transferred tissue. Whereas the development of a flawless technique using the laboratory model forms an essential basis for further apprenticeship, a sound microsurgical acumen relies on the appreciation of the careful and specific need for preoperative planning that free tissue transfer surgery entails.

CAUSES OF FAILURE

The single event that finally causes the demise of every free flap is an interruption of blood flow within the transferred tissue. Compression of the pedicle or thrombosis at one or more of the anastomotic sites results in "no-flow ischemia" in the flap's microcirculation, which initiates the beginning of a secondary ischemic insult.[28] Attempts at revascularizing the flap once vascular compromise is detected are often thwarted by the paradoxic effects of reperfusion injury,[17] which is at present not effectively reversible in the clinical setting. It is the duty of the surgeon to identify each factor that may enhance the likelihood of flap failure and to adopt an effective and reproducible system by which to avoid it.[29]

Preoperative Factors

Patient Selection

The diversity of techniques that have been proposed to reconstruct bony defects of the head and neck attest to the complexity of the problem and underscore the fact that no one option may be regarded as suitable for all defects.[10] Thus, although free vascularized bone grafting represents the most advanced form of oromandibular reconstruction,[30] the potential morbidity of this method prohibits its use outside a clearly defined set of indications.[16] It is always regrettable to see a free flap fail, but the failure becomes inexcusable if the reconstructive goals could have been achieved by other, more simple methods.[31] A variety of classifications of bony and soft tissue defects of the mandible have been proposed in order to identify the role of free tissue transfer in reconstruction, which serve as a useful basis for preoperative planning.[3, 11, 15]

As the natural history of oral cancer entails, a significant proportion of patients undergoing oromandibular reconstruction are elderly and may suffer from an impaired cardiorespiratory reserve.[32] It is essential to keep in mind the strain that free tissue transfer surgery may impose upon these patients and to remember that several "major" interventions may be necessary during a short time. Particular attention should be paid to optimizing the preoperative status of nutrition, electrolyte balance, and pulmonary function.[33, 34] The benefits of employing a multidisciplinary approach to the assessment of oromandibular defects are well established[35], and the highest possible level of communication with the anesthetic team should be established from the very beginning. Contrary to previous opinion, concurrent systemic illnesses such as diabetes, hypertension, and peripheral vascular disease do not appear to threaten free flap survival.[33] There is a direct association between smoking and an increased risk of partial necrosis in soft tissue flaps. However, there is no direct correlation between smoking and an increased risk of flap failure.[32, 36] The presence of an underlying hypercoagulable state in some patients clearly raises the risk of microvascular thrombosis[32] but is fortunately rare and usually not preoperatively screened against.

Donor Site Selection

On the basis of the rationale that almost any part of the musculoskeletal system can be transferred to another site if its vascular geometry allows for reanastomosis, an increasingly wide array of donor sites have been suggested in the literature to be suitable for the transfer of vascularized bone, including ilium, fibula, scapula, radius, ulna, humerus, metatarsus, and rib.[1, 2] It is essential to become familiar with both the common anatomy and the variations in vascular patterns that may occur with each considered donor site.

Cadaver dissections and angiographic studies have proved invaluable in identifying these patterns[37, 38] and in determining the extent of tissue that can safely be transferred based on the vascular territory of individual arteries.[39, 40] Thus, the iliac crest flap has four contributory vessels to its arterial supply—the superficial and deep circumflex iliac, the superior deep branch of the superior gluteal, and the ascending branch of the lateral circumflex femoral arteries—but only the first two are suitable for transfer of composite flaps from this region.[2, 38, 41]

With the design of composite flaps, the surgeon must maintain the anatomic relationships among the different constituent parts, as the exigencies of recreating intraoral defects may place undue strain on the flap vasculature. Sustaining the orientation of the cutaneous paddle in iliac crest free flaps by using it to recreate external skin defects thus helps to avoid partial flap necrosis.[42]

One of the most significant factors in choosing a donor flap is selection of an appropriate pedicle. Table 22–1 summarizes the characteristics of some of the more commonly used bone flaps. A flap with pedicle vessels of large diameter (scapula, fibula, radial forearm) is likely to be associated with fewer intraoperative difficulties,[6, 29] and a longer flap pedicle makes the choice of recipient vessels in the neck more flexible.[6] Pedicle length should be planned to be excessive, not adequate, and although the use of vein grafts should be avoided, it is wise to have patient consent obtained and the patient surgically prepared for the possible harvesting of autologous vein grafts.[43] Atheromatous disease is frequently encountered in larger vessels such as the external iliac and femoral arteries,[44] but it rarely constitutes a problem in the smaller arteries that are used to create the flap pedicle.[45]

The choice of whether the ipsilateral or contralateral donor site should be used for harvest of the flap depends on its desired final position and its subsequent relationship with the vascular anatomy in the recipient region. Thus, the reconstruction of a right hemiman-

Table 22–1. Pedicle Characteristics of Commonly Used Free Flaps in Oromandibular Reconstruction

Flap	Pedicle Length (cm)	Pedicle Diameter (mm)	Pedicle Rating*	Accessibility for Two-Team Approach	Donor Site Morbidity
Ilium	6–8	1.5–3.5	3	4	3
Scapula	4–6	2–3	4	2	3
Metatarsus	5–8	2–3	4	4	2
Ulna	6–8	2.0–2.5	4	4	2
Radius	8–10	2.0–3.0	4	4	2
Fibula	5–8	2.0–2.5	4	4	4

*4 (excellent) to 1 (poor).

dible demands the use of an ipsilateral iliac crest free flap if the pedicle is planned to enter the flap at the angle of the neomandible, and of the contralateral side if it better matches recipient vessels nearer the mental symphysis. The anatomy of the fibula makes the ipsilateral leg the better choice if the recipient vessels are chosen on the same side of the neck, and contralateral leg if the flap is planned to be revascularized from the side opposite the lesion.[46] Several intraoperative maneuvers have been described that allow for flexibility in designing the fibula flap pedicle.[47, 48]

A final and highly requisite part of flap design is the provision for alternative wound coverage in the event that the planned reconstruction is unsuccessful. Prolonged primary ischemia, iatrogenic injury to the pedicle, failure to adequately cover the defect, and "unexplained" absence of reflow immediately after revascularization are only some of the potential causes of on-the-table flap failure, which must be foreseen and considered in the preoperative planning.[29] The solution may be in the form of local or regional pedicled soft tissue flaps or of another vascularized bone free flap performed at the same time.

Choice of Recipient Vessels

The importance of choosing recipient vessels of large diameter is regarded by many as the single greatest factor in reducing flap failure rates in recent years. In this respect, it is essential that the surgical team performing the resection be aware of the vascular requirements for the reconstruction.[35] Such decisions mostly affect the planned venous pedicle, because the resection of large veins in the neck may have a bearing upon the design of the tissue transfer.[46] Selecting the recipient arterial pedicle generally poses less of a problem, with the facial, transverse cervical, external carotid, and superior thyroid arteries being the more popular choices.[46] Careful arrangement of pedicle geometry is an important factor in all free tissue transfers to the head and neck that may greatly affect flap performance. Urken and associates[49] suggest that an ideal configuration requires the recipient vessels to lie along the longitudinal axis of the neck, which lessens the likelihood that the pedicle may become kinked or occluded with every turn of the patient's head. On this basis, they recommend the transverse cervical artery and external jugular vein as the nutrient vessels of choice for most oromandibular reconstructions.[49]

Careful consideration should be given to the inflammatory vascular injury that results from previous radiation therapy or surgery in the operative field and to how this affects the selection of recipient vessels. In cases in which the nutrient pedicle appears scarred, it is essential to have the preoperatively planned opportunity to harvest vein grafts from an upper or lower limb.

Reconstruction of certain oromandibular defects is made optimal by the combination of separate bone and soft tissue free flaps, which when placed together afford a more accurate restoration of premorbid anatomy than is achievable using composite flaps.[50] Thus, the thin, supple neurofasciocutaneous soft tissue of a radial forearm flap provides excellent coverage of vascularized bone supplied by a free iliac crest flap and renders a better definition of sulcular anatomy.[51] Although the radial forearm can readily be used as a flow-through flap to perfuse its bony counterpart, it is advisable to avoid the potential loss of two flaps by choosing an individual pedicle for each flap.[50, 51]

Operative Factors

Preanastomotic Factors

The attainment of a sound microsurgical technique in a laboratory model is an obvious prerequisite that need not be repeated here in detail. However, a firm grasp of the fundamental principles of microsurgery commonly offers the best solution to problems that are encountered intraoperatively. Thus, strict adherence to the guidelines for maximizing the performance of fine motor skills is imperative, and appraisal of the importance of preoperative psychological preparation and early recognition of microsurgical fatigue helps to eliminate impatience and confusion.[52] The extra few minutes taken to rearrange the microscope and surgical personnel are usually time well spent if they contribute to providing a wider exposure of the operative field and better comfort for the surgeons.

Following the resection or harvesting of the flap, a "stepping down" in surgical pace is necessary, because the careful dissection of the recipient pedicle requires an appropriate adaptation of surgical technique. Meticulous attention should be given to the gentle handling of vessels and the judicious use of bipolar diathermy,[53] and thought should be given to preserve a protective soft tissue "cuff" around the pedicle in certain cases.[14] Thus, a fringe of iliacus and transversus abdominis muscles are taken when the deep circumflex iliac artery pedicle supplying the iliac crest flap is dissected, in order to protect against the vascular trauma and spasm that follow skeletonization of the vessels. Once the pedicle is dissected, it should be handled atraumatically, and instruments should be used to protect it from injury during the harvest and trimming of the bony fragment. It is advisable, for the most part, to secure the bony component of the flap before commencing microsurgery, because trauma to the pedicle is easily incurred during maneuvers necessary to achieve any method of internal fixation.[23]

Anastomotic Factors

Poorly executed anastomoses are most often not to blame for flap failure.[54] More commonly, it is an overall error in operative decision-making or a failure in designing pedicle geometry that is responsible for circulatory compromise within the transferred tissue. Nonetheless, the tenets of a sound microsurgical technique adhere, and it is essential to maintain meticulous standards during the completion of all anastomoses. A wide range of factors have been identified that adversely affect the patency of repaired microvessels,[55] which all involve stripping of the endothelium to expose the strongly thrombogenic subendothelial matrix.[54] It suffices to say that all efforts should be directed at maintaining the integrity of the endothelial cell layer during anastomotic repair and to recognize the danger of operating within the so-called zone of injury that surrounds a traumatic or postinflammatory defect.[54]

A variety of methods have been proposed by which to coapt microvessels, but primary suturing probably still represents the most versatile technique. Laser-assisted anastomoses are reported to decrease operating time and to attain high patency rates because of a reduction in foreign material.[56] They may be associated with a greater tendency to late anastomotic stenosis, however,[57] and require the purchasing of expensive equipment. Other nonsuture techniques include the use of stapling devices, which maintain high patency rates in the experimental setting but require extra mobilization of vessel ends, which should be of similar diameter.[58] In spite of the reported benefits of these other methods, the exigencies of pedicle design associated with head and neck tissue transfers weigh largely in favor of using primary sutures for anastomosis.

Experimental studies suggest that an optimal balance between obtaining a good anastomotic seal and minimizing intimal injury is achieved with the placement of eight sutures per anastomosis,[59] although a general move toward using larger vessels may mean that more sutures are necessary. Opinions differ about the benefit of using continuous rather than interrupted sutures: The former offers the advantage of expediency, but this advantage is outweighed by the higher risk of suture entrapment and breakage,[60] and has been reported to cause a pursestring-like constriction of venous anastomoses.[61] Similarly, the "sleeve-like" telescoping of vessels, as originally described by Lauritzen,[62] has found fewer advocates following reports of its lower patency rates in the experimental setting.[63, 64]

A continuing debate exists as to whether anastomosing vessels end-to-side (ETS) is more reliable than suturing them end-to-end (ETE). In theory, the former method is associated with higher rates of flow,[65] but patency rates are similar for the two techniques when used with vessels of similar caliber. Although the revision of ETS anastomoses is more complex, and the deposition of atheroma in large vessels may make it technically more difficult, it is to be preferred when the diameter of the recipient vessels exceeds that of the flap pedicle.[58] This is frequently the case with tissue transfer surgery of the head and neck.

In cases in which it is not possible to approximate the flap pedicle to recipient vessels because of insufficient length, autogenous veins are the most commonly used form of microvascular graft.[58] They should be planned to be 35% longer than the measured gap,[66] and care should be taken that they do not become twisted before commencing of the second anastomosis. In spite of their reported high patency in the experimental setting, it is generally accepted that the use of autogenous veins is associated with a higher incidence of microvascular complications. The decision as to how many veins to reconstruct depends largely upon available anatomy and personal experience; many would favor the use of two veins wherever possible.

The addition of heparin to irrigating solutions used in microvascular surgery is now almost universal, and experimental studies show that a maximum antithrombotic effect is seen at a concentration of 100 IU/mL.[67] Similarly, the use of topical antispasmodics is useful during the dissection of a pedicle or the preparation of vessel ends for anastomosis. Vasospasm prevents a clear view of the vessel lumen during suture placement and, if prolonged, causes significant endothelial damage. Popular drugs include xylocaine (which has an optimal spasmolytic effect at a concentration of 20%[68]), papaverine, and verapamil.

Postanastomotic Factors (Figure 22–1)

Once the flap is revascularized and set into the recipient bed, one must arrange the pedicle so that its geometry lays at minimal risk of distortion during the postoperative period. Sharp kinks over bony ridges should be avoided, as should any course by which the vessels come to lie in a soft tissue "tunnel," which may then become compressed with postoperative edema. In cases in which simultaneous brachytherapy is given, the position of the afterloading catheters should be planned so as to avoid impingement upon the pedicle vessels.[69] Great care should be taken in the placement of drains in the wound, with particular attention to avoid placing suction drains in the immediate vicinity of anastomoses.[36] Penrose and other open drains should be dependent and also should be directed away

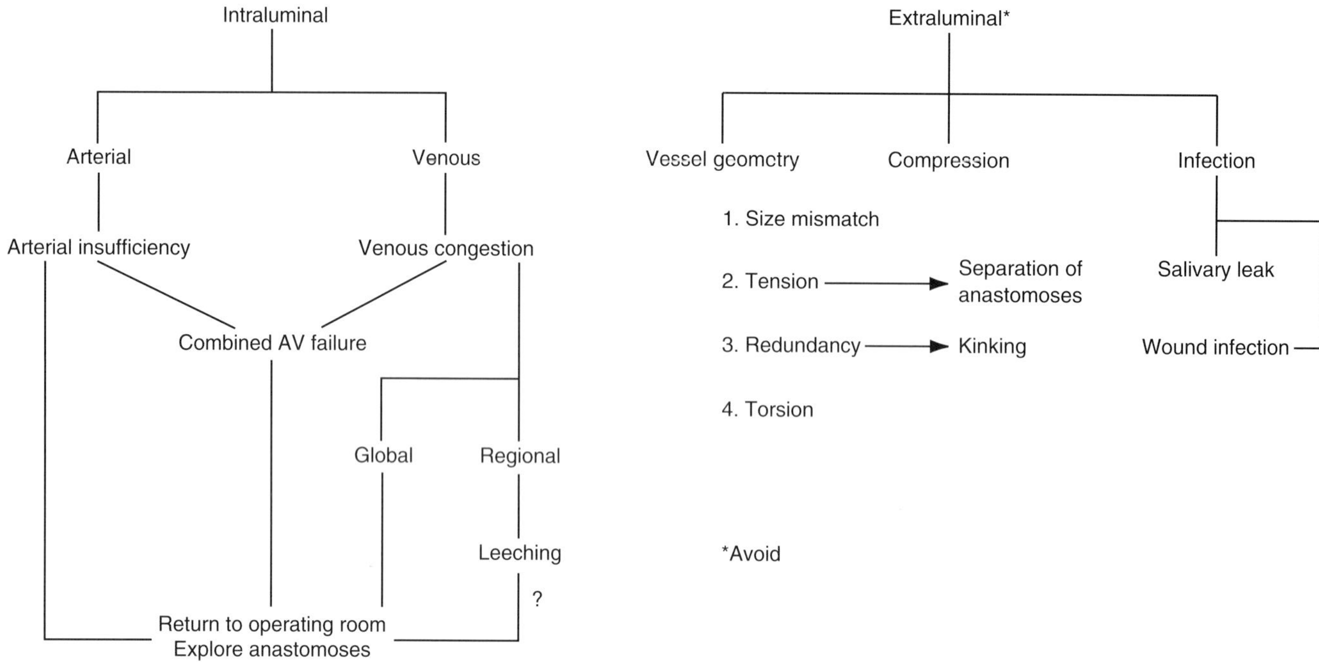

Figure 22–1. Sequence of events of failing flaps.

from all microsurgical sites. Wound closure should be accomplished with careful surveillance of the flap, because it may be found to compromise venous drainage. In such cases, part of the suture line may be left open or loosely tacked until postoperative edema subsides, when it may more safely be closed. It is commonly desirable to know the location of the pedicle in the neck for the purposes of postoperative monitoring, and a reference mark can be made on the overlying skin to facilitate the location of an ultrasound probe.

A minimum of dressings is necessary with oromandibular reconstructions, because any constriction will likely embarrass the flap circulation. In addition, good access to the flap surface is required for repeated clinical observation. It is of paramount importance to maintain good communication with the nursing staff, who should strive to maintain the postoperative conditions that are favorable for microvascular success as indicated by the reconstructive team.[29] A semisupine patient position of 30 to 45 degrees with slight head tilt is preferable, and sandbags may be used to restrict excessive side-to-side movements of the head.

There is no universally accepted regimen of antithrombotic therapy for routine uncomplicated free tissue transfers, and personal choice varies widely among microsurgeons.[58] Aspirin consumption is discouraged preoperatively but is of value in the early postoperative period at a low dose (3–5 mg/kg). Dextran 40, a polysaccharide that was initially used as a volume expander, was subsequently found to have significant antiplatelet and antifibrin properties. It has been associated with high rates of microvascular patency in a recreated thrombogenic experimental setting and is widely used clinically during the first 24 to 72 hours following tissue transfer.[58] Hypersensitivity may occur, and it is recommended that a test dose always be administered first.

Heparin remains one of the purest and most potent anticoagulant drugs available, and its application in microsurgery has been widely investigated. The major anticoagulant action of heparin is to augment the inhibition of several coagulation factors (IIa, Xa, IXa, and XIIa) by antithrombin III.[70] At higher concentrations, heparin catalyzes the inhibition of thrombin by heparin cofactor II, and it has been shown to stimulate the release of tissue plasminogen activator.[71] As well as preventing the formation of new fibrin and its subsequent integration into thrombus, heparin may facilitate flow by lowering the viscosity of blood.[72]

The main disadvantage of its use is bleeding, and many believe that its risks outweigh its benefits in an uncomplicated microsurgical case.[58] However, this agent has no direct thrombolytic activity[73] and is more commonly used when delivered selectively[74] or systemically[75] in attempts to salvage a failing flap during the postoperative period.[20]

Although autonomically denervated, a free flap remains under the vasoactive influences of its recipient bed arterial supply. It is desirable to maintain a high rate of flow through the flap microcirculation in the early, "thrombogenic" postoperative period (3–5 days). Hypovolemia, hypotension, and hypothermia all compromise peripheral circulation, and a combination of high-volume fluid replacement in a warm environment is required to optimize perfusion in free tissue transfers.[19] Moderate hemodilution enables the maintenance of a high cardiac output and a low peripheral resistance, and a combination of crystalloids to replace insensible fluid loss and synthetic colloids to replace plasma constituents is preferred.[76]

Close attention should be paid to the early diagnosis of wound hematomas, as even relatively inconspicuous collections may compromise the vascular geometry of the pedicle.[77] Although the release of a suture line may suffice in some cases,[11] most hematomas are more appropriately dealt with in the operating room.

The development of venous congestion in flaps used for oromandibular reconstruction is not uncommon,[11] and the value of medicinal leeches in decompressing the microcirculation is well documented (Fig. 22–2).[78,79] Oral antibiotics (e.g., ciprofloxacin) should be used to cover against *Aeromonas hydrophila,* an organism commensal to the leech, inhabiting its intestinal system. Bleeding continues from the site following the removal or engorgement of the leech, owing to the secretion of hirudin in its saliva, which inhibits the thrombin pathway.[79]

The majority of cases of "late" thrombosis in oromandibular flaps are secondary to other complications, namely, infection[22,24,80] and salivary fistulas.[77,78,81] The adverse effect of sepsis on the thrombogenicity of anastomoses has been documented both experimentally and clinically, although the exact mechanisms are not entirely clear.[82] A change in conformation in the reactivity of the vessels seems to be the primary cause, and a relative thrombocytosis may also be involved.[83] Although an early wound infection that does not involve the anastomoses may be managed conservatively, any evidence of spread to tissues that neighbor microsurgical sites should prompt an immediate reexploration. Similarly, salivary fistulas bathing a microvascular repair should be drained or diverted surgically at the soonest possible opportunity.[77]

The monitoring of free tissue transfers used in oromandibular reconstruction is traditionally imprecise and frequently includes the need for a cutaneous paddle to be incorporated into the design of buried bone flaps. The reliability of this paddle may be questionable with some flaps (e.g., fibula),[45] which has prompted the modification of flap design to include septocutaneous perforators situated at the upper aspect of the donor site.[84] Although repeated clinical assessment remains the gold standard method for detecting vascular compromise within the transferred tissue, other, adjunctive technologies may also be of use (Fig. 22–3). External ultrasound monitoring of a subcutaneous pedicle is a popular technique for monitoring surface and buried flaps[44,46,48,85] but is of limited value in diagnosing venous obstruction. Bone scintigraphy may be useful in the first week after surgery[81,86] but is seldom performed routinely because the data it provides are noncontinuous.[46] In particular, the measurement of tissue oxygen tension, whereby flexible microcatheters are implanted into the flap, seems to hold promise for the future.[87,88] This method provides an index of tissue viability that is rapidly responsive to circulatory change and reliable in the experimental setting. Clinical trials are currently under way to evaluate its application to the monitoring of buried flaps in oromandibular reconstruction.

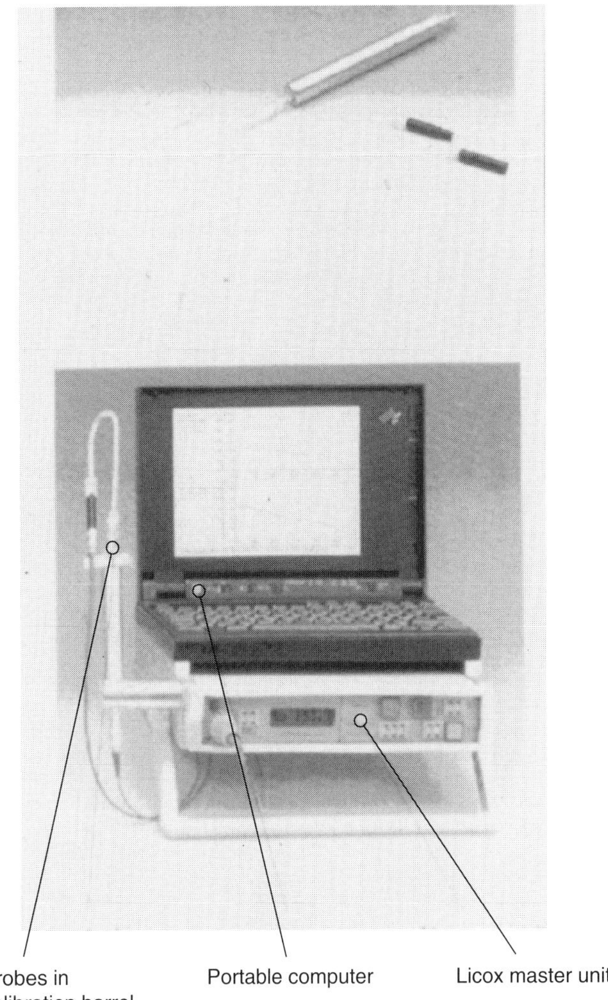

Figure 22–3. TiO_2 Monitor for free tissue transfer. (Courtesy of Licox Medical Systems Corp., Greenvale, NY.)

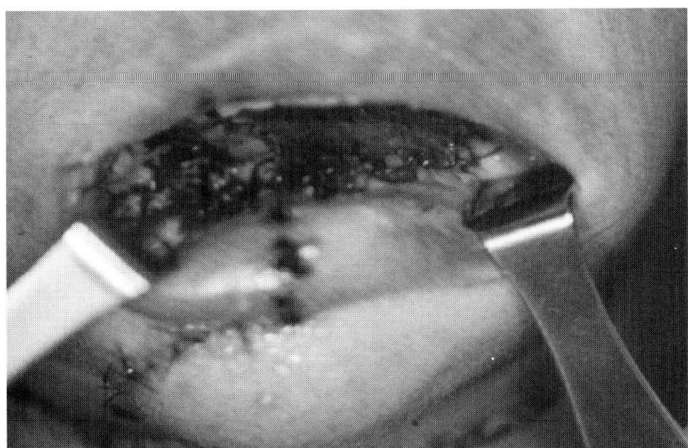

Figure 22–2. Failing flap demonstrating venous congestion.

References

1. Moscoso JF: Mandibular reconstruction. Curr Opin Otol Head Neck Surg 1994;2:337.
2. Urken ML: Composite free flaps in oromandibular reconstruction: Review of the literature. Arch Otolaryngol Head Neck Surg 1991;117:724.

3. David DJ, Tan E, Katsaros J, et al: Mandibular reconstruction with vascularized iliac crest: A 10-year experience. Plast Reconstr Surg 1988;82:792.
4. Mirante JP, Urken ML, Aviv JE, et al: Resistance to osteoradionecrosis in neovascularized bone. Laryngoscope 1993;103:1168.
5. Duncan MJ, Manktelow RT, Zuker RM, et al: Mandibular reconstruction in the radiated patient: The role of osteocutaneous free tissue transfers. Plast Reconstr Surg 1985;76:829.
6. Boyd JB, Rosen I, Rotstein L, et al: The iliac crest and the radial forearm flap in vascularized oromandibular reconstruction. Am J Surg 1990;159:301.
7. Urken ML, Buchbinder D, Weinberg H, et al: Primary placement of osseointegrated in microvascular mandibular reconstruction. Otolaryngol Head Neck Surg 1989;101:56.
8. Riediger D: Restoration of masticatory function by microsurgically revascularized iliac crest bone grafts using enosseous implants. Plast Reconstr Surg 1988;81:861.
9. Shenaq SM, Klebuc MJA: The iliac crest microsurgical free flap in mandibular reconstruction. Clin Plast Surg 1994;21:37.
10. Kroll SS, Schusterman MA, Reece GP: Costs and complications in mandibular reconstruction. Ann Plast Surg 1992;29:341.
11. Urken ML, Weinberg H, Vickery C, et al: Oromandibular reconstruction using microvascular composite free flaps. Arch Otolaryngol Head Neck Surg 1991;117:733.
12. Urken ML, Buchbinder D, Weinberg H, et al: Functional evaluation following microvascular oromandibular reconstruction of the oral cancer patient: A comparative study of reconstructed and non-reconstructed patients. Laryngoscope 1991;101:935.
13. Hidalgo DA: Aesthetic improvements in free-flap mandible reconstruction. Plast Reconstr Surg 1991;88:574.
14. Kroll SS, Schusterman MA, Reece GP: Immediate vascularized bone reconstruction of anterior mandibular defects with free iliac crest. Laryngoscope 1991;101:791.
15. Jewer DD, Boyd JB, Manktelow RT, et al: Orofacial and mandibular reconstruction with the iliac crest free flap: A review of 60 cases and a new method of classification [see comments]. Plast Reconstr Surg 1989;84:391.
16. Wenig BL, Keller AJ: Microvascular free flap reconstruction for head and neck defects. Arch Otolaryngol Head Neck Surg 1989;115:1118.
17. Kerrigan CL, Stotland MA: Ischemia reperfusion injury: A review. Microsurgery 1993;14:165.
18. Jones NF: Intraoperative and postoperative monitoring of microsurgical free tissue transfers. Clin Plast Surg 1992;19:783.
19. Khouri RK: Avoiding free flap failure. Clin Plast Surg 1992; 19:773.
20. Salemark L: International survey of current microvascular practices in free tissue transfer and replantation surgery. Microsurgery 1991;12:308.
21. Davies D: A world survey of anticoagulation practice in clinical microvascular surgery. Br J Plast Surg 1982;35:96.
22. Sullivan MJ, Baker SR, Crompton R, et al: Free scapular osteocutaneous flap for mandibular reconstruction. Arch Otolaryngol Head Neck Surg 1989;115:1334.
23. Boyd JB, Mulholland RS: Fixation of the vascularized bone graft in mandibular reconstruction. Plast Reconstr Surg 1993;91:274.
24. Urken ML, Weinberg H, Buchbinder D, et al: Microvascular flaps in head and neck reconstruction: Report of 200 cases and review of complications. Plast Reconstr Surg 1994;86:492.
25. Godina M: Early microsurgical reconstruction of complex trauma of the extremities. Plast Reconstr Surg 1986;78:285.
26. Harashina T: Analysis of 200 free flaps. Br J Plast Surg 1988;41:33.
27. Serafin D, Sabatier RE, Morris RL, et al: Reconstruction of the lower extremity with vascularized composite tissue: Improved survival and specific indications. Plast Reconstr Surg 1980;66:230.
28. Kerrigan CL, Daniel RK: Critical ischemia and the failing flap. Plast Reconstr Surg 1982;69:986.
29. McKee NH: Operative complications and the management of intraoperative flow failure. Microsurgery 1993;14:158.
30. Stern JR, Keller AJ, Wenig BL: Evaluation of reconstructive techniques of oropharyngeal defects. Ann Plast Surg 1989;22:332.
31. Woods JE: Reconstruction in head and neck cancer: A place for conservatism. Ann Plast Surg 1987;18:209.
32. Al-Quattan MM, Bowen V: Effect of pre-existing health conditions on the results of reconstructive microvascular surgery. Microsurgery 1993;14:152.
33. Bonawitz SC, Schnarrs RH, Rosenthal AI, et al: Free-tissue transfer in elderly patients. Plast Reconstr Surg 1991;87:1074.
34. Mohr DN: Estimation of surgical risk in the elderly: A correlative review. J Am Geriatr Soc 1983;31:99.
35. Markowitz BL, Calcaterra TC: Preoperative assessment and surgical planning for patients undergoing immediate composite reconstruction of oromandibular defects. Clin Plast Surg 1994;21:9.
36. Al-Quattan MM, Boyd JB: Complications in head and neck microsurgery. Microsurgery 1993;14:187.
37. Taylor GI, Townsend P, Corlett R: Superiority of the deep circumflex iliac vessels as the supply for free groin flaps. Plast Reconstr Surg 1979;64:595.
38. Gong-Kang H, Hu R, Miao H, et al: Microvascular free transfer of iliac bone based on the deep superior branches of the superior gluteal vessel. Plast Reconstr Surg 1985;75:69.
39. Morris SF, Taylor GI: Predicting the survival of experimental skin flaps with a knowledge of the vascular architecture. Plast Reconstr Surg 1993;92:1352.
40. Taylor GI, Minabe T: The angiosomes of the mammals and other vertebrates. Plast Reconstr Surg 1992;89:181.
41. Taylor GI, Watson N: One-stage repair of compound leg flaps defects with free, revascularized flaps of groin skin and iliac bone. Plast Reconstr Surg 1978;61:494.
42. Urken ML, Weinberg H, Vickery C, et al: The internal oblique–iliac crest free flap in composite defects of the oral cavity involving bone, skin, and mucosa. Laryngoscope 1991;101:257.
43. Flemming AF, Brough MD, Evans ND, et al: Mandibular reconstruction using vascularised fibula. Br J Plast Surg 1990;43:403.
44. Robb GL: Free scapular flap reconstruction of the head and neck. Clin Plast Surg 1994;21:45.
45. Urken ML: Reconstruction of the mandible following resection for head and neck cancer. Adv Otolaryngol Head Neck Surg 1991;8:301.
46. Hidalgo DA: Fibula free flap mandibular reconstruction. Clin Plast Surg 1994;21:25.
47. Wei FC, Seah CS, Tsai YC, et al: Fibula osteoseptocutaneous flap for reconstruction of composite mandibular defects. Plast Reconstr Surg 1994;93:294.
48. Hidalgo DA: Fibula free flap: A new method of mandible reconstruction. Plast Reconstr Surg 1989;84:71.
49. Urken ML, Vickery C, Weinberg H, et al: Geometry of the vascular pedicle in free tissue transfers to the head and neck. Arch Otolaryngol Head Neck Surg 1989;115:954.
50. Wells MD, Luce EA, Edwards AL, et al: Sequentially linked free flaps in head and neck reconstruction. Clin Plast Surg 1994;21:59.
51. Urken ML, Weinberg HW, Vickery C, et al: The combined sensate radial forearm and iliac crest free flaps for reconstruction of significant glossectomy-mandibulectomy defects. Laryngoscope 1992;102:543.
52. Daniel RK, Terzis JK: Reconstructive Microsurgery. Boston, Little, Brown, 1977.
53. Caffee HH, Ward D: Bipolar coagulation in microvascular surgery. Plast Reconstr Surg 1986;78:374.
54. Lidman D, Daniel RK: Evaluation of clinical microvascular anastomoses—reasons for failure. Ann Plast Surg 1981;6:215.
55. Acland R: Thrombus formation in microvascular surgery: An experimental study of the effects of surgical trauma. Surgery 1978;73:766.
56. Sartorius CJ, Shapiro SA, Campbell RL, et al: Experimental laser-assisted end-to-side microvascular anastomosis. Microsurgery 1986;7:79.
57. Flemming AF, Colles MJ, Guillianotti R, et al: Laser assisted microvascular anastomosis of arteries and veins: Laser tissue welding. Br J Plast Surg 1988;41:378.
58. Tittle BJ, English JM, Hodges PL: Microsurgery: Free tissue transfer and transplantation. Select Read Plast Surg 1993;7:1.
59. Colen LB, Gonzales FP, Buncke HJJ: The relationship between the number of sutures and the strength of microvascular anastomoses. Plast Reconstr Surg 1979;64:325.
60. Hamilton RB, O'Brien BM: An experimental study of microvascular patency using a continuous suture technique. Br J Plast Surg 1979;32:153.
61. Chen L, Chiu DTW: Spiral interrupted suturing technique for microvascular anastomoses: A comparative study. Microsurgery 1986;7:72.

62. Lauritzen C: A new and easier way to anastomose microvessels: An experimental study in rats. Scand J Plast Reconstr Surg 1978;14:65.
63. Sully L, Nightingale MG, O'Brien BM, et al: An experimental study of the sleeve technique in microarterial anastomoses. Plast Reconstr Surg 1982;70:186.
64. O'Brien BM, Morrison WA, Gumley GJ: Principles and techniques of microvascular surgery. *In* McCarthy JG (ed): Plastic Surgery. Philadelphia, WB Saunders, 1990, p 412.
65. Acland RD: In discussion: Bas L, May JW, Jr, Handren J, Fallon J: End-to-end versus end-to-side anastomosis patency in experimental venous repairs. Plast Reconstr Surg 1986;77:449.
66. Mitchell GM, Zeeman BJ, Rogers IW, et al: The long-term fate of microvenous autografts. Plast Reconstr Surg 1988;82:473.
67. Braam MJ, Cooley BC, Gould JS: Topical heparin enhances patency in a rat model of arterial thrombosis. Ann Plast Surg 1995;34:148.
68. Ohta I, Kawai H, Kawabata H, et al: Topical use of xylocaine for relieving vasospasm: Effect of concentration. J Reconstr Microsurg 1991;7:205.
69. Moscoso JF, Urken ML, Dalton J, et al: Simultaneous interstitial radiotherapy with regional or free-flap reconstruction, following salvage surgery of recurrent head and neck carcinoma: Analysis of complications. Arch Otolaryngol Head Neck Surg 1994; 120:965.
70. Rosenberg RD: Actions and interactions of antithrombin and heparin. N Engl J Med 1975;292:146.
71. Marckwardt F, Klocking HP: Heparin-induced release of plasminogen activator. Haemostasis 1977;6:370.
72. Mahadoo J, Hiebert L, Jaques LB: Vascular sequestration of heparin. Thromb Res 1977;12:79.
73. Holemans R, Adamis D, Horace JF: Interaction of heparin with fibrinolysis. Thromb Diathes Haemorrh 1963;9:446.
74. Yajima H, Tamai S, Mizumoto S, et al: Vascular complications of vascularized composite tissue transfer: Outcome and salvage techniques. Microsurgery 1993;14:473.
75. Knight KR: Review of postoperative pharmacological infusions in ischemic skin flaps. Microsurgery 1994;15:675.
76. Sigurdsson GH: Perioperative fluid management in microvascular surgery. J Reconstr Microsurg 1995;11:57.
77. Moscoso JF, Urken ML: Why free flaps fail. Oper Tech Otolaryngol Head Neck Surg 1993;4:169.
78. Coleman JJ 3d, Wooden WA: Mandibular reconstruction with composite microvascular tissue transfer. Am J Surg 1990;160:390.
79. Dabb RW, Malone JM, Leverett LC: The use of medicinal leeches in the salvage of flaps with venous congestion. Ann Plast Surg 1992;29:250.
80. Chandrasekhar B, Lorant JA, Terz JJ: Parascapular free flaps for head and neck reconstruction. Am J Surg 1990;160:450.
81. Boyd JB, Morris S, Rosen IB, et al: The through-and-through oromandibular defect: Rationale for aggressive reconstruction. Plast Reconstr Surg 1994;93:44.
82. Luk KDK, Zhou LR, Chow SP: The effect of established infection on microvascular surgery. Plast Reconstr Surg 1987;80:423.
83. McLean NR, Ellis H: Does remote sepsis influence the patency of microvascular anastomoses? Br J Plast Surg 1988;41:395.
84. Schusterman MA, Reece GP, Miller MJ, et al: The osteocutaneous free fibular flap: Is the skin paddle reliable? Plast Reconstr Surg 1992;90:787.
85. Lyberg T, Olstad OA: The vascularized fibular flap for mandibular reconstruction. J Craniomaxillofac Surg 1991;19:113.
86. Bos KE: Bone scintigraphy of experimental composite bone grafts revascularized by microvascular anastomoses. Plast Reconstr Surg 1979;64:353.
87. Hofer SOP, Timmenga EJF, Christiano R, et al: An intravascular oxygen tension monitoring device used in myocutaneous transplants: A preliminary report. Microsurgery 1993;14:304.
88. Hjortdal VE, Awwad AM, Gottrup F, et al: Tissue oxygen tension measurement for monitoring musculocutaneous and cutaneous flaps. Scand J Plast Reconstr Surg 1990;24:27.

INDEX

Note: Page numbers in *italics* refer to illustrations; page numbers followed by (t) refer to tables.

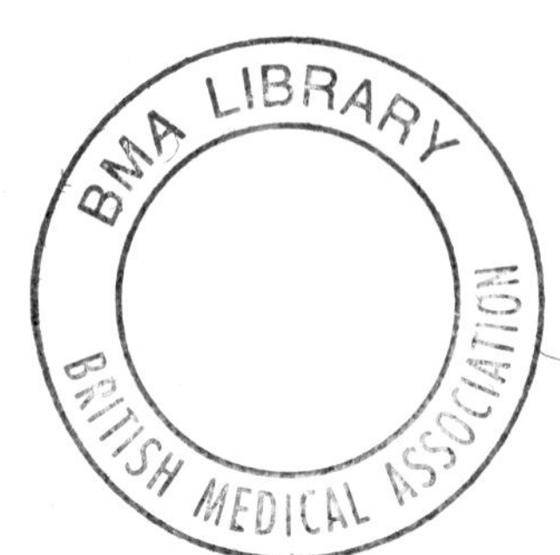
BMA LIBRARY
BRITISH MEDICAL ASSOCIATION

ISBN 0-7216-4861-4